Springer
Berlin
Heidelberg
New York
Barcelona
Budapest
Hong Kong
London
Milan
Paris
Santa Clara
Singapore
Tokyo

Spinal Meningiomas

A. Pansini

F. Lo Re - P. Conti - R. Conti

E. Montali - G. De Luca

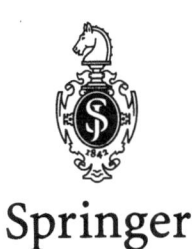

Springer

ARNALDO PANSINI MD, Professor of Neurosurgery

Director of the Department of Neurological and Psychiatric Sciences
Director of the Department of Neurosurgery
University School of Medicine of Florence- Italy

FULVIO LO RE MD, Professor of Neurosurgery
PIERO CONTI MD, Professor of Neurosurgery
RENATO CONTI MD, Professor of Neurosurgery

Department of Neurological and Psychiatric Sciences
Department of Neurosurgery
University School of Medicine of Florence- Italy

ENRICO MONTALI MD, Professor of Genetics

Department of Clinical Pathophysiology
University School of Medicine of Florence- Italy

GIOVANNI DE LUCA MD, Professor of Neurophysiology

Department of Neurological and Psychiatric Sciences
Department of Neurosurgery
University School of Medicine of Florence - Italy

ISBN 978-88-470-2262-1   ISBN 978-88-470-2260-7 (eBook)
DOI 10.1007/978-88-470-2260-7

Die Deutsche Bibliothek – CIP-Einheitsaufnahme
Spinal Meningiomas: A. Pansini ...
- Berlin; Heidelberg; New York: Springer, 1996
ISBN 978-88-470-2262-1
NE: Pansini, Arnaldo

© Springer-Verlag Italia, Milano 1996
Softcover reprint of the hardcover 1st edition 1996

Cover design by Marco Vaghi

Preface

This volume follows an earlier collection of cases from the Institute of Radiology at the University of Florence entitled *"Early Diagnosis of Myeloradicular Compressions, X-Ray, CT, MRI,"* (A. Pansini, P. Conti and Collaborators, 1987) which dealt with the diagnosis not only of spinal tumours but also of compressions of other natures. There we expressed the view that the new diagnostic techniques available today for the early diagnosis of medullary compressions should by no means exclude other diagnostic procedures. After presenting in the previous volume the most common radiographic and myelographic aspects for the diagnosis of spinal tumours, we now evaluate the diagnostic capabilities of computed tomography (CT), myelo-CT and magnetic resonance imaging (MRI) which reveal the importance of these most recent methods of investigation. In our first publication, the comparative study of various methods was not restricted to the diagnosis of spinal tumours but extended also to compressions of other natures.

The experience we acquired in evaluating the various diagnostic investigations in medullary compression cases, prompted us to use a similar approach in examining a series of meningiomas. In contrast to tumours which show an early onset of symptoms, meningiomas, among the primary intrarachidian tumours, are particularly subject to a delayed development of symptoms.

We cannot stress enough the importance of a plain X-ray of the rachis in the diagnosis of meningiomas. This is considered as being the fundamental neurological procedure to be performed before all others, as it provides the basis for identification of characteristic details which assist in reaching an early diagnosis of medullary compressions from tumours.

In addition to the images supplied by CT and MRI, we have stressed the importance of myelo-CT features and the axial scans produced with an iodine contrast medium introduced by means of lumbar puncture, which very clearly identify the borders of pathological tissue and the internal structures of the rachis.

There are 125 cases of meningiomas in this monograph, derived from the surgical treatment of 125 cases of meningiomas operated on between 1962 and 1994. In recent years surgical techniques have undergone a gradual evolution, making the removal of any form of meningioma safer than it was in the past.

Our intention in presenting these experiences in the diagnosis of meningiomas is to expand our knowledge of the techniques available and of the respective roles which they can play in reaching an early diagnosis, thereby improving surgical results.

My own deepest gratitude goes to my junior neurosurgeons and to my Associate Professors F. Lo Re, P. Conti and R. Conti who have collaborated in clinical diagnoses, and complete surgical activity, and to the assistance of patients at the Neurosurgical Clinic of the University of Florence which I have had the honour of directing since 1970. This monograph has been completed with their valuable assistance, during the course of the years, by keeping rigorous accounts of all clinical observations over this period, evaluated from an evolutionary perspective and with the addition of comments added immediately after each operation.

We wish to thank our colleagues in the Department of Genetic Medicine at the University of Florence, who worked in close collaboration with the Neurosurgical Clinic and participated in this study from a cytogenetic point of view, paying special attention to chromosomic anomalies of some tumours with particular emphasis on spinal meningiomas. Our gratitude is extended to Prof. E. Montali and to Dr. L. Papi who have recorded data of their experiences in the chapter on genetics. We also wish to thank our neurophysiopathology assistant, Prof. G. De Luca, who handled the recordings of pre-, intra- and post-operational evoked potentials, and who contributed to the chapter on neurophysiopathology.

Dr. A. Franchi from the Institute of Anatomy and

Pathological Histology at the University of Florence dealt with and closely examined all the histopathological material on the 125 menigiomas, classifying them according to the WHO criteria. Our sincere thanks we express to him, particularly for the meticulous work which he carried out in the preparation of the staining methods.

Our gratitude also goes to all of our radiologist and neuroradiologist colleagues and particularily to Prof. G. Dal Pozzo, G. Pellicano and to Dr. S. Mangiafico who carried out the necessary neuroradiological investigations on the clinical material which we supplied and helped us to identify the exact location and nature of the lesions.

Sincere thanks to the young assistants and to those specializing in neurosurgery, who have worked with dedication and competence on the study of clinical material, on the elaboration of all statistical data and on postoperative checks. These include Dr. P. Bono, Dr. P. Gallina, Dr. F. Cioffi, Dr. J. Buric, Dr. S. Carnesecchi, and Dr. S. Romoli.

Thanks also to the technicians of the Radiological Service: Maurizio Galli and Riccardo Lombardo.

We are also indebted to Professor G. Staderini, Director of the Didactic Television Centre at the University of Florence, and to his collaborators G. Guidi and his technicians who produced the long-distance images taken during surgery, allowing us to demonstrate the highlights of the surgical techniques employed. These were recorded on video tape and were recently presented at the European Congress of Neurosurgery in Berlin.

Our gratitude and sincere thanks we also extend to the distinguished publisher Springer-Verlag for their interest shown and for the collaboration in the preparation and editing of this monograph.

A. Pansini

Contents

Contents

1 General Considerations

The traditional division of primary intradural-extramedullary spinal tumours, intramedullary and epidural tumours is still used today to describe tumours on the basis of location. However, one must also consider that a meningioma can grow towards the inner spinal dura and in the epidural site, thereby becoming extrameningeal at the same time. The various forms of development are associated with the histological nature of the tumour; benign characteristics and transformation processes towards malignancy, which brings about an alteration in the dimension of the tumour although the tumour attachment remains well defined.

Meningeal tumours are referred to as meningioma, the term proposed originally by Cushing. This refers to a particular type of tumour characterized by the same elements that constitute the connective tissues of the meninges, to such a degree that it becomes easy to distinguish the major fibre component in the histological classification. These are distinguished from tumours that undergo transformation of a degenerative or other nature which may develop into neoplasm and, especially, those that show distinct signs of dysembryogenetic development.

The spinal meningioma inserts itself on the spinal dura and is a well-defined tumour, varying in consistency in each case, subject to a variable progressive course but frequently a very slow formation. The morphological appearance of meningiomas is described as encapsulated by a dense connective tissue formation under which the intrinsic tissue of the tumour may appear friable, haemorrhagic, soft or otherwise dense, fibrous, strident in the excision phase, not very haemorrhagic, of a yellowish white colour and granular due to its calcifying transformation. Other forms have a hard, compact consistency similar to bone tissue. Normally when a diagnosis is reached the tumour shows an exclusively intradural development and has the size of a cherry.

There are other forms, however, which are much larger, especially when the meningioma becomes particularly elongated, being both intra- and extrarachidian at the same time. It is important to note at the beginning that its structure together with its histological variants is identical to cerebral meningioma, and the spinal meningioma is sometimes clinically confused with a neurinoma or neurofibroma, not only in structure but also because both undergo a slowly progressive course of development and show similar initial symptoms. When the lesion syndrome is minimal and motor impairment is slight, manifest by the swaying motion of the lower limbs, one is reminded of the numerous types of cord syndromes. However, the presence of constant pain leads to perplexity in diagnosing noncompressive root syndromes; radicular coinvolvement at the lumbar level, often on one side only, or with some contraradicular sensitivity, suggests a possible painful cauda syndrome which is not of tumourous nature. In cases in which the meningioma is completely extradural and extends out of the vertebral canal through the intervertebral foramen, the initial pattern of sensitive disturbance is the same as that of the neurofibromas with hourglass appearance. This sensitive disturbance is also frequently found at the level of the dorsal spine.

In the forms with the level syndrome restricted to the grey matter of the cervical spine in the initial phase of meningiomatous compression one must consider myelopathy, especially in the presence of arthrosis alterations on the cervical tract of the spine, which may also account for the symptoms of second motor neuron involvement. These simple caveats, which are not the only ones, have been evaluated in recent publications on the progressive course of meningiomas. We draw attention to the various possible diagnoses to underline the fact that a meningioma is a tumour which delays in showing recognizable signs of a compression, misguiding the clinical discussion to other pathologies.

Diagnosing intrarachidial compression simply with the help of the patient's medical history and clinical signs already present, frequently proves too late in the case of a suspect tumour to request neuroradiological confirmation. In many forms of tumours this delay could influence surgical results, particularly when the preoperative semiological picture expresses bilateral involvement of the cord, affecting movement in a way resembling severe paraparesis tending towards paraplegia.

At the October 1988 Turin Congress on "Primary Tumours of the Spinal Cord" we were indebted to Pagni for presenting the most valuable and up-to-date information ever collected on this pathology. This Congress also discussed experimental research and genetics as these areas may in future prove crucial in the search for means to modify and improve acute or chronic damage to the central nervous system.

This monograph examines a series of 122 meningioma cases operated on by the same group of neurosurgeons from the University of Florence between 1962 and 1994. The data include those from the period (1962-1980) when neuroradiological diagnosis depended solely upon myelography performed suboccipitally. The subsequent introduction of computed tomography (CT) and magnetic resonance imaging (MRI) has allowed us to consider many additional clinical-anatomic factors. The vast literature that has accumulated over the past 10 years is reviewed but without neglecting previous fundamental work on this subject, including particularly diagnostic aspects and therapy.

The impressive set of statistical data collected by Pagni from the most important neurosurgical centres of the world has been an enormous help to us. We have included references from this work and used a similar methodology in order to produce a significant contribution from a neurodiagnostical point of view, with the addition of some innovative details regarding the techniques that we use.

We also include here our considerations after each operation as these observations, together with the explanatory and schematic diagrams of the relationship between tumours and the myeloradicular structures, may contribute to much more accurate interpretation of the anatomical-clinical picture. This was made possible by the operative microscope and by microneurosurgery, which has improved our surgical techniques.

This monograph concludes with an evaluation of the various elements regarding spinal meningiomas and the problem of early diagnosis, which continues to be of fundamental importance in obtaining optimal results.

2 Historical Origins of Embryology

A. Pansini - P. Conti

Following the pioneering research by His (1890), Salvi (1897) and Kolliker (1896) on the differentiation of the neural tube, many researchers studied particular aspects of cellular development in neuroepithelium. According to His' theory, the neuroepithelium is heterogeneous in nature, and the spongioblasts in their ventricular site gradually move away from one of the bordering membranes and assume the cellular nature of astroblasts, astrocytes, oligodendroblasts or oligodendrocytes. The spongioblasts which remain connected to the internal membrane form the future ependymal cells.

Salvi (1897) used the term primitive meninges for all the layers between the cord and the vertebral primordium. However, this mesenchyma constitutes the meninges and the endorachis, and Sterzi (1915) referred instead to the perimedullary mesenchyma, which later divides into two layers: one adhering to the vertebrae and forming the endorachis and the other surrounding the cord forming the early primordium of all the meninges. This is the only feature which could properly be termed primitive meninges. According to Sauer (1935, 1936), the neuroepithelium during the very early phases of development is formed by a homogeneous grouping of cells whose proliferation and differentiation stabilize eventually at a specific point to form the matrix or ventricular layer. This layer is formed by cells with a particular selective potential of differentiation and is considered responsible for the origin of all the elements that form the adult nervous system. Sauer's theory has been confirmed by numerous researchers, including Watterson et al. (1956), Sidman and Coll (1959), Fujita (1963) and by Hinds' ultrastructural studies (1971).

Neuroblasts originate from the pluripotent cells of the ventricular area and are destined to various layers of the cerebral cortex and to the medullary neuroblasts. Further insight into cellular dynamics, the differentiation and maturity of distinct groups of cells present in the adult spinal cord and the behaviour of neuroblasts have been provided by Levi-Montalcini (1950, 1967), Hamburger (1952), Harris (1965) and Romanes (1951, 1964).

In young embryos the outline of the cord shows an irregular oval shape; as seen in a cross-section, the lateral sides are thick while the ventral and dorsal sides are thin, leading to their being termed lamina. The ventral side is called the basal lamina and the dorsal side the tegmental lamina. In a cross-section of a 1-month-old embryo the cavity of the cord resembles a fissural lumen, such as a great vertical axis. In embryos older than 1 month the lateral sides of the cord present increased thickness and a sagittal sulcus in the interior wall (bordering sulcus) that separates a higher and thicker ventral portion which is shorter and thinner and is known as the wing lamina. On each side on the surface of the fundamental lamina the anterior and lateral cords of the white matter differentiate and the anterior grey horns, from within the lamina, give rise to the anterior spinal root. Peripherally from the wing lamina, the posterior white cord differentiates from the deep grey horn, from which arises the posterior spinal root medially.

In this phase the exterior of the spinal cord appears in cross-sections as a triangle with a large base situated ventrally and the rounded apex rising dorsally. The cavity still appears in the shape of a vertical fissure as a great axis. The bordering sulcus enlarges the fissure as it joins two-thirds of its length ventrally and one-third dorsally. The cavity of the cord which represents the future ependymal cavity then declines in height as the posterior portion, which corresponds to the wall of the wing lamina, gradually disappears to form the posterior septus on the median line. The remaining portion of the cavity gradually transforms into the central canal of the spinal cord.

In cross-sections we can distinguish three layers in the spinal cord. Peripherally and under the meningeal sheath there is a white thin layer called the marginal veil which at first appears as a thin border corresponding to the external surface of the fundamental and wing laminae.

A. Pansini et al.
Spinal Meningiomas
© Springer-Verlag Italia 1996

In a later phase the marginal veil appears also peripherally to the basal lamina and gradually presents axons or axis cylinders within its chain-like structures which run vertically along the length of the spinal cord. Below the marginal veil there is a thick mantle, or neuroblastic layer, presenting more closely packed cells in the fundamental lamina than in the wing lamina. The greater volume of the mantle layer corresponds to the ventral portion of the fundamental lamina, and for this reason the cord, in cross-section, appears to have an irregular triangular shape at the base. The deep cellular stratum is that enclosing the canal. Embryo cells that are in full karyokinetic activity constitute a germinative centre of neuroblasts which gradually move into the medial or mantle layer.

The innermost elements, those that line the cavity, transform into the ependymal cells of the central spinal cord. The ependymal elements of the basal plates with their high protoplasmatic border reach a significant height and face the lumen of the canal, while the nuclei push outwards, i.e. towards the surface of the meninges. These form the so-called ependymal cone. Apart from the ependymal elements of the basal plates, the neuroblasts do not undergo a densifying process, nor does the marginal veil become thicker. This medial portion stops developing while the ventral portion of the fundamental laminae advances at the sides, where the production of neuroblasts is very active; the anterior medial fissure of the spinal cord is thus outlined.

The mass of neuroblasts of the fundamental laminae gradually form the anterior horn, and among smaller neuroblastic elements the great anterior cells (the anterior horn's motor cells) differentiate early. The axons push forwards and horizontally and thereby emerge from the surface of the cord to form the anterior roots of the spinal nerves. The wing lamina transforms at a slower rate. The tegmental lamina disappears with the loss of the dorsal portion of the cavity and becomes part of the median line of the connection link which forms the posterius septum. The medial layer of the neuroblasts transforms very slowly into the posterior horns. The elements of the dorsal extremity of this layer remain small, but numerous, and develop into Roland's jelly-like substance. In the marginal veil, at the sides of the posterior sect, the two bundles of the posterior cord develop: the gracile and cuneate bundles.

As some of the elements that form the neural tube transform into the neuroblasts which gradually become the nerve cells of the spinal cord, other elements differentiate, such as spongioblasts which become elements of the ectoglia. As the neuroglia is of ectodermal origin the mesoglia must be considered of a similar origin because mesenchymal elements of the primitive meninges enter into the neural substance via the blood vessels and disperse within, forming the characteristic cells of mesoglia.

With the closure of the posterior neural groove, the cells corresponding to this point migrate laterally and rapid growth occurs. At each end of the neural tube a continuous vertical band forms called the ganglia crest which is detached from the neural tube. Later the crest begins to fragment into various segments, lying neatly one after the other and forming the primordium of the spinal ganglia deep in the mesenchyma of the primitive meninges. The cells of the ganglia outlines later differentiate into neuroblasts and lemnoblasts. The neuroblasts transform into opposite-polar cells which become the characteristic T-shaped nerve cells of the spinal ganglia. The lemnoblasts form the elements of the pericellular capsule. The ganglia capsule forms from the mesenchyma of the primitive meninges. The ganglia neuroblasts extend early towards the neural tube, which forms the posterior root of the cord and a peripheral dentritic extension, similar to an axon, which later forms the sensitive fibre of the spinal nerve.

The sympathetic paravertebral chain appears in human embryos after the beginning of the second month of gestation. The origin of the sympathetic elements is still a matter of discussion. Experimental research (Levi-Montalcini 1950) on chicken embryos with large damaged areas in the cord suggests that the sympathetic system is formed without medullary influence. The problem remains unresolved. The majority of embryologists still believe that these outlines are derived from the cord by migrate cells from the ganglia crests.

During the embryonic stage, when the neural tube is surrounded by mesenchymal tissue, the formation of the cells in thin rows can already be seen. These internally form the outline of what will become the perimedullary covering, i.e. the leptomeninges. From the outermost mesenchymal layer originate the spinal meninges, peridural tissues and perichondrium of the respective somites. The external layer delimits a space in which the blood vessels run parallel to the respective nerve root course and particularly to the spinal ganglion. The spinal ganglion arises from a more ventral position (ectodermal origin) before reaching its permanent position in relation to the future intravertebral foramen (Figs. 1, 2).

In the mesenchymal tissue which surrounds the neural tube (Pansini 1950) the arachnoid is the last to develop. From the outermost layer of the same mesodermal layer originates the spinal dura, which during the differentiation phase maintains a thicker external layer than the innermost layer. During the development stage the blood vessels which form the blood system of the future spinal dura maintain their position within the dura, while those of the thinner interior mesenchyma remain below the arachnoid in relationship with the pia mater and the perivascular septum within the cord. Research by Schachenmayr and Friede (1978) on morphological cellular relationships of the encephalic meninges confirmed that the arachnoid, like the cord, develops from the internal part of the mesodermal layer.

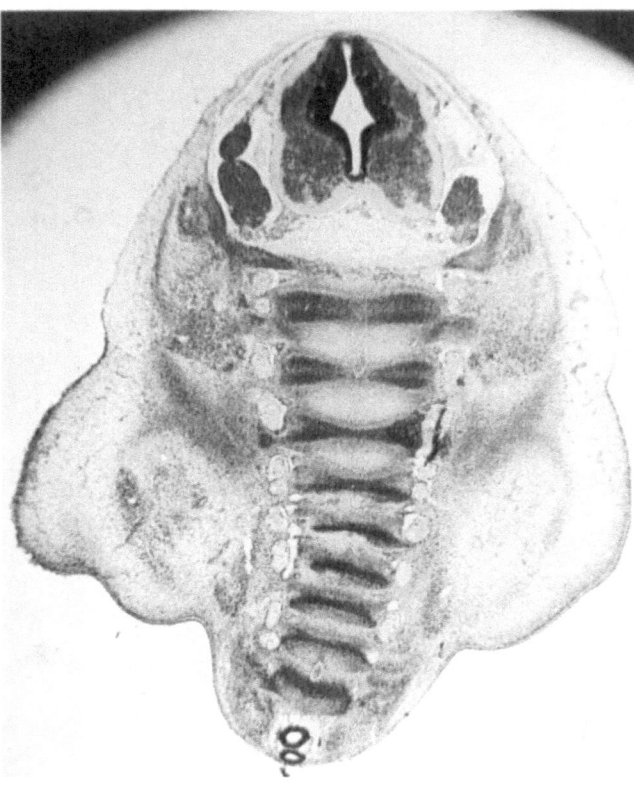

Fig. 1. Lumbar cross-section of spinal cord, with sequence of frontal views of the sacral to the coxygeal vertebral bodies. The caudal extremity of the cord appears twice on the cross-section due to the oblique cut. (Human embryo, 45 days old)

On the basis of the primary perineural mesenchyma differentiation we determined that once a laminectomy is performed and the spinal dura divided into two thin membranes coagulation can be performed of the blood vessels that form the vertebral or aortic system and reach not only the rachidial structures but also the meningioma of mesodermic origin. This preparation of the spinal dura facilitates the removal of a meningioma either with subarachnoidal development or when found lying between the arachnoid and the internal dural plane.

The microsurgical technique that we use includes: (a) millimetric incision performed in a longitudinal direction on a horizontal plane (patient in a lateral decubitus) or in the vertical plane (patient in the sitting position), (b) delamination of the spinal dura by splitting of the external dural layer from the internal layer using a spatula, and (c) anchorage of the external dural layer to the paravertebral muscles. This preparation ensures: (a) visibility of the vascularization in the dural thickness, (b) progressive coagulation of blood flow afferent to tumour before opening the deep dural plane of the spinal dura in continuity with the attachment of the meningioma, thus facilitating surgical excision, and (c) minor bleeding before opening the deep dural strata and then the arachnoid.

Mallory (1920) and earlier still Weed (1917) conducted important research on the mesodermal origins of the meningioma. At that time it was generally believed that the arachnoid was of epiblastic origin and derived from the neural crest. Cushing (1922) put an end to the classification of meningiomas as arachnoidal fibroblastomas and termed them meningiomas as he was convinced that meningocytes and fibroblasts are of mesenchymal origin. It took almost 50 years to confirm Cushing's interpretation. This was achieved by Shuangshoti et al. (1971) who demonstrated that fibroblasts and Schwann cells are able to produce reticulin, verifying that meningocytes and fibroblasts are derived from the mesenchyma. This histogenetic association had been reported by Penfield (1927) and by Tarlov (1940).

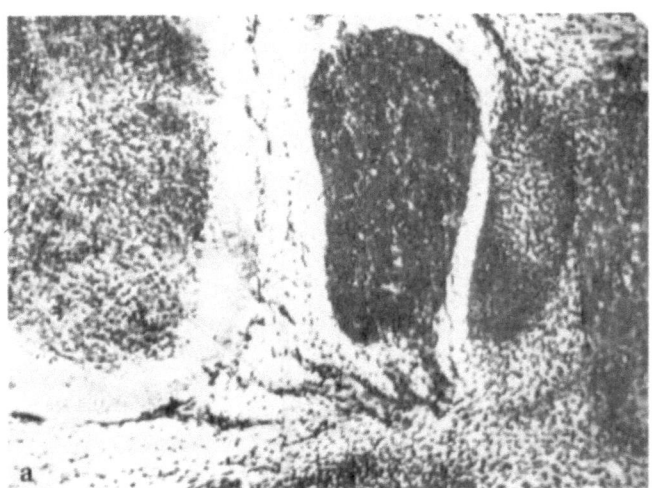
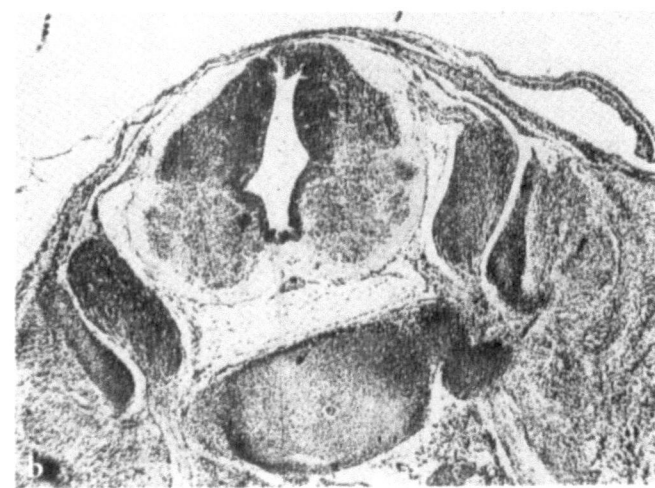

Fig. 2. a Cross-section of thoracic segment of the spinal cord. The outline of the vertebral laminae lie laterally to the spinal ganglia. *Below*, the anterior roots place themselves by the side of the emerging fibres of the ganglion's distal pole. Gradual stretching of the posterior roots simultaneously with the gradual migration of the ganglia towards the intravertebral foramen. b A magnified view of the anterior root of one side joining below the efferent fibres, from the distal pole of the ganglion. Note the wide lumen and very thin walls of the blood vessels in the mesenchyma

3 Genetics

E. Montali

Meningiomas are generally sporadic and solitary tumours, but some rare cases have been known to be hereditary (Memon 1980; Conti et al. 1981; Ferrante et al. 1987). They occur particularly in patients affected by type 2 fibromatosis (NF2; Pansini et al. 1991). NF2 is a hereditary autosomal-dominant syndrome characterized by the occurrence of multiple tumours in the central nervous system, such as acoustic neuromas, meningiomas, ependymomas and gliomas. The NF2 gene, mapped to the long arm of chromosome 22 in 1986 (Seizinger et al. 1986), has been recently identified (Trofatter et al. 1993; Rouleau et al. 1993). Meningiomas are the most studied forms of tumours *from a cytogenetic* point of view. Chromosomic analysis performed on neoplastic tissue has shown the presence of chromosomic anomalies in the majority of cases. Among these, the total (monosomy) or partial loss of chromosome 22 constitutes a specific marker (Zang 1982; Casalone et al. 1987; Al Saadi et al. 1987). The complete monosomy of chromosome 22 has been observed in 20%-50% of cases documented in the literature, while deletion of the long arm of 22 (22q) with consequent partial monosomy is much rarer. It must be mentioned that normal karyotic meningiomas do exist, and that chromosomes other than 22 are sometimes involved (either in the presence or in the absence of monosomy 22). In the latter case the nonrandom involvement of chromosomes 8, 14, X and Y in numeric anomalies has been demonstrated, while chromosome 1 is involved in structural anomalies (Casalone et al. 1986; Al Saadi et al. 1987). The involvement of chromosome 22 in meningiomas has been confirmed in a molecular genetics study which demonstrated (by analysing the loss of heterozygosis of 22q with probe) that the partial or total loss of the long arm of chromosome 22 is a specific anomaly present in approx. 60% of these tumours (Seizinger et al. 1987; Dumanski et al. 1990; Wolff et al. 1992).

The demonstration that the partial or total loss of chromosome 22 is a specific anomaly of meningiomas gave rise to the theory that their development depends on the loss of one or more regulating genes located on 22q. For this reason Knudson's hypothesis (1985), which states that neoplastic development is due to the mutation of so-called oncosuppressors was applied also to meningiomas. According to this theory these genes would have the function of controlling cell growth, in an inhibitory sense, and their loss would cause uncontrollable growth. Therefore the oncosuppressor genes would have to be recessive, as the homozygosis of the genetic defect would be indispensable as a clinical sign. According to Knudson's theory, the neoplastic transformation occurs in two successive phases. The first mutation would not cause neoplastic transformation because the other allele is still working; the second mutation deactivates the remaining allele and therefore allows tumour growth. The first mutation can be verified in the germ line in the case of hereditary tumours and in somatic cells in sporadic tumours; the second occurs in both cases, in somatic cell carriers of the first mutation.

These theories have been proved correct in tumour cases affected by NF2, where the gene, as noted above, is located on the long arm of chromosome 22. These patients are carriers of the first germ mutation (present in all the cells of the body), and tumours develop starting from a cell where the complete or partial loss of chromosome 22 leads to inactivity of the only functional allele of the gene present in these cases (Rouleau et al. 1993). These mechanisms have been confirmed even in sporadic neurinoma cases (Twist et al. 1994), but in these cases both the first and the second mutation occur in the somatic cell where the tumour originates.

Meningiomas as a characteristic anomaly involve chromosome 22 and as these frequently occur in patients affected by NF2, the gene NF2 has been considered the gene responsible for the development of sporadic meningiomas. Somatic mutations of the NF2 gene have indeed been demonstrated (Ruttledge et al. 1994; Twist et al. 1994),

A. Pansini et al.
Spinal Meningiomas
© Springer-Verlag Italia 1996

thus confirming involvement of the NF2 gene in the pathogenesis of these tumours. It is interesting to note that mutations involving the NF2 gene have been found only in those meningiomas which present a total or partial loss of chromosome 22, suggesting that the mechanisms of this gene correspond to those of an oncosuppressor. Mutations in the NF2 gene occurring in tumours which lose chromosome 22, either totally or partially, lead us to ask whether meningiomas not showing a loss in the sequence of chromosome 22 are caused by punctiform mutations of the gene (and therefore not easily identifiable) or by the mutation of another gene localized on chromosome 22 or some other chromosome. Future research will attempt to solve this problem.

4 Vascularization of the Spinal Cord and Variations in Myelitic Blood Flow

A. Pansini - P. Conti

Following the classical descriptions of Adamckiewicz (1882), Kadyi (1889), and Tanon (1908), Suh and Alexander (1939) and Lazorthese (1957), the last 30 years have seen advances in the knowledge of medullary circulation together with the problems associated with vascular myelitic pathologies. Significant advances have been made thanks to the research of Garcin, Lazorthes, Zulch, Corbin, Gillian, Alajouanine, Castaine, Lhermitte, Sarteschi, Giannini, Gruner, Poules, La Presle, Godlewski, Rondot and Zadeh.

According to Lazorthes, there are three great arterial territories of the spinal cord. The first is the uppermost cervicodorsal area from C1 to D3 where the arterial supply is particularly plentiful and derives from numerous arteries originating directly from the vertebral artery. There is a distinct difference in the blood supply between the upper and lower tracts of this territory; the arteries of a major calibre are those that run along the roots of the brachial plexus from C4 to C8, the most important being the sixth cervical root. There is less blood supply to the cord from C1 to C4 than in that of the intumescentia cervicalis. In the second arterial territory there is reduced arterial supply in the medial dorsal tract from D4 to D8 because the circulation to these segments derives from an artery of lesser calibre which acts as a junction between the upper and lower vascular territories. The third territory is the inferior or dorsolumbar territory, which corresponds to the intumescentia lumbalis and to the last dorsal metameres. Vascularization is plentiful in this medullary tract as it derives from an artery of greater calibre which originates from one of the first lumbar arteries leading from the thoracic-abdominal aorta; this is Adamkiewicz's great anterior radicular artery, which Lazorthes termed the artery of the intumescentia lumbalis.

This artery sometimes runs parallel to an artery of small calibre which originates at a lower level. It usually reaches the cord from below the intumescentia lumbalis along the 10th, 11th and 12th dorsal nerves or along the 1st and 2nd lumbar nerves. In its division into anterior and posterior radicular arteries it reaches the anterior surface of the cord and then divides into two ramifications. The thinner ascending branch supplies the lower dorsal myelomeres, and the descending branch, which is a major artery, reaches the entire intumescentia lumbalis and the medullary cone. At the level of the medullary cone the circulation of the anterior spinal artery anastomizes with that of the posterior spinal artery, forming a reticular surface layer.

The radicular arteries vary in calibre. The anterior arteries are of greater calibre while the posterior ones are of lesser calibre and are more homogeneous; consequently their contribution to the blood flow is generally more uniform (Lhermitte and Corbin 1960). However, this also requires the participation of each side of the posterolateral spinal artery (of a lesser calibre) which runs laterally to the blood flow of the two posterior spinal arteries and contributes to the anastomatic network of the coronal vessels.

The anterior and posterior pial network to the cord's surface layer is less subject to haemodynamic variations because it is nearer to the radicular arteries. According to Charpy (1921), this arterial network extends along the entire length of the spinal cord, providing a blood supply to maintain uniform pressure and supplementing in the absence of the radiculars. The principal arterial systems derive from the perimedullary network and are distributed vertically with collateral arteries running horizontally. Adamckiewicz recognized three groups of arteries in these collaterals: (a) arterial branches for the white superficial columns, (b) deep-lying arteries also for the white matter, and (c) arterial trunks reaching peripheral zones of the posterior horn's head. According to Lazorthes, these arteries distribute almost entirely to the white matter or, better, to cord systems of sensory conduction. The major part of the grey structures, on the other hand, are under

A. Pansini et al.
Spinal Meningiomas
© Springer-Verlag Italia 1996

the control of commissural sulcus arteries; the commissural system along the entire length of the cord provides some branches to Turk's fasciculus before extending centrally to the grey horns.

According to Kadyi (1889) and Suh and Alexander (1939), two arteries supply the commissural sulcus, branching out at the sides into arteries for the grey matter of the anterior horns circulation, for the bases of the posterior horns and for the deep cordal portion, corresponding to the pyramidal pathway. The exact morphology of the vertical anastomosis which reach the medullary segments is as yet not well-defined; however, the commissural arteries are of major calibre and are closer at the cervical and lumbar levels. In the greater extention of the lumbar tract the arteries are at a great distance from each other (Lazorthes).

Herren (1939) and Suh (1939) agree that at the intumescentia lumbalis level, the left and right collateral arteries deriving from the commissural artery originate from a single trunk of an important calibre. Lazorthes agrees with this. The artery supplying the sacrolumbar tract has been described by Desproges-Gotteron (1955) and noted by Guillaume et al. (1955) in paralysing sciatica. This artery extends to the cord, parallel to the fifth lumbar or first sacral root. Consequently we can find a central arterial supply and a peripheral supply in the cord. Charpy's concept (1921), which considered the central arteries as the vascular motor territory, and which separated the peripheral arteries responsible for the sensory system, is no longer accepted. Some arteries from the central territory pass beyond the grey matter, diffusing deeply into lateral cord tracts. The same applies to some surface arteries, especially in the posterior portion, which in addition to being responsible for vascularization of the posterior and postolateral tracts of the white matter reach the great crossed, pyramidal tracts territory (Gillian 1957; Figs. 3, 4).

The most modern micro-angiographic studies show that the whole central and peripheral arterial system within the cord is composed of a network of capillaries which are more numerous in the grey matter and along Clarke's column, thus confirming the report of Suh and Alexander in 1939. Despite the lack of anastomoses between the various central and peripheral arteries the entire capillary network maintains a continuity in the marginal tract of the white and grey matter. The veins originate distally from the capillary network and maintain the same route as the arteries, the only difference being that the peripheral veins are fewer (Fig. 5). The venous circulation of the perime-

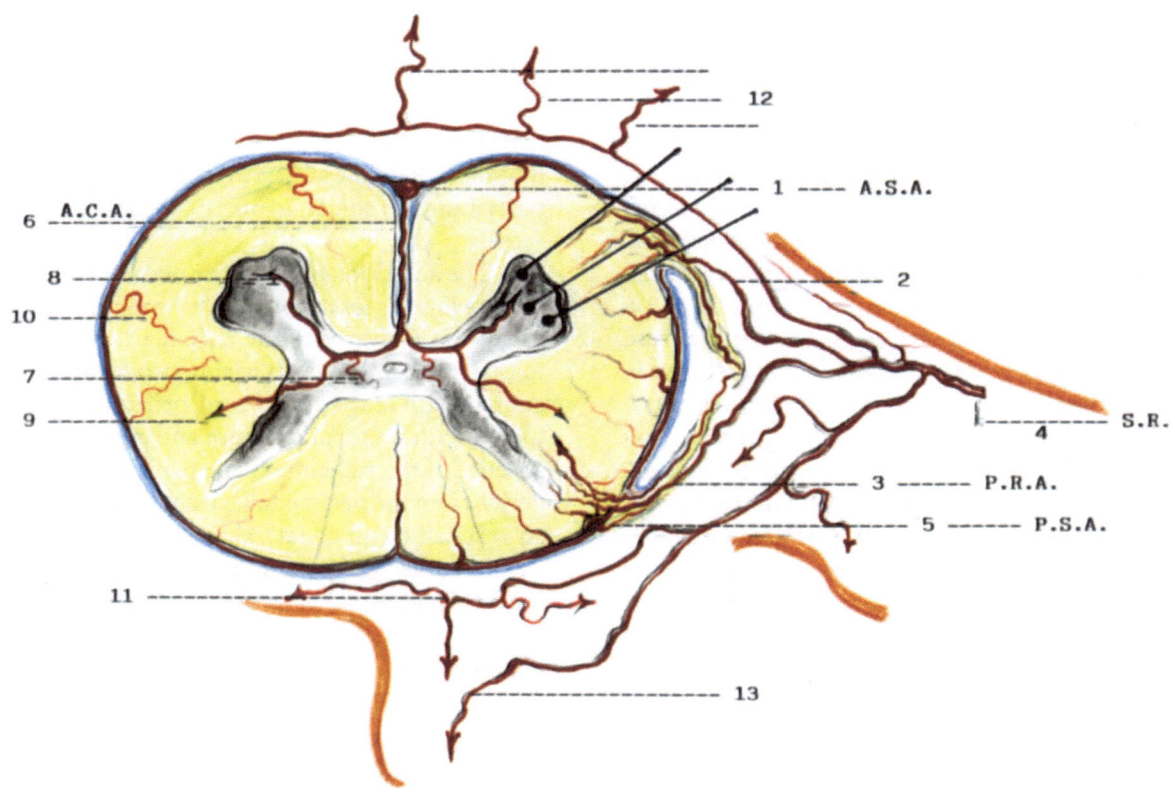

Fig. 3. *1, ASA,* Anterior spinal artery; *2, ARA,* anterior radicular artery; *3, PRA,* posterior radicular artery; *4, SB,* spinal branch; *5, PSA,* posterior spinal artery; *6, ACA,* anterior central artery; *7,* commessural artery; *8,* grey matter branch; *9,* pyramidal tract branch; *10,* white matter branch; *11, PL,* prelaminar branch; *12, PC,* postcentral branch; *13,* dorsal branch

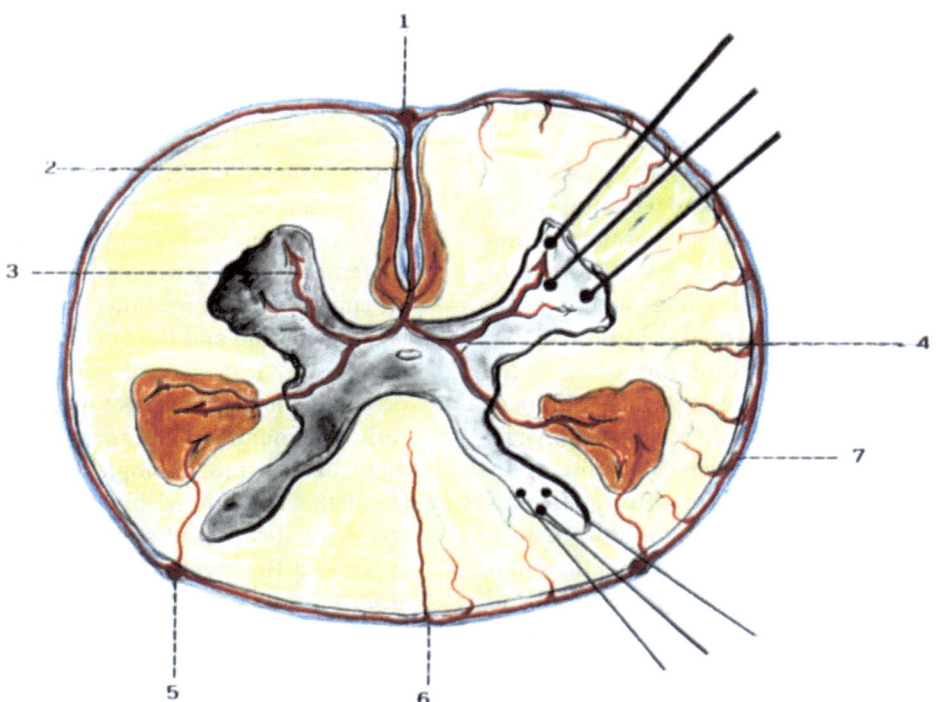

Fig. 4. *1*, Anterior spinal artery; *2*, commessural artery; *3*, grey horn's collateral artery; *4*, crossed pyramidal tract branch; *5*, posterior spinal artery with collateral branch for the crossed pyramidal tract; *6*, posterior sect artery; *7*, coronal blood vessels

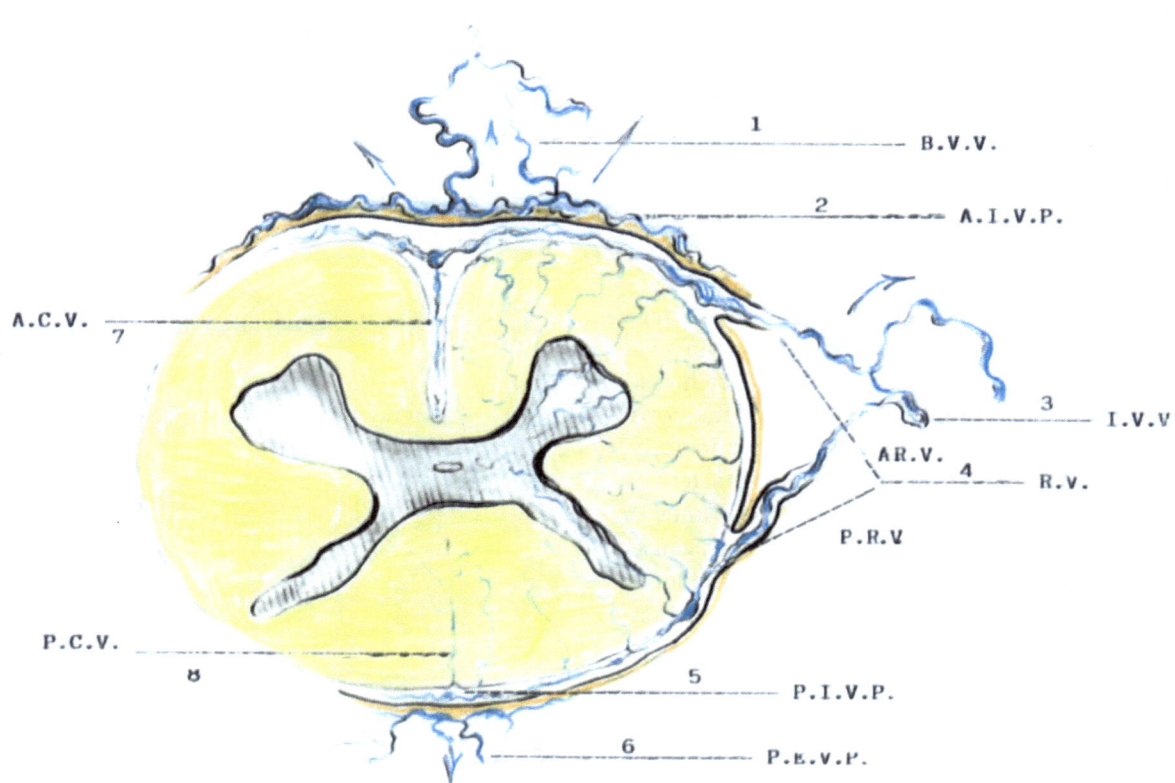

Fig. 5. *1, BVV*, Basal vertebral vein; *2; AIVP*, anterior internal vertebral plexus; *3, IV*, intravertebral vein; *4, RV*, radicular vein; *ARV*, anterior radicular vein; *PRV*, posterior radicular vein; *5, PIVP*, posterior internal vertebral plexus; *6, PEVP*, posterior external vertebral plexus; *7, ACV*, anterior central vein; *8, PCV*, posterior central vein

dullary pia mater, via the arterior and posterior radicular veins, is in relationship with the spinal veins and therefore with the vertebral-epidural and vertebral veins. The radicular arteries do not correspond to the number of spinal roots, and the veins follow a similar pattern.

According to the various interpretations by Lazorthes (1958), Gilligan et al. (1958), Sarteschi and Giannini (1960) and Corbin (1960), the exact "territorial" vascularization within the depth of the cord still remains uncertain. At the dorsal neuromere level where the white matter is prevalent there is a major supply of coronal vessels or, better, of arterial branches, which lead within the cord systems from the perimedullary pial plexus. The vascularization of the cord is not, however, uniform in the various segments. Based on Suh and Alexander's research (1939), the circulation descends in the upper part of the cord and ascends at the lower level. With this supply of blood flow there is a confluence zone in which the anastomotic circulation is not sufficient to connect the vascular territory above and below the upper dorsal tract. The results of the studies carried out by Suh and Alexander have been confirmed by Zulch (1961) and Lazorthes (1957).

Fazio (1938) was of the opinion that a pathogenetic mechanism is involved in ischaemic disturbances in medullary pathologies, very similar to that in encephalic vascular insufficiency. There are areas in the cord which are more exposed to complications of an ischaemic nature. These areas are further away from the arteries' origin and are found in the neighbouring areas between two territories with different vascularization. According to Zulch (1962), the segment lying between the two territories C6-C7 and D9-D10 and the segment L1, is that more probably affected by a haemodynamic variation when the original trunk of D9-D10 is insufficient. Another neighbouring zone lies between the central and peripheral intramedullary vascularizations, although the latter is also reinforced by the large anastomotic premedullary network, with the contribution of the posterior spinal arteries lying beside the posterolateral arteries along the posterior surface of the cord. It is probable that the rich vascular supply in the peripheral most part of the cord prevents insufficiency of ischaemic nature, particularly at the various posterior and posterolateral myelitic levels, whereas insufficiency in the central system of the anterior spinal artery and the commessural arteries can cause damage, more frequently due to a reduction in the blood supply. According to Zulch (1962) the critical area is that at the fourth dorsal myelomere, where the blood flow is reduced from above and at the same time reaches the extremely thin ascending branch derived from Adamckiewicz's great radicular artery. This interpretation was confirmed by experimental studies on Tanon's cadaver (1940), where circulation of the upper dorsal tract failed to manifest itself when a coloured solution was injected into the lumbar circulation.

Present knowledge about the morphological disposition of the medullary vascularization has been confirmed by the neuroradiological studies of Djindjian (1967), who demonstrated pathological aspects of vascular malformations and spinal tumours with selective medullary angiography (Fig. 6). Many anatomical-clinical aspects of functional features of the myelitic vascularization have yet to be resolved, although in ischaemic types of strokes we tend to identify the major contribution of the anterior spinal artery in relation to the anastomatic perimedullary circulation and the posterior spinal artery's circulation. Today it is still difficult to determine the actual pathogenetic mechanism of myelitic vascular disturbance. Although meningiomas are affected by ischaematic-type disturbances, morphological features of the superficial circulation remain variable, as seen in the operating microscope. Verification of a cordal ischaemic process of the surface at the level of the tumour suggests that in an almost asymptomatic case, with a neuroradiological picture showing a meningioma almost completely occupying the rachidian canal, all supplementary supplies to the perimedullary vascular network are well tolerated in an initial phase and also tolerant to resistance from the anterior spinal artery and the commissural fissure. However, these

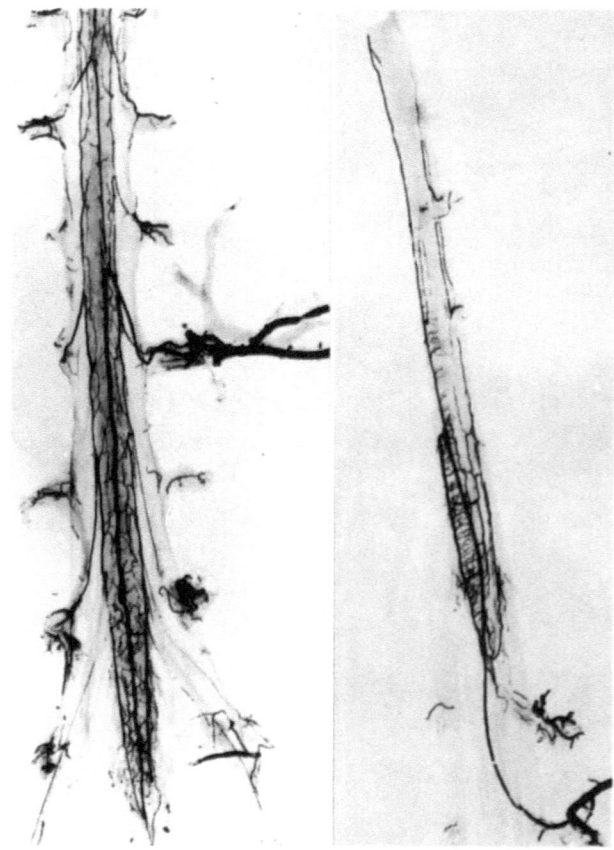

Fig. 6. Anatomical preparation of Adamkiewicz's arterial circulation, derived from the second lumbar artery level. (From Djindjian 1966)

remain the most vulnerable in relation to the posterior spinal arterial system and run the risk of being affected by an ingravescent decompensation condition. The anatomical-clinical picture and symptoms of lateral, posterior and posterolateral meningiomas differ considerably from those with premedullary development in which the mechanical action from the beginning is exerted on the anterior spinal artery circulation.

Corbin (1961) recognized major vulnerability at the C1 level with premedullary meningiomas lying between two territories which depend on different vascular blood supplies. The major vascular disturbance in the dorsal tract at D4, defined by Schneider and Crosby (1959) as the "central" irrigation zone, has a precise relationship with the anatomical-clinical plane because a compression at a lower cervical level can cause upper thoracic myelitic disturbance, and vice versa. Zulch (1962) observed that at this level the blood flow from the cranial-caudal direction is reduced to a minimum and is not compensated by the lower blood supplies. Multiple factors intervene in the haemodynamic variations of the medullary vascularization in meningiomas. One should not forget the polimorphic vascularization of tumours and therefore be capable of recognizing poorly vascularized meningiomas from others which present hypervascularization in the

tumoral tissue and in all the rachidian and extrarachidian region where the tumour has developed.

Another factor concerning major and minor vascular participation of the territory in which the meningioma is located is the positive morphological variations, probably of a congenital nature, of the surface and radicular arteries. The haemodynamic arterial alterations during the slow growth of the meningioma depend on physiopathological factors associated with the particular territorial supply of the medullary vascularization. These conditions worsen in various ways due to the compression of the tumour on the venous epidural system.

We would not be able to explain the surprising surgical results achieved in patients suffering from total paraplegia without considering the reversible nature of the vascularization. This clinical syndrome, even in the most acute form, must never be considered a contraindication for surgery. In spinal meningiomas with pathogenesis of an ischaemic nature and an area of major vulnerability in the cord, we believe that it is indispensable to reduce and control haemorrhages deriving from the intrinsic system of the neoplasm and from the dura as far as possible during surgical removal, thus impeding any possible variation in the blood supply responsible for vascular damage of the neural structures.

5 Case Reports

P. Conti

The series of primary intrarachidian tumours observed at the Neurosurgical Clinic of Florence University between 1962 and 1994 included 432 patients with neoplasms, 206 men (48%) and 226 women (52%), aged between 1 and 89 years. In the youngest we found an intramedullary glioblastoma in the cervical tract of the spine, and in the oldest a dorsal meningioma. Table 1 presents the distribution of neoplasms by histological type.

Meningiomas are tumours found at the rachidian level with considerable frequency. According to some reports, in fact, they are actually more prevalent than neurinomas (Table 2). In our series there were 125 meningiomas, which accounted for 29% of all operated medullary compressions.

Table 1. Histological distribution of the spinal neoplasms

Histological types	n	%
Intrarachidian-extramedullary tumours (n=378, 87.5%)		
Neurinoma and Neurofibroma	156	41.27%
Meningioma	123	32.54%
Ependymoma	50	13.22%
Dermoid and epidermoid cysts	15	3.97%
Haemangioma	14	3.70%
Lipoma	7	1.85%
Chordoma	10	2.64%
Aneurysmal cysts	1	0.27%
Angiolipoma	1	0.27%
Melanosarcoma	1	0.27%
Intrarachidian-intramedullary tumours (n=54 cases; 12.5%)		
Ependymoma	13	24.08%
Astrocytoma	10	18.52%
Lipoma	6	11.11%
Spongioblastoma	5	9.26%
Glioblastoma	4	7.41%
Haemangioma	4	7.41%
Dermoid and epidermoid cysts	4	7.41%
Neurinoma	3	5.55%
Meningioma	2	3.70%
Ependymoblastoma	1	1.85%
Astroblastoma	1	1.85%
Teratoma	1	1.85%

Table 2. Relative prevalence of meningiomas and neurinomas: review of the literature

Reference	Meningiomas		Neurinomas	
	n	%	n	%
Cornil and Mosinger (1933)	22	24.1	19	20.8
Elsberg (1941)	73	26.5	65	23.6
Puech (1947)	19	24.3	19	24.3
Von Muralt (1949)	24	19.8	34	28.1
Broager (1953) (Bush's series)	86	35.5	44	16.5
Paillas (1954)	27	33.7	14	17.5
Pais and Mastragostino (1955)	23	27.7	34	40.9
Rowbotham (1955)	14	23.3	22	36.6
Sassaroli and Chimenz (1955)	16	20.7	11	14.2
Torma (1957)	338	30.2	263	23.5
Arseni and Ionesco (1958)	114	31.4	130	35.9
Lang and Bridge (1959)	50	16.8	67	22.5
Pertuiset et al. (1960)	72	26.8	39	14.5
Cassinari and Bernasconi (1961)	44	23.6	52	27.9
Tucker et al. (1962)	49	29.3	55	32.9
Umbach (1962) (Riechert's series)	25	13.0	40	20.8
Agnoli et al. (1963)	23	31.9	9	12.5
Arjundas (1963)	20	10.8	48	26.0
Lombardi and Passerini (1964)	82	26.2	87	27.8
Sloof et al. (1964)	338	25.5	383	28.9
Guidetti et al. (1964)	45	20.2	53	23.8
Kloss et al. (1965)	42	13.9	45	14.9
Scaglietti et al. (1971)	55	19.9	132	47.8
Ausin (1972)	70	22.3	48	15.3
Nittner (1976) (Tonnis's series)	116	22.6	108	21.0
Niebeling and Hohrein (1978)	150	37.5	80	20.0
Cheng (1982)	204	12.4	767	46.1
Wen-Qing et al. (1982)	331	14.6	1110	47.1
Pagni et al. (1985)	39	24.0	18	10.7
Pansini (1994)	125	29.0	159	36.8

A. Pansini et al.
Spinal Meningiomas
© Springer-Verlag Italia 1996

We observed 18 meningiomas in men (14.4%) and 107 in women (85.6%). All case reports show a clearly higher prevalence among women, from a minimum of 66.7% (n=40) in Learmouth's series (1928) to a maximum of 100% (n=12) in that of Selosse and Granieri (1968) with Katz et al. (1981) and Umbach (1962) reporting prevalences of 70% (n=31) and 88% (n=22) respectively.

Only 65 cases have been reported that affected patients in the first 15 years of life (Table 3). The oldest

patient to undergo surgery was an 89-year-old who had a dorsal meningioma in D-12. Hossmann and Zulch (1966) report only one patient aged over 80 years as undergoing surgery. Table 4 presents the age distribution of our patients with meningiomas; here one sees that the neoplasm occurs more frequently in women and prevails in older age. Table 5 presents the distribution of meningiomas in our patients in terms of location. The corresponding data from other studies is shown in Table 6.

Table 3. Meningiomas in childhood (until 15 years of age): review of the literature

Reference	Total Meningiomas	Meningiomas in childhood
Ingraham (1938)	-	2
Hamby (1944)	185	10
Guillaume et al. (1949)	-	1
Ford (1952)	19	1
Hoff and Weingarten (1952) (with cases of Hoff and Potzl)	9	2
Ross and Bailey (1953)	13	1
Pais and Mastragostino (1955)	-	1
Grant and Austin (1956)	23	5
Gaist and Piazza (1957)	4	1
Haft et al. (1959)	30	1
Klein (1960) (with cases of Lefebvre)	35	1
Rand and Rand (1960)	48	2
Kozlowski and Michalski (1962)	3	1
von Geisler and Schuck (1963)	5	1
Romagnoli and Dal Monte (1964)	13	3
Iraci and Pellone (1965)	19	1
Arseni Maretsis (1967)	35	2
Matson (1969)	122	3
Till (1970) (with cases of Richardson and Till)	43	2
Intrau and Usbeck (1971)	10	2
Friedmann et al. (1972) (with Nittner's cases)	46	2
Ekelund and Cronqvist (1973)	8	1
Koos et al. (1973)	73	3
Rougerie (1973)	58	3
Grote et al. (1975)	83	2
Farwell and Dohrmann (1978)	21	1
De Sousa et al. (1979)	70	3
Pansini and Conti (1981)	270	2
Liu et al. (1985)	-	1
Tomita et al. (1988)	-	1
Chen et al. (1992)	-	1
Shuangshoti et al. (1992)	-	1
Fournier et al. (1993)	-	1

Table 4. Age distribution (years) of meningioma patients

	0-10	11-20	21-30	31-40	41-50	51-60	61-70	71-80	81-90
Men	1	-	-	1	3	5	6	2	-
Women	1	-	6	2	8	27	37	22	4
Total	2	-	6	3	11	32	43	24	4

Table 5. Location of meningiomas

Level	Men	Women	Total	%
Cervical	2	18	20	16.0
Dorsal	12	86	98	78.4
Sacrolumbar	4	3	7	5.6

The duration of symptoms among our patients was generally long, up to 50 years, but with a minimum of 1 month. The average was 6 years and 9 months. The onset of symptoms is analysed in terms of the location of meningiomas: cervical, dorsal and sacrolumbar. The symptoms observed include paraethesias, pain, loss of motility, sphincter disturbances and ataxia. Furthermore, each patient was examined to determine whether the disturbances corresponded to the level of the lesion or to supra- or sublesional sites. In many cases other disturbances may have been associated with the lesion that we had initially identified, but only the latter had been taken into account in the anatomical relationship between meningioma and spinal cord (as observed in the operating theatre). Due to certain anatomical-clinical aspects, seven cases were excluded from the concluding report: one of meningioma in double location, three meningosarcomas, two intramedullary meningiomas and one neurofibromatosis.

In the 432 primary intrarachidian tumours only twice was a meningioma in an intramedullary location identified. This is indeed an exceptional finding. To the present day only four cases have been reported in world literature (Table 7). In each case the intramedullary meningioma was located at cervical tract level, such as the cases reported by Pagni (1985) and by Salvati (1992). Both of these patients were men, 40 and 60 years old respectively, who had suffered from a very slow clinical course lasting over 30 years. The first case, where the neoplasm extended from C3 to C6, presented a distinctly improved postoperative clinical picture, while the patient in whom the lesion was located at C1-C2 level died due to respiratory insufficiency 2 months after surgery.

There were 9 cervical meningiomas (n=20; Table 8) whose initial symtomatology arose with motor deficit. In eight cases pain was the initial symptom (six ventroilate-

Table 6. Location of meningiomas: review of the literature

Reference	n	Cervical n	%	Dorsal n	%	Lumbar n	%
Elsberg (1916, 1925)	73	10	13.7	59	80.8	4	5.5
Busch (1935)	26	4	15.4	22	84.6	-	-
Antoni (1936)	18	3	16.6	15	83.4	-	-
Rasmussen et al. (1940)	140	23	16.4	115	82.2	2	1.4
Brown (1941)	130	24	18.0	101	78.9	5	4.0
Oddsson (1947)	48	4	8.4	42	87.4	2	4.2[a]
Bull (1953)	59	5	8.4	54	91.5	-	-
Broager (1953)	86	9	10.4	73	84.8	4	4.6
Pais and Mastragostino (1955)	23	2	8.6	14	60.8	7	30.4[a]
Guillaume et al. (1957)	70	19	27.0	49	70.0	2	3.0[b]
Arseni and Ionesco (1958)	114	15	13.0	99	87.0	-	-
Kolle (1959)	45	4	8.9	40	88.9	1	2.2
Pertuiset et al. (1959)	57	5	8.7	51	89.4	1	1.7
Cassinari and Bernasconi (1961)	44	5	11.3	39	88.6	-	-
Umbach (1962)	25	6	24.0	17	68.0	2	8.0
Lombardi and Passerini (1964)	82	9	10.9	73	89.0	-	-
Becker (1965)	86	26	30.2	60	69.8	-	-
Hossmann and Zulch (1966)	68	16	23.5	48	70.5	4	5.8[c]
Selosse and Granieri (1968)	12	1	8.3	9	75.0	2	16.6
Iraci et al. (1971)	94	22	23.4	69	73.4	3	3.1[a]
Scaglietti et al. (1971)	55	18	32.7	35	63.6	2	3.6
Bret et al. (1976)	60	8	13.3	47	78.3	5	8.3
Nittner (1976)	86	26	30.2	60	69.7		-
Katz et al. (1981)	44	10	22.7	33	75.9	1	2.2
Grellier et al. (1982)	42	3	7.1	38	90.4	1	2.3
Levy et al. (1982)	97	17	17.9	73	73.0	7	7.0
Wen-Qing et al. (1982)	165	36	21.8	115	69.6	14	8.4[a]
Pagni et al. (1985)	39	2	5.1	36	92.3	1	2.5
Solero et al. (1989)	174	26	14.9	144	82.7	4	2.4
Pansini (1994)	125	20	16.0	98	78.4	7	5.6[a]

[a] Extended to the sacrum.
[b] None below L2.
[c] Two sacral.

Table 7. Reported cases of intramedullary meningiomas

Reference	Age, sex	Level	Clinical course	Operation	Symptom	Result
Pansini (1981)	40, M	C4-C6	10 years	Total	Tetraparesis	Improvement
Pansini (1981)	60, M	C1-C2	37 years	Total	Tetraplegia	Death
Pagni et al. (1985)	47, F	C5	7 months	Total	Tetraparesis	Improvement
Salvati et al. (1992)	67, F	C2-C4	10 years	Total	Tetraparesis	Improvement

ral; one posterolateral; one posterior). Three patients complained of sole paraesthesias as initial disturbances (two ventrolateral; one posterolateral). In 11 patients the initial symptoms corresponded to the level of the lesion, in 9 to a level below that of the lesion. Sphincter disturbances affected two patients only, and one complained of ataxic gait.

Dorsal meningiomas were the most frequent in our series (n=98; Table 9). In 49 pain was the typical element occurring at the onset of symptoms (also occurring in association in 14 others). The neoplasm was posterolateral in 26 cases, ventrolateral in 8, anterolateral in 6 and posterior in 4. Paraesthesias were the initial symptoms in 27 patients (in 39 associated with other factors): 10 ventrolateral, 7 posterolateral, 5 posterior and 5 anterior. Twenty-two patients complained of motor impairment in the initial stage of symptoms (reported by 65 other patients in association with other symptoms); in 11 cases the meningioma was posterolateral, in 6 posterior, in 4 ventrolateral and in one anterior. The symptom mani-

Table 8. Cervical meningiomas

C1	1[a]
C1-C2	3
C2-C3	2[a]
C2-C6	1
C3-C4	1
C4	1
C4-C5	3[b]
C4-C6	1
C5-C6	2
C7	1
C7-D1	4

[a] The meningioma in C1 is one of the two meningiomas observed in C2-C3. They were located in an intramedullary site.
[b] A case in an extradural location.

Table 9. Dorsal meningiomas

D1	3
D1-D2	11
D2	4
D2-D3	9
D3-D4	3
D4	5
D4-D5	1
D4-D6	1
D5-D6	8
D5-D7	1
D6	2
D6-D7	9
D7	3
D7-D8	5
D8	2
D8-D9	5
D9	1
D9-D10	6[a]
D10	2
D10-11	5[a]
D11	3
D11-D12	5
D12	2
D12-L1	2

[a] One case in D9-D10 and one case in D10-D11 had a completely extradural location.

ally reported in five and paraesthesia disturbances in one. Only two patients presented sphincter disturbances.

Figures 7-11 illustrate meningiomas in the various locations, and Table 11 summarizes the locations of the 125 meningiomas, excluding the two with intramedullary locations and the one with intrarachidian location. This

Table 10. Sacrolumbar meningiomas

L1	1
L1-L2	1[a]
L2	1
L2-S1	1
L3-L4	1
L5-S1	1
S1	1

[a] The meningioma observed in L1-L2 had intra- and extradural location.

summary demonstrates that a greater percentage of these tumours are of anterolateral or posterolateral development (21.1% and 28.4% respectively); these data confirm the surgical experience that meningiomas are located very close to the motor roots or, more frequently, to the sensory roots.

In three cases of our series (2.4%) the location of the meningioma was entirely extradural while one case (0.8%) showed predominantly extradural development. According to Pagni et al. (1987), 9.7% of cases show epidural development (the completely extradural plus the predominantly extradural). However, the incidence of extradural locations in meningiomas varies in different case reports. In Henschen's case report (1955), it reaches 20%, while other authors (Rasmussen et al. 1940; Guillaume et al.

fested itself below the level of the lesion in 56 patients, at the level of the lesion in 38 and above the level in two. Various degrees of sphincter disturbances occurred in 24 patients, and ataxia was observed in two of these.

Lumbar and sacral meningiomas are relatively rare, and we observed only seven cases in our series (Table 10), all of which presented with a painful onset. In relation to the spinal cord, two occurred in posterolateral sites, one anterior, one anterolateral, and one occupied the rachidian canal completely. Motor deficit was addition-

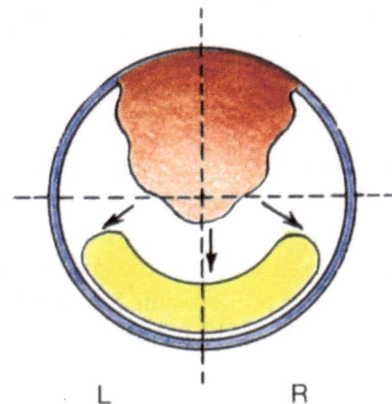

Fig. 7. Anterior view. In our series this location was identified 12 times at dorsal level and only once at lumbar level

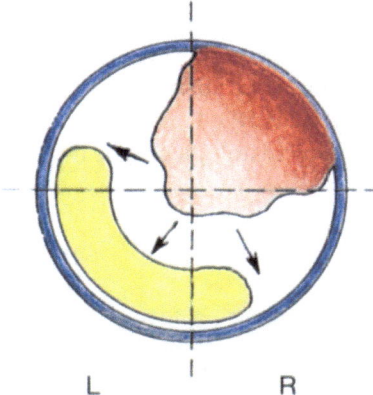

Fig. 8. Anterolateral view. The most frequently identified meningiomas in this location are located dorsally. In our series there were 26 of these, against 10 cervical and 1 lumbar

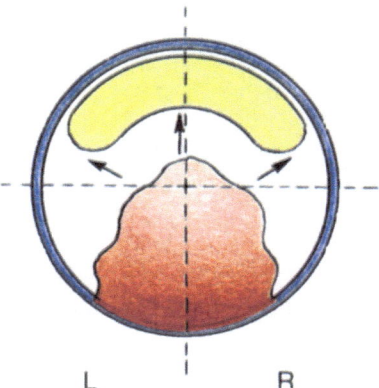

Fig. 11. Posterior view. There are 15 posteriorly located meningiomas, 14 dorsal and 1 cervical

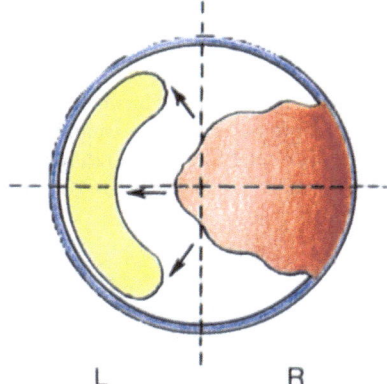

Fig. 9. Lateral views. Eight meningiomas were identified in lateral locations, all of which were located dorsally

Table 11. Summary of locations of meningiomas

Location	Cervical		Dorsal		Lumbar	
	n	%	n	%	n	%
Anterior (n=13)	0	0	12	92.3	1	7.7
Anterolateral (n=37)	10	27	26	70	1	3
Lateral locations (n=4)	0	0	4	100	0	0
Posterolateral (n=41)	4	9.8	35	85.4	2	4.8
Posterior (n=15)	1	6.6	14	93.4	0	0

1957; Becker 1965; Levy et al. 1982) report none. In only one case did we observe a double location of a meningioma. A second observation concerned a patient suffering from type 2 neurofibromatosis. Multiple locations of meningiomas are rare. Pagni et al. (1990) report 22 cases from a review of the literature. More recently other sporadic cases have been reported (Roda et al. 1992; Spinas and Beninia 1992; Makiuchi et al. 1993; Chaparro et al. 1993).

Table 12 presents the results of diagnostic rachicentesis performed in 86 of the 125 meningiomas observed in our series. Rachicentesis was not performed in cases presenting a clinical picture of severe medullary pain and where the withdrawal of fluid could have contributed to aggravation of the neurological syndrome. The values of the protein levels in the fluid suggest that cytological albumen dissociation is more frequent the lower the fluid block. The changes in the protein doses were 68.75% in cervical meningiomas, 85.07% in dorsal meningiomas and 100% in lumbar meningiomas. These differences are statistically significant although the numbers of cases considered, at least in the lumbar tract, are low.

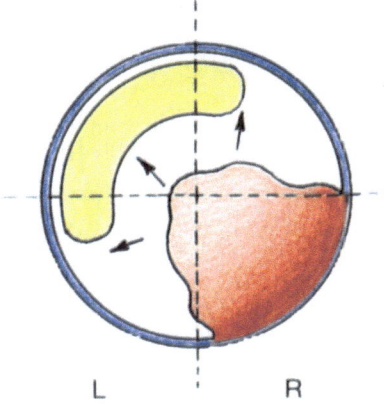

Fig. 10. Posterolateral view. Of the 41 meningiomas under observation 35 were located dorsally, against 4 cervical and 2 lumbar

Table 12. Results of cerebro spinal fluid test in 86 meningiomas

	Cervical	Dorsal	Lumbar	Total	%
Abnormal (prot. tot. >40 mg/100 ml)	11	57	3	71	82.6
Normal (prot. tot. <40 mg/100 ml)	5	10	-	15	17.4

Each case in this series was examined histologically by colleagues at the Institute of Anatomy and Pathological Histology, University of Florence. In examining the various meningiomas we abided strictly by the classification specified by the WHO. Table 13 presents the distribution of our cases by histological type (Figs. 12-20).

Table 13. Frequency of the different histological types of meningiomas

	n	%
Transitional	55	44
Psammamatous	21	16.8
Meningothelial	18	14.4
Fibroblastic	15	12
Nonclassified	7	5.6
Sarcomatous	4	3.2
Calcified in toto	3	2.4
Syncytial	1	0.8
Angioblastic	1	0.8
Total	125	

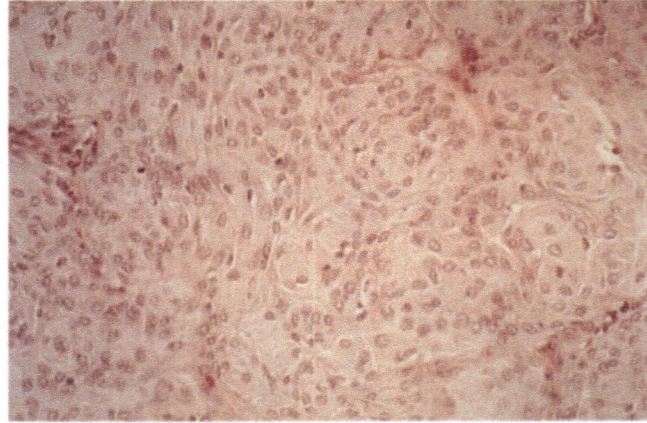

Fig. 12. Meningothelial meningioma. The neoplastic cells, arranged in a layer, have an ample and slightly eosinophil cytoplasm and undefined margins. The nuclei are moderately large and located centrally. H&E, 40

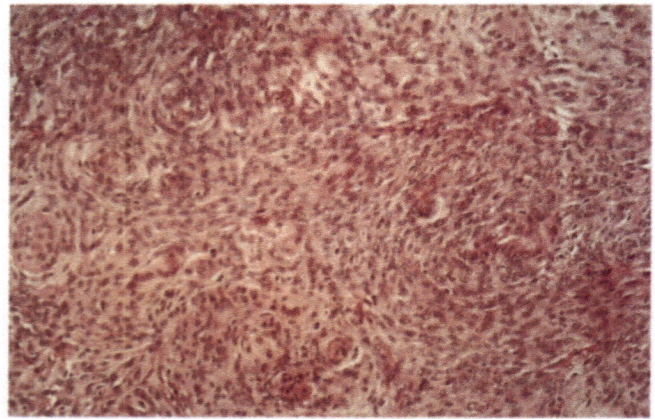

Fig. 13. Transitional meningioma. The neoplastic cells have a polygonal, spindle-shaped appearance and are arranged in a layer or in a vortex. H&E, 40

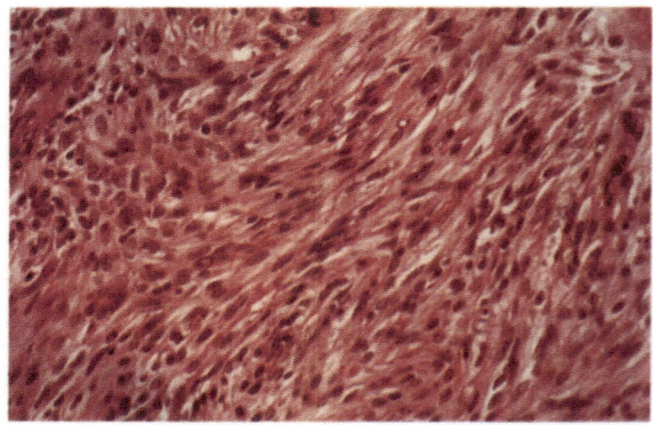

Fig. 14. Fibroblastic meningioma. The neoplastic proliferation derives from bundles of spindle-shaped cells. H&E, 40

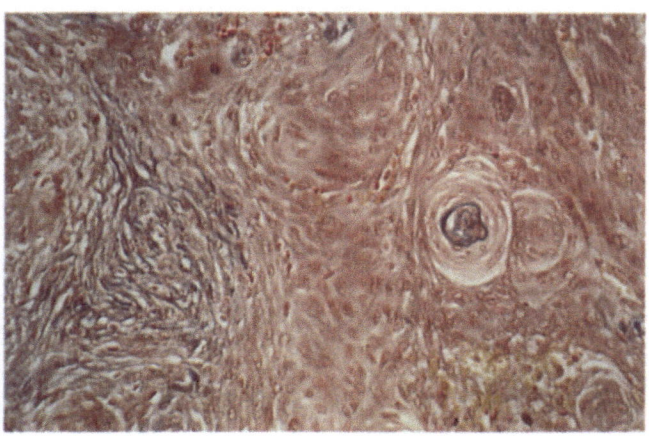

Fig. 15. Transitional meningioma. The trichromatic colouring (according to Masson) enhances the presence of collagen fibres between the neoplastic cells and the central part of a vorticoide structure

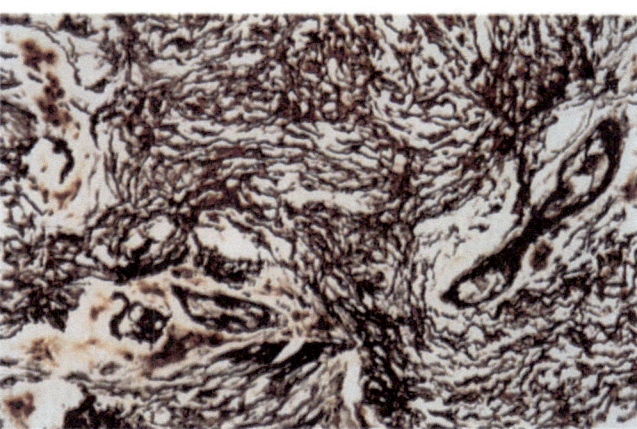

Fig. 16. Transitional meningioma. The silver staining shows an abundance of reticular fibres around the neoplastic cells and in the walls of blood vessels 25

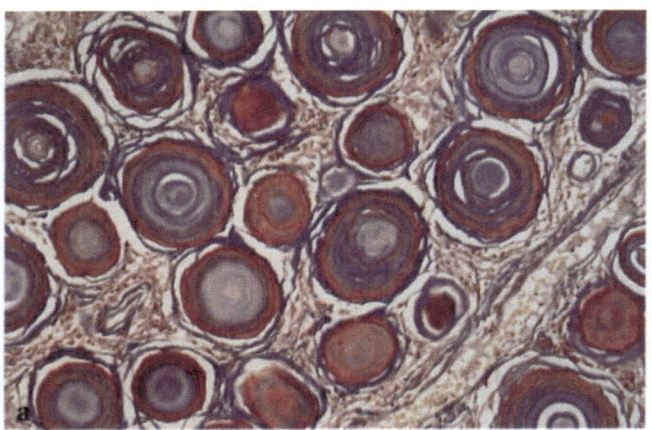

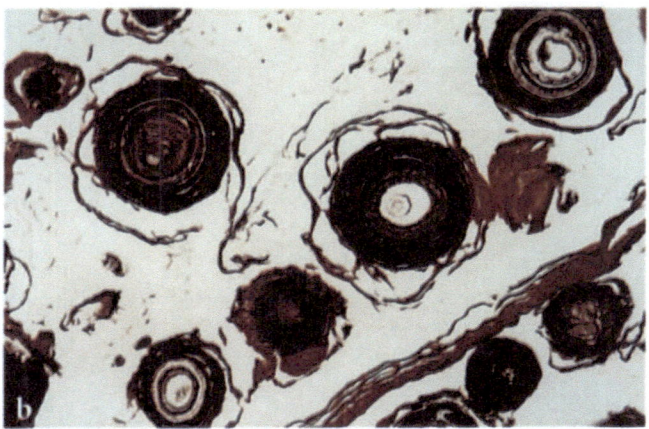

Fig. 17a,b. Psammomatous meningioma. Psammomatous bodies enhanced by trichromatic colouring, according to Masson (a; × 25) and by silver staining for the reticular fibres (b; × 40)

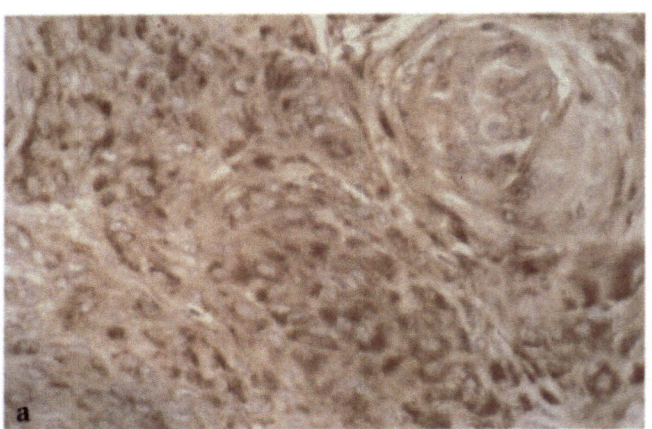

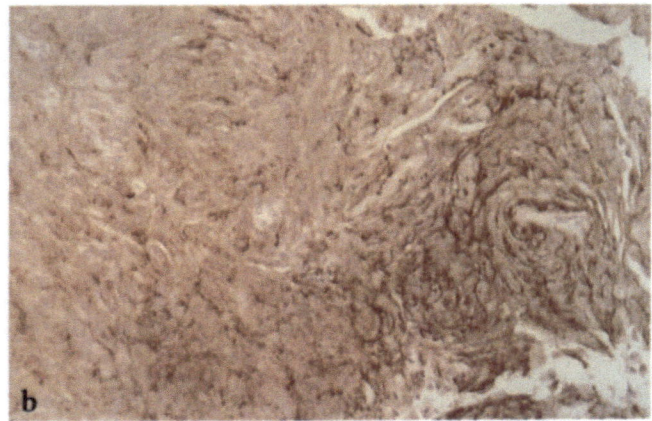

Fig. 18a,b. Transitional meningioma. The immune histochemistry test shows a diffused positivity of the neoplastic cells for Vimentin (a; × 40) and for the epithelial membrane antigen (H&E: b; × 40)

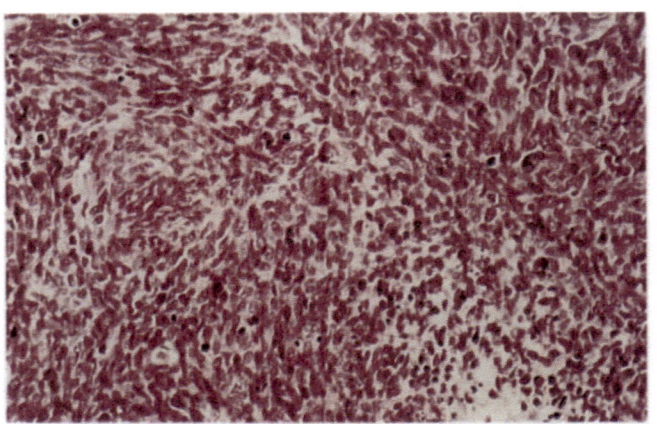

Fig. 19. Malignant meningioma. Neoplastic proliferation formed by closely packed cells. There are numerous mitotic elements and a necrotic area (H&E: × 25)

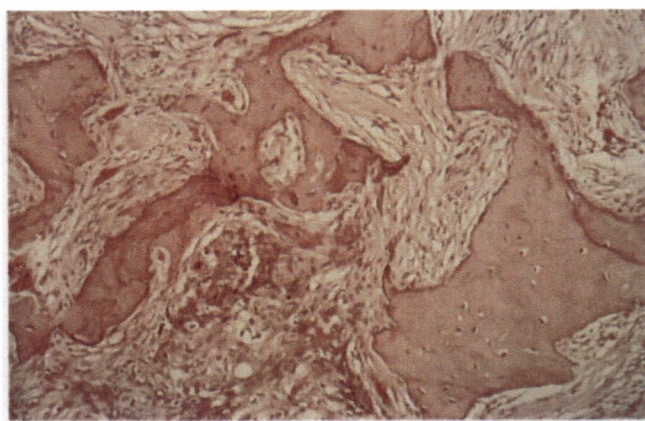

Fig. 20. Transitional meningioma, with a widespread ossified area (H&E: × 40)

6 Clinical Symptoms

A. Pansini - F. Lo Re - P. Conti - R. Conti

The course of clinical symptoms in cases of spinal meningioma is generally characterized by a variable period of time, pain, and later by a phase in which cord disturbances seem to stabilize. The symptoms of the irritative pain syndrome are due to direct initial compression of the mengioma on one or more nerve roots. We retrospectively studied the clinical reports of our patients from 1962 to 1994 and collected data useful in identifying anatomical-clinical features and the beginning of the syndrome.

Descriptions in the literature regarding the onset of this compression concern the sensory and motor lesion syndrome, beginning from the alterations in the roots by the side of the spinal cord which are followed by sublesional signs, both motor and sensory, due to functional damage to the columns of the cord. These characteristics constitute the clinical picture of many meningiomas, which after a variable length of time from the onset of symptoms establish a pathological condition known as myelitic affection, which results from the mechanical action of compression affecting vascular variations.

The semiological picture is established shortly after the irritative symptoms begin or by an uncertain course lasting months or even years, therefore making early diagnosis of the tumour very difficult. A clinically suspected meningioma is even more difficult because after an initial phase, signs of medullary disturbances do not appear for a long time, and results of the neurological examination are almost always negative. In comparison to other compressive forms of various etiology, the characteristic features of a meningioma are a very slow developmental course and the ability of the cord to adapt, being enclosed and compressed against the meningeal walls inside the rachidian channel. These features are found particularly in benign juxtamedullary tumours such as neurinomas. In these compressions there is evidence of resistance by the medullary neural structures, which accounts for the long

asymptomatic period and rapid functional decompensation of the medullary cord tracts by a mechanism consisting of a segmental or sublesional vascular insufficiency. Chapter 9 examines the morphological alterations caused by meningiomas on the neural structures of the cord and the meningeal sheaths which are detectable with the operating microscope, and we also examine ischaemic processes in the anterior and posterior arterial territories. The radicular arteries undergo compression during the formation of the meningiomas.

Since the clinical symptoms of myelitic disturbance can occur at a very late stage and develop into a serious and irreversible condition if not identified before serious vascular damage takes place, we studied the subjective symptoms reported by patients before the appearance of neurological symptoms. We observed that when clinical signs persist for decades the first symptom was not radicular pain but simply back pain. The pain associated with the rachis reported by patients is located in the rachidian tract where, on the basis of other symptoms the diagnosis of levels was formulated, without well-defined characteristics and still corresponding to the region in which the meningioma developed. The dorsal tract was found to be definitely more frequently affected.

6.1 Regionally Localized Pain

The pure form is extremely rare on the cervical tract and is hardly ever present on the occipito-atlantoid passage in meningiomas in C4 or in lower sites. In one case of meningioma in C2 with a clinical course lasting 22 years, back pain of a transitory nature was accompanied by contractions of the paravertebral muscles, thereby reducing voluntary lateral movements and flex extensions of the head (see case no. 68; Figs. 21-25).

A. Pansini et al.
Spinal Meningiomas
© Springer-Verlag Italia 1996

Case No. 68: Transitional Meningioma

An 82-year-old woman (1988). Right anterolateral extramedullary-intradural meningioma in C2.

Clinical Course. 22 years. Slight cervical pain from the age of 60 years. One year before hospitalization painful paraesthesias appeared distally on both hands. In a few days progressive sensory loss imped-

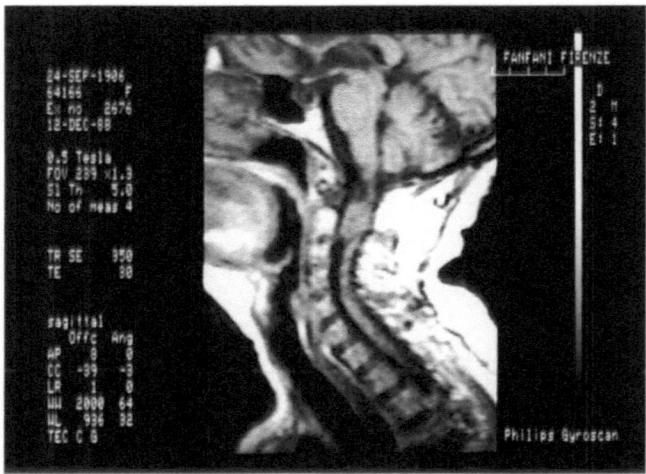

Fig. 23. MRI, multiplanular, cervical study. In T1, an isohyperdense ovoidal lesion located behind the vertebral body of C2. The antero-laterally located meningioma compresses the cord posteriorly and on the left

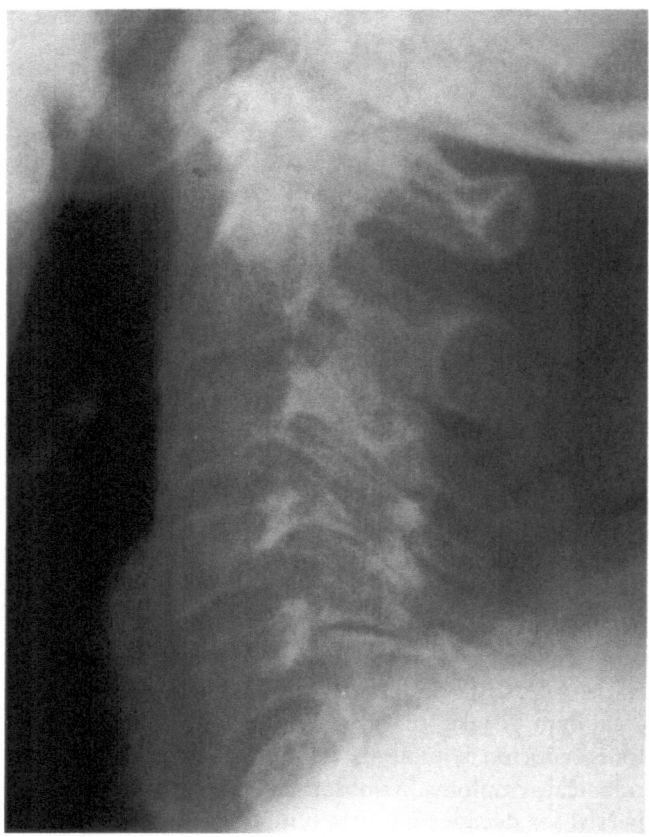

Fig. 21. X-ray of cervical rachis. The lateral projection produces an image showing a calcified thickening corresponding to the lamina of C2 and C3

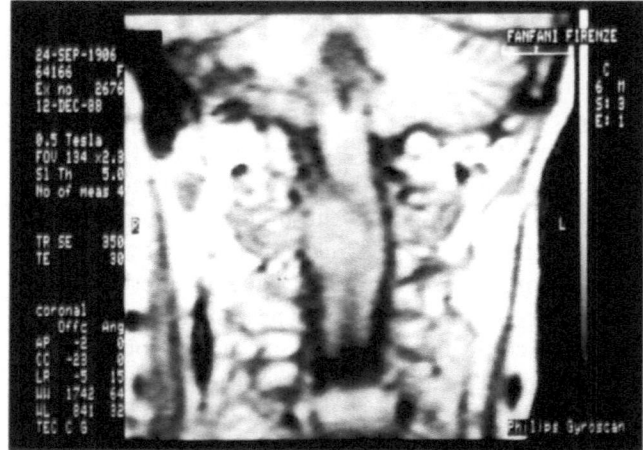

Fig. 24. MRI, coronal projection

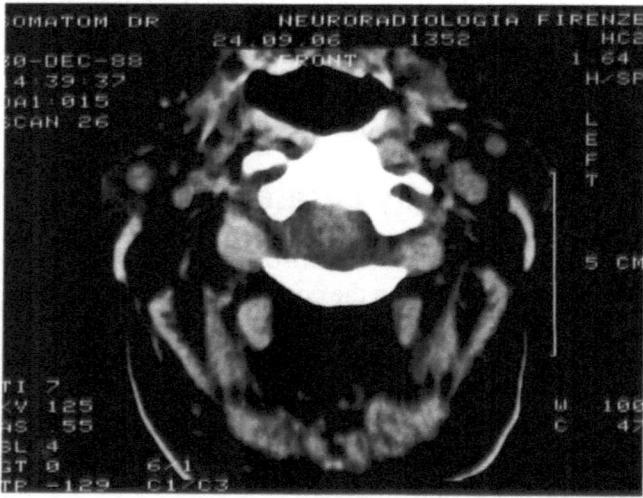

Fig. 22. Myelo-CT. A small thickening stands out on the right near the intravertebral foramen, which probably represents the meningioma's base of attachment

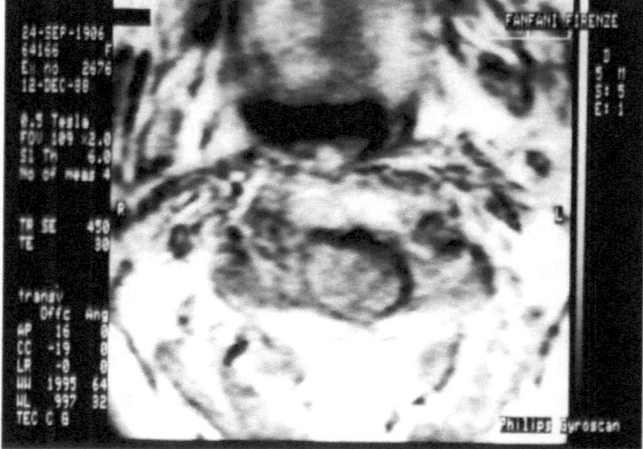

Fig. 25. MRI, axial projection

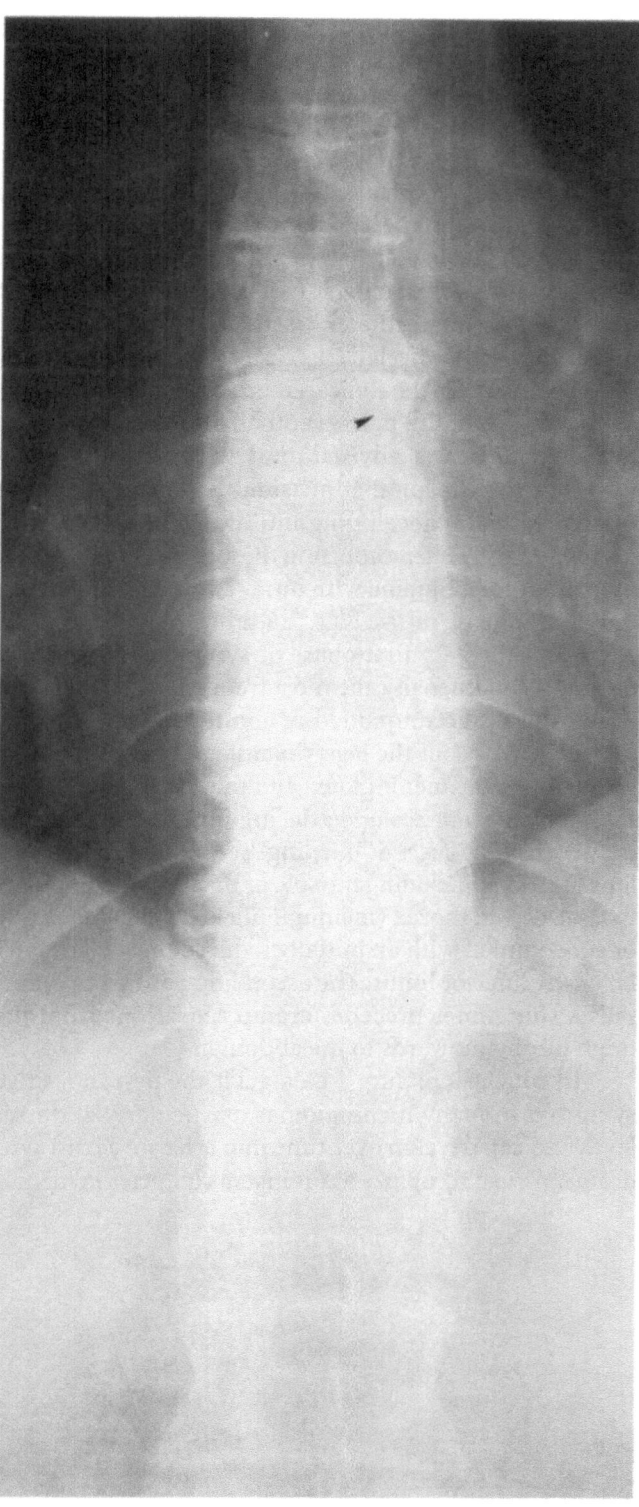

Fig. 26. X-ray of dorsal rachis. Anteroposteriorly the erosion of pedicles in D8-D9 is observed and is more evident on the left *(arrow)*

ed movement of the fingers. Rigidity felt at lower limbs with difficulty in moving.

Neurological Examination. Spastic tetraparesis mainly on the right. Evident impediment in movement of the fingers. Band of hyperaesthesia on C2, bilaterally with hyperaesthesia below.

Rachicentesis. 0.55 g protein per thousand.

X-Ray of Cervical Rachis. Laterally a slight increase in distance from vertebral body of C2 to base of spinous process, of the space at C2-C3 level; anteroposteriorly an irregular, roundish image of a calcified appearance.

Myelo-CT. Hyperdense lesion in relation to cord in C2-C3 which occupied three-fourths of the canal anterolaterally and on the right pushing the cord contralaterally.

MRI. In T1 an isohyperintense ovoidal lesion located behind vertebral body of C2. The meningioma in an anterolateral site displaced the cord posteriorly and to the left.

Surgical Treatment. On opening the dura the whitish coloured cord, due to poor superficial blood supply, seemed to be pushed towards the left. After performing a large opening in the arachnoid near the right cervical root, slight traction on the cord showed a brownish red meningioma. Without performing a posterior radicotomy, attempt to incise capsule of the tumour. The hard consistency of the meningioma prevented surgical removal by fragmentation. The meningioma was removed en bloc after tilting it against the internal dural wall. Coagulation of the well-defined base of the tumour.

Results. The immediate postoperative course showed signs of recovery of the motor deficit. After a further 40 days there was improvement in the neurological picture and walking without support.

The symptomatic triad consists of back pain, contracture and the reduction in movement which occurs in many compressions with intramedullary development.

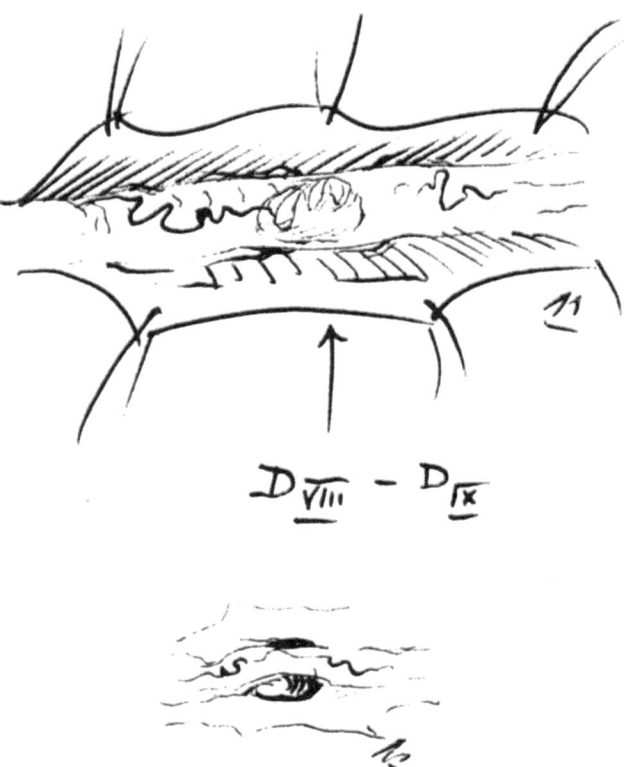

Fig. 27. Drawing of the operative field

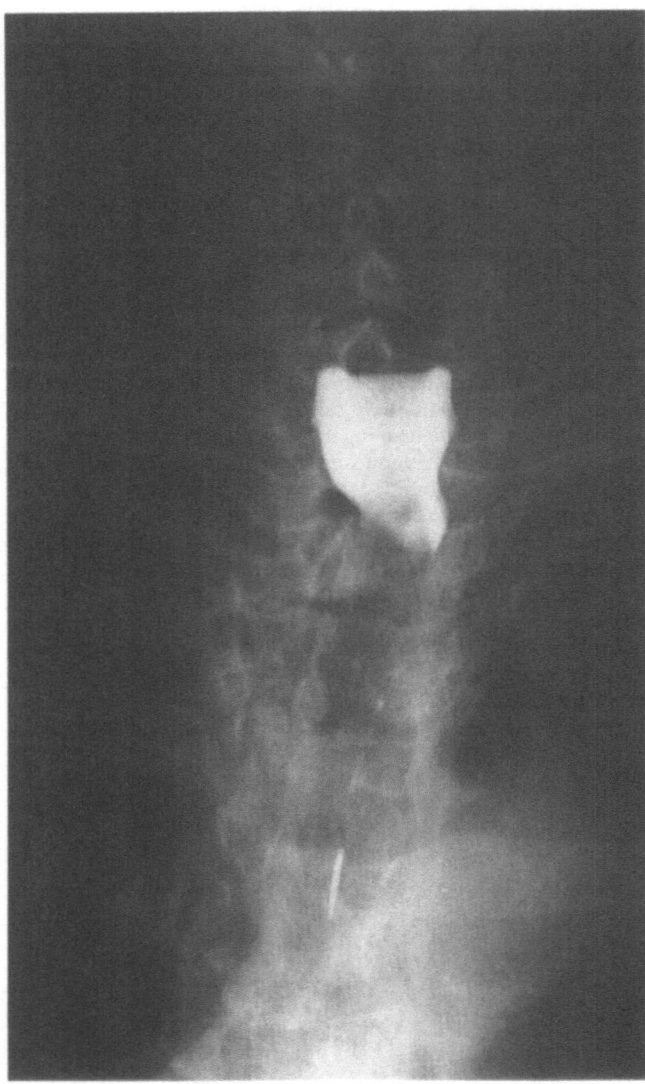

Fig. 28. Suboccipital myelography. Total block in D2, producing a doubtful diagnosis for meningioma. The tumour is definetely located on the left

When cervical pain occurs, it is very early in meningiomas and is subject to a variable duration. It occurs more frequently in dorsal locations (19 cases) and produces signs of simple back pain or a form of pain affecting shoulder and head movements, not necessarily constant or intermittent, but when it is constant the pain is accompanied by a paravertebral numbness of the skin. In one case the clinical course lasted 15 years (see case no. 27; Figs. 26, 27). The intensity varies; when it persists, it is associated with slight paravertebral paraesthesia, particularly if the superior dorsal segment is affected (see case no. 55; Figs. 28, 29). In one of our patients the clinical course of the syndrome lasted 41 years, and the pain eventually became so intense that the patient was advised to use a spinal cast. Only 3 years prior to hospital admission the back pain led to intercostal pain, developing into the painful root syndrome, typically interscapular in the same territory (psammomatous meningioma with intra- and extradural development. See case no. 55; Figs. 28, 29).

After the very first phase of symptoms, variable in duration and intensity, the most frequent signs are distal paraesthesias accompanied at about the same time by motor weakness of the legs, first affecting the leg on the same side as the meningioma and then the other. Paraesthesia to the feet rises up to the inguinal region (see case no. 71). In some cases a "burning" sensation is felt in various locations, including the sole of the foot (meningioma in D5-D6) and thorax (meningioma in D1-D2) preceding or concomitant with an initially reduced muscular tonicity of the inferior limbs. The ascending nature of paraesthesia sometimes precedes cramp sensations from the thigh leading upwards to the abdomen.

In conclusion: pure rachialgia is the first subjective symptom in many meningiomas, particularly at dorsal level, and can develop over time into a sensory cord syndrome. We can recognize a contingent character in menin-

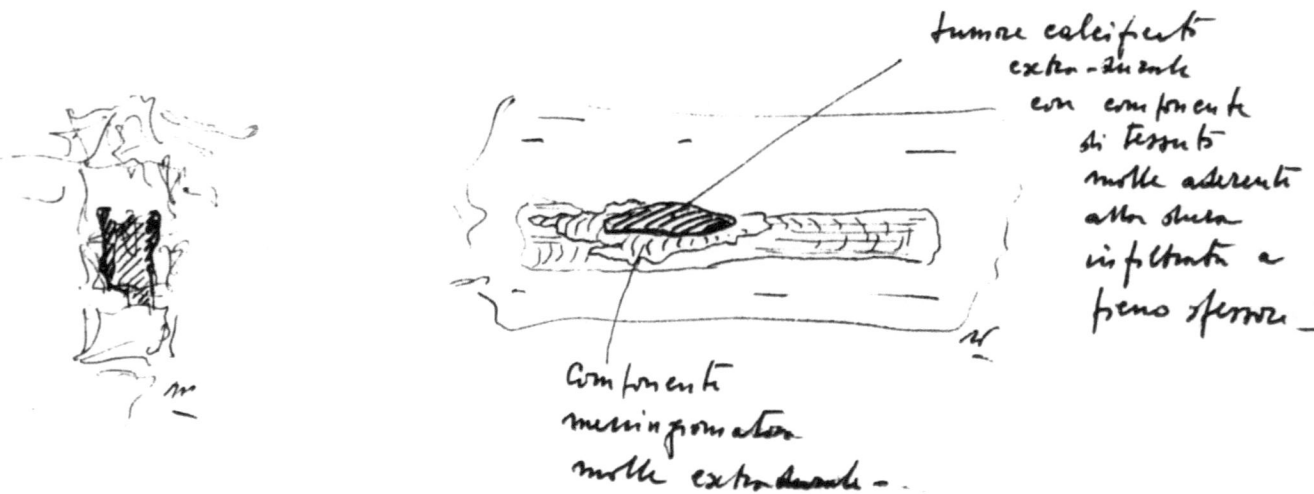

Fig. 29. Drawing of the myelography and of the operative field

gioma when distal paraesthesia occurs before the onset of radicular signs. In all cases except one (case no. 51) the clinical course of the syndrome, with back pain, lasted between 5 and 50 years. In this one case lower dorsal pain continued for 40 years and the meningioma in D12 was diagnosed after 50 years; the first irritative radicular symptom to the right hip appeared only after the patient had suffered 40 years of back pain (see case no. 43; Figs. 30, 31).

Case No. 43: Transitional, Psammomatous Meningioma
A 75-year-old woman (1978). Premedullary-extramedullary-intradural meningioma in D12.
Clinical Course. 50 years. Pain in lower dorsal tract. For 10 years an accentuation of dorsal pain with irridiation to the right hip; then cutaneous numbness and paraesthesia distally to the feet. Irridiation to the posterolateral side of the thigh and the leg up to the external malleolus, bilaterally and occasionally to the heel, prevalently to the right, for 3 years. Difficulty and instability in walking for 1 year. Sphincter disturbances in the form of incontinence. In the 3 years previously she was able to walk with support.
Neurological Examination. Spastic paraparesis with hyperreflexia. Hypertrophy of the lower third of the femoral quadricep on the left. Ataxic gait without support. Hypoaesthesia from L1 on the left and from L2-L3 on the right.
Rachicentesis. 0.30 g per thousand.
X-Ray of Dorsolumbar Rachis. Scoliosis with peaks of acute spondyloarthrosis. Erosion of left pedicle of D12 and of posterior margin of vertebral body, with enlargement of the interlaminal space, due to erosion of the lamina.

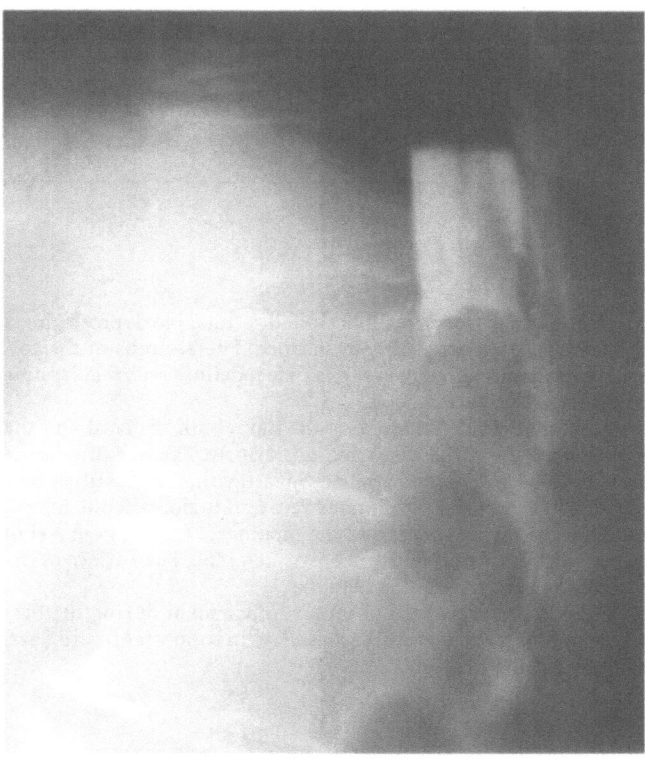

Fig. 30. Suboccipital myelography. Total block laterally producing a dome-shaped image with irregular margins in D12. The subarachnoidal space above is wide anteriorly

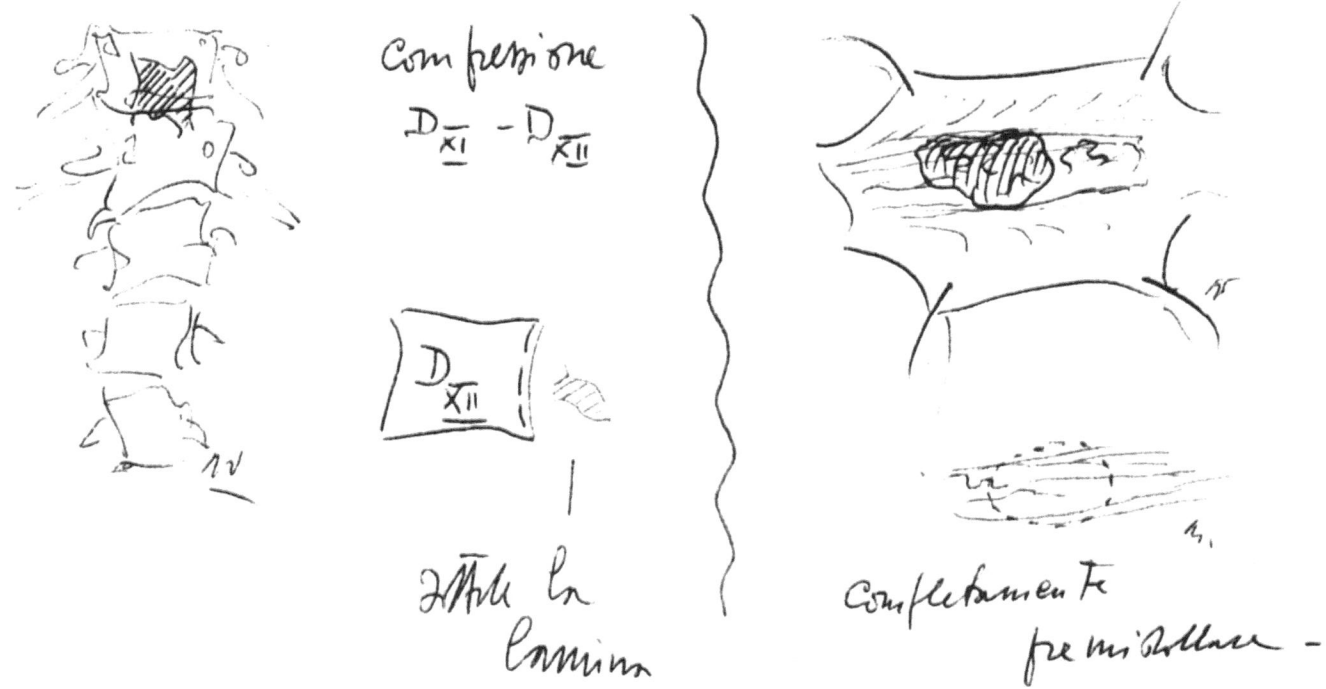

Fig. 31. Drawing of the myelography and of the operative field

Table. Length, in years, of symptomatology, affecting patients with an onset of back pain.

Years	0.5	1	3	5	8	10	12	15	20	30	41	50
N	1	2	2	3	1	3	1	2	1	1	1	1

Mean	=	10 years
Average	=	12 years, 10 months

Myelography (performed suboccipitally). Total block producing a dome-shaped aspect. Anteroposteriorly, lateral limbs of the column spread and the central filling defect defines an irregular area in the form of a cluster.

Surgical Treatment. On opening the dura, both the cord and the spinal roots appeared displaced posteriorly. The opening of the arachnoid allowed a premedullary investigation to identify a neoplasm adhering to a large lumbar vein and to the 12th dorsal root on the right, corresponding to the meningeal funnel. Removal of adherent process and of the neoplasm en bloc. The surface of the tumour presented a calcified lamina.

Results. Gradual recovery of motor impairment during the first week, and the patient was able to walk with support. After 10 days, normal ambulation.

The above table shows the various durations of the clinical course in compressive syndromes of the meningioma with an onset of back pain.

6.2 Sensory Radicular Symptoms

The clinical development of the meningioma is in every way similar to juxtamedullary compressions with an involvement of a posterior root. Radicular pain or pain distributed in a lateral band is considered to be the first symptom affecting the level of the irritative monoradicular symptoms. There is not always involvement of a single root; this depends on the vertical extent of the meningioma. It seems clear that the particular vertical extention of a lateral meningioma affects the symptomatic picture and in time causes an irritative action or compression on more than one root.

After the initial phase of radicular symptoms the adjacent nerve cordal structures are affected by compression, varying at different times in relation to the volume of the tumour. The course and sequence of symptoms varies from case to case. In every form of meningioma there is a precise anatomic correspondence between the site of tumour and nearby neural structures; however, the alterations to the arterial reticular surface-layer circulation and the intrinsic vascular network to the cord cause symptoms at a distance from the compression site. *During the course of the symptoms there are therefore early sensory root syndrome cases followed by cordal disturbances (see case report no. 54, Fig. 32); alternatively,* the latter may precede the irritative-compressive root syndrome.

Case No. 54: Psammomatous Meningioma

A 70-year-old woman (1976). Ventral and lateral intradural-extramedullary meningioma on the right in C4-C6, invading near the motor root in C5 on the right.

Medical History. Surgery at the age of 20 years for a fibroid. Bronchial asthma, recurrant phlebitis to lower limbs and cardiopathy.

Clinical Course. 10 years. Pain to margin of ulna on the right hand. For 2 years suffered from motor claudication with sudden loss of strength at the knees, and consequent paraplegia.

Neurological Examination. Spastic tetraparesis characterized by loss of strength distally to the hands, in particular to the right hand. Lively patella reflexes with bilateral foot clonus and bilateral Babinski sign. Impossible for the patient to stand upright or walk. Hypoaesthesia from C6-C7, pronounced distally. Sphincter disturbances in the form of retention.

Rachicentesis. Protein 6 g per thousand.

X-Ray of Cervical Rachis. Cervicodorsal kyphosis with enlargement of canal in C4-C5.

Myelography (performed suboccipitally). Total block with lateral flow and a lateral left filling defect area in C4.

Surgical Treatment. On opening the dura, the cord appeared reduced in volume, displaced and curved to the left; the sensory roots of C5-C7 appeared elongated and wound around the tumour. A radicotomy of posterior sensory root of C6 and removal of the meningioma en bloc, cutting the motor component of C5 enveloped by the tumour.

Results. After an initial improvement in flex-extension movements of lower limbs, on the fifth day the patient was affected by bronchial pnuemonia; fell into a coma, and death followed.

The root syndrome sometimes develops only at a later stage. Major or minor myelitic damage often causes sublesional cordal signs which assume certain characteristics, distinguishing these signs from other forms of compression. The effort to identify for every tract of the rachis the most frequent symptoms of the various sites at onset has lead us to add a detailed description of cases that show a very particular neurological picture. When the meningioma is located at a low cervical tract pain usually irridiates to the upper limb, in contrast to the upper dorsal forms in which the pain affects the thorax and extends to the abdomen. In meningiomas with sacrolumbar development (particularly rare forms: 7 of 125) the symptoms almost always show characteristics of monoradicular pain or, from the beginning, pluriradicular pain that is similar in every way to that identified in cauda syndromes of other forms. The so-called "radicular" pain does not always develop in the same way because the pain

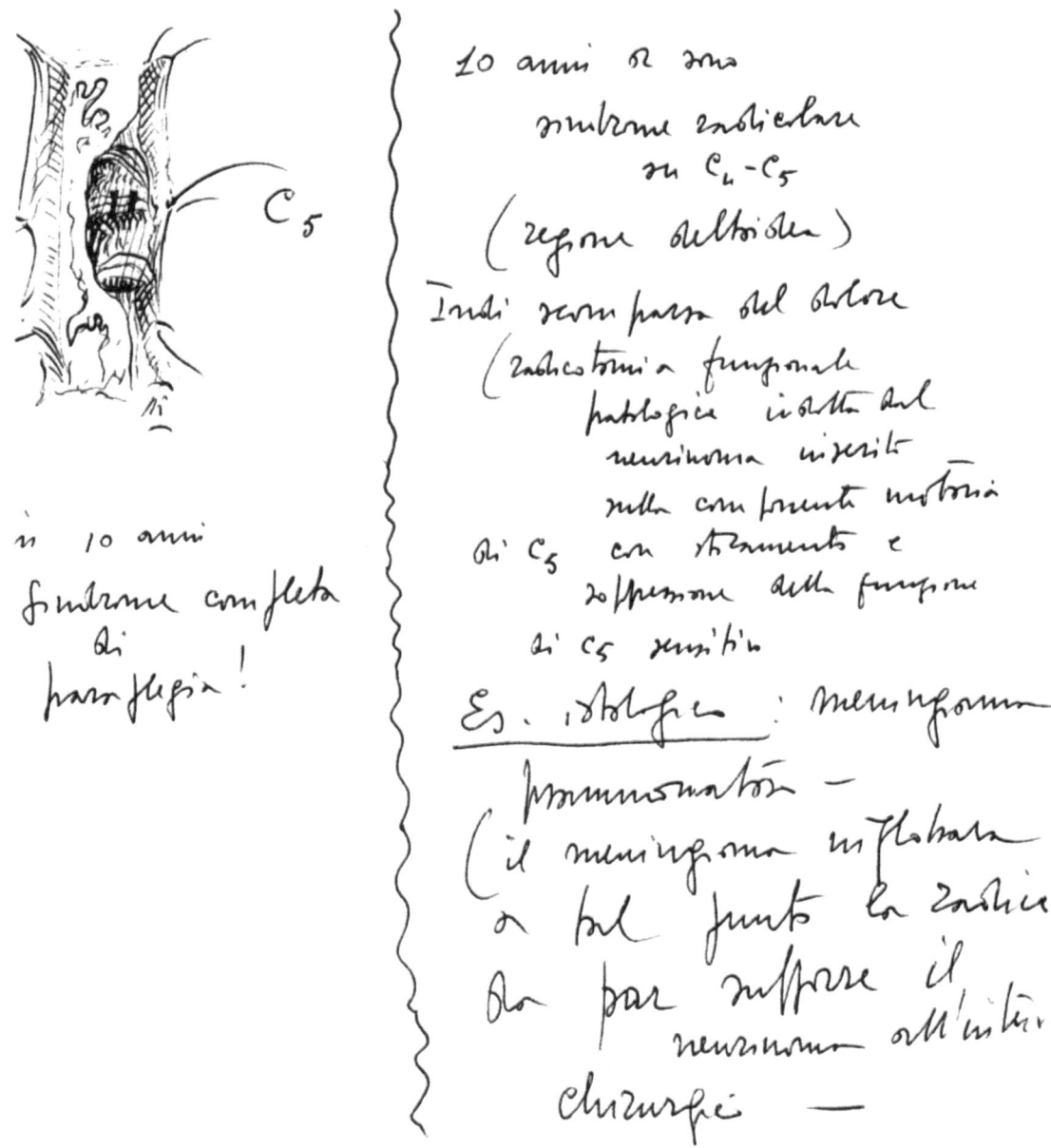

Fig. 32. Drawing of the operative field

in the dorsal region along a particular dermatomere can be traced to the single vegetative fibre component of the cord. It is difficult to define the source of the pain, as it is described as producing uncomfortable deep "internal" sensations located in a deep, muscular area or producing a feeling of constriction or of burning. These ailments are never anteroposterior as in cases affecting the sensory roots where the pain is in the thoracic region and is sometimes restricted to the precordial site (see case no. 105, Figs. 33-36).

Case No. 105: Psammamatous Meningioma

A 69-year-old woman (1981). Posterolateral intradural-extramedullary meningioma on the left in D1-D2 adhering to the root D2 on the left.

Clinical Course. 30 years. At the age of 34 years the patient was affected by at intervals irradiated pain in the suprascapula and left mammary region. In recent years the pain appeared more frequently until it became finally constant. Four months before she came under observation both inferior limbs were affected by hypostenia and progressive difficulty in walking.

Neurological Examination. Spastic paraplegia with slight hyperreflexia without clonus or Babinski signs. Slight instability in walk-

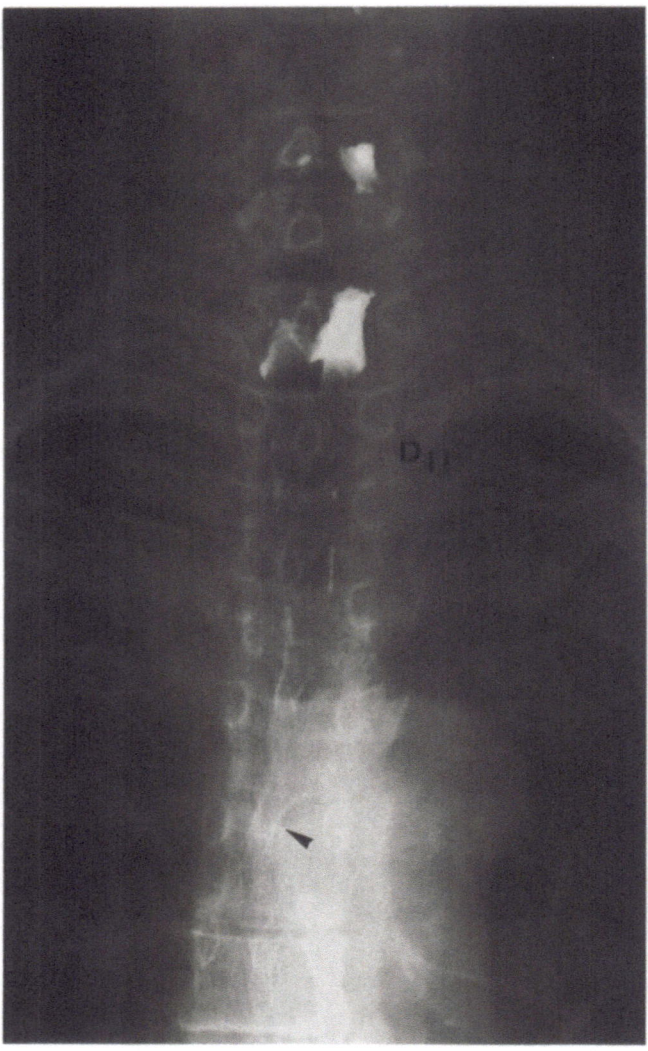

Fig. 33. Suboccipital myelography. Total block in D1-D2, predominantly on the left, producing a curvilinear aspect with irregular margins and defining an expansive intradural-extramedullary lesion. Slight right-convex scoliosis and anomalies of the spinous processes (*arrow*)

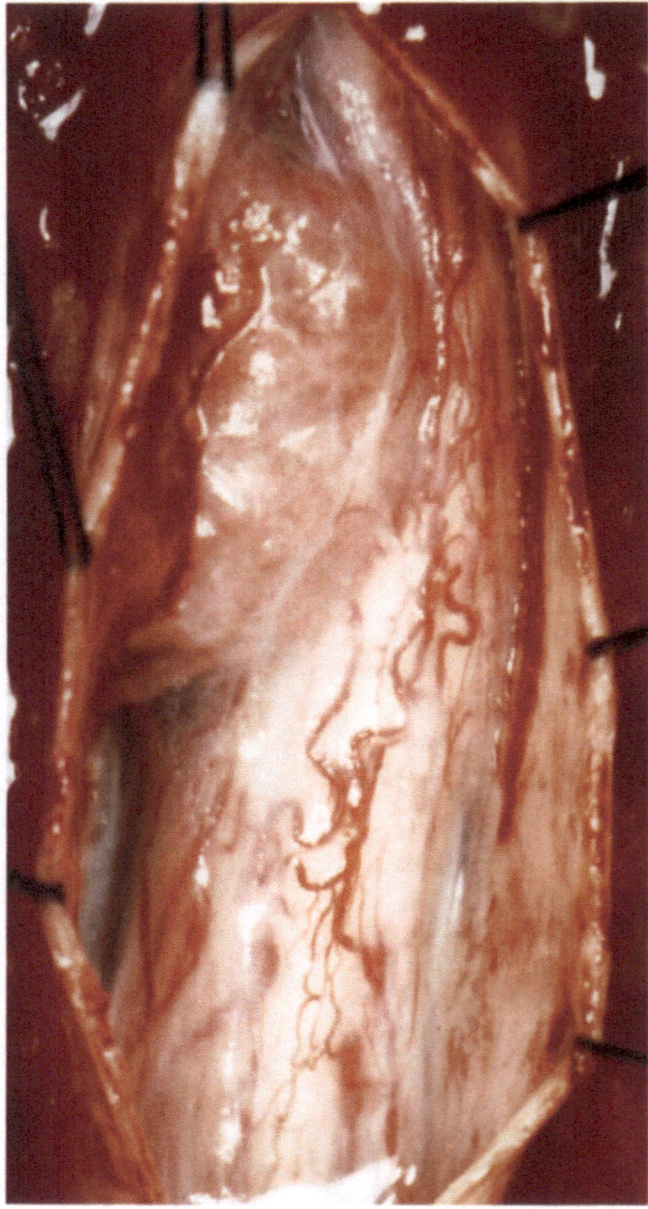

Fig. 34. The meningioma is covered by an arachnoidal process. The insertion to the internal dural surface is clearly visible, with infiltration of the dural plane

ing. Hypertrophy on the left thigh. Hyperaesthesia on D1-D2 on the left.

Rachicentesis. 0.40 g protein per thousand.

X-Ray of Dorsal Rachis. Slight left convex scoliosis.

Myelography (performed suboccipitally). Partial block producing a dome-shaped filling defect corresponding to the space D1-D2.

Surgical Treatment. On opening the dura, the spinal cord was pushed to the right by a small meningioma the size of a peanut. Opening of the arachnoid and freeing the tumour below from the root D2, which was removed in toto. The enlarged cord transversely showed signs of ischaemia 2 cm below the tumour. Coagulation at the base of the attachment.

Results. Total disappearance of pain and after a few days complete recovery from paraparesis. Still no disturbances after 10 years. Seven years after the surgery a small meningioma on the left side of one falx in the frontal region was found.

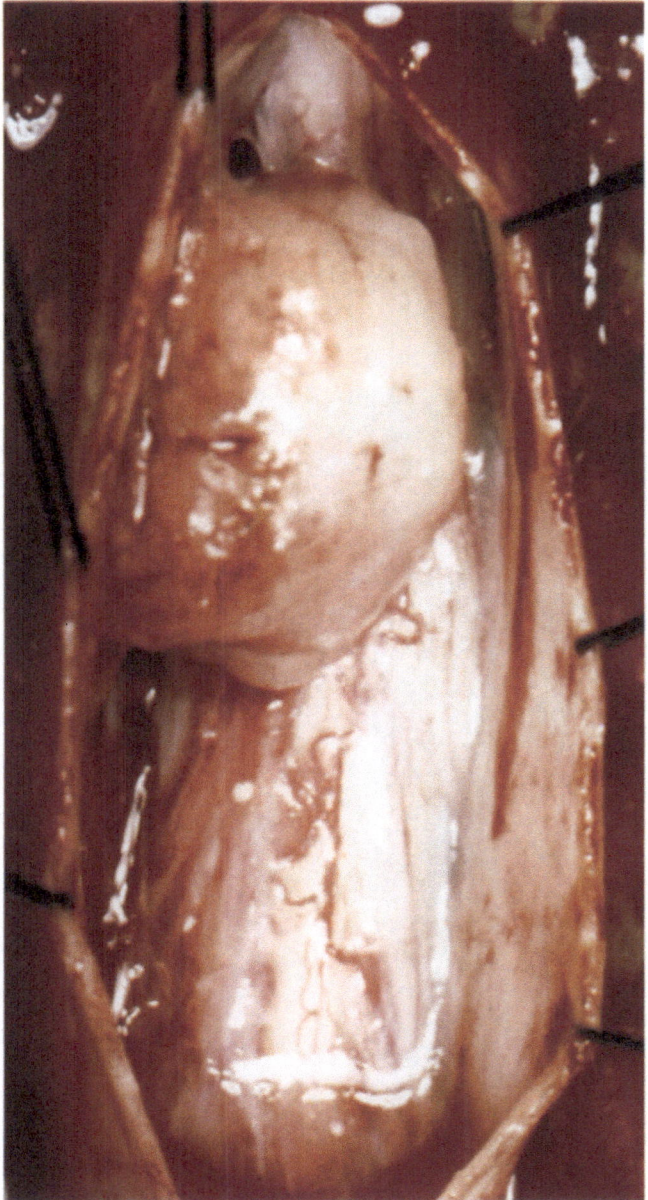

Fig. 35. The meningioma appears freed from the arachnoidal covering. Below on the left it appears in close connection to the second dorsal root in proximity to the ventral part of the tumour. Dilatation of the plial circulation with widespread ischaemic areas. The cord seems flattened below the tumour

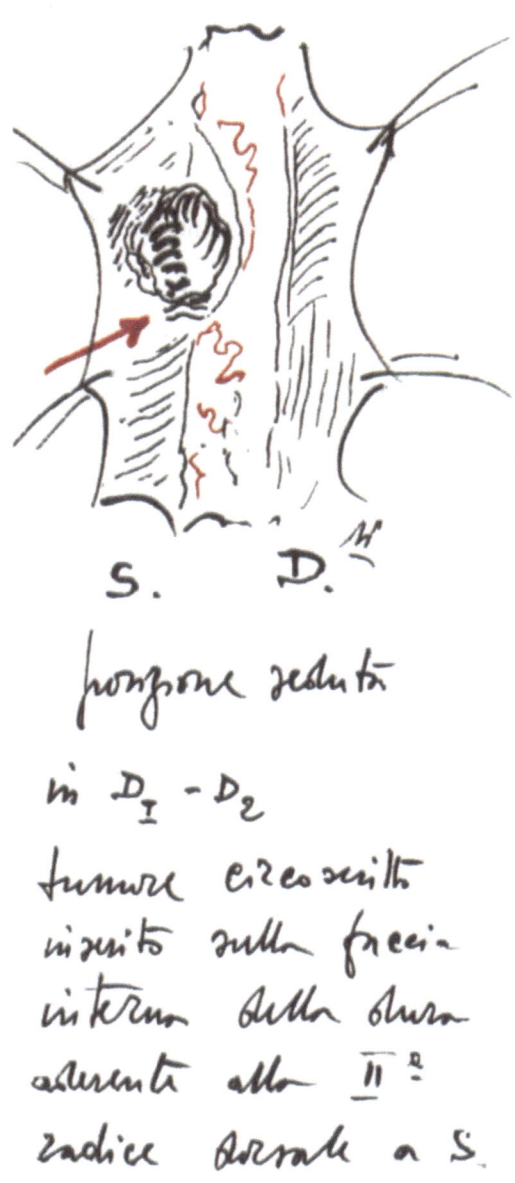

Fig. 36. The meningioma insertion occupies the whole thickness of the dura (dashed line)

6.3   Cervical Root Syndrome

Radicular pain in our 20 patients was located from onset at the distal region of the upper limbs. The pain seemed to be more intense at the proximal level of the arms and in the paravertebral site. The forms and the development of cervicobrachial pain (see case nos. 2, 21) were characterized by motor impairment, in one case of the hand which was later rapidly affected by monoplegia, while another case was affected only by a simple sensation in the legs. In two cases, in C2-C3 and in C4-C6, the entire development of the clinical syndrome was prolonged: in one patient it lasted 22 years and in another 10 years. In the latter case the pain (of an intermittent nature) remained within the margin of the ulna and the upper limb for 8 years with subsequent motor impairment "claudication" to the lower limb (see case nos. 68 and 54).

6.4 Dorsal Root Syndrome

Dorsal root syndrome was found in 20 cases (20.83%) in relationship to the rachidian level and distributed as follows: from D1 to D5 in the upper dorsal tract in five patients, from D6 to D9 at the medial dorsal tract in eight and from D9 to D12 in seven. Upper dorsal pain may affect the supramammary region spreading to the underarm and subscapula regions (meningioma in D2; see case no.

112). The initial unilateral pain is generally located at the middle dorsal level from D7 to D10 (see case no. 57, Figs. 37-41) and presents a bilateral distribution before the appearance of myelitic symptoms.

Case No. 57: Transitional Meningioma
A 56-year-old woman (1986). Lateroposterior intradural-extramedullary meningioma in D8-D9 on the right.
Clinical Course. 6 years. Dorsal pain on medial tract irradiating

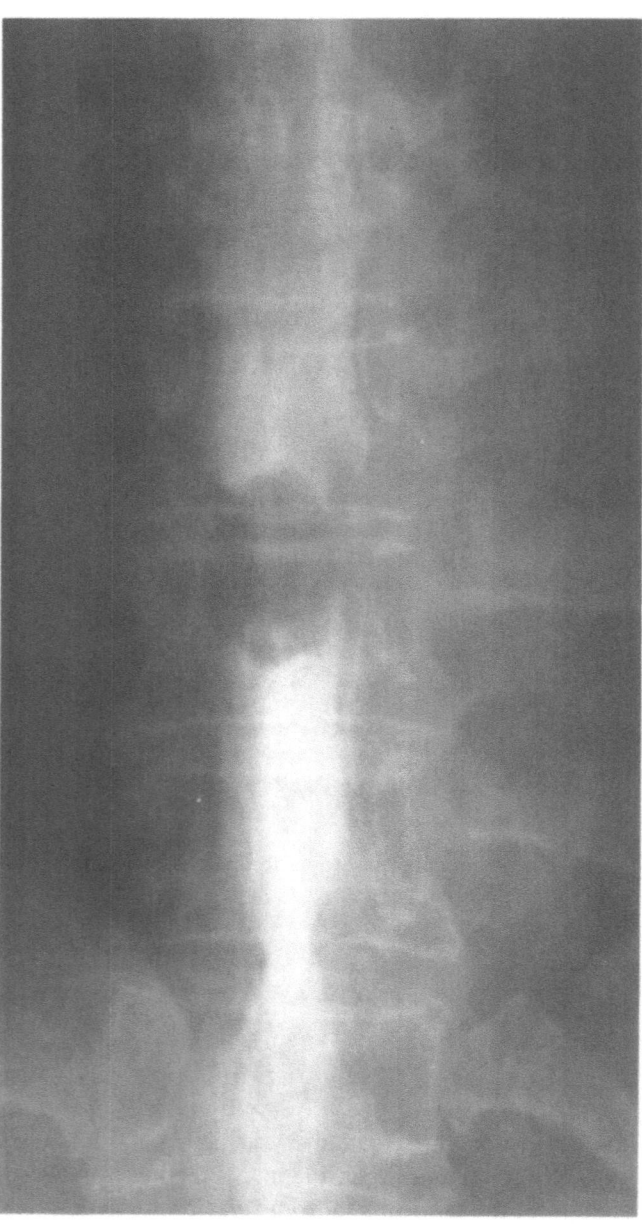

Fig. 37. Myelography via lumbar puncture. The contrast medium stops flowing temporarily at D9 level, defining an oval-shaped filling defect which extends to the lower border of D8 on the right. The cord is displaced contralaterally. Below this block in D10-D11 the dural sac has an hourglass appearance which, as seen in a lateral projection, is due to the posterior compression by the apophyseal arthrosis

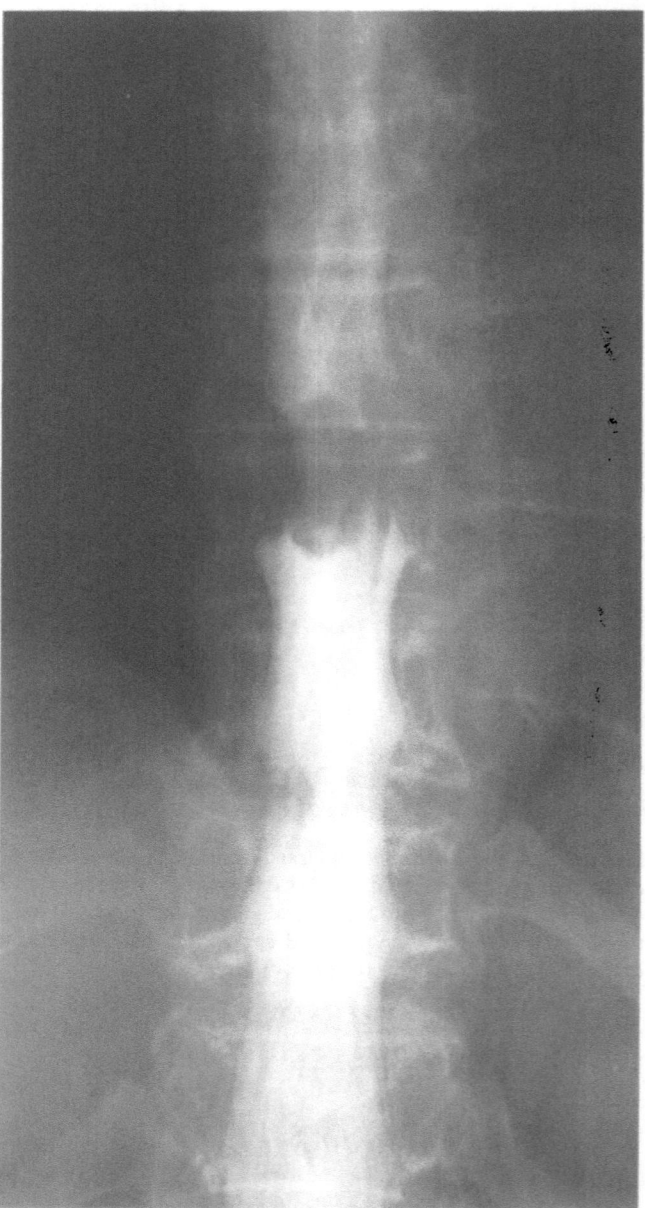

Fig. 38. The presence of the contrast medium is seen better at the inferior margin of the meningioma. The root outlets are dilated on the right side

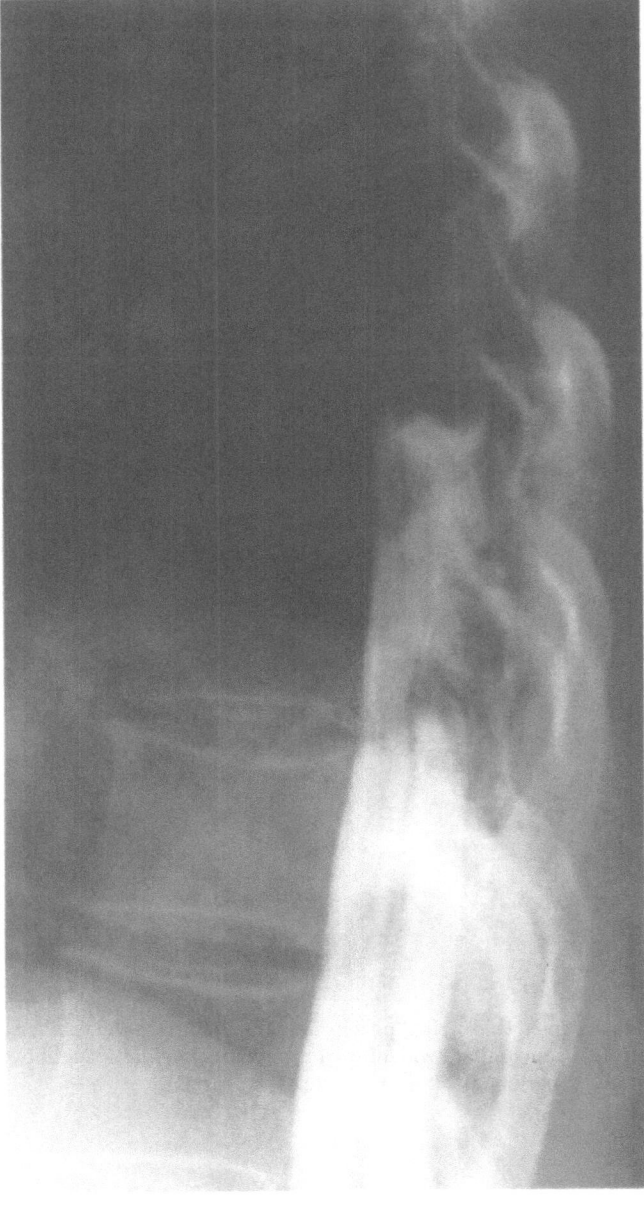

Fig. 39. The contrast medium shows an irregularity at the bottom of the meningioma corresponding to the double bumping of the tumor

and worsened by coughing. The pain stopped spontaneously after a few months but started again on the right hemithorax and was still affecting the patient. Impediment to the lower limbs, affecting the right limb in particular, with loss of strength. Paraesthesia, as a tingling sensation to the lower right quadrant of the abdomen and to the soles of the feet. Hot and cold type of dyaesthesias affecting the lower limbs. The symptoms presented gradually ingravescent characteristics until 1 month prior to hospital admission, when the motor deficit grew rapidly worse, presenting coordination impairment that made walking impossible.

Neurological Examination. This showed the presence of cutaneous angiomas in the abdomen region. Hypotonia of the femoral quadricep and right leg. Deficit of leg flexation to the thigh. Deficit of dorsal and plantar flexation of the foot, bilaterally and predominantly on the right. Flaccid left patella; lack of ankle jerk. Walking was impossible without support. Tactile, temperature/pain hypoaesthe-

sia from D9, becoming anaesthesia from D11. Sphincter disturbances in the form of retention of urine.

Rachicentesis. 0.70 g protein per thousand.

X-Ray of Dorsal Rachis. Slight, segmental scoliosis. Erosion of the vertebral pedicles in D7-D8 on the right. Stenosis of the rachis canal in D10-D11.

Myelography (via lumbar puncture). Total block in D9, with oval-shaped and irregular filling defect; a slight flow passed the block on the left. Anterolaterally the corridor corresponded to the displaced cord on the left.

Myelo-CT. This confirmed the irregularity of the subarachnoidal space, which identified the morphological aspect of the neoplasm.

Surgical Treatment. The dural surface appeared stretched. The dura was opened, showing the reddish coloured meningioma adhering to the dural surface. Stasis of the arterial circulation. The right root at D9 was wrapped round the meningioma as a band. Gradual splitting of the tumour, lifting it upwards and pressing it to the left. Excision and coagulation of the dural layer of the attachment. The cord presented a mark left by the neoplasm.

Results. Gradual recovery and progressive regression of sensory disturbances. All movements involving the lower limbs recovered except for flexion of the right leg to the thigh. Notable recovery of plantar and dorsal flexion of the right foot and the disappearance of sphincter disturbances. After 3 months walking became possible with the aid of a support. Slight paraesthesia persisted at the feet. In inferior dorsal meningiomas the pain retained similar characteristics to the pain associated with neurinomas.

In this location the attacks of variable intensity can be of a paraosseous nature and only later rapidly deteriorate; the pain is described by patients as intolerable under strain, when coughing and during defecation, and with the typical characteristic intense peaks of pain at night which occur more frequently in neurinoma cases. The accentuation of pain occurring in the variations of the decubitus position is also typical of the neurinoma syndrome, with the difference that patients suffering from meningiomas are incapable of finding a comfortable position. However, the pain is less constant. These symptoms were found in four cases and only once in a dorsal meningioma in D5-D6 (see case no. 60, Figs. 42, 43; and case no. 120).

Case No. 60: Psammomatous Meningioma

A 62-year-old woman (1982). Right anterolateral intradural-extramedullary meningioma in D5-D6.

Clinical Course. 1 year. Pain at dorsal level with band-like irradiation affecting predominantly the right, brought on by coughing or with strain. Gradual sensory impairment mainly on the right with motor impediment. Sphincter disturbances started 1 month previously.

Neurological Examination. Spastic-ataxic paraparesis mainly on the right with bilateral foot clonus and Babinski sign. Hypoaesthesia from D7.

X-Ray of Dorsal Rachis. Modification of vertebral body in D5 due to slight decalcified area in the lower right lateral portion.

Myelography (performed suboccipitally). Total block on the right in D5-D6. The iodine column became thicker, producing a dome-shaped image. A slight flow passed the block, defining an oval-shaped filling defect.

Surgical Treatment. The cord appeared curved towards the right, where the surface of a neoplasm was seen. The sensory root was wrapped around it. After opening the arachnoid, the capsule was

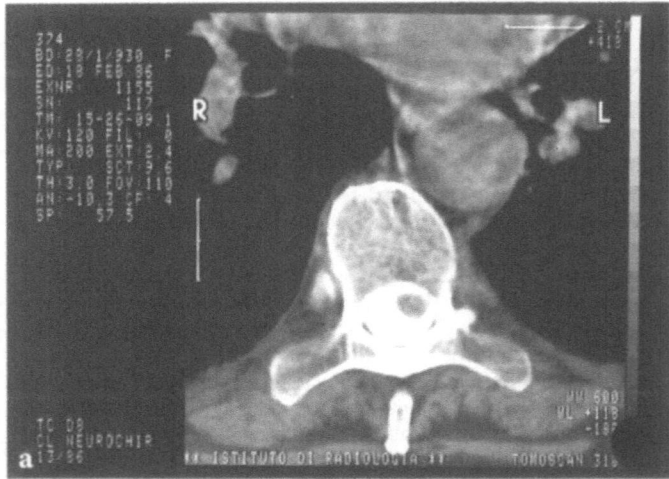 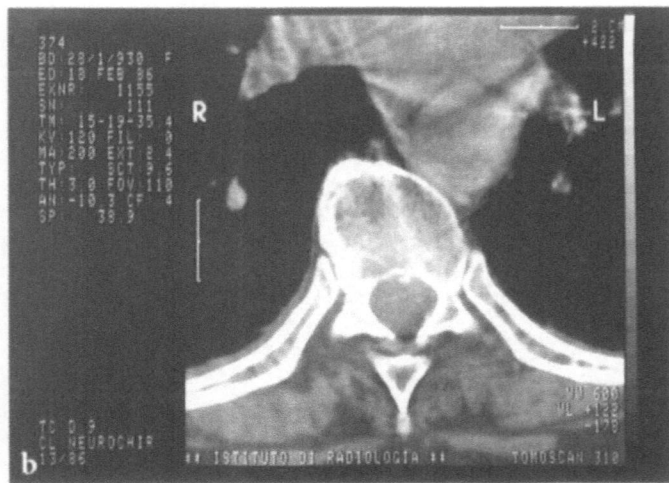

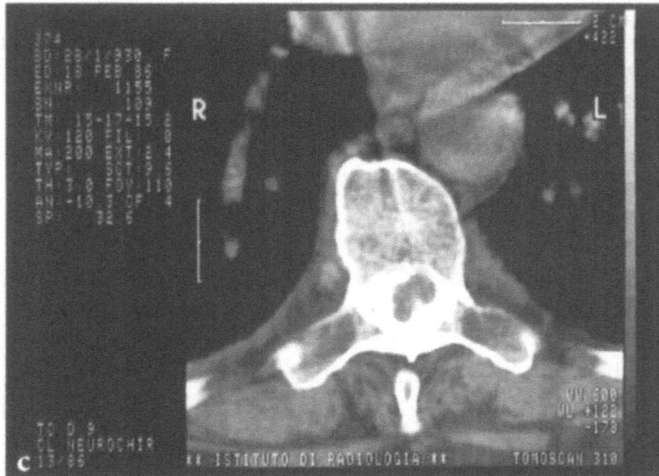 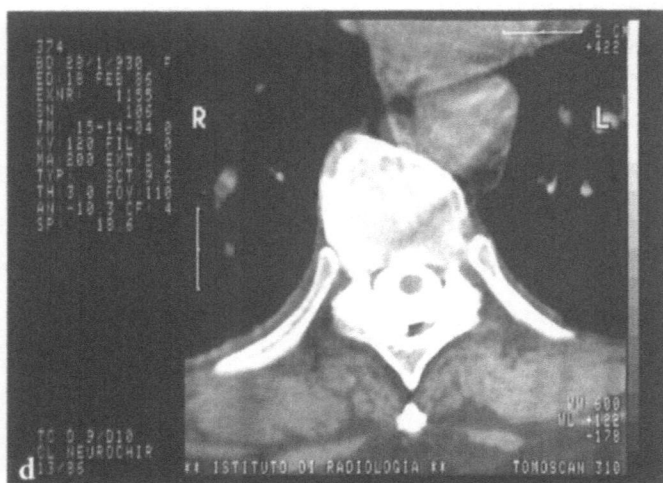

Fig. 40a-d. Myelo-CT. At D8-D9 level the vertebral canal is almost completely occupied (b) by right posterolateral, intradural solid, isodense lesion at the spinal cord, which is compressed and displaced towards the left (c). Concomitant widening of the subarachnoidal space above (a) and below the lesion (d). In D10 the yellow ligaments are calcified and leave a mark on the posterior side of the dural sac

incised, and the tumour was debulked, which facilitated the removal of adhering structures between the neoplasm and anterolateral surface of cord. The cord's surface blood system appeared greatly narrowed.

Results. Walking began within 15 days and became normal in 3 months. The patient's condition remained stable after 1 year. Occasional slight pain in the submammary region on the right.

At the initial stage of every painful dorsal syndrome the pain is localized in a particular area but eventually spreads, following a pattern typical of radicular syndromes. Irradiation at the beginning may appear incomplete, but it can become band-like bilaterally and sometimes occurs with greater intensity on one side. In lower thoracic sites (D11-D12) pain appears to affect a very unusual topography. The pain along one hip is accompanied by paraesthesia, with a saddle-like supply in sublesional zones (see case no. 35). The clinical course in one of our patients

lasted 10 years. Radicular pain can regress almost totally after reaching peak intensity. This is an exceptional condition and has been reported only once, together with peripheral paresis to a lower limb; the meningioma in L2 followed a rapid course of 6 months. In this case the meningioma was malignant and underwent a sarcomatous change (see case no. 22). In one case the painful syndrome, still at dorsal level, was accompanied by herpes zoster; compression was suspected when sublesional cordal signs appeared. The meningioma was located in the territory which corresponded to the cutaneous involvement (see case no. 34, Fig. 44).

Case No. 15: Meningothelial Meningioma

A 66-year-old woman (1982). Right posterolateral intradural-extramedullary meningioma in D6-D7.

Clinical Course. 15 years. Dorsal pain. Three years before hospitalization the patient was affected by constricting band-like irradia-

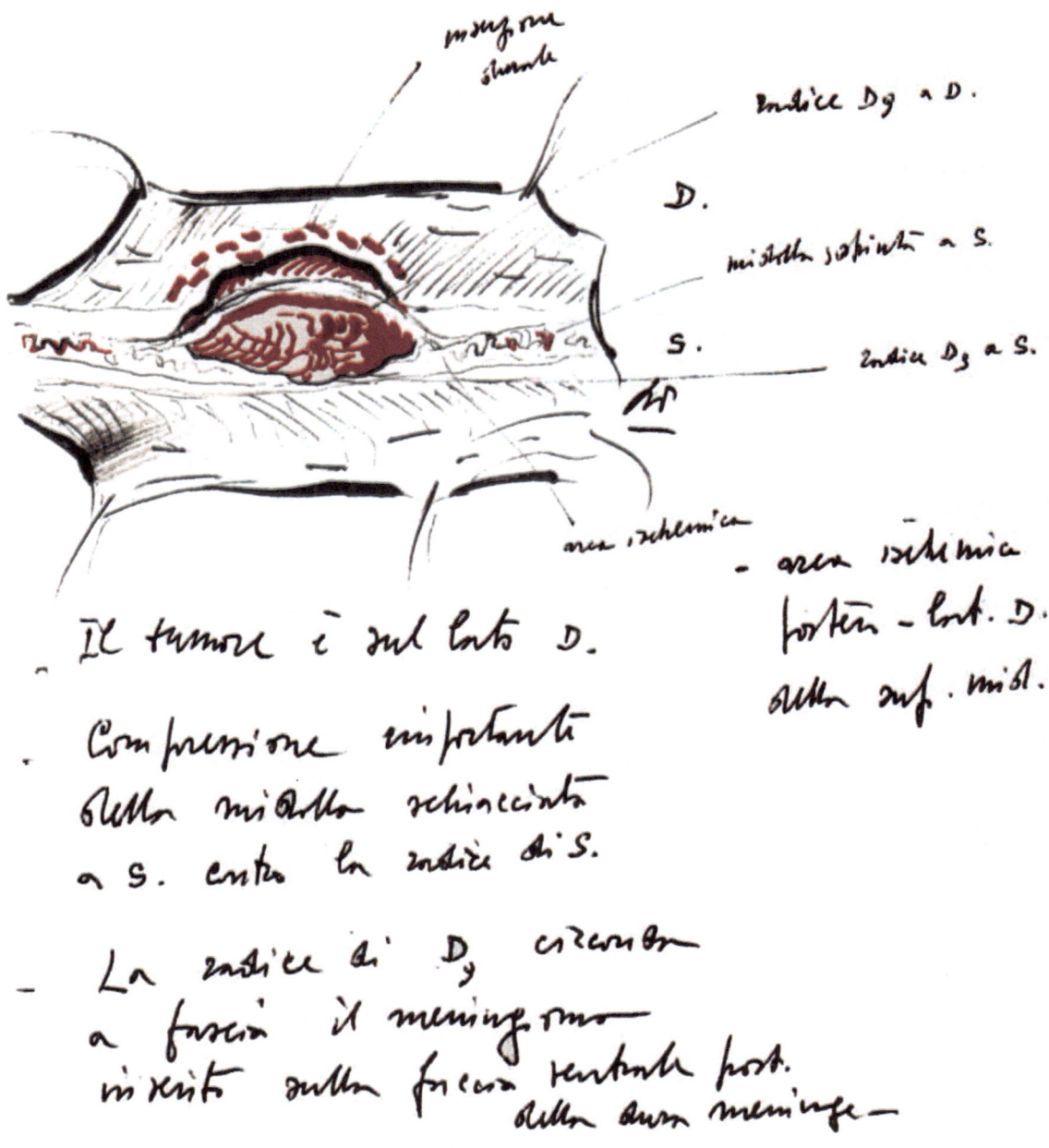

Fig. 41. The dashed line on the internal surface of the dura mater equales to the major extension of the dural insertion of the tumor

tion to the thorax and paraesthesias in the form of a burning sensation to the lower right limb and then to the left. One year before hospitalization a sensation of stiffness was felt in the legs, impeding walking and motor claudication and causing the patient to fall. One month before hospital admission the patient was affected by cutaneous herpes in D6-D7 on the right.

Neurological Examination. Spastic paraparesis. Ataxic gait. Hyperreflexia of patella. Tactile hypoaesthesias from D7 on the right, and from D10 to the left. Painful hypoaesthesia from D7 bilaterally.

X-Ray of Dorsal Rachis. Grave scoliosis of level with spondyloarthrosis.

Lumbar Myelography. Performed in another hospital. Partial block and identification, after tilting the lower and upper pole of the neoplasm in D6-D7, of greater development on the right.

Surgical Treatment. On opening the dura, the immediate view of a reddish wine coloured tumour with posterolateral invasion on the right. The cord appeared greatly compressed contralaterally. Excision after fragmental debulking of the tumour. The posterolateral invasion on the right had a granular and calcified appearance.

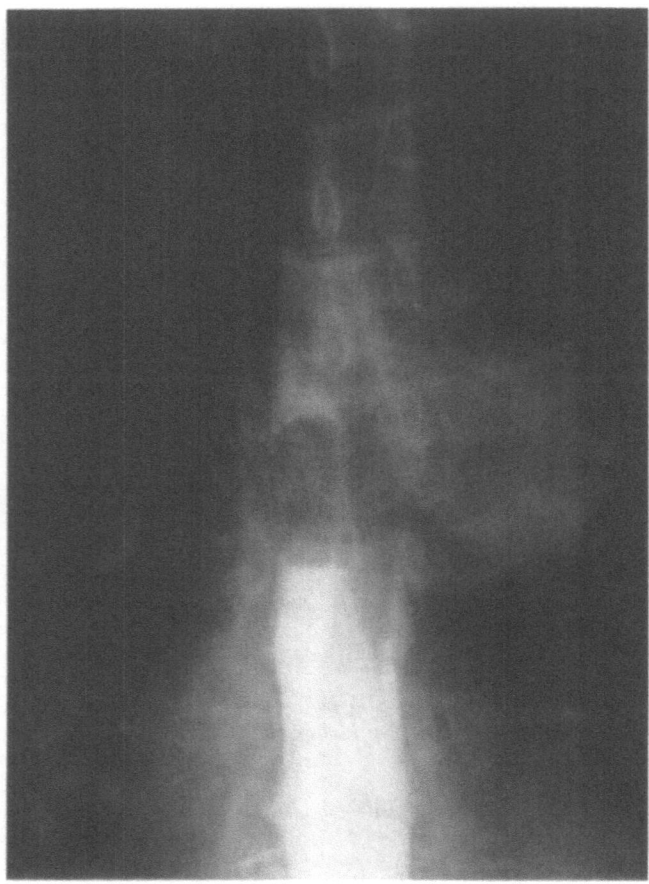

Fig. 42. Myelography via lumbar puncture. An oval-shaped filling defect defines an area inside the enlarged subarachnoidal space in D5-D6 on the right, which displaces the cord towards the left

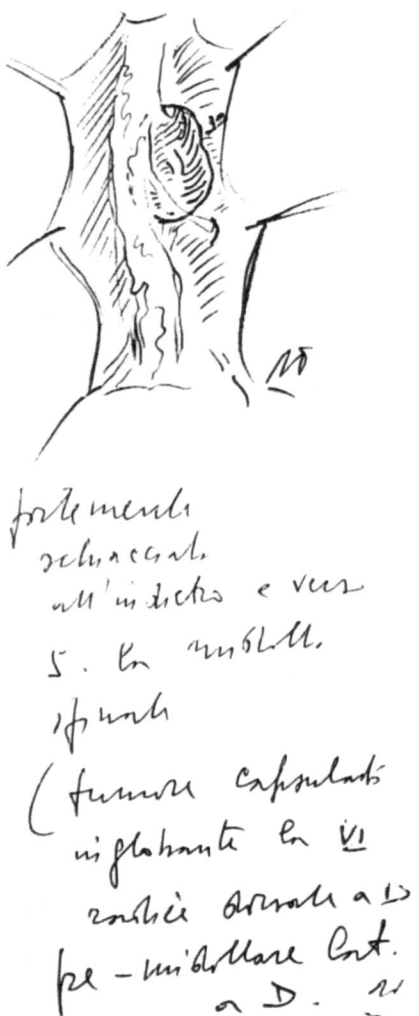

Fig. 43. After opening of the dura mater, the spinal vessels near the tumor are seen filiform. The spinal surface, near the root enclosed in the tumor, is ischemic

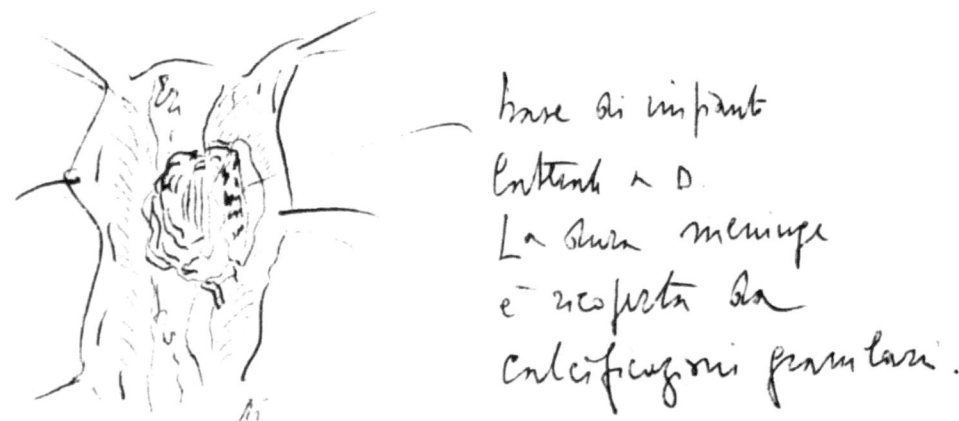

Fig. 44. The right-sided base of attachment is inserted against a sensory root. During the removal of the meningioma granular calcifications along the internal dural surface are observed

6.5 Lumbar Root Syndrome

Meningiomas of the rachidial tract from L1 to L5-S1 are extremely rare. In our series we observed only six (in L1, L1-L2, L2, L3-L4, and L5-S1). In the sixth case, a child aged 2 years 3 months, a large meningioma surrounded the filum terminale from L2 to S1. (See case no. 72, Chap. 6). The clinical development is typical of simple lombago at the dorsal lumbar passage; subsequently a monoradicular involvement begins at the third medial part of the thigh and upwards to the inguinal area. The pain follows a slow progressive course, spreading to one side only and becomes bilateral in the course of months or years. The mono- or bilateral pain in successive phases is identical to the neurinoma (see case no. 62, Chap. 8). When pain is followed by distal paraesthesias to the lower limbs, the peripheral motor deficit is more evident in the side where the pain originated (see case no. 69, Chap. 8). Apart from the case of malignant transformation of the meningioma and the meningioma located on the filum terminale in the child patient aged 2 years 3 months, the clinical course of the syndrome generally lasted a particularly long time, from 15 to 30 years. In one of our patients whose clinical course lasted 30 years, pain persisted for over 20 years before being affected by paralysis of the right foot, parietal deficit on the left 5 months before hospitalization and sphincter disturbances a week before hospitalization.

The clinical irritative syndrome on more than one root followed by a peripheral paretic type of deficit resembles other compressions with variations; however, the course of symptoms is in relation to the various extentions and morphological characteristics of the tumour. It is difficult to define or foresee a differential diagnosis for the neurinoma of the canda in this work. A large vertical extension with invasion on the filum terminale is considered exceptional in meningioma cases. It is very rare to find a meningioma located on the lower lumbar tract in L5-S1, we found only one in our series. This was a compression with a bilateral lumbarsciatical picture and the tumour was partly intra- and partly extradural. It finally proved to be a meningeal sarcoma.

6.6 Sensory Cord Syndrome

The symptoms that patients report as paraesthesia affect areas distant to the location of meningioma development. These symptoms sometimes precede pain and the onset of radicular pain. Paraesthesias can semiologically be traced to a functional disturbance of conduction at an upper compression level and has appeared 23 times: 3 times (15%) at the cervical tract from a total of 20 meningiomas and 20 times (20.8%) in 98 dorsal meningiomas. In all these cases they began in the lower limbs as a burning sensation on one or both sides. Two cases presented a progressive ascending supply (see case no. 64). A meningioma in C5-C6 presented a minimal irritative sensation distal to the upper limbs for 40 years (see case no. 93).

Distal irritative disturbance to the lower limbs reflects the topographical pattern of the sensory long fibres of the anterolateral tracts of the cord. The most external layers, and therefore the more superficial, are in relationship to the fibres of the territory in lower locations, while the deeper fibres, and therefore nearer to the base of the anterior and posterior grey horns, correspond to the upper limb territory. The burning sensation at the feet and paraesthesia-type sensations such as "needles", "stinging" and a sort of "numbness" are frequent but inconstant. They have been referred to in upper meningioma cases in D1-D2 and in lower medial dorsal meningiomas in D10-D12. Irritative manifestations in the form of spontaneous electric shocks while bending the trunk are more rare. These cord signals are very similar to those described by Lhermitte (1960) in extradural compressions in discoarthrosis and in central or lateral intraforaminal cervical hernias. They usually appear after the pain syndrome and after sublesional signs.

In meningiomas of the medial dorsal tract some forms of distal paraesthesias to the feet also present irritative sensations affecting the upper side of the thigh or subjective band-like constrictions which spread to the thorax and thus indicate myelitic level coinvolvement. The period of time from the initial paraesthesia syndrome until motor impairment is sometimes short, lasting a few months (see case no. 103), but in some cases sensitive distal cord manifestations last for many years (see case no. 79) and with a precise location corresponding to the area between the lateral paraesthesias and the site of the meningioma.

6.7 Motor Cord Syndrome

In 1917 Cushing reported that motor impairment and sensory contralateral disturbances followed an initial period of pain in the clinical course of 18 patients affected by spinal meningiomas. His series demonstrated the set of fundamental elements in compressive syndromes: radicular level syndrome, sublesional cordal signs and paraparesis leading to paraplegia. These symptoms are still taken as those identifying the progressive phases of this type of compression, as well as the cord disturbances affecting the motor system, which leads over a very variable length of time to complete paralysis of the lower limbs. At a clinical level this occurs constantly and in many cases while others may present very unusual manifestations. The symptoms of the pyramidal pathways may follow a similar pattern to that of the painful symptoms, and one can recognize different forms during the progressive course of compressions. The motor deficit may not appear for months or years and then only in the form of a simple "impediment" while walking, or motor claudication when back pain is of long standing. In the vertebral pain phase the neurological examination of a simple modification of a deep reflex response indicates motor impairment and suggests a further search for a slight hypoaesthesia, a hyperaesthesia zone or loss of temperature, pain and oscillating sensitivities. In the cervical tract it is possible to identify sensory and motor radicular coinvolvement at the topographical level, but in the dorsal tract only myelitic disturbance leads us to conduct an interrogation of the patient as this can help to assess an initial coinvolvement of the pyramidal pathways and whether there is a sudden loss of tonicity of an intermittent nature affecting the two lower limbs, a vague sense of loss of agility at the legs, fatigue when walking or slight muscular stiffness. These symptoms of an asymmetric nature may be expressed simply by "tiredness", "heaviness", or slight incoordination but are all signals of motor impairment. The onset of acute motor deficit is rare.

Cushing reported a case of acute hemiplegia in a patient suffering from diabetes: "Oct. 3, 1917. Admission of Mrs. B., 63 years of age, with the history of an injury to the back received 15 years previously, followed by a progressive right hemiparesis. She was transferred to the medical service for treatment of her coincidental diabetes mellitus to which she succumbed in coma on Jan. 26, 1918. At autopsy an unsuspected tumour was disclosed in the upper thoracic level. The sketch shows the posterior (surgical) view of the lesion lying largely lateral to the cord. It proved to be a moderately psammomatous meningioma and a section taken through the dural attachment showed it to be infiltrated by the growth." In 1957 Guillaume et al. reported an acute paraplegic syndrome during a very brief clinical course of a meningioma in a dorsal site. These cases are exceptional but point out, in the mechanism of motor damage, a sudden vascular disorder in the slow course of a compressive syndrome.

We have noted motor disturbance to be the first sign in the alternating progression of the symptoms of the syndrome. In 24 patients 4 had cervical meningiomas and 20 dorsal meningiomas. Regarding the site of the meningioma, they occur more frequently in the medial dorsal tract from D5 to D8 (10 cases) than in the tract from D1 to D4 (5 cases) or lower dorsal tract (5 cases). Only one tumour was located between the upper dorsal tract and the medial dorsal tract (D4-D6), with the medial dorsal tract proving the location of most of the meningiomas.

According to Lazorthes' (1958) description of medullary vascularization, there is a clear clinical-anatomical relationship between minor arterial vascular supply and motor damage. Compared to the morphological variations in the calibre of the radicular arteries of the med-

ial dorsal tract, the intrinsic medullary network supplying the pyramidal pathways is less important because it is supplied by the anterior spinal artery, which is particularly reduced in calibre. Although the posterolateral tract of the pyramidal pathways reaches the posterior spinal arterial branches, these are usually compressed with posterior and posterolateral meningiomas. The most unusual symptoms are various topographical features of motor damage. Cases of variable progression and asymmetric nature sometimes spread in an ascending manner.

In cervical locations we have noted hemiparetic development (see case no. 114, Chap. 8). In one patient the meningioma in C1-C2 had a predominantly premedullary development that was more pronounced on the right, and in another the motor impairment affected all four limbs simultaneously following only a feeling of minor weakness at the right hemisome which had been present for years. Considering the initial back pain, the clinical examination must be made on the spine at the level where the discomfort is felt by the patient. Low cervical rachidian rigidity is easily identified because the dorsocervical passage tract is the most flexible. The clinical examination uses simple flexion and lateral movements of the head to determine whether paraesthesias appear in the form of diffused electric shock sensations to the lower limbs. These paraesthesias should produce similar sensations to those which the patient feels without undergoing any particular movement or without strain. Pressure on the spinous processes helps the patient to locate the pain level without provoking the intense discomfort that generally occurs in lesions involving invasion of the bone.

Scoliosis is frequently present in the medial dorsal tract, particularly in patients aged over 65-70 years. This presents as a slight malformation that is often accompanied by a kyphotic component in dorsal curvature. In patients with a kypho-scoliotic attitude the malformation may be of long standing and have caused no disturbance before the initial regional pain.

6.8 Brown-Sequard Syndrome

Following the initial observations of Cushing (1917), Learmonth (1927) and Christiansen (1932), it was reported that the Brown-Sequard syndrome does not always follow the common patterns. In Cushing's series of 18 cases this was the case in six. In 1976 Nittner found this 37 times (42%) in 88 cases and noted that the symptom does not always manifest itself completely. Pyramidal disturbances are pronounced on the side of the tumour, with incomplete sensation signs on the opposite side. Guillaume et al. (1957) observed this in 16% of 70 cases, while in the report of Pertuiset et al. (1960) 9 of 57 meningioma patients were affected (15.8%).

The presence of minor or major manifestations of sensory damage to the anterolateral semilunar fascia of Dejerine depends on the degree of lateral compression caused by the meningioma, provoking a more or less diffuse hemimedullary disturbance on one side and leading to a conduction disturbance of the ascending, crossed sensory fibres on the side opposite to the motor damage. In the very slow development course of the meningioma cord disturbances are slow. The frequency of the syndrome varies in the various reports depending on the observation period. In the mechanisms of sensory and motor cord damage the vascular alterations differ depending on the location of the compression. When this is lateral the medullary hemisyndrome is more frequent and varies in relation to the consistency and volume of the tumour. In the past, without the aid of modern diagnostic tools, a clinical diagnosis was probably reached when the compressions were already at a late stage. Although myelitic damage in the syndrome continues to be a clinical entity today, it is less common (Harkey and Crockard 1991). In our series there were only three cases of Brown-Sequard syndrome (2.46%).

The association of radicular level signs on the side of the tumour with radicular involvement to a lesser degree on the opposite side may indicate that the motor cord hemisyndrome on the side of the meningioma has an initial, partial contralateral sensory and motor cord involvement affecting the "hot" and "cold" fibres, without affecting superficial tactile sensitivity when the others are well perceived. In the incomplete Brown-Sequard syndrome sensory disturbance does not reach the site of the tumour and stabilizes two or three dermatomes below. Harkey and Crockard (1991) note that the pain-temperature fibres continue several segmental levels before intertwining into the contralateral spinal talus tract.

In addition to mechanical-vascular causes, it must be noted that in the pathogenesis of the syndrome variations in the pressure of the fluid in the subarachnoidal space are pronounced above the meningioma and are sometimes distributed very differently near the upper pole than near the lower. Pagni (1989) reported an "inverse" Brown-Sequard syndrome, with painful anaesthesia ipsilateral to the tumour with contralateral motor disturbance attributed to medullary compression on the opposite side of the tumour against the bony wall of the canal. These symptoms demonstrate the polymorphic nature of myelitic damage and its relationship to the various causes mentioned above.

6.9 Clinical Signs in the Development of Meningiomas

The principles of general semiology apply to the various rachidian tracts, as the criteria used for evaluating the initial signs during neurological examination vary in relation to the rachidian tract where the compression with juxtamedullary development is located.

6.9.1 Cervical Tract

A precise account of the symptomatic picture supplied by the patient is essential for diagnosing tumours in the cervical tract. Meningiomas located in the first cervical segments present rachidian symptoms that are more complex than pain in the dorsal tract. The patient complains of rigidity of the neck, noticeable during examination and with passive movements of the head. On examination the patient shows signs of muscular contraction and keeps the head inclined to one side, finding it difficult to hold the head upright because it is resistant to passive movements. Sensory examination for C1-C2 segments shows an initial area of hypoaesthesia which usually extends beyond the occipito-atlantoid passage. For these locations clinical development signs appear long before cord signs. Motor disturbance and the diffusion of sensory disturbance increase considerably, as in the expansive intramedullary forms. For this reason no feature seems helpful for a differential diagnosis in the various expansive processes. We note here that one of our meningioma cases (C1) was intramedullary and completely calcified; perhaps we could have identified the first clinical signs 3 years previously (see case no. 73, Chap. 6).

The literature also reminds us of torcicollis attacks, during which the patient complains of increased intensity of paraesthesia and accentuation of muscular contracture. Paraesthesias presents in an upper bilateral paravertebral pattern which spreads from the margin of the trapezius muscle to the posterior border of the sterno-cleidomastoid muscle, in the direction of the submamillary region. Meningiomas in C1 with an upward development and occupying the posterior tract of the foramen magnum present sublesional symptoms including cerebellar signs, cerebellar-spinal disturbances and the functional modification of nerves together with coinvolvement of the descending branch of the phrenic nerve. The development of pain is more contingent in relation to paraesthesias of a meningioma in C1-C2, presenting more intense pain than one along the great occipital nerve territory. The first motor and sublesional sensory signs are very similar. Cushing (1938) described a set of symptoms revealing a gradual alteration of nerve centres and nerve bundles due to the mechanical action of the tumour. We are reminded that post-operative progress in these cases is exceedingly delicate as attacks of respiratory insufficiency may occur.

Brachial-cervical compressions in locations from C5 to D1 were the second most frequent in our series (11 cases). The clinical signs here are more manifest because they correspond to the involvement of the upper, medial and lower radicular groups. The nature and course of symptoms may be unusual when a meningioma develops substantially in extension and causes damage to the myelomeres and to the lowest of the intumescentia cervicalis (see case no. 123, Chap. 8).

Meningiomas located in the first cervical segments are less frequent than those located between C5 and D1. These progressively affect certain muscular regions over a variable length of time and affect the osteotendinous reflexes. Some early symptoms help to identify the compression level. Asymmetry of reflexes is the general rule even in the presence of excellent voluntary movements and without loss of strength. Here the examination of muscular atrophy of the hand is very important if carried out in connection with the pattern of sensory radicular symptoms. Often the symptoms are interpreted as neuritis, rheumatism or arthrosis when the initial symptoms can indicate only a location of the lesion corresponding to the posterior roots.

In the same dermatome in which the patient feels spontaneous pain, sometimes corresponding to the innervation territory of a posterior root, the examination shows a considerable reduction in muscular eminence of the hand or reduced tonicity in minor flexation and extension movements of the fingers without other alterations in strength and motility. In juxtamedullary meningiomas in C3-C4 there is reduced tactile sensitivity on only one side of the territory up to the thorax and in the proximal tract of the shoulder. This sign defines the innervation margin of the fourth cervical root. Another sign for identifying the level is lack of deltoid reflex of one side, while reflexes below are normal or pronounced to one side. When the last four cervical roots are affected sensory coinvolvement affects the area along the distal tract of the arm in C5-C8. When the first dorsal root is involved pain spreads not only to the underarm region but also to the highest part of the thorax.

A particularly large vertical extension of the tumour does not affect the course of symptoms regarding cord disturbances. An exceptional case has been reported in the literature of a tumour developing along the whole length of the cervical tract and up beyond to the posterior fossa (Sawa et al. 1993). For 8 years this patient complained only of bilateral pain at the shoulder and difficulty in abducting the arms. Even in these forms there may be an initial and almost completely asymptomatic period before the appearance of signs indicating the compression. A more precise localization of the lesion is permitted when the mechanical compressive action and vascular disturbance show clear signs of sensory deficit accompanied by the modification of reflexes.

The causes of functional disorders of the spinal tracts remain uncertain. Every symptom in the pathogenesis of *compressive syndromes is to be equally related* both to mechanical and vascular factors. Some authors maintain that the compression is caused by demyelination with

neuronal morphological recovery after removal of the tumour. Together with Harkey and Crockard (1991), however, we do not believe this but consider instead a possible functional recovery of the vascularization once the meningioma has been removed. On the basis of vascular disorder one can understand the sometimes rapid recovery of the deficiency syndromes shortly after an operation. The same functional disorders far from the site of the meningioma, corresponding to a disturbance of the grey horns and the motor and sensory tracts, lead to a certain vascular pathogenesis. We must add here that in some forms the meningioma is associated with malformative alterations in the superficial medullary circulation (see case no. 73, Chap. 6). Vascular disturbances at points far from the site of the lesion may be eased by the latter condition and are not to be excluded. Some authors refer to pathogenetic factors caused by the compressive action in relation to the variability of neurological signals; these remain important, but always in relation to vascular weakness which varies from case to case. Davis and Washburn (1972) report a relationship between the medullary level and vertebral location in 80% of their cases. Tumours in a premedullary site often show a vertebral-dermatomeric difference of about three levels.

6.9.2 Dorsal Tract

When one or more posterior roots are affected the irritative pain syndrome has an intercostal location with ingravescent characteristics. Nearly always the pain is more intense at the ipsilateral side of the tumour but can also be associated with minimal contralateral pain. According to Learmouth's (1927) and Christiansen's (1932) set of symptoms in dorsal meningiomas, medullary compression symptoms appear after radicular pain symptoms, but in some cases the development of motor disturbances is not preceeded by sensory signs. Clinical symptoms in 20 patients (20.4%) of our series began with motor weakness accompanied by instability; two patients suffered fractures (an instep and a femur) as a consequence of falls (see case nos. 56 and 32). The motor disturbance is manifested by simple hyperreflexia of the lower limbs and may appear initially either on one side only or on both. The side affected by motor deficit is always that of the tumour. In upper dorsal tract locations (D1-D6) the subjective motor deficit is reported to be a simple initial instability while walking due to the weakness of one limb. The course is always slowly deteriorating, over a period lasting from a few months to 1-2 years.

In one of our patients with a meningioma in D6-D7 a slight asthenia to the lower limbs lasted for 10 years. In this case we delayed diagnostic examinations for a suspect tumour because the patient suffered from diabetes and had been intoxicated by mercury. The motor impairment was attributed to the above problems but later developed into severe paraparesis (see case no. 11). In another meningioma case in D7 the simple motor instability had lasted 10 years and the clinical course became rapid, leading to paraplegia in the course of a year (see case no. 115, Figs. 45-49).

Case No. 115: Psammomatous Meningioma

A 49-year-old woman (1972). Left anterolateral intradural-extramedullary meningioma in D7.

Clinical Course. 3 years. At the age of 46 years the patient was affected by progressive hypostenia in the lower limbs with a deteriorat-

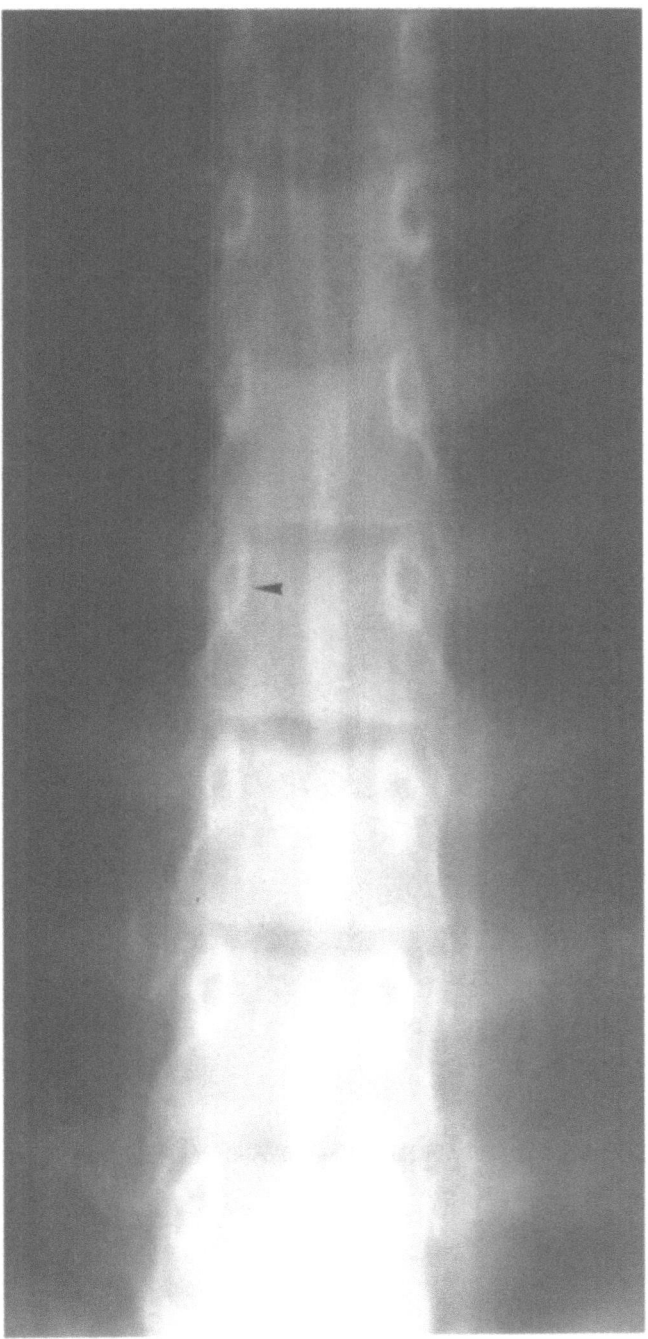

Fig. 45. X-ray stratigraphy of anteroposterior area showing thinning of the right pedicle in D7 (*arrow*)

ing form of muscular contracture. During the year before the examination motor impairment developed into paraplegia. Sphincter disturbances in the form of incontinence.

Neurological Examination. Paraplegia flexion attitude (Levy grade 4). Level of anaesthesia at D7. The presence of severe ulcers resulting from decubitus in the sacral region and at the heels.

Rachicentesis. 2.5 g protein per thousand.

X-ray of Dorsal Spine. Left convex scoliosis with wide angle. The right articular facets in D5 and D6 were thinned.

Myelography (performed suboccipitally). Block corresponding to the upper margin of D7, with slight curved flow, defining the left outline and lower pole of the neoplasm.

Surgical Treatment. The cord presented normal pulsations and appeared narrowed and curved posteriorly. The arachnoid was opened and a radicotomy performed posteriorly at D8 on the right, and by reclining the cord a premedullary meningioma of hard consistency was shown. The tumour with a calcified attachment was seen to invade the internal ventral surface of the dura. Removal was possible only when the meningioma was pressed against the dura. Coagulation of the haemorrhagic attachment of the meningioma.

Results. During the postoperative course there was a reduction in flexion contractures with passive mobilization. When the patient was under general anaesthetic, the thighs and knees were extended with force. After 2 months of physiotherapy there was a partial recovery of the flex extension of the voluntary movements of the lower left limb. After 3 months the patient could take a few steps with support and keeping the right limb in a brace. For 4 months a bilateral support was necessary for walking. Slight flexion disturbance persisted in the right lower limb. After 8 months the patient was able to walk with the aid of one support only.

The major manifestations of cord disturbances are generally due to dorsal meningiomas in D6-D8 (see case no. 122, Fig. 50) but may also be due to one in lower sites (D9, D10; see case no. 83). During the course of their development pyramidal disturbance is frequently a slow process (see case no. 14). In dorsal locations in D7-D9 an examination of the superficial abdominal reflexes can identify the level of the lesion: lack of the epigastric reflex in D7, mesogastric reflex in D9 or D10 and hypogastric reflex in D11 or D12. When the meningioma is located in D10-D11, D11-D12 or L1 the symptoms are more precise. Motor deficit is often preceded by an irritative pain syndrome or by a typical radicular disturbance which resembles those associated with neurinomas; hemigirdle or girdle-like pain predominantly on one side, and intermittent pain that increases when coughing located at the lumbodorsal passage level. Sometimes the patient complains of paraesthesias in the form of sublesional electric shocks alternatively with radicular pain. The pain can last for many years (see case no. 33). In one case the rachicentesis diagnosis showed a pain syndrome contralateral to the site where the pain had initially begun (see case no. 15). In some cases severe lumbago attacks begin initially and transitionally with phases of major intensity and associated with paraesthesias below the umbilicus line. Clinical diagnosis is very difficult in these forms because the range of symptoms does not exclude a herniation of the upper lumbar disc (see case nos. 38 and 16). In the locations D11-D12 the pattern of pain without any particular vari-

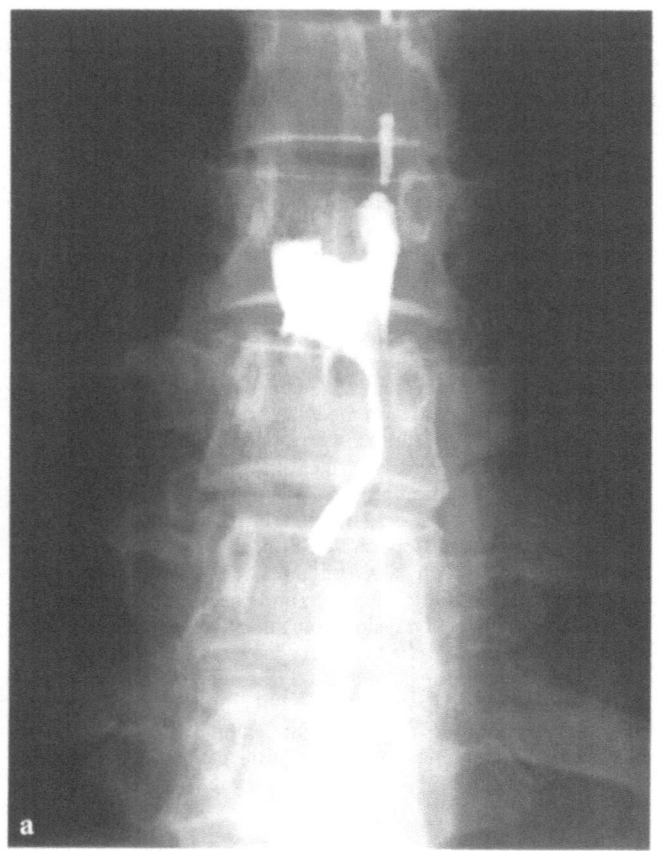
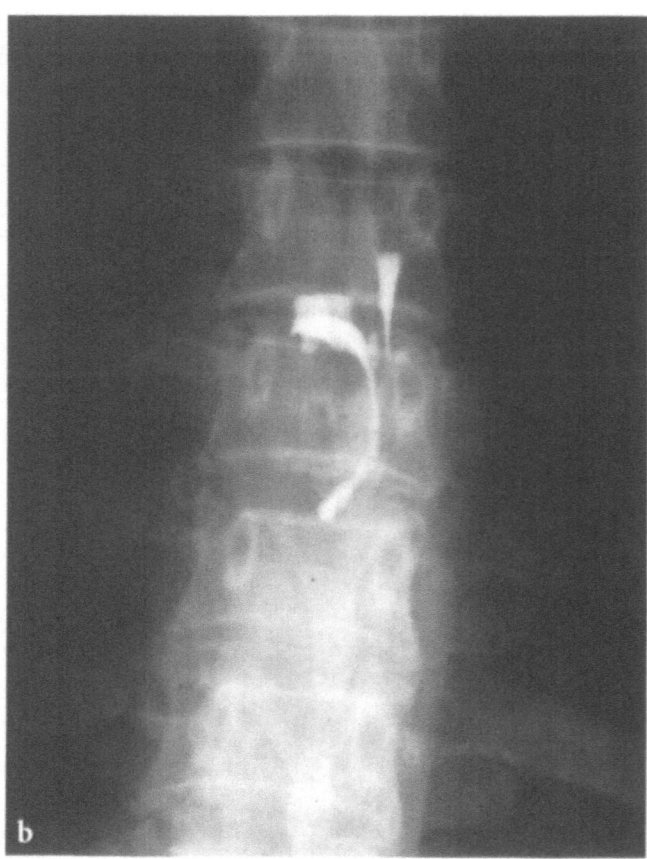

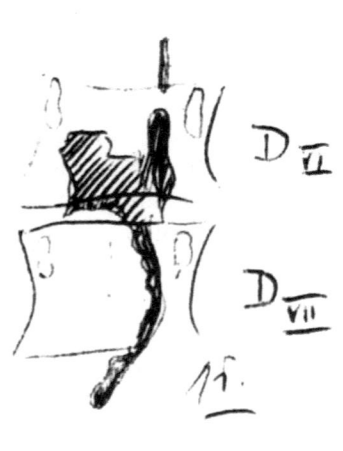

Fig. 46a-c. Suboccipital myelography. Total block at upper margin level of D7 and partial curvilinear passage of contrast medium on the left which presents slight irregularities on the internal margin

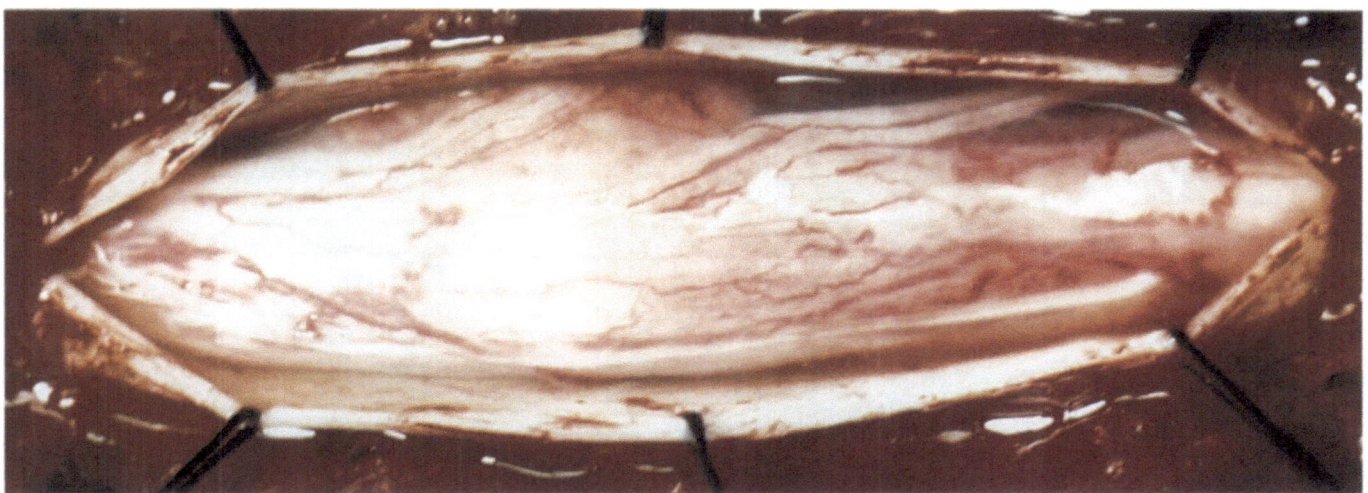

Fig. 47. The dorsal spinal cord with its roots completely covers the tumor that can just minimaly be seen on the right side

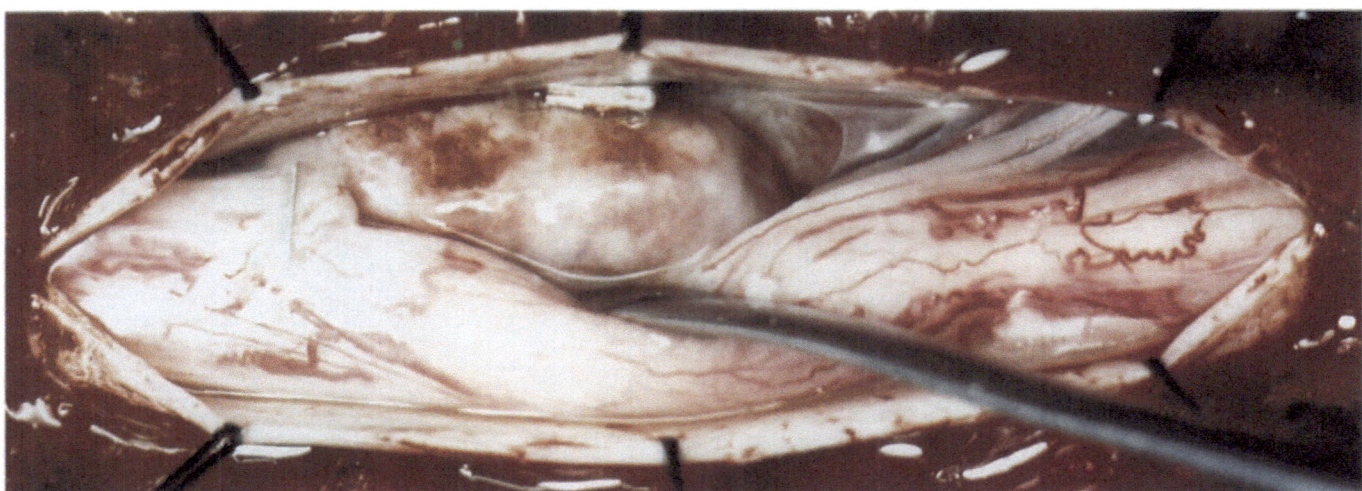

Fig. 48. The vessels at the level of the tumoral compression are reduced while those below are dilated

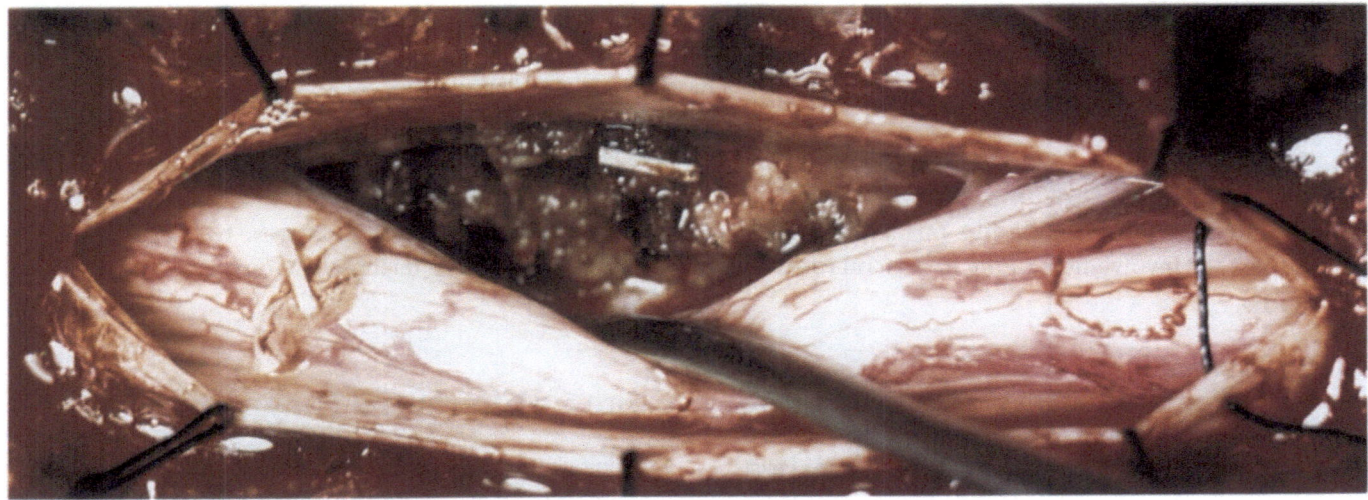

Fig. 49. In this case piecemeal removal of the tumour after performing a radicotomy using a silver clip

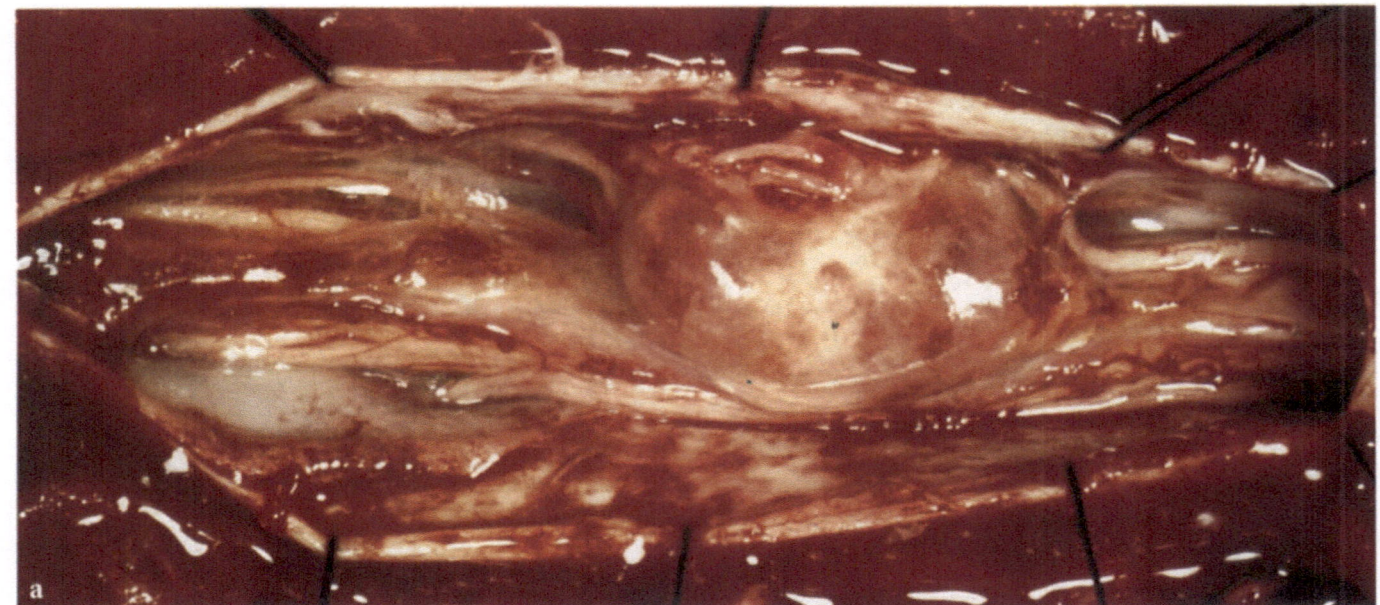

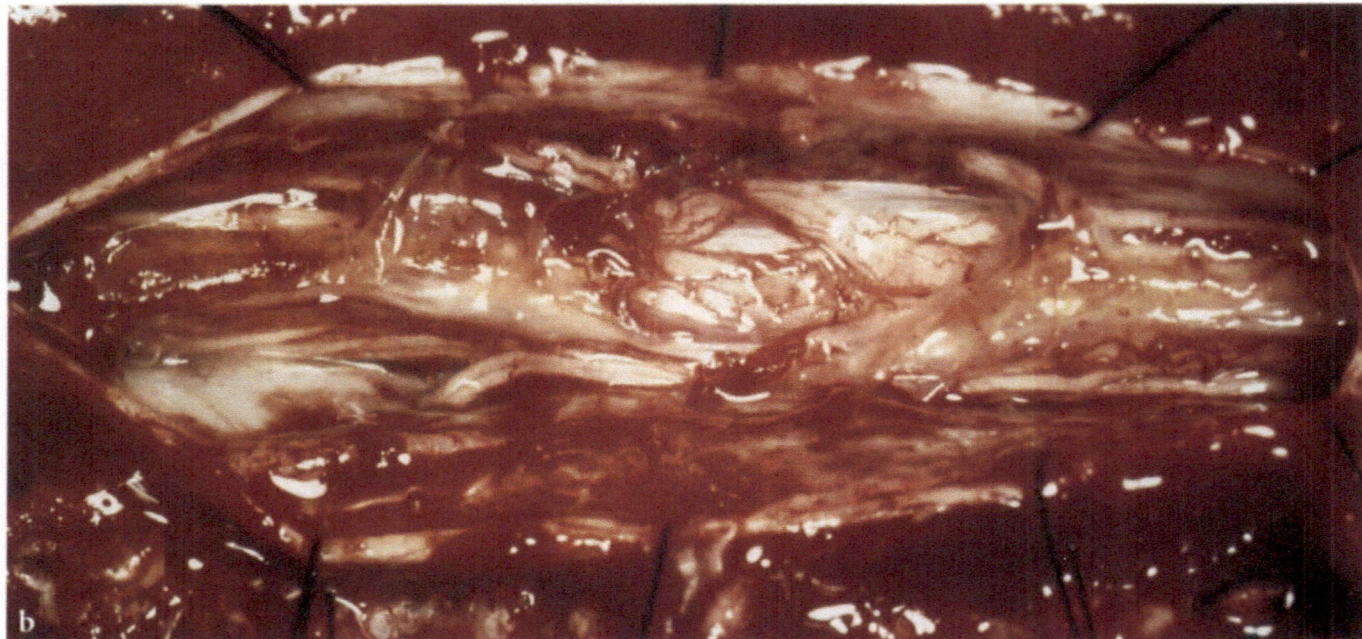

Fig. 50. a Great dilatation of the arterial circulation near the roots above and below the compression. **b** Persistence of the arterial dilatation but an evident whitish ischaemic area is seen at the ventral side of the already removed meningioma

ation in intensity has a saddle-like formation and one may suspect the involvement of the first sacral roots (see case no. 35).

6.9.3 Lumbar Tract

Pluriradicular motor and sensory caudal disturbance produces very rare conditions. When it is present it resembles other compressive forms (ependymonas, epidermoid cysts, neurofibromas, leptomeningeal dysembriogenetic cysts). By general clinical criteria meningiomas on the lumbar tract are extremely rare. There were two cases of meningiomas at the filum terminale in our series.

6.10 Differential Diagnosis

Specific symptoms of meningioma do not exist; however, some features are important for a differential diagnosis of neurinoma: (a) the onset of radicular pain is more intense with neurinoma than with meningioma; (b) radicular pain is often early with neurinoma and from the beginning tends to have a more constant dermatomeric pattern; (c) sublesional paraesthesias far from the development of the lesions, either on the cervical or dorsal tract, seem more frequent with meningioma and have a subjective nature, as reported by the patient, in the form of distal electric shocks in the lower limbs accompanied by dyaesthesias, such as burning sensations, and intense cold felt at the feet.

There does seem to be a relationship between the clinical picture and the location of the tumour. On the basis of 100 neurinomas and 100 meningiomas in our series we evaluated the initial occurrence of radicular and cord symptoms and found that in the neurinomas cases these tended to be radicular symptoms (81% of cases) while in meningiomas they tended to be cord symptoms (71%). When the clinical aspect of the syndrome is a paretic-ataxic type, it is probably meningiomatous. It is very difficult to apply any diagnostic criteria for the nature of compressions in the Brown-Sequard syndrome. Women are more affected by meningiomas than by neurinomas. 83% of spinal meningiomas are located at dorsal level; these are thus seven times more frequent than those located at cervical level (Harkey and Cockard 1991). In our series the relationship was 4.8 to 1. Meningiomas generally occur during the sixth or seventh decade of life while neurinomas usually occur at a younger age (Namer et al. 1987). The foraminal site with intra- and extrarachidian development is more frequent in neurinoma cases and is exceptional in meningioma cases. In comparison to the paraesthesias of the discouncusarthrosis and slight cervical spondylolisthesis, the "Lhermitte sign" seems less important in meningiomas but is always located on the distal tract of the lower limbs. This symptom has an early discoarthrotic nature. The acute onset of cervicobrachial pain is more frequent together with mono- or bilateral motor deficit to the lower limbs.

Neurinomas in lumbar sites develop in a central position between the caudal roots producing pluriradicular symptoms, while meningiomas, often in anterolateral or posterolateral sites, yield a more lateral compressive clinical picture. When the onset of symptoms is monoradicular with lumbocrural or lumbosciatic characteristics, no particular symptoms can indicate the diagnosis. The rachidian rigidity in neurinomas seems greater than in meningiomas. In cases of fibromatosis (5 cases of 156 neurinomas) and in those in which meningiomas are associated with neurinomas, the peripheral sensory-motor involvement of one or more roots varies depending on the site and volume of the lesions. Peripheral symptoms appear earlier than myelitic disturbances in small meningiomas at dorsal sites. The varying periods of development in meningiomas and neurinomas in neuofibromatosis syndromes make it difficult to apply any useful sem-

iological criteria in the diagnosis (see Sect. 6.14).

When the neurinoma extends transversally instead of vertically and compresses the posterolateral surface of the cord indirect mechanical action may lead to contralateral radicular involvement at the same level. This condition seems rare in meningiomas. The compressive syndrome of the intra- or extrarachidian hourglass neurinoma, either in a dorsal or in the lumbodorsal passage, is homologous with the meningioma form. In some cases the characteristic image produced by plain radiography raises doubts as to the saddle-shaped neurofibroma versus the intra- and extraforaminal meningioma (see case no. 9). When the radicular syndrome is preceded by regional back pain there are no specific differences to a histological type of tumour. At the onset of symptoms it seems that motor deficit with hemiparesis characteristics is rarer in neurinomas, though it has been reported in meningiomas at upper cervical level (see case no. 114).

Some authors (e.g. Guidetti et al. 1964) have tried to identify in other oncotypes the particular initial symptoms that would help in a differential diagnosis between an intramedullary and extramedullary tumour. Pagni (1989) reported the results of several such studies, including those of Broager (1953), Brown (1941), Cassinari and Bernasconi (1961), Giudetti et al. (1964), Nittner (1976), Grellier et al. (1982). In these studies, however, he found no features of definite diagnostic significance. According to Guidetti et al. (1964) the onset of symptoms in various tumour compressions such as vertebral, radicular and cord pain do not differ significantly between intramedullary and extramedullary tumours. These authors noted that pain frequently appears on a single side rather than on both sides in neurinomas but on both sides in gliomas and in malignant tumours with extradural development. We agree that cord disturbances occur more frequently in gliomas and meningiomas than in neurinomas and believe that these symptoms appear earlier in gliomas than in meningiomas.

Patients can sometimes be diagnosed for other pathologies during the initial phase of a compression. In the cervical tract one must remember myeloradicular disturbances due to disc herniation, with ingravescent characteristics, discoarthrosis (see case no. 28) and syringomyelia, without evident signs of atrophy in the upper limbs and incomplete sensory associations. In the dorsal tract some signs of neuritis, arthritis and pleura disturbances may be noted during the initial phase before suspecting medullary compression. In the lumbar tract alterations of a congenital stenosis type can raise diagnostic doubts with a meningioma in the dorsolumbar passage (see case no. 80). In the first lumbar segments a lumbosciatica with peripheral motor deficit on one side only may arouse suspicion of a pathologically rapid course of disc herniation.

6.11 Causes of Diagnostic Error and Delay

Positive X-ray of the cervical tract, discoarthrosis and a clinical picture of radicular level involvement may obscure the presence of a meningioma above the exostosis in a persisting asymptomatic phase. We present one of our patients who was twice suspected of radicular disturbance in C5-C6, in a marked marginal posterior discoarthrosis picture (see case no. 28, Fig. 51). Only after two operations to remove the radicular symptoms did an initially ingravescent cord motor weakness appear at the legs. We therefore performed a myelography which revealed a total block in C2 due to a meningioma. The meningioma was removed, and the patient recovered totally. Her condition remained stable for 9 years. This was an obvious case of

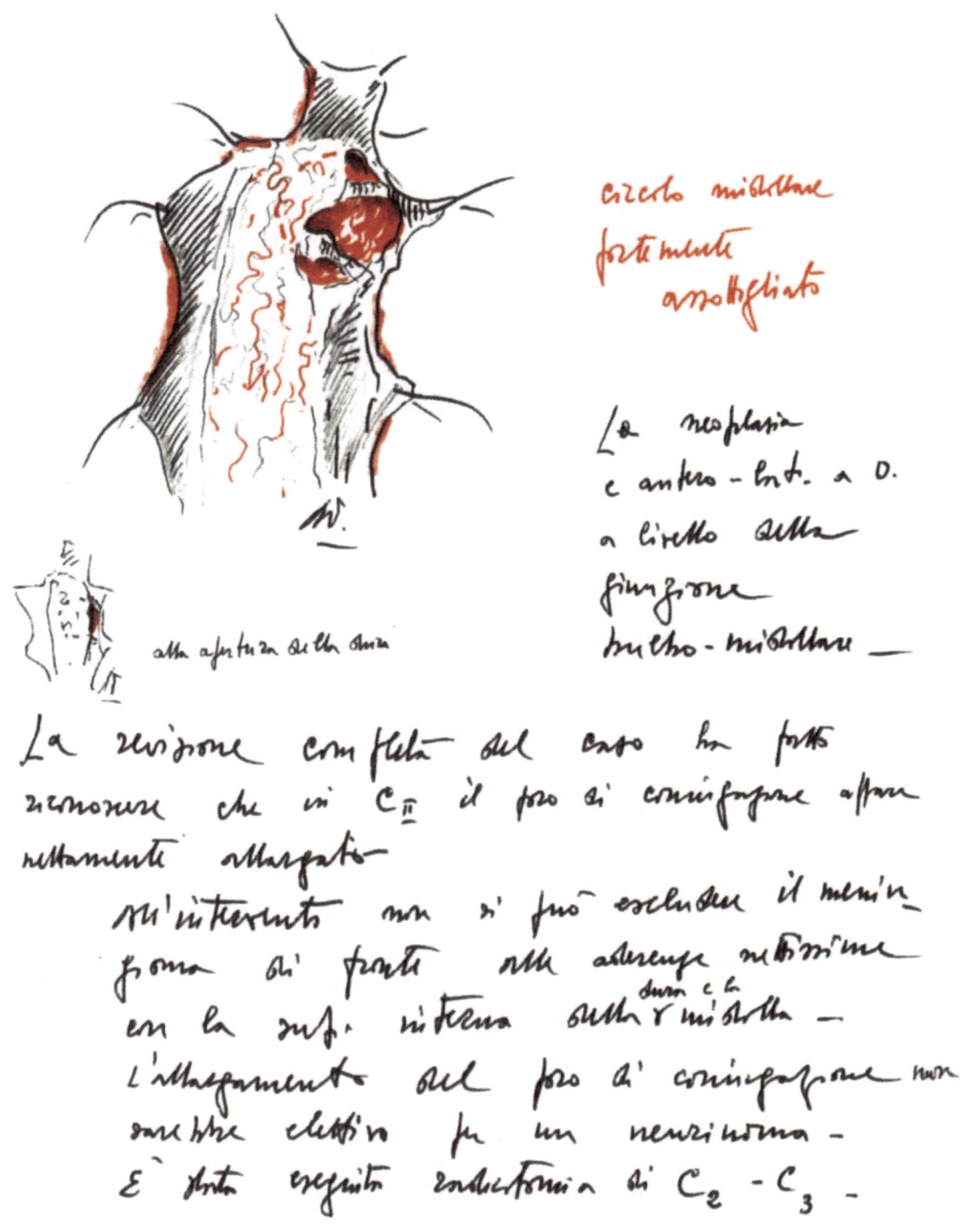

Fig. 51. Mainly anterior meningioma in C2 with intraforaminal development

delayed diagnosis, together with two different pathologies. An upper cervical meningioma may facilitate an irritative syndrome below the discopathy, with marginal posterior exostosis. This case comfirms the observation of Bailey and Craig (1950) that when faced with any diagnostic doubt involving affections of the spinal nervous system it is indispensible that one first exclude a compression. In the literature there are many references to diagnostic errors during the course of meningiomas, including Hanlon et al. (1956), Huffman (1956), Udvarheliy et al. (1966), Nassar and Correll (1968), Davis and Washburn (1972) and Katz et al. (1981). The association of a meningiomatous compression with an evident vertebral pathology of a stenosis type with lumbar spondyloarthrosis, can give rise to another erroneous diagnosis. In this context we present case no. 80 (Figs. 52-56).

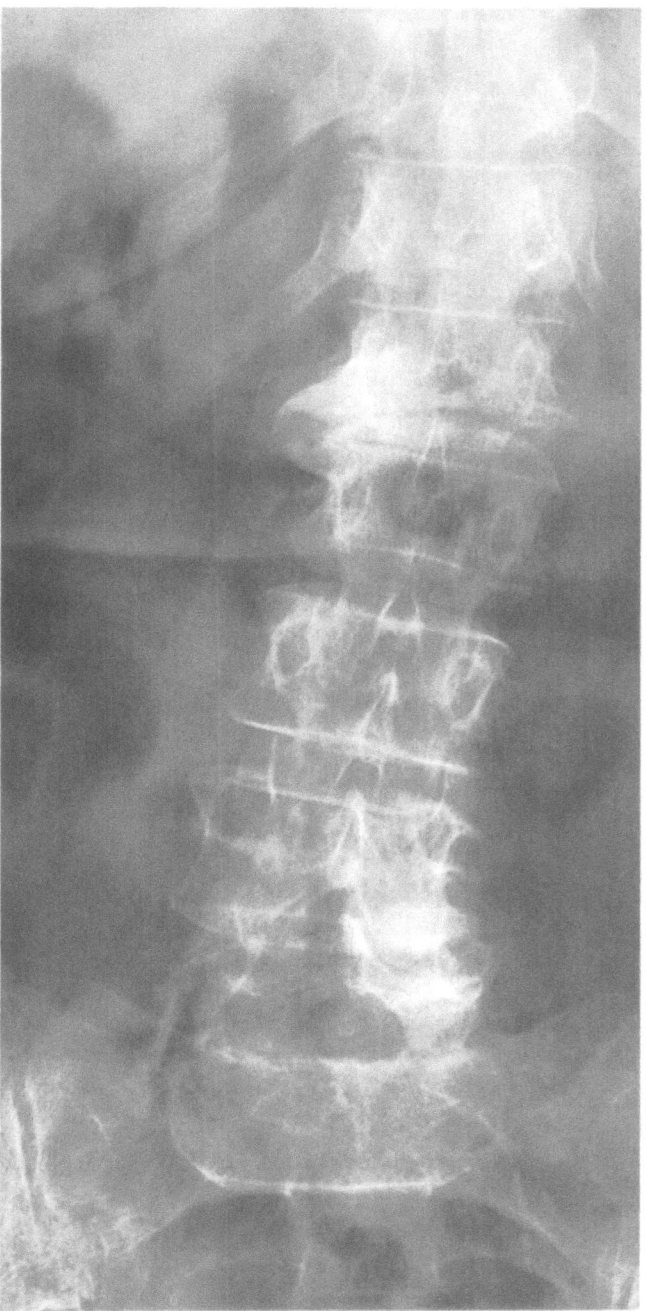
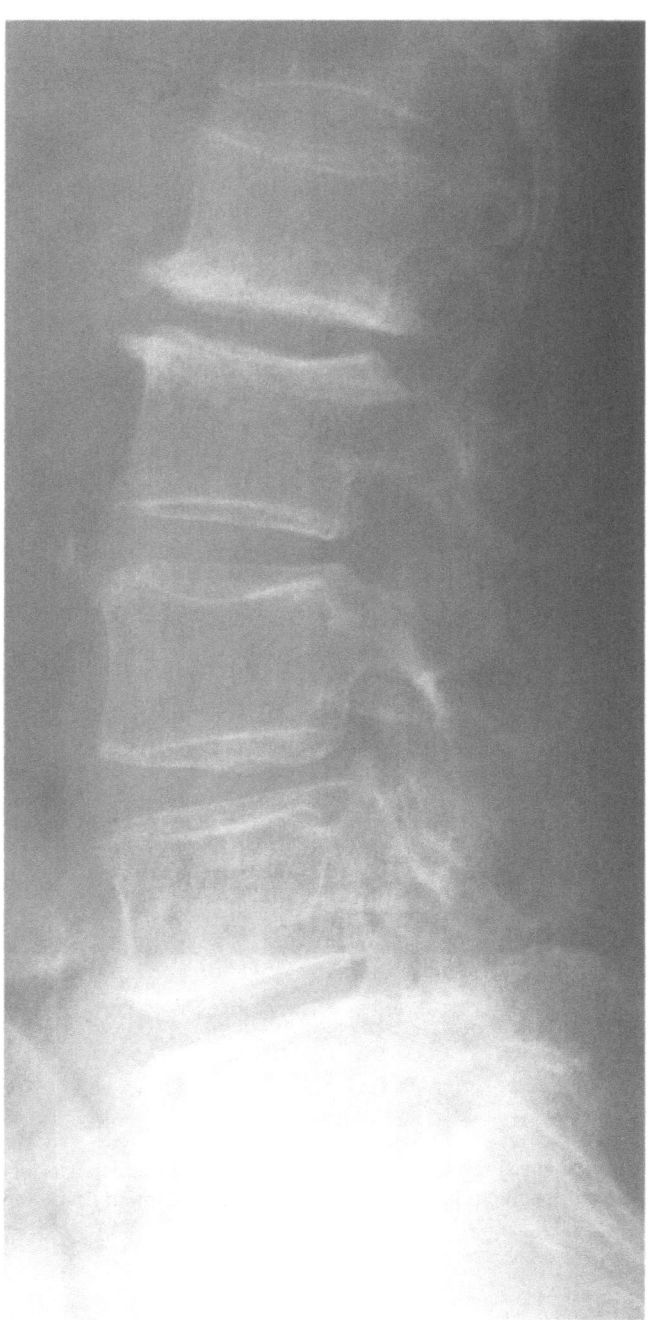

Fig. 52. X-ray of anteroposterior and lateral lumbar rachis. Scoliosis with osteoporosis. Evident exostosis in L1-L2 and L4-L5. The lateral projection shows articular apophyseal degenerative process

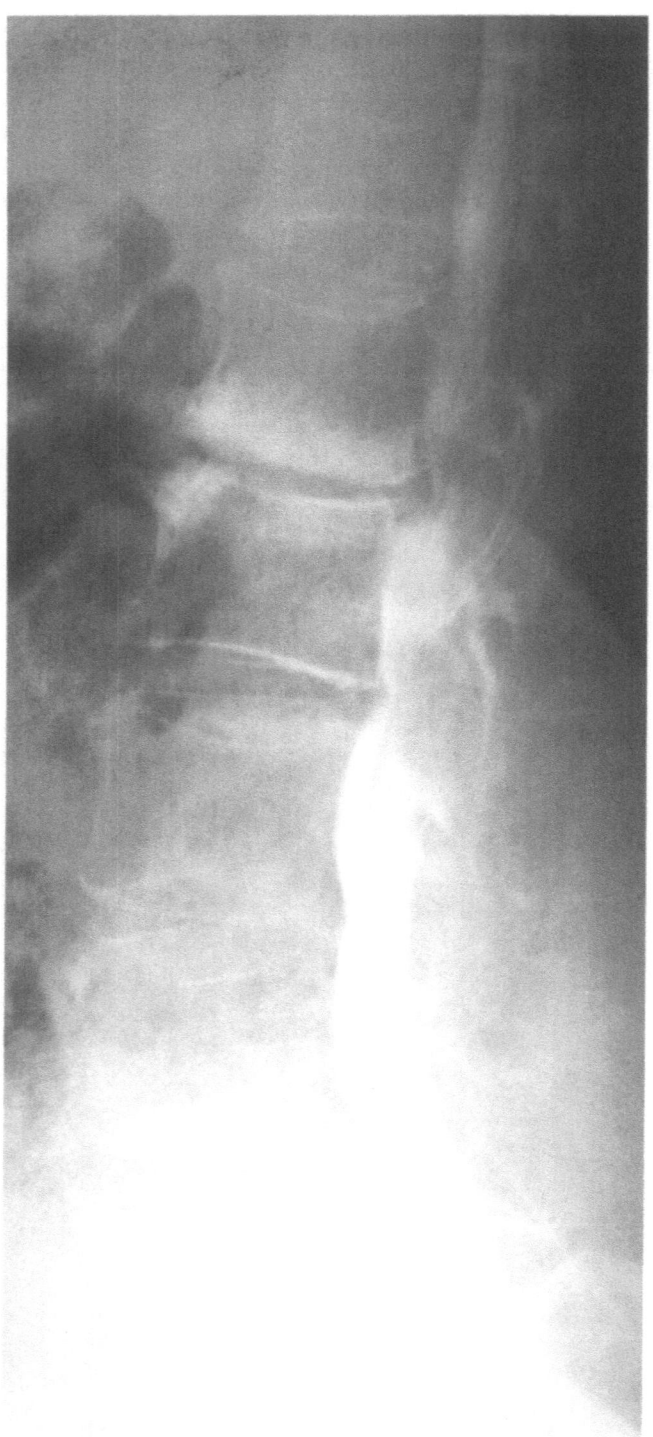 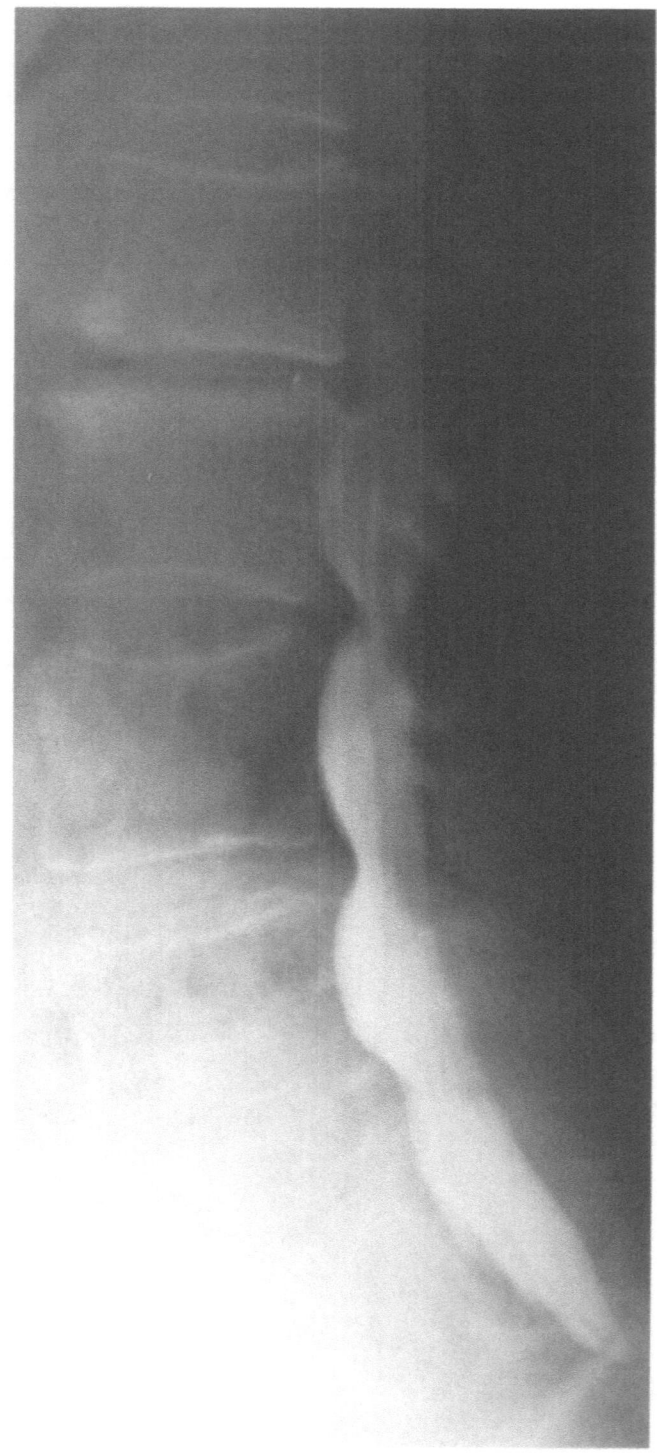

Fig. 53. Lateral myelography. Slight filling defect in the posterior subarachnoidal space reveals stenosis in L1-L2 and L2-L3. A shadow on the anterior profile is produced by the discal projection in L2-L3 and by exostosis in L1-L2

Case No. 80: Transitional Meningioma
A 69-year-old woman (1993). Right posterolateral intradural-extra-medullary meningioma in D10-D11.
Medical History. The patient underwent hystorectomy for a neo-plasm in the uterus at the age of 30 years. She underwent surgery for an intestinal polyp at 63 years.
Clinical Course. 20 years.

Pathological History. Pain at the lumbar tract. For 6 years she had suffered crural-type pain radiating on the left and at the dorsal side of the foot. She wore an orthopaedic corset for 1 year and 3 months before hospitalization, she was affected by motor claudica-tion predominantly on the right and distal paraesthesias to the right lower limb with peripheral deficit at the foot.
Neurological Examination. Motor and sensory, peripheral deficien-

cy syndrome, mainly on the right, with hypertonia and hypotrophy of a third of the inferior femoral quadricep. Slow flex extension of right foot. Flaccid patellas, lack of ankle jerk on the right. Hypoaesthesia on L3, L4 and L5 on the right.

Rachicentesis. 0.03 g protein per thousand.

X-Ray of Lumbar Tract. Severe scoliosis in spondyloarthrosis, and decalcification of the articular pedicles in L3 and L4. On the basis of the clinical picture and from the radiculographic images, which

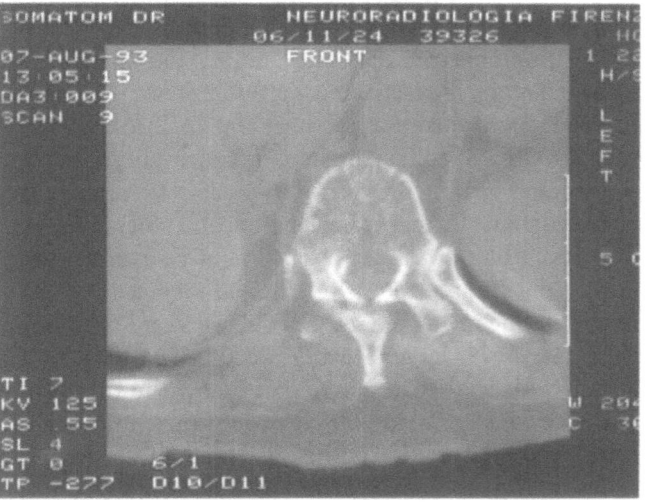

Fig. 54. Dorsal CT. Small calcification inside the canal on the right in D10-D11

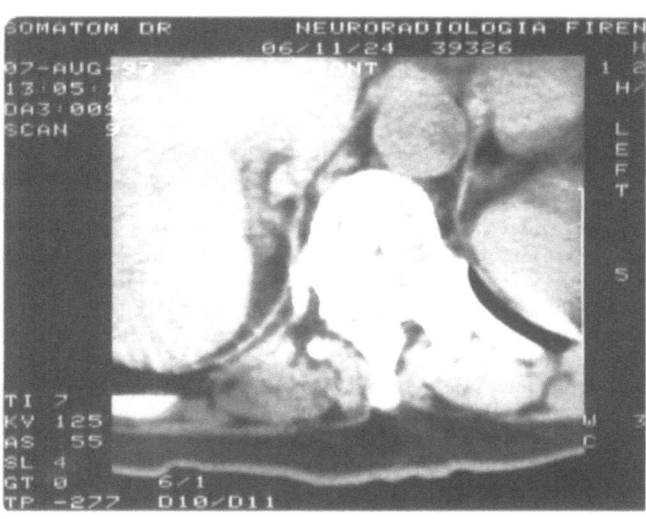

Fig. 55. In three-quarters of the posterior vertebral canal the tissue appears far denser than that in the spinal cord

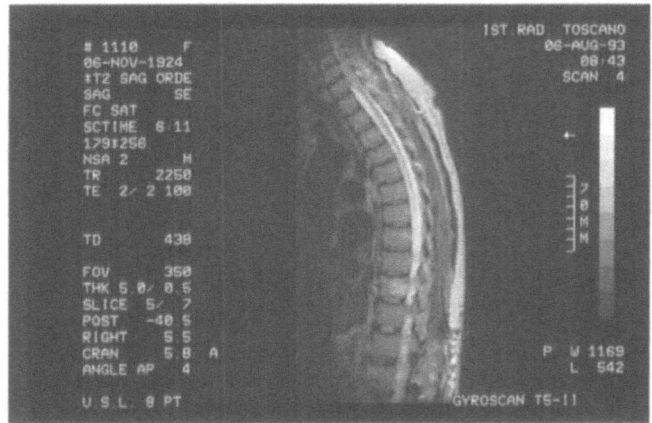

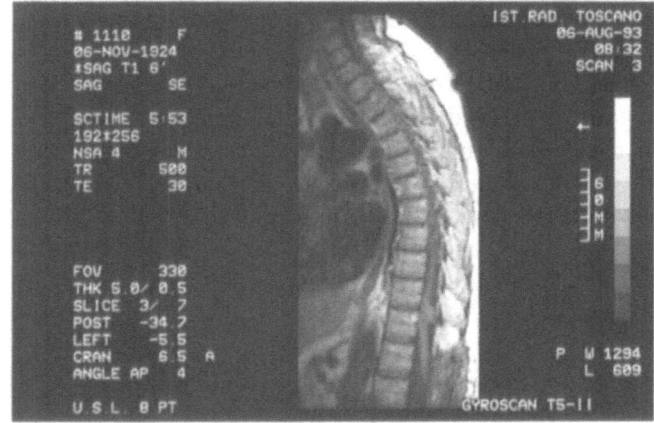

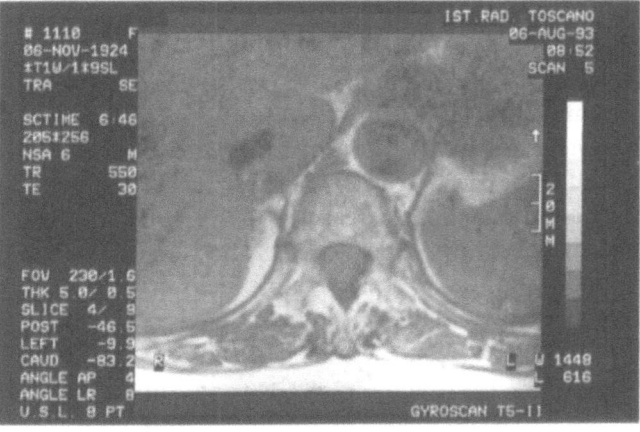

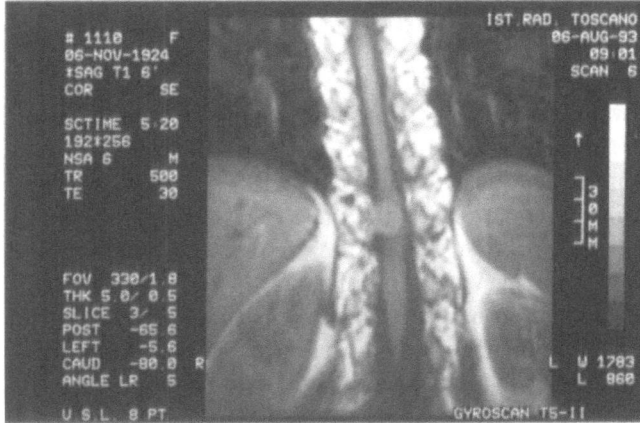

Fig. 56. Sagittal projection T1 (TR 500 and TE 30) and T2 (TR 2250 and TE 100), axial projection and coronal T1. At D10-D11 level the roundish lesion isointense to the spinal cord which is pushed forwards. The vertebral body of D11 presents an angiomatous vertebral area

showed stenosis in L1-L4, patient operated on for stenosis. After the operation her walking gradually improved as she recovered from paralysis of the right foot. Two months later, stiffness appeared to the left lower limb with loss of strength. Over the following 15 days her motor condition rapidly deteriorated.

Neurological Examination. Total paraplegia. Only a minimal degree of flex extension in the feet. Marked hyperaesthesia in D10-D11 on the left. Pallaesthesia below the right knee and to the left malleolus.

MRI. D10-D11. Expansive posterolateral intradural-extramedullary development on the right which displaced the cord contralaterally. Evident widening of the arachnoidal space above and below the lesion.

Plain CT and with Contrast Medium. D10-D11. The contrast medium slightly enhanced the tumour. Small lamina calcifications on the right.

Surgical Treatment. The dura appeared taut and presented a dilatated surface circulation. The delamination of the dura and coagulation of the vascularization between the two layers reduced the arterial supply to the neoplasm. Once the dura was opened, the tumour was seen adhering to the dura which appeared to have a friable consistency and was brownish red in colour. After removing the arachnoid and the adherent peritumourous structures the meningioma was lifted and removed en bloc together with the deep dural layer where the tumour was attached.

Results. On awakening, the reappearance of some slight flexion movements to left inferior limb. After 24 h there was a slow recovery of voluntary leg movements. Over the following 10 days walking was possible with bilateral support. After 3 months with one support only but affected with slight ataxia.

After the first operation, the postoperative rate of progress was so favourable that a relationship between the postoperative clinical syndrome and vertebral stenosis was not to be excluded in this case. The observations regarding delayed diagnosis can be applied to this case of cervical meningiomas associated with discouncusarthrosis below (see case no. 122). However, it is not to be excluded that during an asymptomatic phase the presence of a meningioma can facilitate a vascular disturbance at a lower level when the vertebral canal appears narrow.

6.12 Supra- and Sublesional Symptoms

The presence of supra- and sublesional symptoms has always created a problem in initial evaluations. The pattern of sensory disturbance superior and inferior to the compression was discussed by Elsberg (1923). Neri and Pais (1951) expressed the view regarding pathogenetic mechanisms that supralesional symptoms are associated with upper cervical tumours and the less frequent forms of lower tract tumours. These appear frequently in dorsal compressions. From the observations reported in the literature no deductions can be made with certainty because the oncotype of the tumour is not always specified.

Two mechanisms are involved: (a) block of the fluid which would exclude resorption at spinal nerve root level and (b) medullary oedema caused by venous stasis above the tumour. According to Pagni (1989) these explain the fluctuating nature of the symptoms. Pagni mentions the "distortion" of the structures above the tumour which may account for the ascending type of myelitic disturbance. The observations made in the operating theatre regarding morphological alterations to the adjacent structures of the meningioma cannot exclude, among the various pathogenic factors, the ischaemic vascular factor. Alterations in medullary vascularization vary depending on the tumour site. Medullary oedema is more pronounced in the lesions invading the cord than those in extramedullary compressions. In these the cord becomes narrower and the surface blood vessels present a reduced calibre ipsilateral to the compression site. The pathogenesis of oedema occurring in defined intramedullary forms of tumours is understood. Oedema occurs in the long tract of the greatly enlarged cord above and below the tumour. In upper cervical premedullary locations the clinical symptoms above the lesion can be explained by the apparent reduction in the spinal artery circulation at the point where it leaves the vertebral artery in the part of the tract which joins the opposite side. In this context we recall the bulbar syndromes described by Spiller (1908) which correspond less to vascular insufficiency than to complete arterial occlusion in the tetraplegic syndrome. The transitional nature of many sensory and motor disturbances depends on which tract is affected by the mechanical action of the circulation. Carrot et al. (1959) described symptoms of severe paraparesis during the course of repetitive claudication in a patient suffering from a small meningioma which pressed against Adamkievic's great radicular artery.

A vascular ischemic type of disturbance can lead to prolonged compression on the radicular vascularization. This would explain multisegmental damage due to extradural lesions involving more than one root. Lazorthes (1973) insisted on the transitory vascular factor, and in fact a cord with reduced volume recovers complete functional capacity and the symptoms regress once the compression has been removed. Schneider and Crosby (1959) insist on the specific pattern of the intramedullary vascularization and maintain that the posterolateral part of the paramidal tract is irrigated by narrow branches from the posterior spinal arteries. Regarding disturbances connected to the decrease in blood supply Zulch (1961) emphasizes a central vascular weakness at the cord at the juxtaependymal site where the extremely narrow arteries begin to distribute transversally as terminal branches. Krogh (1945) describes the central ischemic damage by anoxia of the anterior horn's great cells. This interpretation would explain the involvement of vertical cord fibres between the medullary segments at a distance from each other. Usually the medullary surface vascularization is described as being two arterial trunks corresponding to the two posterior spinal arteries. The blood supply originates from these two arteries as a double arterial network running vertically and presenting a paramedian pattern, with collaterals running transversally. The surface anastomotic network varies depending on the different calibres of the nerve root arteries. In dorsal medullary segments the calibre of radicular arteries is less than that in other parts and they become extremely narrow. This can explain how juxtamedullary and radicular involvement can lead to a myelitic sublesional disturbance. In some pain syndromes a radicotomy is performed posteriorly, which in addition to saving the arteries, can ensure complete loss of pain and cord insufficiency symptoms. In 1962 Garcin et al. reported on a lesion of the great radicular artery at the dorsolumbar region level that was responsible for multisegmental weakening.

Apart from the variations and alterations in the internal vascularization of the cord and of the surface layer, the gradual venous stasis of the epidural plexus, which is compressed and flattened against the bony walls of the canal, plays an important role in the various syndromes. It is still difficult, however, to explain the almost complete lack of symptoms in the development stages, sometimes lasting 40 years. It is probable that the very slow alteration process of the blood system is accompanied by a compensatory condition which has a stabilizing effect for many years before being interrupted by a rapid disorder of the cord functions. This may explain the ingravescent development stages typical of the syndrome, with intermittent symptoms on one or both sides, cervical meningiomas with hemiparetic characteristics and acute paraplegic syndromes preceded by transitory phases of motor claudication. At the D4 level, depending on the morphology of the medullary vascularization from the upper area, it appears that once the global blood supply is weakened a thoracic lesion may cause myelitic interruption at the upper thoracic level, and vice versa, in which case a lower cervical compression could produce necrosis at the upper thoracic level instead of at the cervical level (Zulch 1961).

6.13 Von Recklinghausen's Disease

The association of neurinomas and meningiomas scattered along the central nervous system and nerve trunks in von Recklinghausen's disease is an extremely polymorphic pathological expression of a complex dysembryogenesis associated with the migration of neural crest cells from various parts of the cord axis along the nerves and nerve roots to several locations, creating various dysgenetic forms such as amartones and tumours of embryonic origin. Regarding the differentiation defect and the possible inclusions during early embryonic development, Bolande (1974) termed this formation defect neurocrist-

opathy. Solitary intramedullary neurinomas or meningiomas are rare. Only 37 neurinomas of this kind have been reported in the literature (Table 14), to which we add our three cases; however, these are not associated with von Recklinghausen's disease. The solitary intramedullary form of meningioma is reported less frequently. Only two of the 432 primary tumours operated on in our Clinic were cervical intramedullary meningiomas (Table 7).

In forms with multiple locations the clinical picture varies considerably regarding the onset of symptoms which identify upper encephalic structure disturbance or repetitive myeloradicular involvement. One of our patients, 20 years before the the appearance of myeloradicular symtoms, was affected by facial paresis due to a neurinoma at the cerebellopontine angle on the right.

The particularly rapid growth and occasionally even the expansive benign nature of encephalic lesions do not always produce signs of intercranial hypertension. Encephalic lesions often of a meningomatous nature may not produce clinical signs for many years. Myeloradicular locations, however, do show signs of an ingravescent nature, thus facilitating the diagnosis.

Case Nos. 76, 77: Fibroblastic and Transitional Meningiomas
A 28-year-old woman (1988; Figs. 57-64). Multiple meningioma in neurofibromatosis.
Clinical Course. At the age of 20 years the patient was affected by peripheral facial paralysis on the right, which partially regressed. Residual synkinesis and facial spasms bilaterally. After 5 years she developed an impediment to neck movements and paraesthesias to the left upper limb, without radicular pattern. Hyperhydrosis of the hand. Initial pain in the medial dorsal tract and paraesthesias as shooting pain to the right hemithorax followed by an impediment to the lower limbs predominantly on the left, with distal dysaesthesias. During this period the patient complained of slight motor weakness in the legs. Before hospitalization sphincter disturbances appeared.
Neurological Examination. Cutaneous neurofibromas in the right paretic site. Slight ptosis on the left, anisoria (left>right), nystagmus on lateral gaze, peripheral facial paresis on the right, bilateral hypoacuity. Romberg test showed left lateral tendency, spastic paraparesis with Babinski sign on both sides. Spastic ataxia (Levy grade 0) present when walking. Superficial and deep hypoaesthesia from C5-C8 on the left and D6, D7 bilaterally, with distal anaesthesia.
X-Ray of Cranium. Hyperostosis of cranium in frontal area on the right.
X-Ray of Rachis. Slight increase in anteroposterior diameter of canal in C1, C2. Irregularity in spinous processes in D8, D9, deflecting to the right. The articular mass of L3 on the left presented blurred outlines. The canal was slightly enlarged transversally in L2, L3.
MRI. At cranium-encephalus level a right frontal-paretic meningioma en plaque and a small roundish cerebellar-bulbar lesion on the left. From the bulbar junction up to C7 the cord appeared wider and presented a homogeneous signal with small hypointense areas in T1 and hyperintense areas in T2 of a cystic nature. After Gd-DTPA, diffused nonhomogeneous impregnated areas. In D4 the spinal cord presented an increased calibre, with modified signal, increased nonhomogeneously especially in T1 with cavernous malformation within. In D7 confirmation of an intradural-extramedullary meningioma. Small nodular, intradural formations at lumbar level; identification of expansive, intradural-extramedullary

Table 14. Intramedullary neurinomas: a review of the literature

Reference	Age, sex	Level	Duration	Symptoms	Operation	Result
Kernohan (1941)	12, M	C	4 years	Cervical, brachial pain	Partial	-
Roka (1951)	30, M	C	10 months	Cervical pain	Laminectomy	-
Riggs and Clary (1957)	60, M	C	3 years	Tetraparesis	Laminectomy	Death
Ramamurthi et al. (1958)	35, M	D	9 months	Paraparesis	Total	Improvement
Lang and Bridge (1959)	25, M	C	1 year	-	Total	Improvement
Scott and Bentz (1962)	35, F	D	12 years	Monoparesis	Partial	Deterioration
Lu et al. (1963)	32, M	C	3 months	Tetraparesis	Laminectomy	-
Lu et al. (1963)	43, M	C	18 months	Cervical pain	Total	-
Guidetti et al. (1964)	57, M	L	2 years	Sciatica	Total	Recovery
McKormick (1964)	-, -	L	-	-	Total	Recovery
Mason and Kreigher (1968)	37, M	D	2 months	Paraparesis	Total	Recovery
Chigasaki and Pennybacker (1968)	75, F	D	7 months	Sciatica	Partial	Paraparesis
Van Duinen (1971)	24, F	C	4 years	Paraesthesias	Total	Paresis
Bharati and Rammamurthi (1972)	55, F	D-L	6 months	Paraparesis	Total	-
Fabres et al. (1972)	26, M	D	13 months	Radicular pain	Total	Paraparesis
Cambier et al. (1974)	60, M	C	11 months	Pain	Total	Hemiparesis
Pansini (1975)	31, F	C	6 years	Tetraparesis	Subtotal	Improvement
Wood (1975)	48, M	C	3 months	Hemiparesis	Radiotherapy	Death
Isu et al. (1976)	30, F	C	6 months	Hemiparesis	Partial	-
Pardatscher et al.(1979)	41, M	Mult.	6 months	Tetraparesis	Partial	Death
Vailati et al. (1979)	40, F	D	1 year	Paraparesis	Total	Paraplegia
Shalit and Sandbank (1981)	21, F	C-D	6 months	Cervical pain	Biopsy	-
Cantore et al. (1982)	54, F	C	2 years	Cervical, brachial pain	Total	Recovery
Pansini (1982)	44, M	D	3 years	Paraparesis	Total	Unchanged
Kang and Song (1983)	47, M	C	1 year	Cervical, brachial pain	Total	Improvement
Lesoin et al. (1983)	45, F	C	6 months	Cervical, brachial pain	Total	Monoparesis
Lesoin et al. (1983)	28, M	L	5 years	Paraparesis	Total	Monoparesis
Rout et al. (1983)	50, F	C	5 years	Cervical, brachial pain	Total	Paraplegia
Young et al. (1983)	33, F	D-L	3 years	Paraparesis	Total	Unchanged
Sharma (1984)	27, M	C	18 months	Tetraparesis	Partial	Improvement
Drapkin et al. (1985)	30, F	C	3 years	Cervical pain	Total	Deterioration
Gonzales et al. (1985)	29, M	C	1 year	Tetraparesis	Total	Paraparesis
Ross et al. (1986)	67, F	C	4 years	Tetraparesis	Partial	Improvement
Ross et al. (1986)	36, M	C	4 months	Tetraparesis	Total	Recovery
Solomon et al. (1987)	69, M	C	4 years	Brown-Sequard	Total	Hemihypoaesthesia
Herrmann et al. (1988)	51, M	C	-	-	Partial	-
Pansini et al. (1988)	28, F	C	3 years	Tetraparesis	Total	Improvement
Marchese and McDonald (1990)	72, M	C	6 years	Paraparesis	Partial	Improvement
Herregodts et al. (1991)	49, F	D	5 years	Paraparesis	Total	Improvement
Jacquet et al. (1992)	44, M	L	5 months	Lumbago	Total	Paraesthesia

processes of spheroid or ovaloid shape, two of which were particularly evident in retromedullary paramedian right sites, one in L1 and the other in L1-L2. A third lesion was present at the upper portion of the body in L3 in the anterolateral site on the left.

CT on Cranium. A clear thickening of the skull was visible on the right. The internal auditory meatus appeared wider on the left. In the left cerebellar-bulbar region a hyperdense image was produced without a mass effect.

Myelo-CT. The cord from C1 to C3 presented an increased calibre and a nonhomogeneous aspect. Small calcified areas in a dural site in C1 and extramedullary in C3 where the laminae were narrowed. In D4 a marked increment of the cord is visible due to intramedullary lesion. In D7 another intradural-extramedullary lesion on the left anterolaterally which displaced and compressed the cord posteriorly to the right.

SEPs. Upper left limb: block in conduction along the proprioception pathways at proximal central level in relation to C6. In the lower left limb, partial slowing down of conduction at roots of the cauda with a block at the level above.

Surgical Treatment. Five operations led to the removal of 14 neurinomas, 2 intrarachidian meningiomas and 1 intercranial meningioma. First operation (16 Sept. 1988): removal of intramedullary cystic neurinoma in C1, C2 and of another meningioma the size of a lentil adhering to the dura in a posterolateral site on the right. In the postoperative stage the patient complained of minor impediment in the lower limbs but gained an almost total recovery from paraparesis. Minimal persistence of slight hypoaesthesia on L4, L5 and S1 with distal hypopallaesthesia. Disappearance of sphincter disturbances. Second operation (28 Sept. 1988): removal of meningioma in D7, with anterolateral dural attachment on the left. The presence of a calcified subarachnoidal lamella. In the immediate postoperative phase a transitional motor impairment of lower left limb that partially regressed in 3 weeks. Third operation (9 March 1989): removal of ten neurinomas on the roots of the cauda. After 2 years an MRI of the encephalus showed four new small formations of a probable meningiomatous nature in sylvian site on the left in the lateral left ventricle in the parasagittal occipital region on the left and cerebellar site on the right. Fourth operation (23 May 1990): removal of a neurinoma in L1-L2 adhering to the conus and two small nodules attached to the roots of the cauda. Motor impairment immediately after surgery which recovered a few weeks later. Persistent deficiency in right foot but walking was possible without support. Fifth operation (30 Jan. 1991): Removal of a frontal paretic en plaque meningioma on the right. A neurological examination 6 years after the first operation revealed good motor recovery. Walking was possible with slight ataxia. The last MRI (Oct. 1994) performed at encephalus level showed increased volume of the sylvian meningioma, the occipital one and the ventricular one on the left. In addition, there were findings of new, small lesions in the hypocampus and paretic site parasagittally on the left. In the dorsolumbar tract tiny nodular lesions varying from a few millimetres mm to 1 cm from D7 to L2.

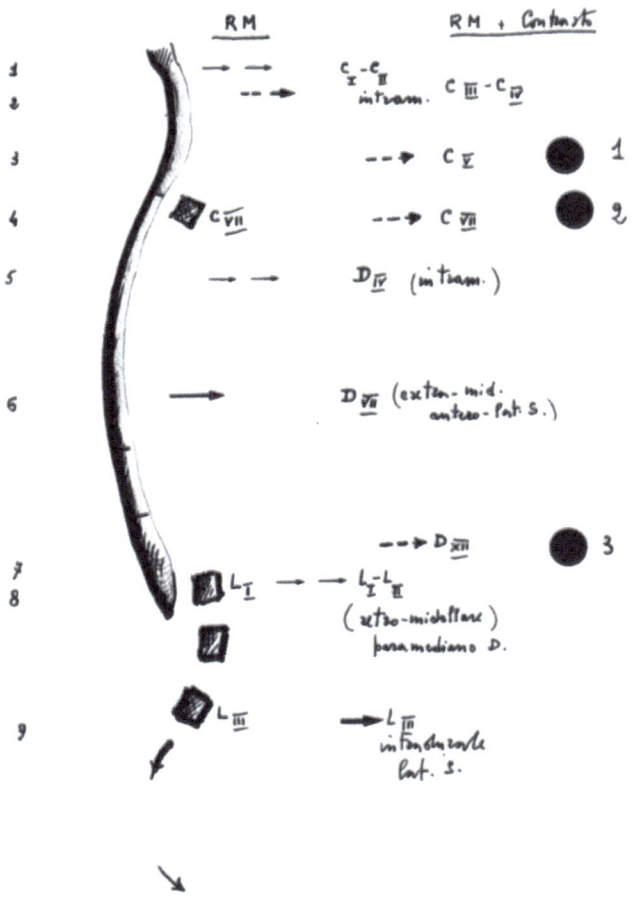

Fig. 57. Various locations of neurinomas and meningiomas in von Recklinghausen's disease. Small meningioma on the internal surface of the dura in C1-C2 on the right (see Figs. 58-64). Altogether 2 meningiomas and 14 neurinomas were removed and a medullary one in C2 was bulging on the surface (see Fig. 58)

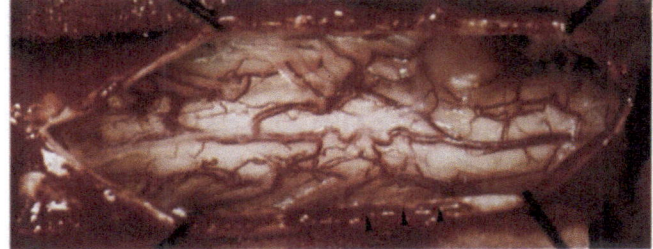

Fig. 59. Left sided antero-lateral intradural extramedullary meningioma in D7

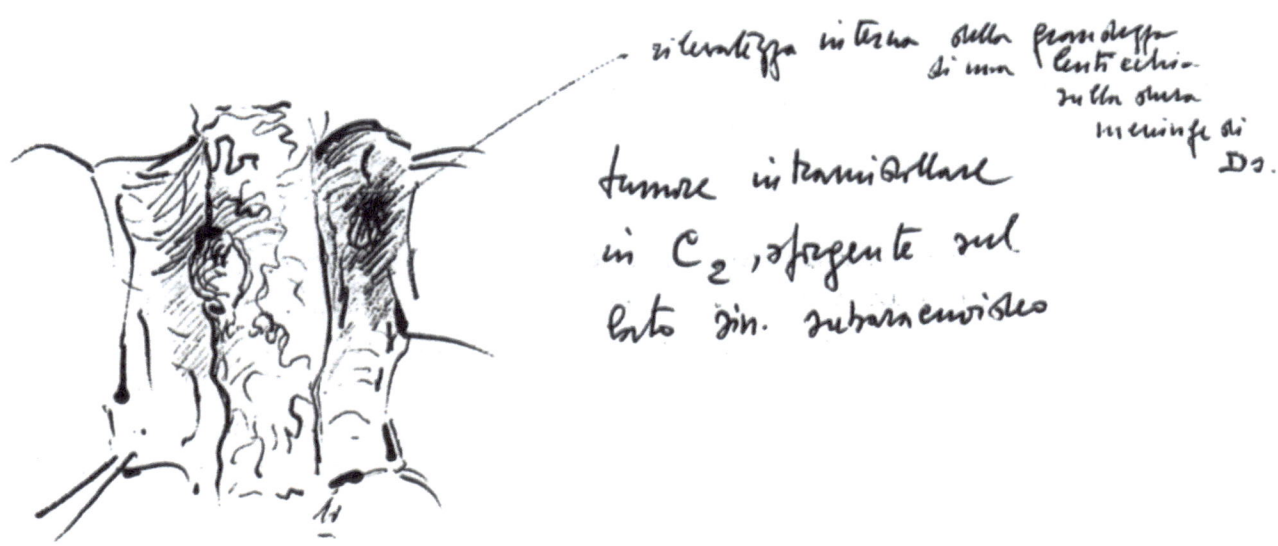

Fig. 58. First operation. Left anterolateral intradural-extramedullary meningioma in D7

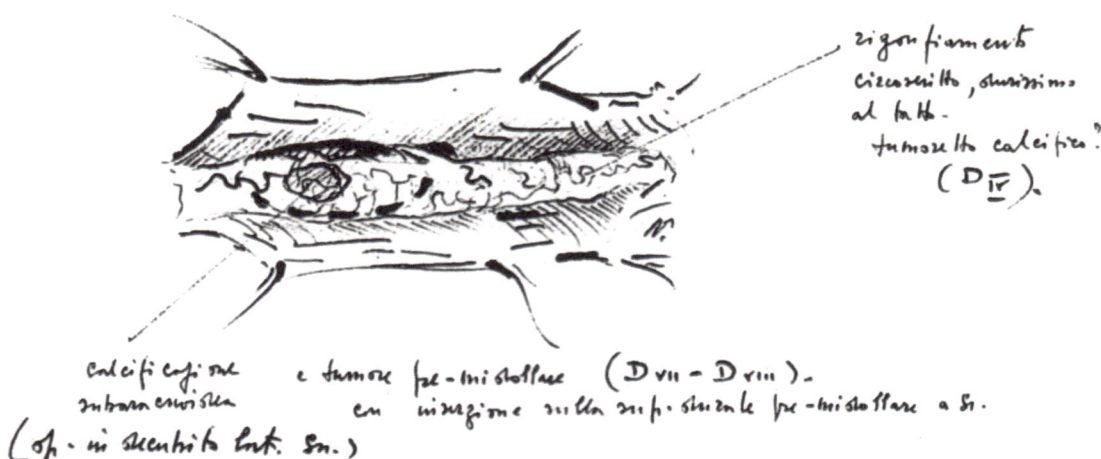

Fig. 60. Second operation

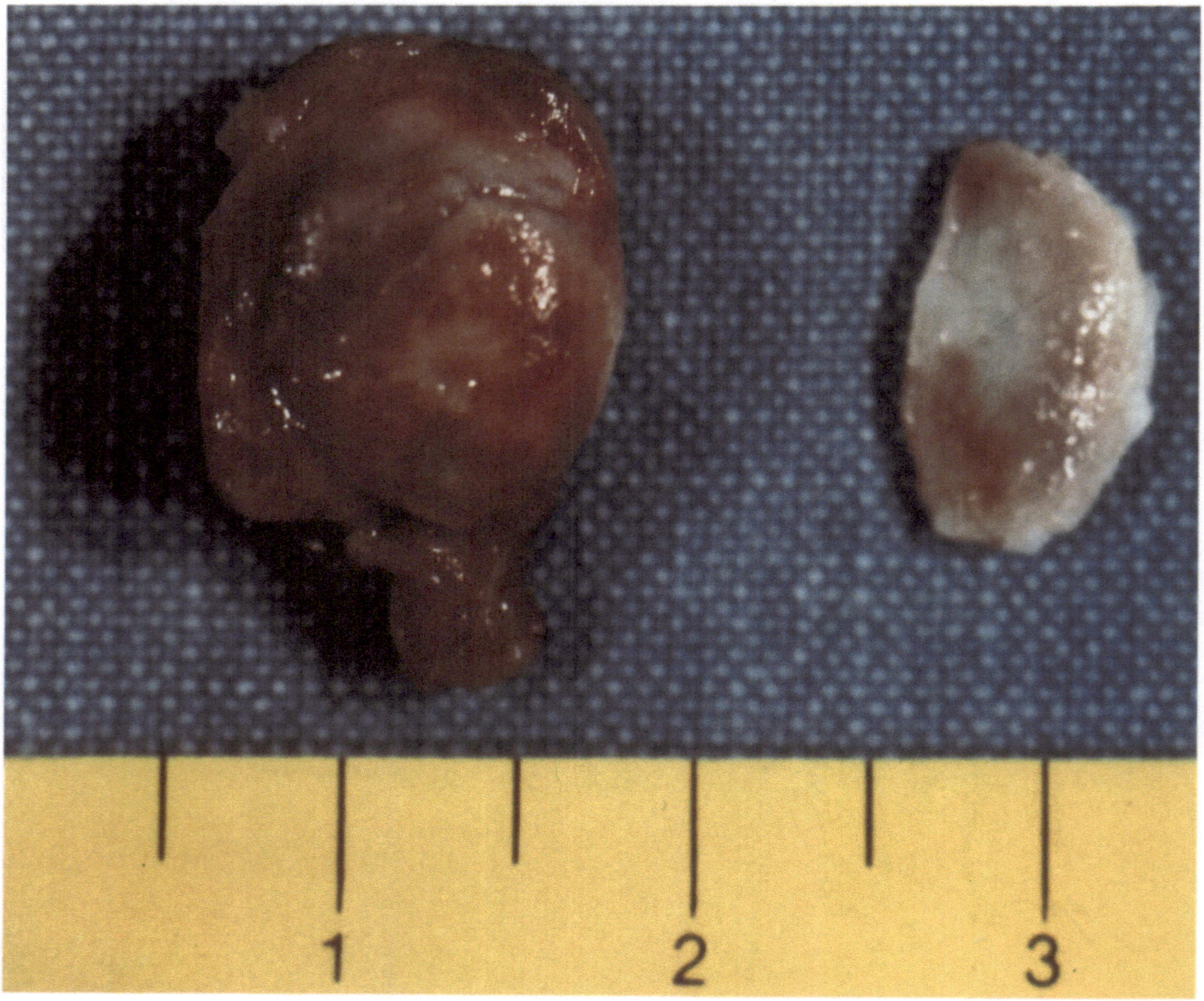

Fig. 61. Tumour and calcified subarachnoidal plate

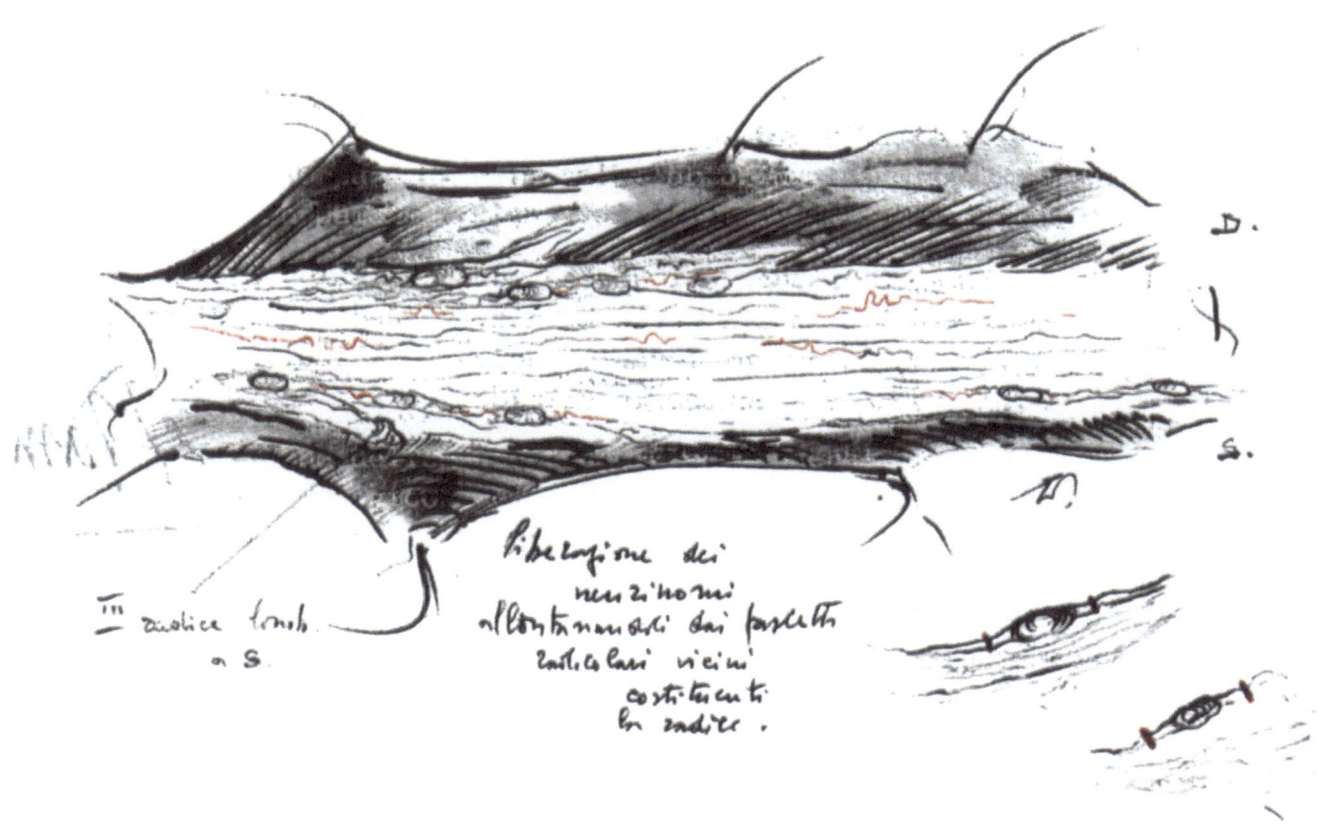

Fig. 62. Third operation

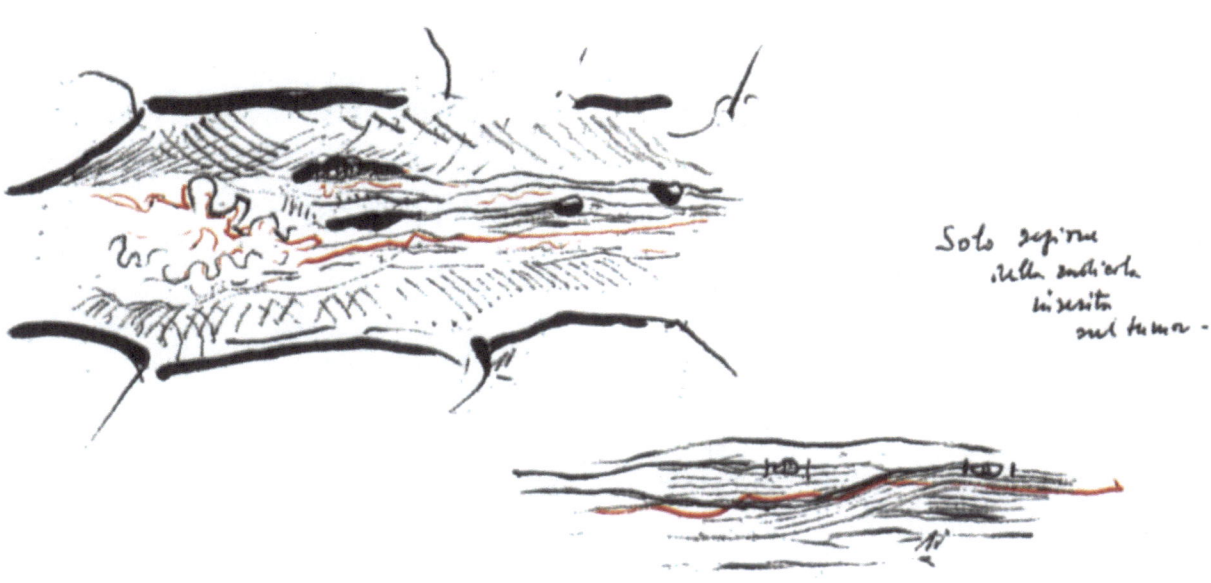

Fig. 63. Fourth operation for the removal of neurinomas in a paramedian right preterminal cone site in L1-L2, and other two neurinomas between the roots below

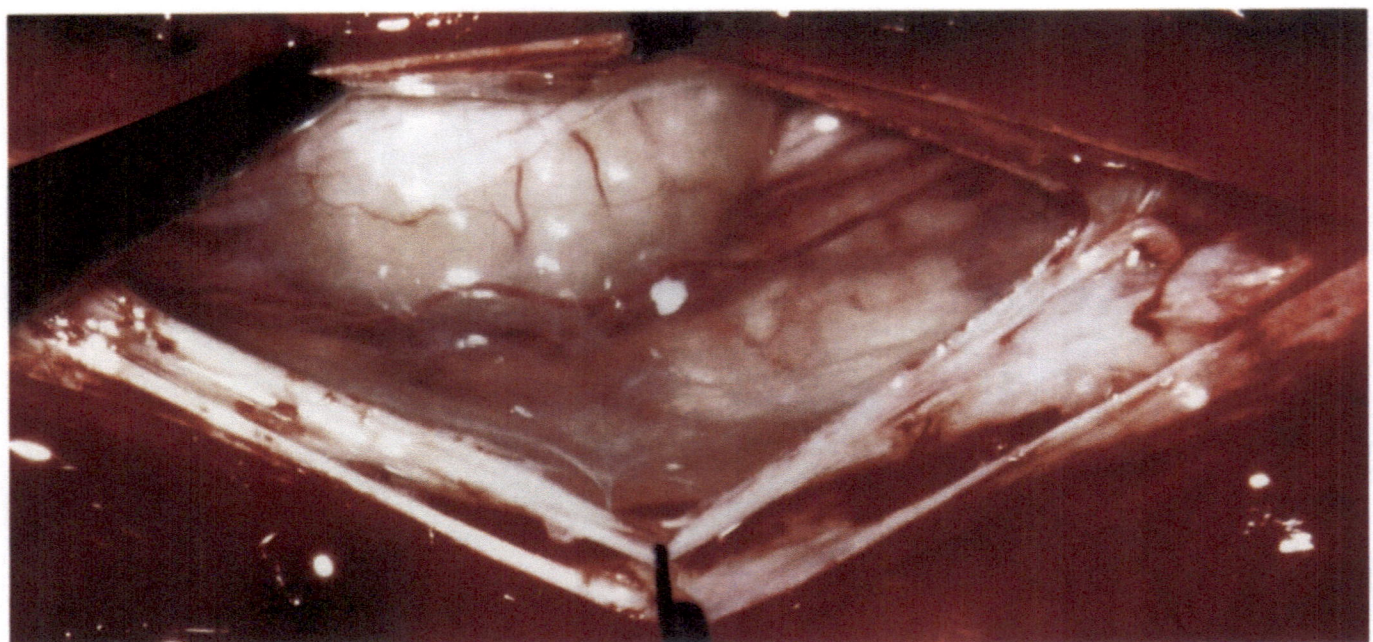

Fig. 64. Postero-lateral neurinoma in L1 - L2

6.14 Rare Cases

The symptoms and anatomical-clinical picture of some rare cases demonstrate a dysembryogenetic nature. We present three cases, two of which are intra- and extramedullary and a particularly exceptional case affecting the filum terminale. With persistent aberrant arachnoidal elements in the vicinity of the neural tube's first cavity, a particularly rare form of meningioma would form inside the spinal cord near the ependyma following the similar process of an embryogenetic defect when the inclusions of arachnoidal cells remain in the vicinity of the primary periencephalic vesicles, evolving into an intraventricular meningioma.

In the first case the ondulating course, similar to motor claudication, suggested a form of demyelination (Figs. 65-68).

Case No. 73: Psammomatous Meningioma
A 60-year-old man (1980). Intramedullary meningioma in C1.
Clinical Course. 37 years. During World War II the patient was affected by cranial trauma in the occipital region; paraesthesias to the hand and right foot with cutaneous numbness throughout the lower limb. Slight motor claudication. Another hospital diagnosed a suspected demyelinized illness. 4 years after the onset of symptoms walking improved and became almost normal for about 20 years. For the following 10 years the patient was affected by a motor impediment distally and in the lower left limb.
Neurological Examination. Forced attitude of the head rotated towards the left. Spastic tetraparesis predominantly on the right with pronounced hyperreflexia and hypertonia. Hypotonia of the right scapula-humerus region. Bilateral Babinski sign. Foot clonus

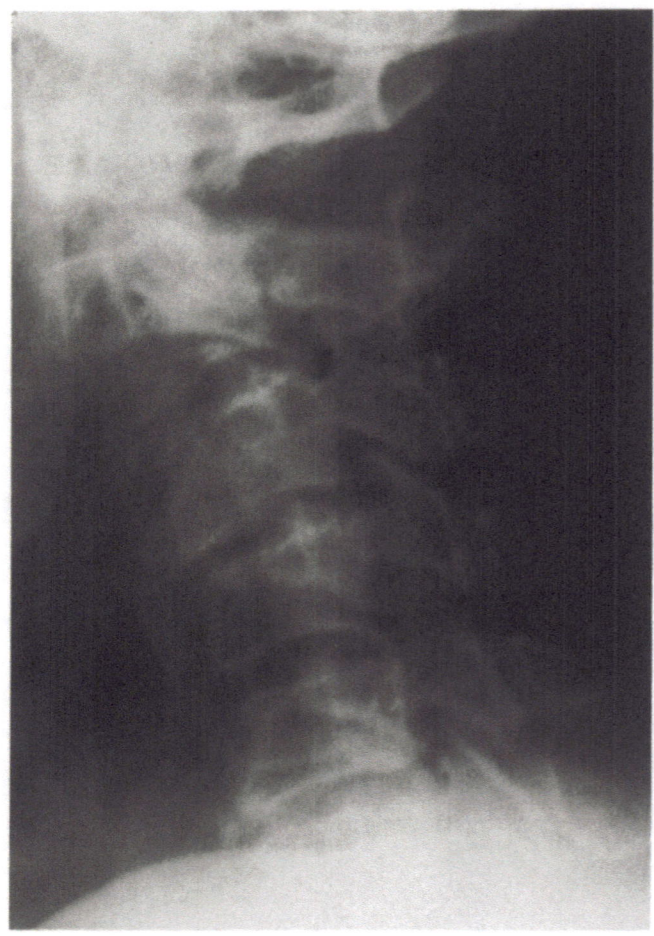

Fig. 65. X-ray. Slight hypoplasia of atlas arch. Mega-apophysis of C2

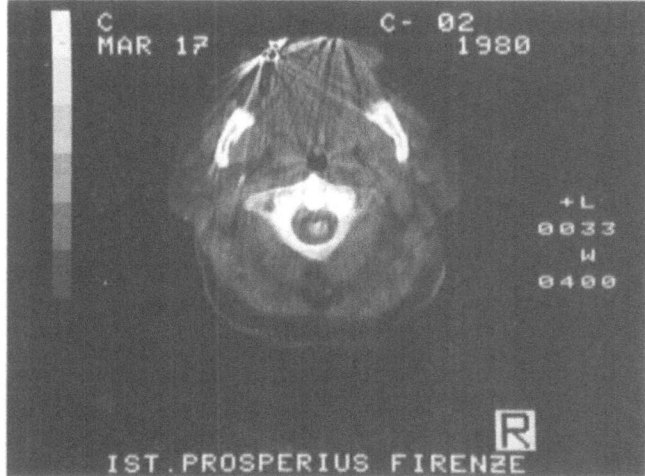
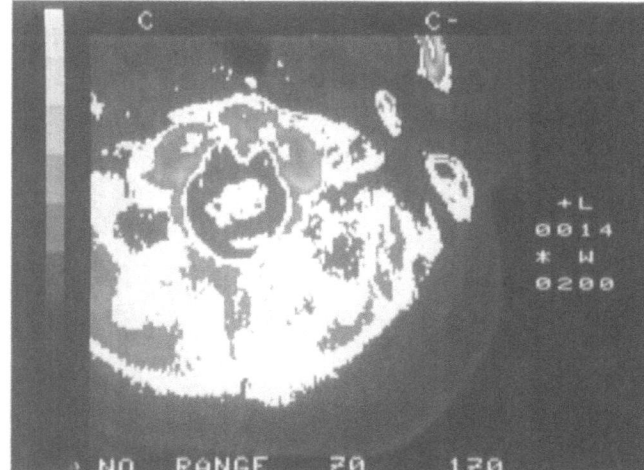
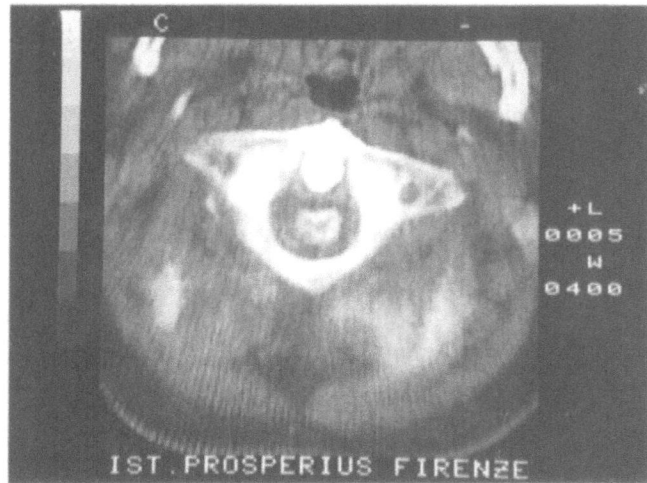
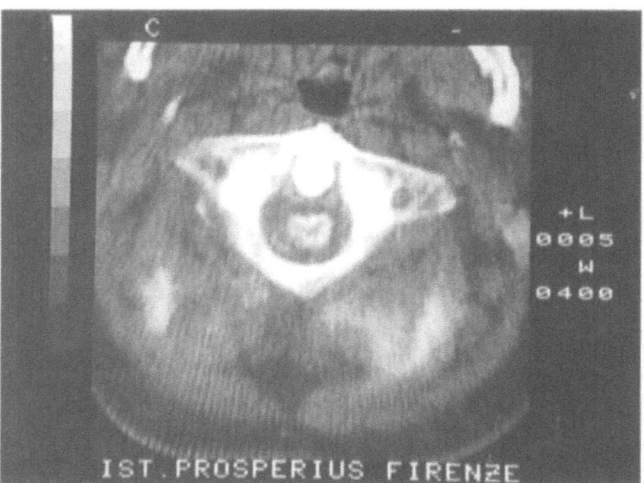

Fig. 66. CT. A large irregular calcified area in the rachidian lumen at the axis level

bilaterally. Thermal and tactile hypoaesthesia at left hemisome. Painful hypoaesthesia only at L1 on the left. Pronounced spastic-paretic type of walking.

X-Ray of Cervical Rachis Tract. Hypoplasia associated with the arch of the atlas, with large spinous processes in C2.

CT of Cervical Tract. Images showed calcified lesion at the level of the medullary-bulbar passage in C1-C2 predominantly to the left.

Surgical Treatment. Extensive laminectomy at upper cervical level and opening the occipital foramen. Opening the dura presented a clear hypotrophy of the cord along 2 cm of its length corresponding to a distinct narrowing of the canal. Once the arachnoid was freed, a medullary enlargement was found below the atrophic tract presenting a yellowish surface layer hard in consistency due to the expansive intramedullary process. A myelotomy was performed limited to the pathological area and followed by the removal of the calcified tumour by fragmentation reaching the central part of the cord. Removal was possible without sacrificing the posterior surface blood system which presented an anomalous flow.

Results. After surgery the patient did not recover spontaneous respiration and died 20 days after reanimation.

The rarity of this case was not only due to the location of the intramedullary psammomatous meningioma in an upper cervical site but also to a bony dysmorphia associated with a lipomatous component in the surface layer of the cord and a malformed circulation along the median line of the posterior columns. The posterior spinal arterial circulation was formed by a single medial trunk running downwards and branching into two paramedian networks. The arrangement of the mesenchyma around the neural tube during the differentiation phase of the future leptomeningeal membranes near the invertebral foramina explains why the arachnoidal elements remain at the depth of the spinal dura near the dural funnel and in the vicinity of the intervertebral foramina, frequently causing the lateral formation of the meningioma rather than in premedullary or posterior sites.

In the second case the meningioma, although intradural and extramedullary, developed on the midline in continuity with an intramedullary cyst (Figs. 69-74).

Case No. 96: Meningothelial Meningioma

An infant, 2 years 3 months old (1972). Posterior intradural-extramedullary meningioma invading the medial raphe in D1-D2.

Family Medical History. The child's mother underwent surgery in

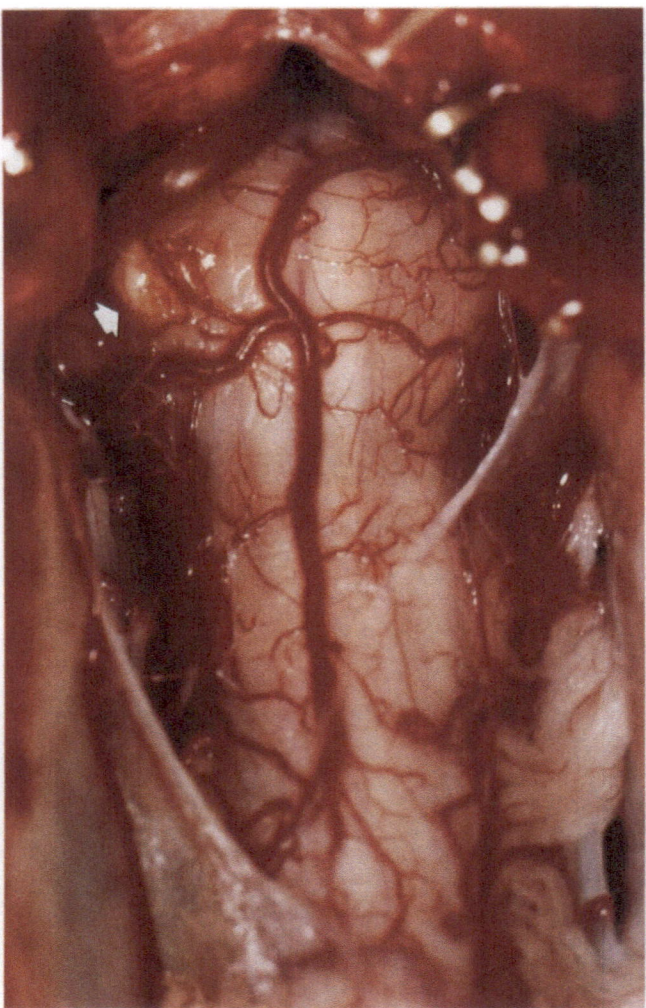

Fig. 67. The posterior columns appear stretched in C1-C2 near the bulbar-medullary junction. A pathological lipomatous area appears on the left (*arrow*). Malformed circulation represented by a single artery from the posterior spinal artery

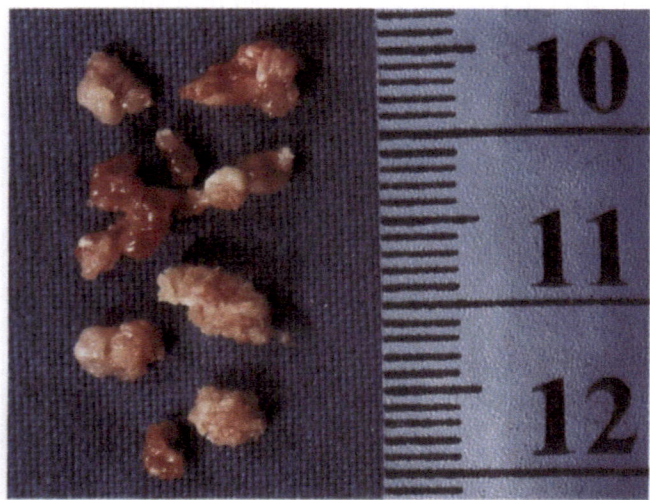

Fig. 68. Fragments of the calcified intramedullary meningioma in C1-C2

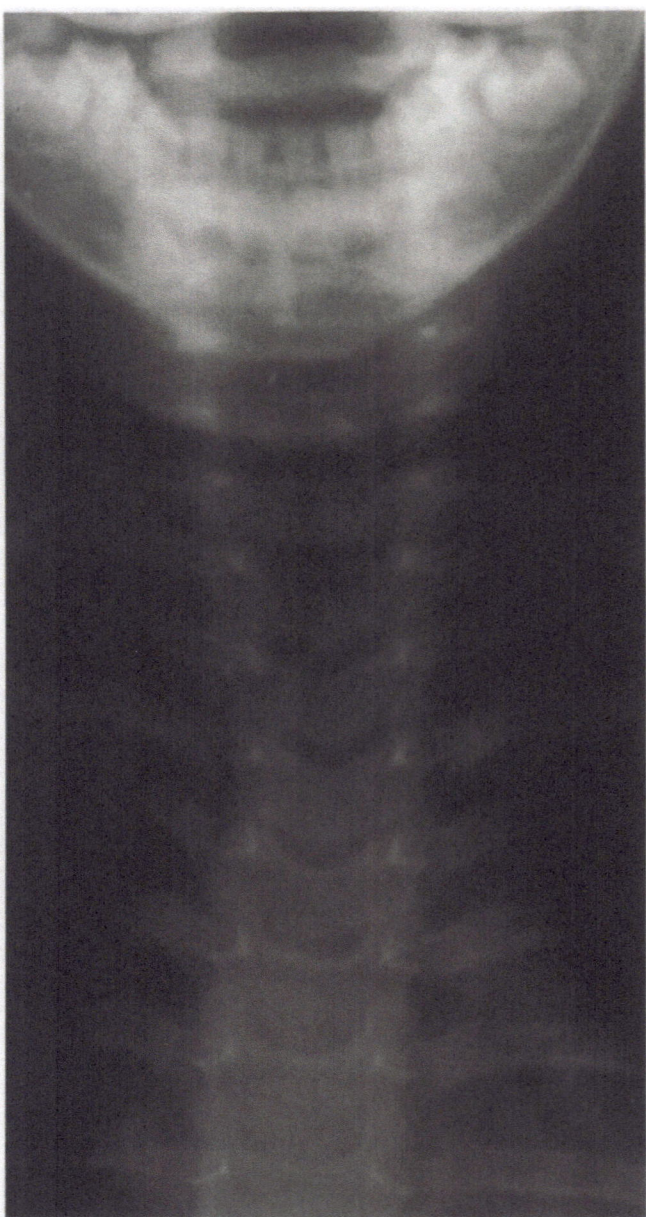

Fig. 69. X-ray of cervicodorsal passage. Anteroposteriorly an increase in the interpeduncular distance at the D1 level demonstrates the presence of an expansive structure inside the rachidian canal

1955 for the removal of a meningioma in the occipital fossa.
Clinical Course. 1 month. The parents reported that the symptoms appeared 1 month prior to hospitalization, consisting of difficulty in walking and evident motor impairment in the lower right limb. Another hospital diagnosed coxitis, for which the patient was treated. After approx. 15 days the motor impairment extended to the lower left limb and made both standing upright and walking impossible. *Neurological Examination.* Spastic paraparesis with hypertonia affecting the lower right limb more seriously than the left. Marked hyperreflexia of the patellas and ankle jerk with bilateral foot clonus. The upright position was impossible. The clinical examination for various sensory forms proved very difficult to perform on the child due to the lack of cooperation; however, we identified an area affected by band-like hypoaesthesia and by pain above the transverse mamillary region.

Rachicentesis. 11 g protein per thousand.
Radiographic Examination of Lumbar and Dorsal Rachis. Slight increase in interpeduncular space in C7 and D1.
Myelography (performed suboccipitally, under general anaesthetic in horizontal position or lateral left decubitus). Overflow of fluid under pressure. Gradual introduction of the iodine medium and adjusting the radiographic table until the patient was in a sitting position. Total block of contrast medium at D1-D2; the image showed an expansive intradural-extramedullary process.
Surgical Treatment. The dura appeared taut and nonpulsating. On opening the dura, a neoplasm was clearly seen in a posterior site, invading the arachnoid of the raphe and adherent to the posterior columns of the spinal cord. The volume of the cord was reduced to half its normal calibre. Once the adherent structures had been removed, the 2-cm-long tumour was removed en bloc. The tumour attachment was along the midline of the perimedullary pia arachnoid. Between the slightly disjointed posterior columns a small intermedullary cyst was seen.
Results. Rapid recovery of voluntary motility. After 1 week the patient was capable of walking a few steps with some help. Two

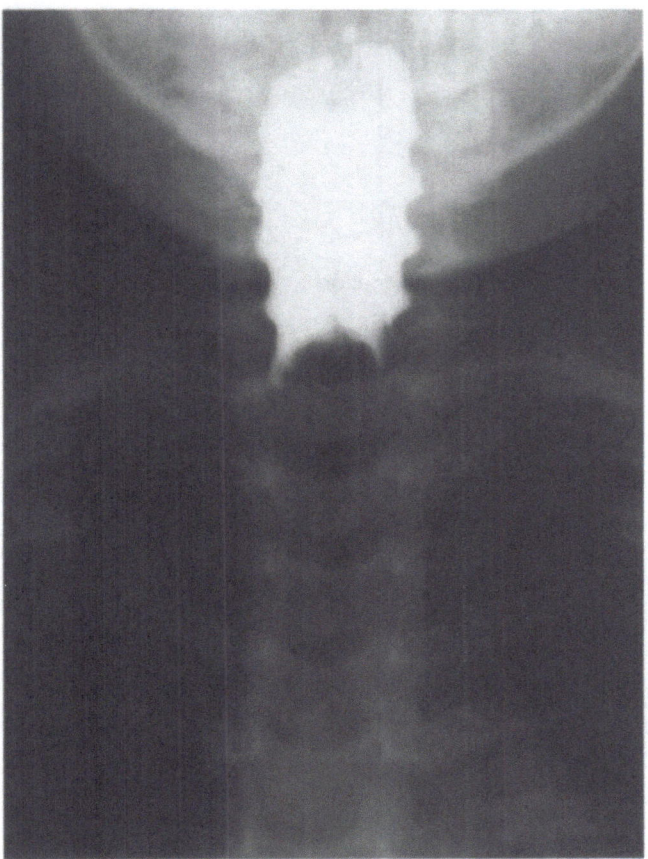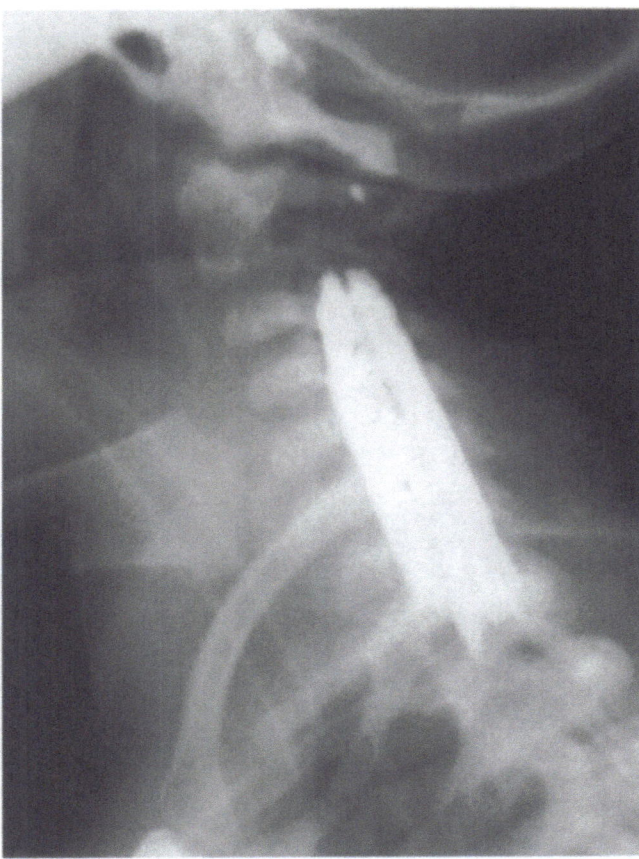

Fig. 70. Suboccipital myelography. Anteroposteriorly a total block at D1-D2 level producing a dome-shaped image shows an intradural-extramedullary lesion. In a lateral projection the block is of an irregular aspect

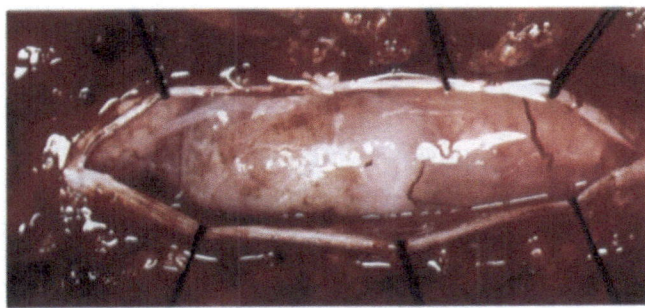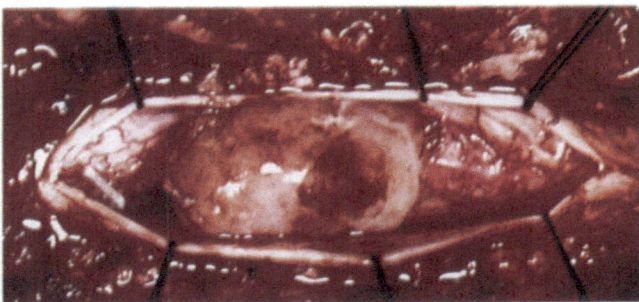

Fig. 71. On opening the dura a well-defined meningioma was seen covered by an arachnoidal process which was thicker at the lower pole level of the tumour. No invasion of the internal layer of the dura. Once the neoplasm removed, its origin identified as being from the deep medial raphe. It is shown associated with a small intramedullary cyst (see Figs. 72-74)

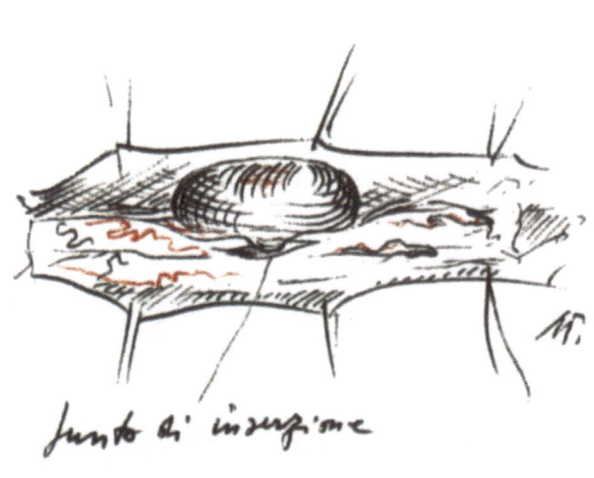

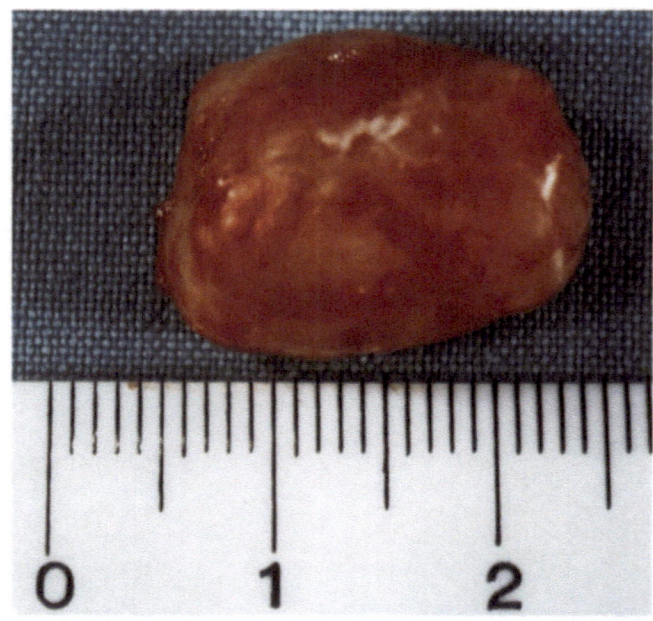

Fig. 72. Intradural extramedullary meningioma developed on the midline in continuity with an intramedullary cyst

Fig. 73. Tumour removed en-block

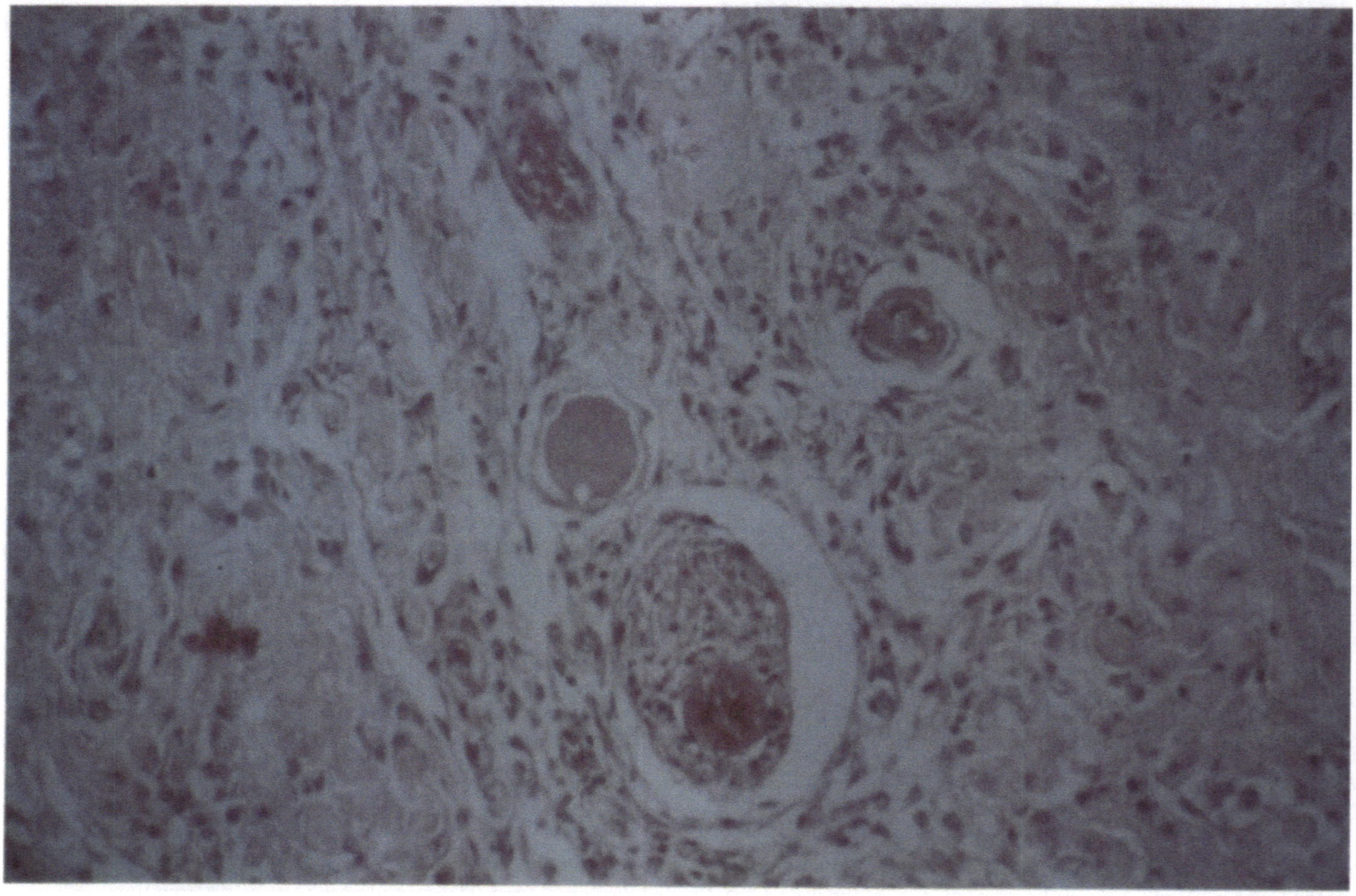

Fig. 74. Meningothelial meningioma

months later walking returned to normal. Surgical recovery was total, even after 20 years; the neurological examination results were completely negative.

In another child also aged 2 years and 3 months the very rare form of meningioma surrounded the filum terminale and presented a small lipomatous component and malformation of the posterior walls of the vertebral bodies, it was of shell-shaped appearance along the entire lumbar tract (Figs. 75-78).

Case No. 72: Meningothelial Meningioma with Lipomatous Component at Lower Pole Level

An infant, 2 years 3 months old. (1972). Extramedullary meningioma at the filum terminale, occupying the entire canal from L2 to S1.

Clinical Course. 3 months. The child's mother reported that the onset of symptoms occurred 3 months prior to hospital admission. The child complained of back pain following a fall (from a chair) and landing on the buttocks, which gradually led to the impossibility of keeping an upright position and walking.

Neurological Examination. Spontaneous response in slight flexation of hips with dorsolumbar kyphosis. The child was unable to walk due to a severe spinal insufficiency and pain spreading to the lower limbs. Passive flexion manoeuvres of the knee and hips and

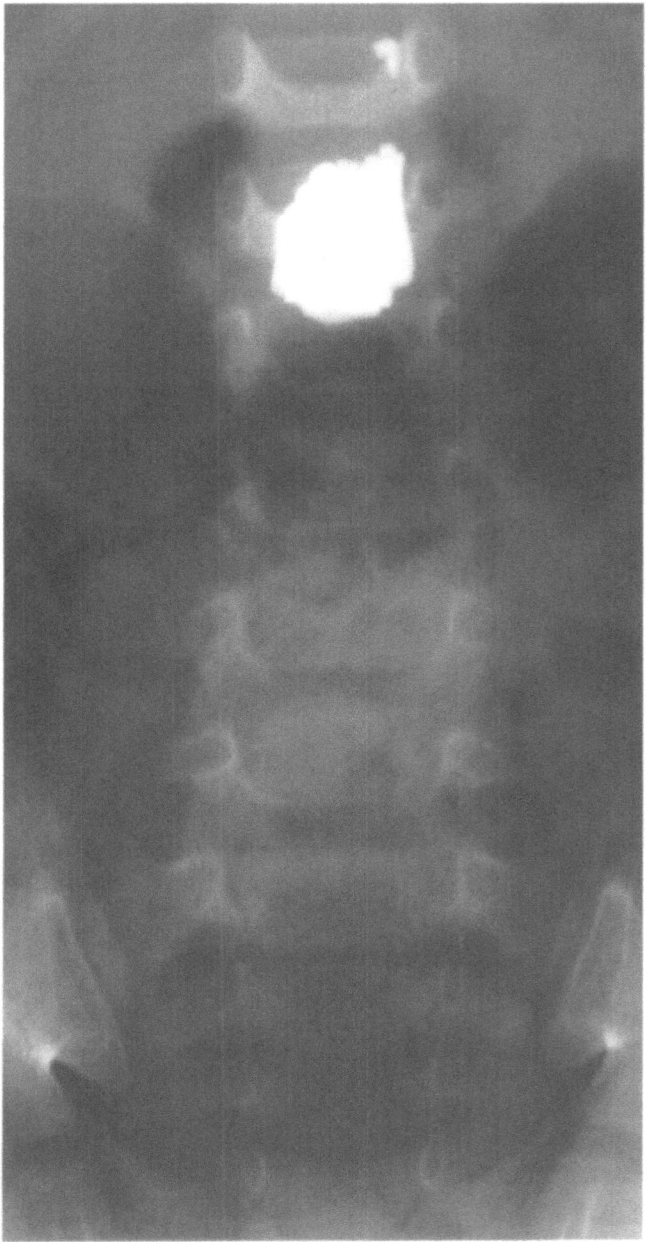
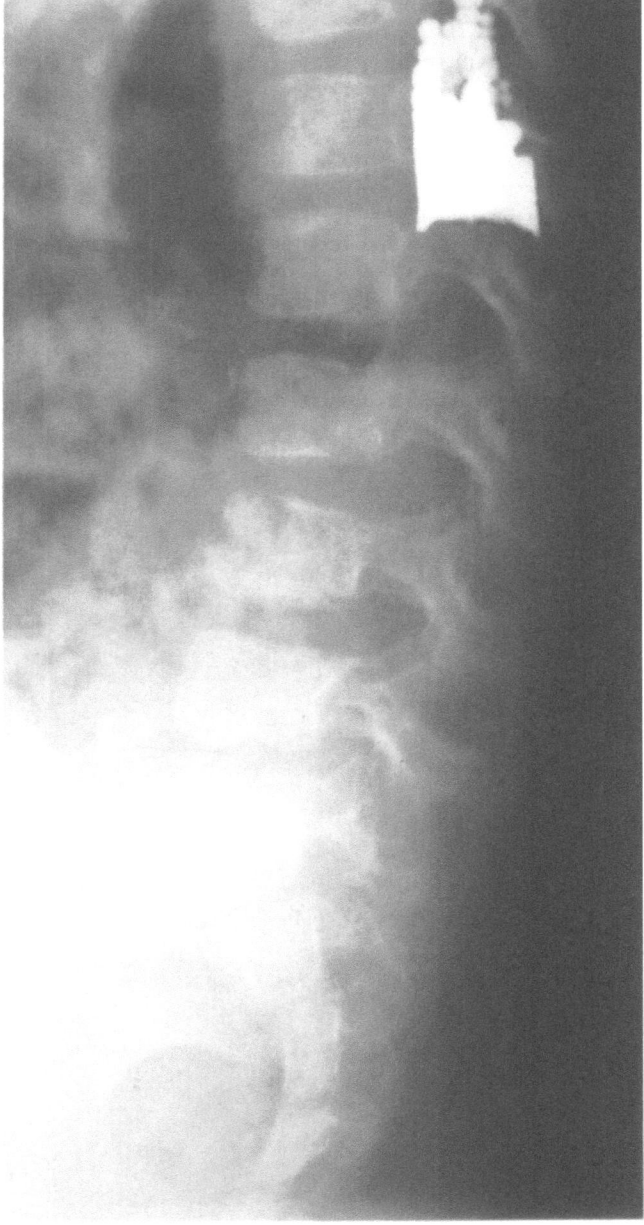

Fig. 75. Suboccipital myelography. Total block in L2 above the modification of the pedicles, mainly in L3-L4

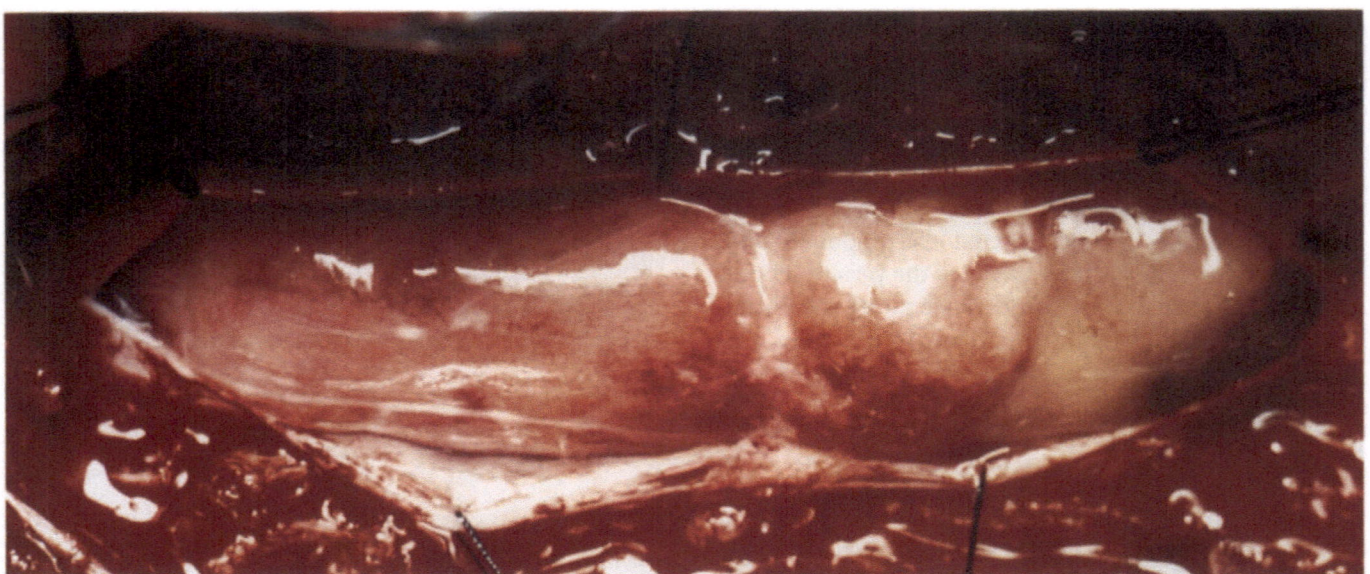

Fig. 76. Photograph of the operating field. The particularly large vertical extension of the tumour shows a lipomatous area at the level of its lower pole (see Figs. 77, 78)

pressure on the spinous processes at the dorsolumbar passage, producing acute pain. Hyporreflexia of patellas and knee jerk. On examining the patient for various sensory forms, hypoaesthesia of the pain form distributed bilaterally on L3-S1.
Rachicentesis. 30.5 g protein per thousand.
X-Ray of Lumbar Tract. In anteroposterior projections the rachidian canal was found enlarged in L2 and the pedicles at the same level were found to be narrowed.

Myelography (performed suboccipitally, under general anaesthetic and in lateral decubitus). Total block at L2 level. The image presented an intradural-extramedullary neoplasm with a rounded upper pole.
Surgical Treatment. The posterior arches from L2 to S1 appeared thinned. The dura was taut and nonpulsating and it was possible to see a compact, tumourous mass occupying the whole lumbar region which tended to appear on opening the dura mater. The large

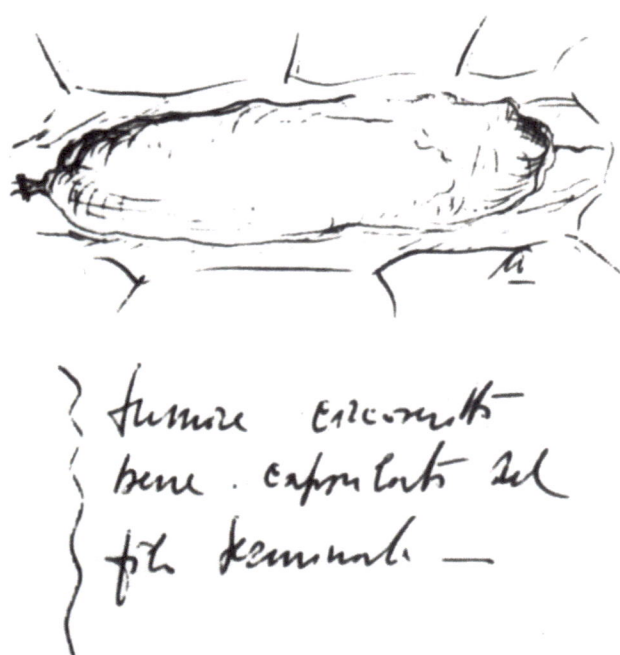

Fig. 77.a Well encapsulated tumour of the filum

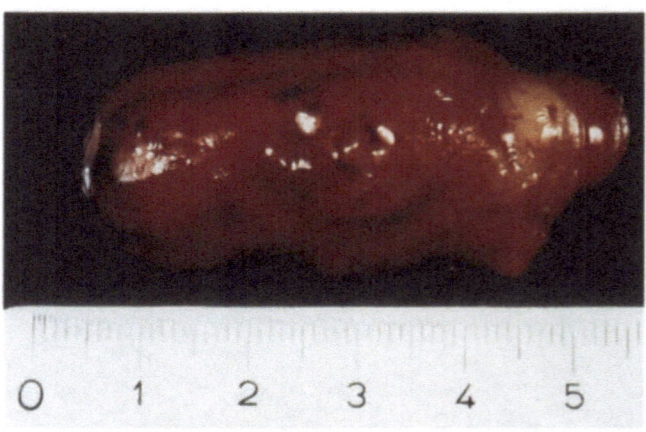

Fig. 77.b Macroscopic view of the lesion

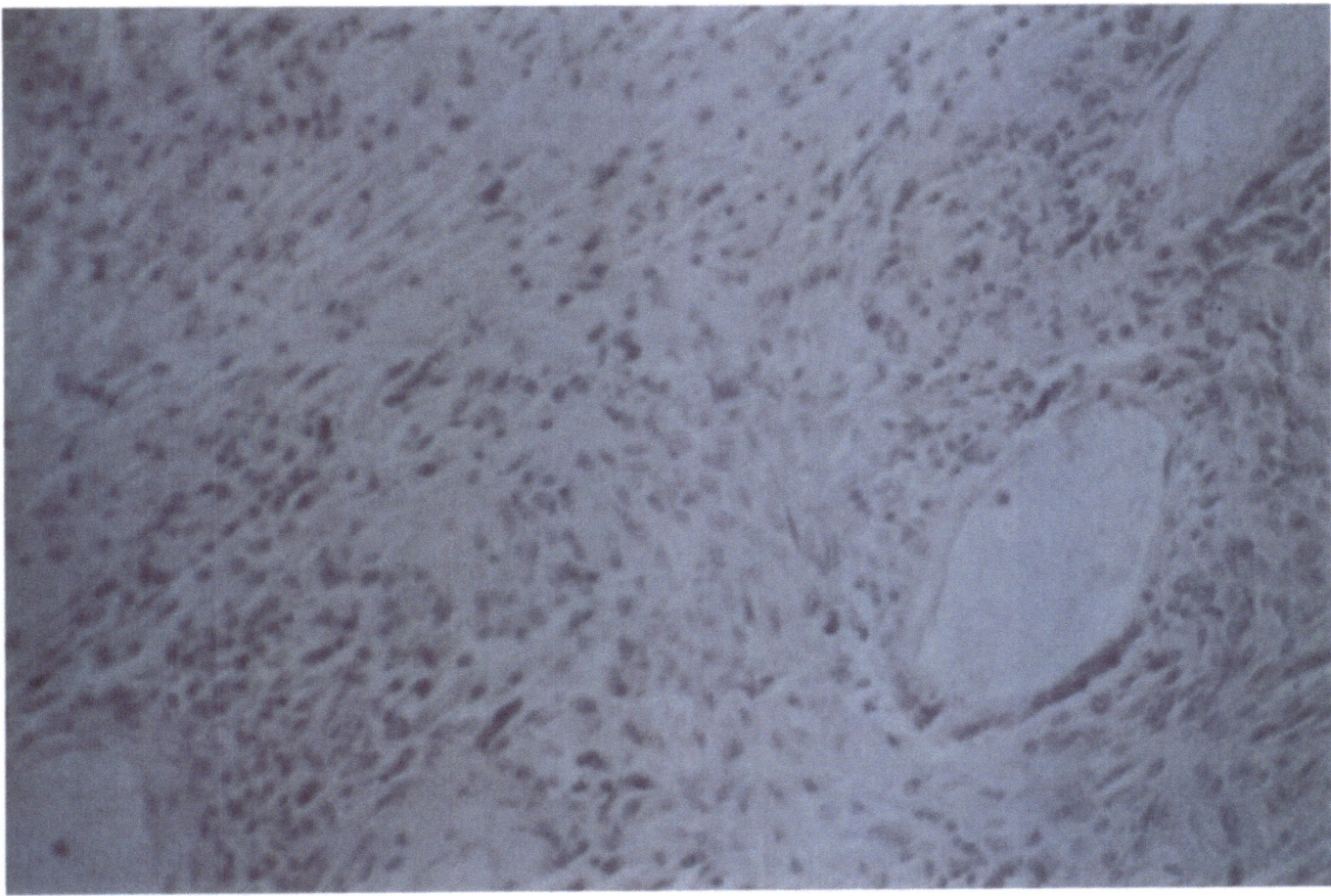

Fig. 78. Meningothelial meningioma

tumour adhered to the thickened arachnoidal membrane. Extensive removal of the arachnoid from the posterior surface of the tumour for about 6 cm. Clipping of the filum terminale near the upper attachment and gradual removal of the neoplasm from the roots of the cauda. Clipping of the filum terminale at the lower pole level. *Results.* During the postoperative phase the patient recovered from the pain syndrome and a gradual recovery of the motility at both lower limbs. Three months after surgery the patient could walk without support. The patient developed normally, and at the age of 20 years dedicated himself to intense gymnastics.

These three cases demonstrate that the presence of differentiation defects accompany the development of a meningioma. This oncotype can manifest itself even in much more complex dysmorphia regarding moments of incomplete formation. In fact, meningiomas can be present in the defective and modified shapes of the primary segments when the somites form from the mesoderma into metameric organs in the same way that occurs at the nerve roots and ganglia, where the lack of the differentiation phase is visible at the midline. In time this may involve even the ectodermal membrane. In this context we describe a case not included in our series which concerns a tumour associated with defective protovertebra formation; the posterior bones did not join and the medial bone spicule surrounded a meningioma, a dermoid cyst and a neurinoma (Figs. 79-83).

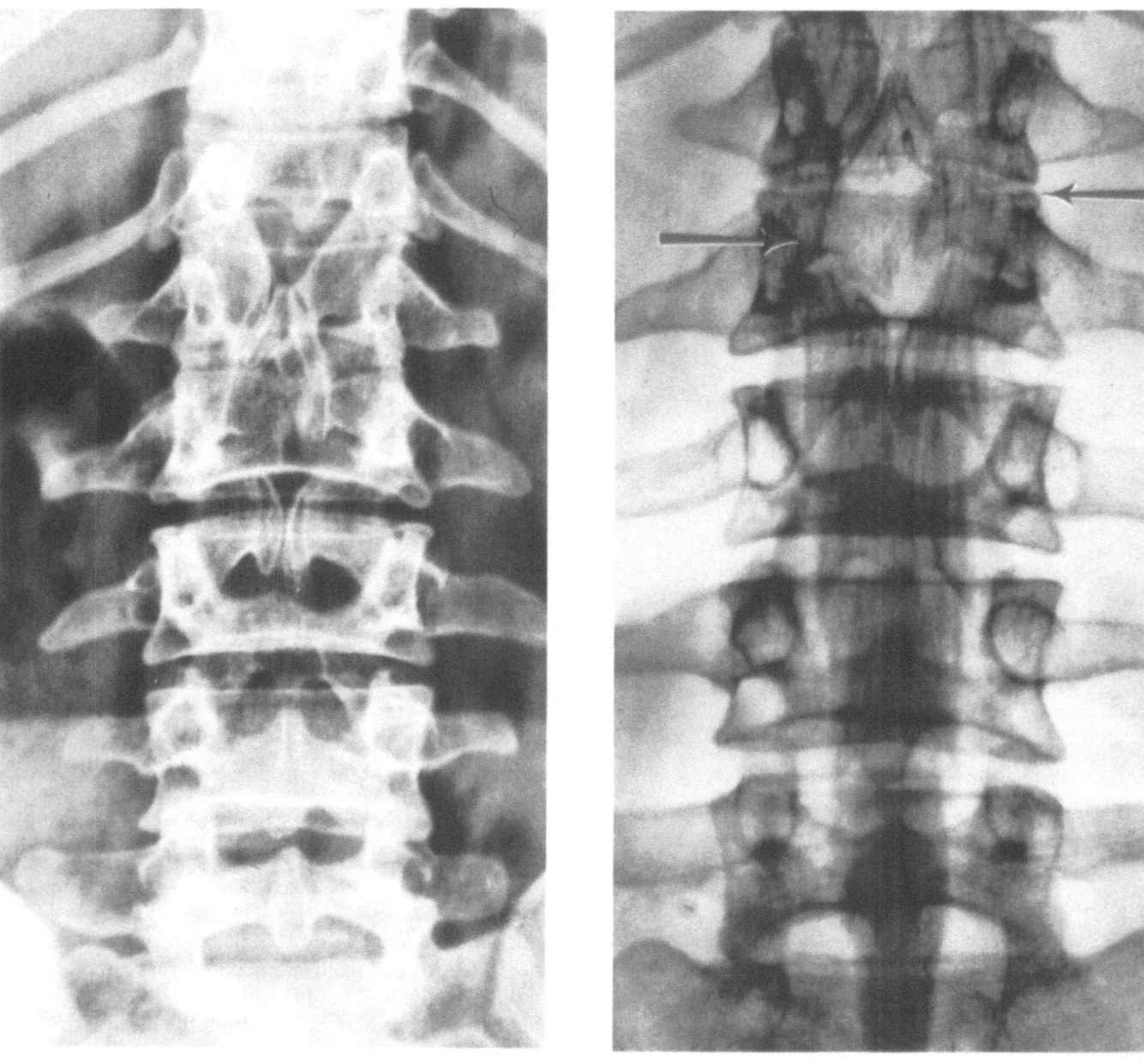

Fig. 79. Osseus modifications in L1-L3 in the form of spinal bifida. Myelography revealed a roundish-shaped filling defect in L2 (*arrow*). The bone spicula in L1-L2 derives from the posterior wall of the vertebral body of L2

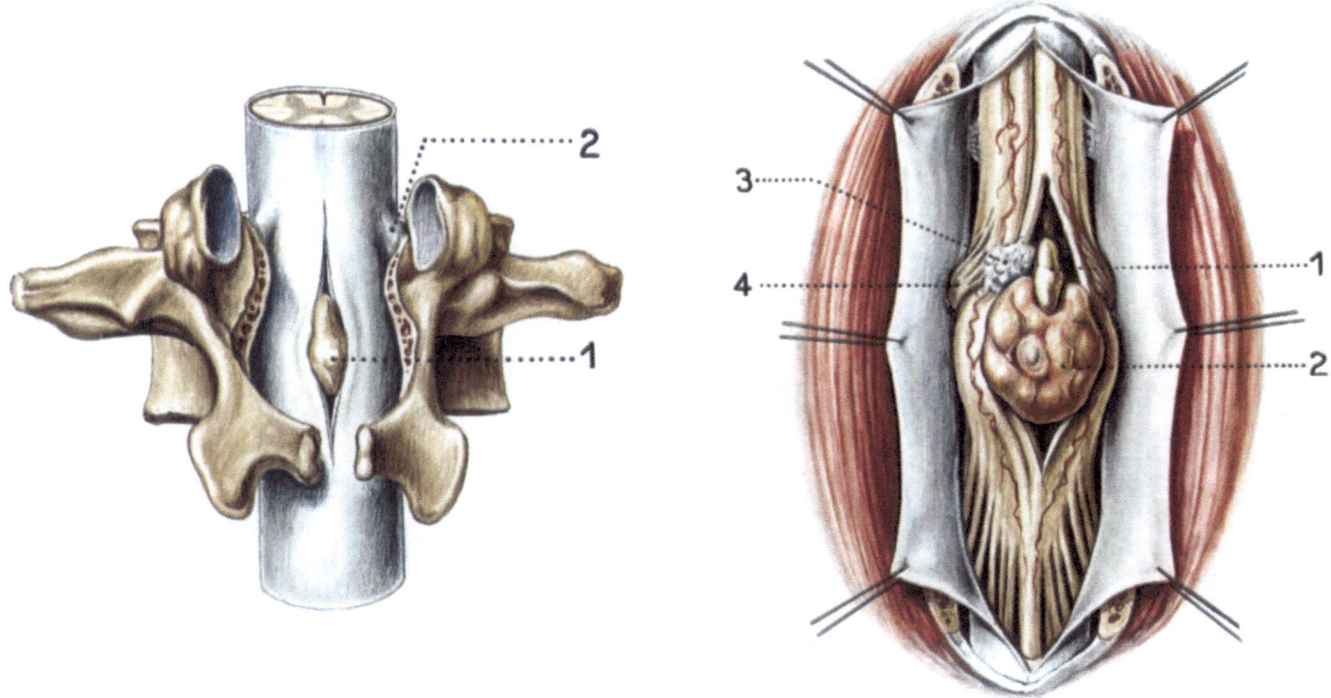

Fig. 80. *1, Left,* schematic diagram of the operative finding. The meningeal sac is divided into two, surrounding the medial bony protrusion invading the posterior border of the vertebral body; *right,* a reconstruction of the operating field after the opening of the dural sac. *2,* Neoplasm inserted on the protrusion. *3,* Collection of colesterin near the XII left dorsal root. *4* Immediately above the terminal cone a dichotomic division of the two medullary columns which reunite near the lower tract of the tumour

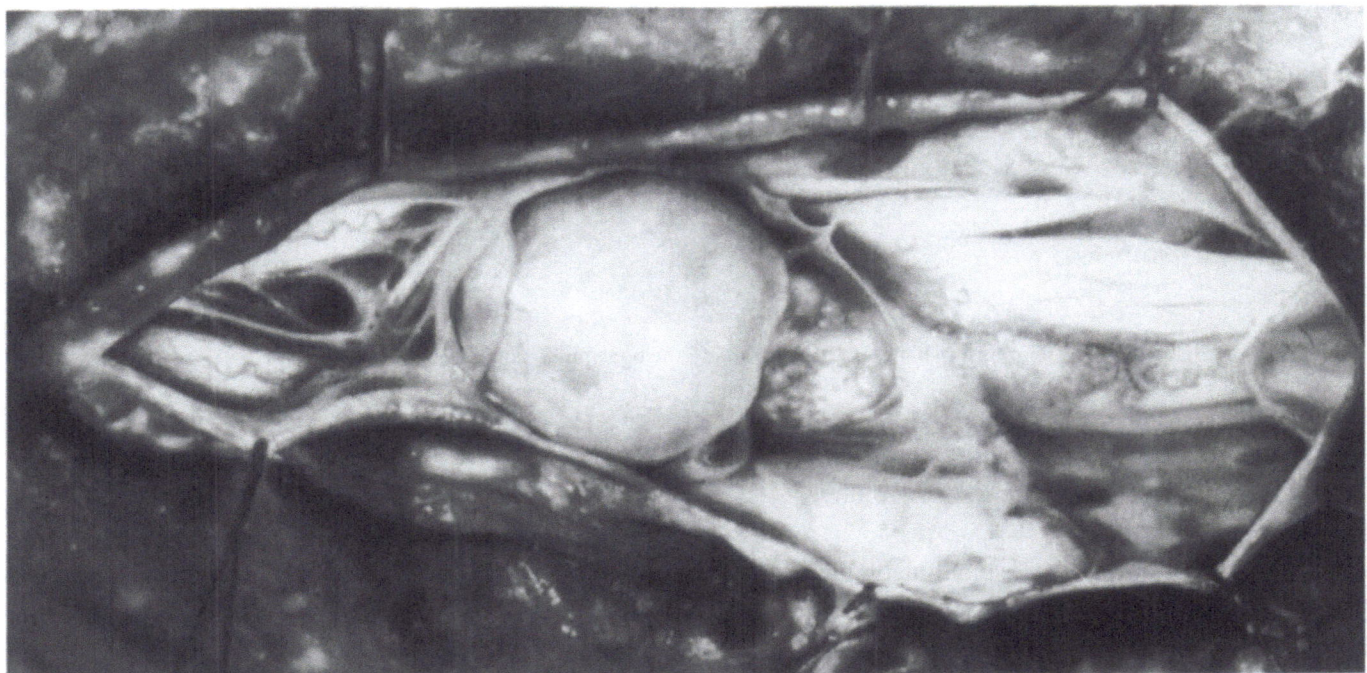

Fig. 81. Photograph of the operative field. On opening the arachnoid, the neoplasm is surrounded by an arachnoidal process against the medullary cone. On the left the two malformed myelic columns are seen

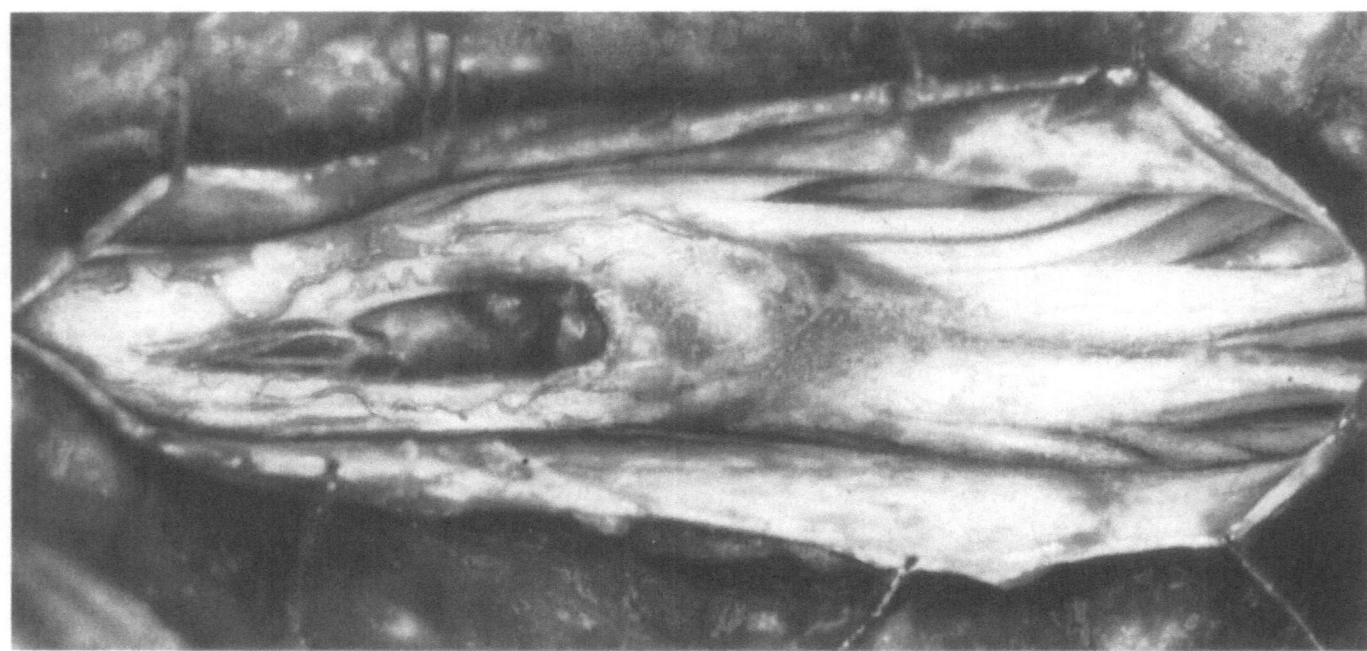

Fig. 82. The division of the medullary columns deep in the terminal cone is clearer. From here the caudal roots appear to separate

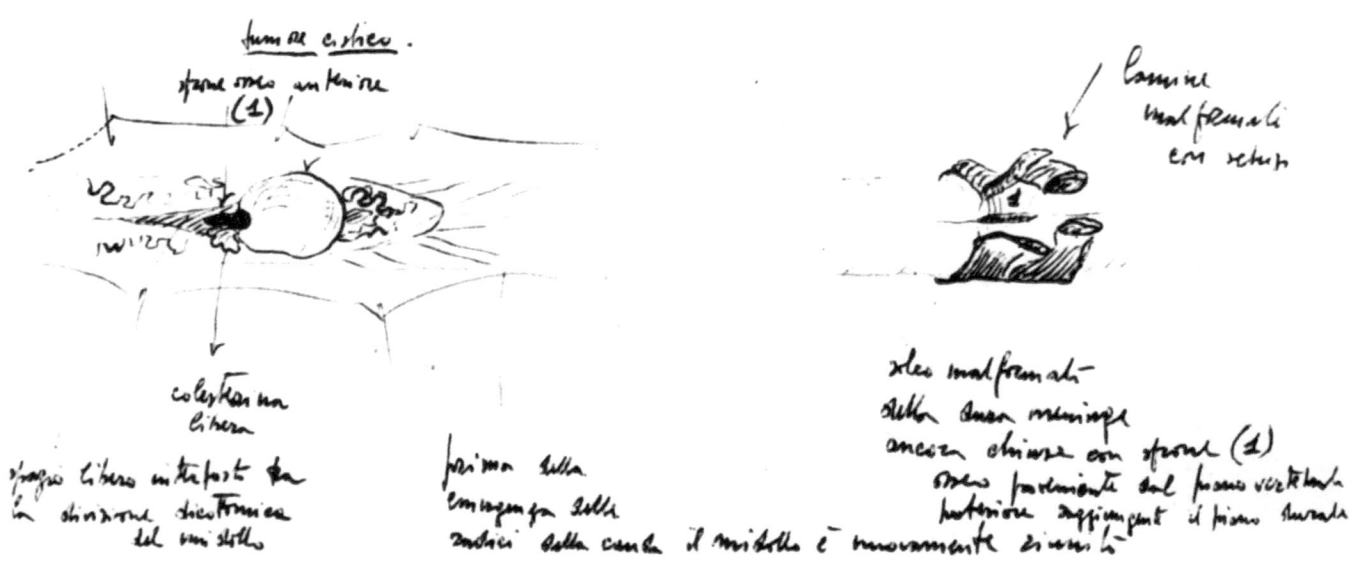

Fig. 83. The diagrams show the relationship between the tumour and the bone malformation

6.15   Conclusions

In 15.73% of our cases of spinal meningioma back pain appears before the initial sensory irritative radicular symptoms. The radicular syndrome can be of a similar nature to other extra- and intradural compressive forms. Usually paraesthesias and dysaethesia signs appear among the symptoms at the same time or before motor and sen-

sory cord disturbances. The course of the syndrome is generally very slow. The time from the appearance of symptoms to diagnosis can vary from a few months to 1-2 years. Paraplegia is the result of vascular disturbance of an ischaemic type. The forms of hemisection of the cord of a Brown-Sequard type are very rare (2.4%). Cases presenting with a clinical onset of motor radicular disturbances showed an incidence of 19.67%. Meningioma cases with cauda symptoms are exceptionally rare (four cases).

Meningiomas are not always accompanied by a cytological-albumen dissociation (92.5%). Sphincter disturbances in meningioma cases appear later than other oncotypes, initially in the form of retention and then of incontinence, often when cord disturbances are already manifest. The symptomatic picture of neurofibromatosis associated with isolated or multiple meningiomas is polymorphic and depends on the encephalus-medullary location. In some cases medullary signs are earlier than those caused by asymptomatic encephalic locations. The Bernard-Horner syndrome recalls the first dorsal myelomere location; however, Cushing (1917) reported one case, and we observed a similar one, in a meningioma in C4. Cases of motor deficit with hemiparetic pattern and acute forms of paraplegia are rare.

For the cases in our series we distinguished three locations of meningiomas in the dorsal tract (excluding cases of neurofibromatosis and double location) and found the following:

- D1-D3: 31 cases; mean duration of symptoms 6 years
- D4-D8: 40 cases; mean duration of symptoms 5.5 years
- D9-D12: 24 cases; mean duration of symptoms 7.9 years

The corresponding evaluation for meningiomas in two locations on the cervical tract (excluding cases of intramedullary tumours and von Recklinghausen's disease) showed:

- C1-C4: 10 cases; mean duration of symptoms 5.1 years
- C5-C8: 7 cases; mean duration of symptoms 9.5 years

These data confirm the findings of Lazorthes and Zulch's reduced arterial vascularization during the peak development phase of the tumour at medial dorsal level in comparison to that present at cervical or lumbosacral level.

7 Neurophysiopathology

G. De Luca

Until the 1960s the neurophysiopathological diagnosis of myeloradicular compressions relied upon electromyography (EMG) and neurography, while neuroelectric examination had been practically abandoned in clinical practice. The possiblity of easily distinguishing muscle diseases from neuropathologies, including peripheral forms from spinal lesions, had largely favoured its use. Nevertheless, the use of EMG for diagnosis of spinal cord neoplasms allowed a valuable functional evaluation of myeloradicular structures only at the level of cervical and lumbar enlargements. The computer revolution over the past 30 years has brought the development of biomedical electronic engineering and improved neurophysiopathological procedures of greater reliability and extent of application.

7.1 Evoked Potentials

The use of evoked potentials (EPs) is based on the fact that various sensitive stimuli, functionally correlated to the afferent pathways and to the specific cortical areas administered to receptors or along nerves, cause an orthodromic diffused action potential that can be registered by electrodes placed on ideal areas of derivation. It is possible to obtain visual (VEP), acoustic (AEP-BAEP) and somatosensory (SEP) EPs. Similarily, regarding motor evoked potentials (MEPs), the electric or magnetic stimulation of the cortical motor areas, the pyramidal pathways or the myeloradicular motor structures cause specific, easily recorded, regional muscle responses (Caton 1875; Beck 1890; Danilevsky 1891; Larionov 1897; Berger 1929; Gasser 1933; Davis 1939; Dawson 1947; Eccles 1951; Bremer 1958; Chang 1959; Bergamini and Bergamasco 1967; Gastaut et al. 1967; Remond 1973-75; Desmet 1980; Vaughan 1975; Lehmann and Callawaye 1978; Aminoff 1979; Low 1979, 1980; Barber 1980; Bodis-Wollner 1982; Courjon et al. 1982; Mauguiere and Fischer 1982; Greenberg and Ducker 1982; Chiappa 1988; Young et al. 1985; Cracco and Cracco 1976; Owen 1990). Other similar signals are called "slow" EPs because they have a longer latency; these are also known as "event-related" slow potentials (ERSP) and are of a principally psycho-physiological interest (Kornhuber and Deecke 1964; Walter 1964; Sutton et al. 1965; Zappoli et al. 1970).

EPs with an amplitude of few microvolts, as registered by surface derivations, are related to all other electric potentials but not to specific stimulation, known as noise (e.g. bioelectric muscle activity, spontaneous neuronal activity, artefacts, environmental electromagnetic fields) that presents with an equal or often higher voltage and can be identified by technical procedures such as spectral filtering and statistical suppression or "averaging" (Damson 1954). Signals are filtered during the acquisition phase to limit the analysis to those potentials having frequencies compatible to those required; a further "clearing" of the recordings may be obtained using digital filters during the post-elaboration phase. Averaging is a procedure in which a computer for each derivation calculates the average point by point of each registered potential amplitude following each stimulus over a period of previously arranged analysis during which the studied bioelectric phenomena appears. The EPs with a constant latancy in relation to the stimulus, while each average index increases, become progressively more evident than occasional potentials with decreased amplitude.

7.2 Somatosensory and Motor Evoked Potentials

The first description of spinal cord SEPs were obtained in experimental feline models by stimulation of sensory nerve roots (Gasser 1933). This procedure was first used in

A. Pansini et al.
Spinal Meningiomas
© Springer-Verlag Italia 1996

humans nearly 20 years after Gasser's observation (Magladery 1951) with epidural needle electrodes (Shimoji 1971; Tsuyama 1978) or subdural needles (Ertekin 1976; Caccia 1976). The current choice of surface SEPs recording is due to the fact that this procedure avoids the most common complications caused by deep derivations without substantially changing the quality of the evoked responses (Liberson 1963; Cracco 1973; Delbeke 1978; Dimitrijevic 1978; Ertekin 1978; Jones 1978; Feldman 1980). SEPs and MEPs represent the neurophysiopathological procedures of choice in all forms of myeloradicular diseases, in particular for compressive pathologies (Giblin 1964; Bergamini et al. 1966; Desmet 1980; Croft et al. 1972; D'Angel 1973; Bricolo et al. 1975; Vaughan 1975; Cracco and Cracco 1976; Hume and Cant 1978; Eisen and Nudleman 1979; Mauguiere et al. 1981; Rossini 1988; Abbruzzese et al. 1988; Chiappa 1988; Vanasse et al. 1988; Kakigi 1988; Crespi et al. 1988; Zentner and Ebner 1988; Ingram et al. 1988; Claus et al. 1988; Ugawa et al. 1988; Lance et al. 1988; Caramia et al. 1989; Macdonell et al. 1989).

Various experimental studies have focused on the type, location and nature of myeloradicular compressions and their haemodynamic effects (stasis, ischaemia) along with variation in SEPs and MEPs (Gelfan and Tarlov 1956; Allen et al. 1975; Cracco 1978; Ducker et al. 1978; Kobrine et al. 1978, 1979; Schramm et al. 1979; Bennet 1983; Cheng et al. 1984; Aki and Toya 1994; Salzman 1986; Nainzadeh and Lane 1987; Machida et al. 1988; Owen et al. 1988, 1989, 1990; Khan et al. 1989; Delamarter 1990; Ghaly 1990; Hitchon et al. 1990; Kai et al. 1990, 1994; Zornow 1990; Ueta et al. 1992). Other research has examined the effects of various drugs, in particular anaesthetics, on SEPs and MEPs (Meinck et al. 1980; McPherson 1985; Gravenstein 1984; Mirimanoff et al. 1985; Sloan and Koth 1985, 1988; Scheepstra et al. 1989; Conrad 1989; Zentner et al. 1989; Keller et al. 1992).

7.3 Intraoperative Neurophysiological Monitoring

Intraoperative monitoring of physiological parameters was first proposed by Cushing (Beecher 1940), but its importance was doubted for many years (Bendixen 1978). Although many of the difficulties with cardiocirculatory parameters that Cushing encountered have now been largely solved, problems persist regarding intraoperative neurophysiological monitoring (EEG and EPs procedures). These are due both to the high cost of equipment and to the lack of qualified technicians able to resolve the frequent problems of recording that arise in the operating room and to correctly understand the results obtained. Nevertheless these procedures allow verification of the functional status of various neuronal systems in the patients affected by coma or under the effect of anaes-

thetics, they are applied as routine only in a few centres, but their use is in fact increasing. This is due to the insurance and legal implications for the surgeon in the event that the absence of neurophysiological monitoring leads to intraoperative neurological complications.

The various EPs are of great value in surgery, particularly neurosurgery. VEPs have been studied during surgery in the optic chiasma and in the temporal and occipital regions, the acoustic and trigeminal responses for temporal, cerebellar, brain stem and cranial nerve pathologies and the SEPs and MEPs for the surgical treatment of epilepsy, vascular, traumatic and neoplastic pathologies and for myeloradicular compressions (Grundy 1988).

Intraoperative SEPs and MEPs monitoring have found wide application in the field of vertebral pathologies, particularly in the treatment of degenerative and traumatic lesions and malformations (kyphoscoliosis) (Domino et al. 1964; Humphrey 1968; Bricolo et al. 1975; Scarff 1979; Lueders 1982; Macon 1982; La Mont 1983; Brown 1984; De Luca 1984, 1991; Milano 1984; Whittle 1984; Keim 1985; Machida 1985; Nashold 1985; Dinner 1986; Herron 1987; Pansini et al. 1987, 1988, 1989, 1990; Heiskari et al. 1988; Jones 1988; More 1988; Whittle 1988; Keith 1990; Cheliout-Heraut 1991; Cioni 1991; Hicks 1991; Jeanmonod 1991; Pelosi 1991; Thompson 1991; Ashkenaze 1993; Epstein 1993; Erwin 1993; Herdmann 1993; Hormes 1993; Owen 1993; Robinson 1993; Tabaraud 1993; Toleikis 1993; Wagner 1993; Kalkman 1994; O'Brien 1994). There are few data in the literature regarding the application of intraoperative monitoring of SEPs and MEPs in myeloradicular compressions (Koht 1985; Mauguiere 1985; Levy et al. 1986; Pansini 1987, 1990, 1991; Landi 1988; Shields 1988; Watanabe 1988; Zentner et al. 1989; Fromme 1990; Morioka 1990; De Luca 1991; Jellinek 1991; Lumenta 1991; Kearse 1993), or regarding meningiomas in particular (Rossini 1988; Long 1987), but various authors agree upon its importance.

The rare occurrence of false-positive or false-negative results (Ginsberg 1985; Kaplan 1986; Lesser 1986; Molaie 1986; Salzman 1986; Chatrian 1988) are often explained by technical or interpretation errors, as reported in reviews of the literature (Friedman 1987; Grundy 1988), thus confirming the efficiency, sensibility and specificity of this procedure.

7.4 Materials, Methods, Case Reports

Since 1988 we have used the Biopotential Analyzer Software Interactive System for Evoked Potentials and Myelography (BASIS EPM) manufactured by ESA-OTE Biomedica (Italy) to perform EMG and SEPs/MEPs monitoring. This equipment has four preamplified floating derivation channels, eight traces of 1024 points, each sampled at velocity of 2 μs per point, videographic memory with a capacity of 131.072 points, on-line fast-averager with a memory of 4096 points for 20 bits, 12-in. oscilloscope screen, two floppy-disk drives, electric, acoustic, visual (flash and pattern) stimulators and a triggered magnetic stimulator, completely managed and controlled via software, thermic printer and x-y plotter.

In agreement with the standards of the Italian Society of Clinical Neurophysiology (Rossini 1988), we use the following parameters for SEPs recording: (a) Upper limbs: time base 50 ms [5 ms/div (1 div=1 cm)], sensibility 5 μV/div (magnified 64 times in postelaboration phase), bandwidth 20-5000 Hz. Stimulation: 200-1000 stimulations over motor threshold of median nerve at wrist level, stimulus frequency 3 Hz, duration 0.1 ms. Derivations: elbow, Erb's point, C6 and primary somatosensory cortex [C3'-C4' (10/20 International System)] with frontal reference (Fpz'); (b) Lower limbs: time base 100 ms (10 ms/div), sensitivity and filters as above. Stimulation: 500-1000 stimulations of the sural or superficial peroneal nerves at ankle level, stimulus frequency and duration equal to those of the median nerve. Derivations: popliteal fossa, LV, C6 and primary somatosensory cortex (Cz') with frontal reference.

Depending on the clinical and neurological findings, stimulation and sources vary in individual patients (ulnar or radial nerves, brachial plexus at axilla or Erb's point, peroneal, sciatic and femoral nerves stimulation; derivations at different levels of the spinal cord: electrospinogram). Intraoperative SEPs monitoring allows, when possible, a direct derivation from the sensory nerve roots or from the posterior spinal cords, in addition to those located centrally and peripherally (Fig. 84). Nevertheless the recording of myeloradicular EPs is of greatest value during surgery, the simultaneous recording of the peripheral responses which assures the orthodromic activation of the sensory fibres, and cerebral responses which guarantees the arrival at this point of somatosensory afferent discharge, is also very important.

Our experience with MEPs is limited to the intraoperative electric stimulation of motor nerve roots and the registration of the muscle responses derived from the relative muscle regions by means of coaxial needle electrodes (Fig. 84). Faradic transcutaneous stimulation of the cortical motor area (Cracco 1986; Rossini 1988) has not proved easy to apply in the clinical study of alert patients because of the disturbing sensations which these stimulations produce. When the appropriate equipment is available we will complete the neurophysiological assay with MEPs by transcranial magnetic stimulation.

We have used SEPs or MEPs in spinal meningiomas in ten women and one man with an average age of 58 years (range, 28-82 years). These cases included three cervical meningiomas, seven dorsal (a double location in the same patient), one lumbar and one neurofibromatosis

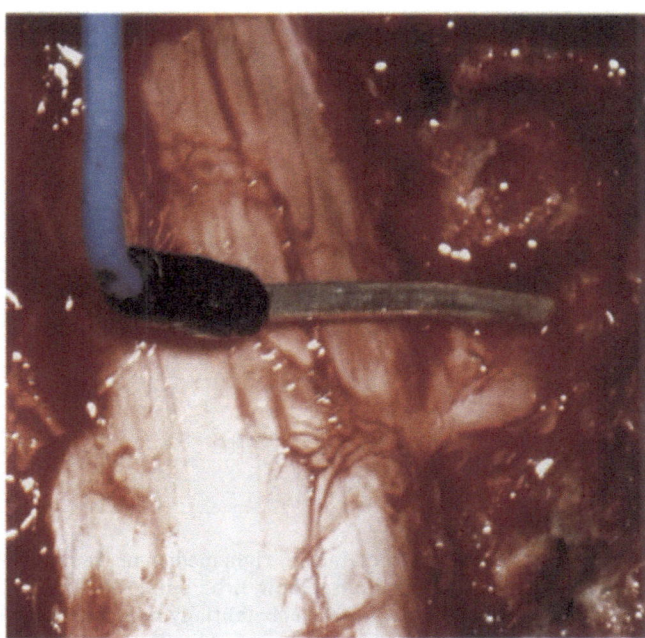

Fig. 84. Photo of operating field taken by surgical microscope showing the silver registration/stimulus electrode placed at radicular foramen level.

with meningiomas located within the brain, at cervical and dorsal levels and multiple neurinomas. Seven patients underwent preoperative SEPs, four had intraoperative monitoring, and nine were submitted to postoperative control. Only one patient underwent intraoperative MEPs, obtained by radicular stimulation. Although our case reports are poorly represented, we have tried to quantify neurological deficits and pre- and postoperative SEPs by means of an average 1-year follow-up to evaluate the correlation between clinical and neurophysiological signs.

Motor deficits were classified according to Levy's scale; SEPs were subdivided into five groups, with an increasing degree of severity and given a score from 0-4: 0, normal; 1, slow conduction; 2, amplitude decrease; 3, slow conduction and decreased amplitude; 4, block in conduction (in categories 2 and 3 the following are considered as pathological: latency increase of more than 3 standard deviations and amplitude decrease of more than 50% of the average or healthy). We then evaluated the presence or loss of the sensory, radicular and cord deficits, besides sphincter disturbances.

Case No. 94:
A 73-year-old woman (1988). Right, ventrolateral meningioma in C4-C5. Tetraparesis, more severe on the right with a distal upper limb paresis and a clear sublesional hypoaesthesia on the other side. Progressive motor improvement on both upper and lower limbs after surgery. Two months later, walking without support and residual flexion deficit of the fingers on the right hand. Preoperative SEPs presented a block in conduction at cervical level, well in terms of the severity of the clinical pattern (Figs. 85, 86).

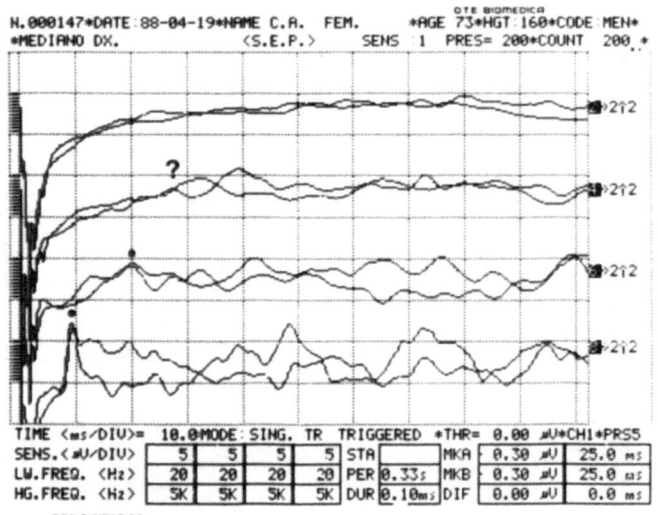

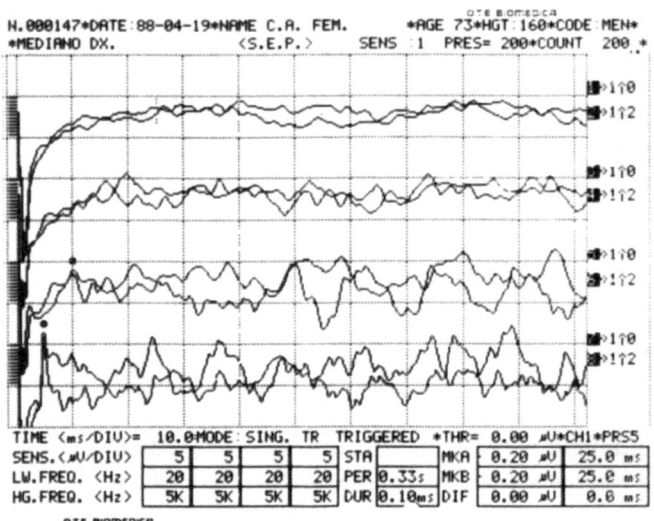

Fig. 85. Preoperative SEPs obtained by right median nerve stimulation at wrist level. Derivations: elbow, Erb's point, C6, C3'/Fpz'. Peripheral evoked responses are substantially normal. Central responses are absent at cervical and cortical levels.

Fig. 86. Analysis of the first 100 ms following the stimulus. A block in conduction at cervical level is confirmed.

Case No. 46:

A 36-year-old woman (1990). Posterior meningioma in T2-T3. Severe spastic-ataxic paraparesis with walking allowed for only small steps, necessarily using bilateral crutches; bilateral hypoaesthesia from T4 and cord dysaesthesias in the lower limbs. The patient showed progressive improvement in the clinical pattern following surgery until recovery which followed 1 year later. Preoperative SEPs, technically incomplete because the patient refused to cooperate (schizophrenia), showed a clear partial block in conduction at medullary level (Fig. 87).

Case No. 28:

A 68-year-old woman (1985). Right ventrolateral meningioma in C1-C2. Before surgery she reported tetraplegia with sphincter disturbances regarded as retention and neurological deficiences within 8 months. Postoperative SEPs confirmed clinical recovery and were normal after 9 years (Figs. 88, 89).

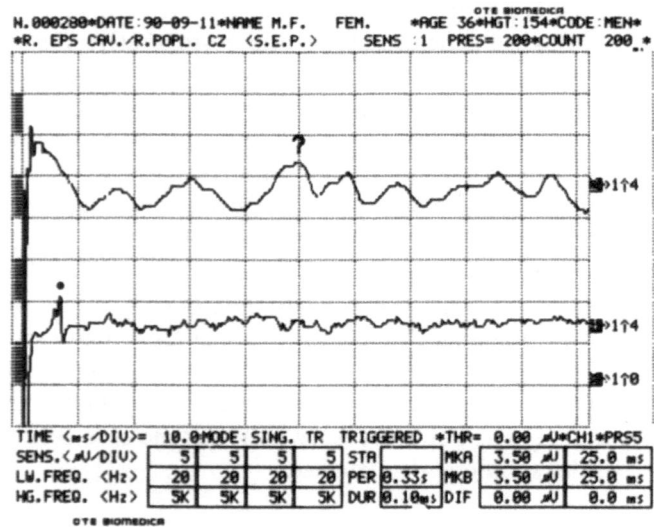

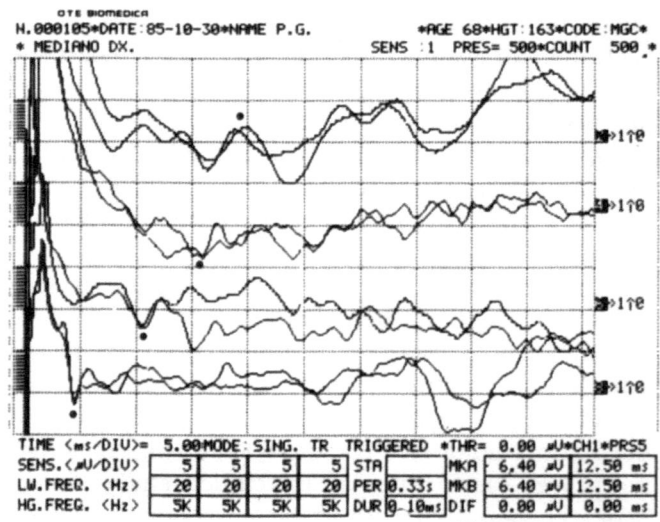

Fig. 87. Preoperative SEPs obtained by superficial peroneal nerve stimulation at the right ankle level and popliteal and vertex derivations. Only the relative responses were registered at a series of 200 stimulations because the patient was very agitated due to her severe psychological disease. The evoked popliteal response is clear, having a normal latency and morphology. The cortical response is dubious due to the impossibility to the overlap of other traces, showing a very low amplitude and increased latency (particularly if correlated with the patient's height, 154 cm).

Fig. 88. Postoperative SEPs (8 months) obtained by stimulation of the right median nerve at wrist level. Derivations: elbow, Erb's point, C6, C3'/Fpz'. The evoked responses are substantially normal, confirming the resettlement of a valid conduction of somatosensory stimuli, both peripherally and centrally (N20 = 20 ms).

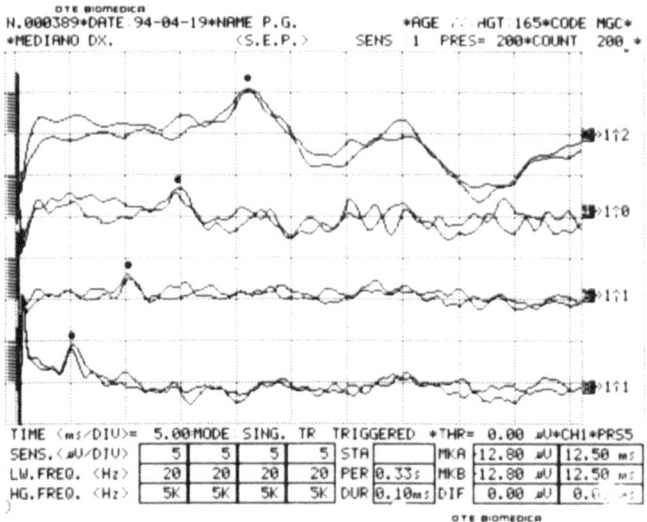

N.000389*DATE 94-04-19*NAME P.G.   *AGE .. HGT 165*CODE MGC*
*MEDIANO DX.   <S.E.P.>   SENS 1 PRES= 200*COUNT 200 .*

Fig. 89. Control SEPs remain normal after 9 years (patient's age 77 years)

Case No. 68:

A 82-year-old woman (1988). Right ventrolateral meningioma in C2. Severe spastic tetraparesis predominantly on the right with walking allowed only by means of crutches; hyperaesthesia band in C2 and hypoaesthesia below this level. Immediate recovery from motor deficiencies resulting from surgery. SEPs performed on 14th postoperative day proved substantially normal (Fig. 90).

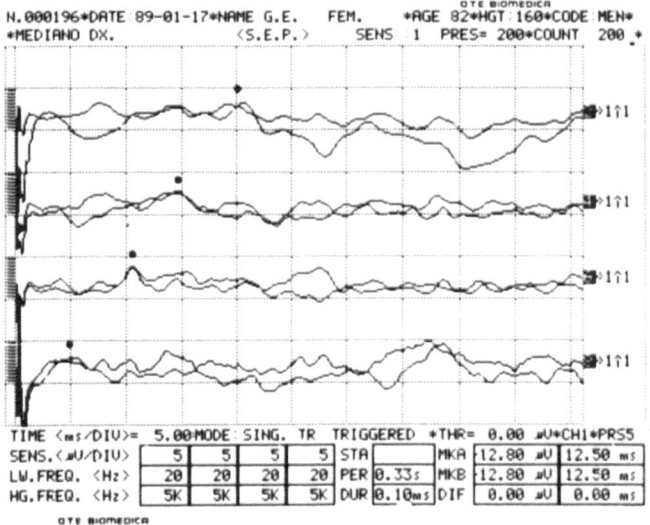

N.000196*DATE 89-01-17*NAME G.E.   FEM.   *AGE 82*HGT 160*CODE MEN*
*MEDIANO DX.   <S.E.P.>   SENS 1 PRES= 200*COUNT 200 .*

Fig. 90. Postoperative SEPs by stimulation of right median nerve at the wrist level. Derivations: elbow, Erb's point, C6, C3'/Fpz'. Evoked responses are clearly seen on every derivation site. Cortical N20 demonstrates a slightly irregular morphology with normal latency (20 ms); nevertheless a nearly 1- ms delay occurred in peripheral conduction.

Case No. 85:

A 72-year-old woman (1993). Left posterolateral meningioma at T-4. The patient presented with spastic paraparesis and required crutches for walking; the level of hypoaesthesia was from T4 on both sides with prevalently right paraesthesias and sphincter disturbances. A nearly complete clinical recovery 1 month following surgery, with a residual subjective hyposthenia at the right lower limb. Postoperative SEPs performed 16 months after surgery were nearly normal, with a slight increase in latency of central responses at upper lesion level (Fig. 91).

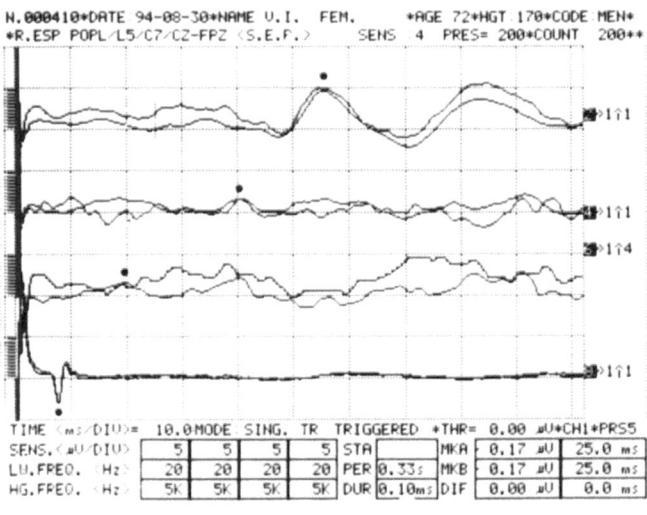

N.000410*DATE 94-08-30*NAME V.I.   FEM.   *AGE 72*HGT 170*CODE MEN*
*R.ESP POPL/L5/C7/CZ-FPZ <S.E.F.>   SENS 4 PRES= 200*COUNT 200**

Fig. 91. Postoperative SEPs obtained by stimulation of superficial peroneal nerve on the right ankle level. Derivations: popliteal fossa, L5, C4, Cz'/Fpz'. Evoked responses are clear and well superimposed on all derivation sites. The popliteal and lumbar evoked responses are perfectly normal. The cervical and cortical responses show slightly increasing latency, with normal morphology and amplitude.

Case No. 62:

A 62-year-old woman (1982). Ventral meningioma in L1. Lumbar crural pain and sciatica on both sides. Spastic paraparesis with sphincter disturbances. Clinical recovery took only 3 months with slight residual dysaesthesia on lower limbs. The results of postoperative electrospinogram and EMG performed 17 months after surgery were normal (Figs. 92, 93).

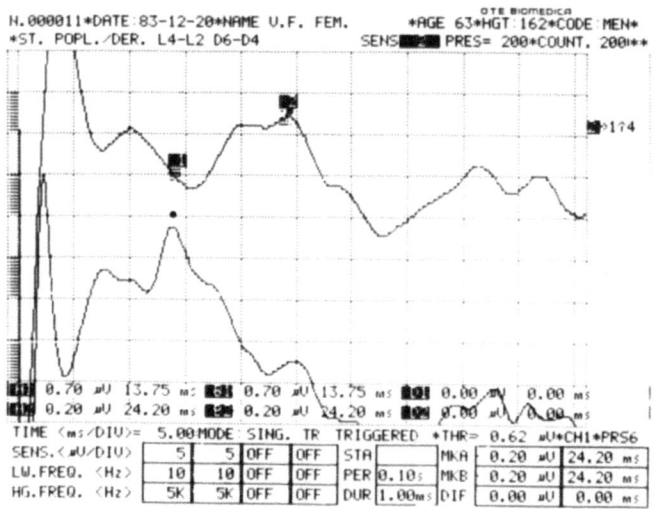

Fig. 92. Electrospinogram obtained by stimulation of left sciatic nerve in the popiteal fossa. Derivation below and above the lesion (L4-T4). The evoked responses show normal amplitude, morphology and latency.

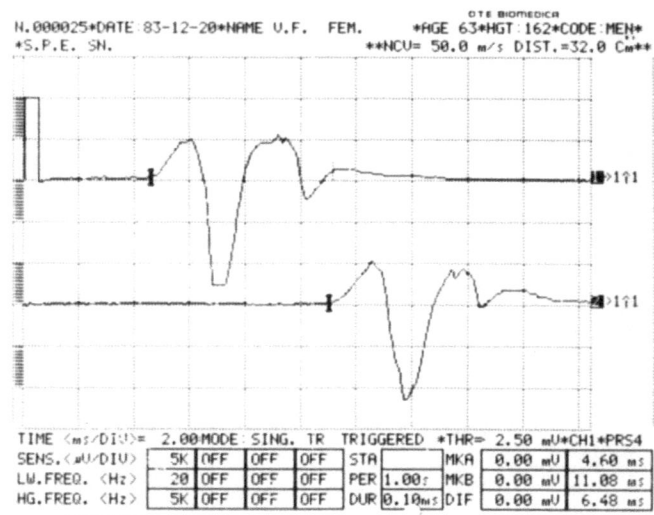

Fig. 93. EMG obtained by means of a needle electrode placed into the left anterior tibial muscle. Muscle responses, obtained by stimulation of popliteal fossa and at the distal level, show normal regarding latency, morphology and amplitude, with well-conserved motor conduction velocity (50 m/s).

Case No. 83:

A 48-year-old woman (1992). Left posterolateral meningioma in T9-10 and another meningioma ventrally on the right in T11. She presented spastic-ataxic paraparesis with sphincter disturbances; dorsolumbar spinal pain which spread to the inguinal region and level of hypoaesthesia in D10, predominantly on the right. A progressive improvement in this clinical pattern was observed after surgery, with complete regression of sensitive and motor deficits within 45 days. Preoperative SEPs showed no EPs at the lesional level and increased latency of the cortical responses (Fig. 94). A check performed 27 months after surgery with the patient asymptomatic showed a significant decrease in this former latency period (Fig. 95).

Case No. 75:

A 53-year-old woman (1994). Right posterolateral meningioma in T4. She presented back pain and cord anaesthesias and dysaesthesias in the perineal region and along the internal surface of the lower limb for 10 years. Three years previously she presented a left sciatic pain syndrome. For 6 months the patient had hyposthenia on the left lower limb, pain, paraesthesias and hypoaesthesia in the lower limbs and perineal region, sphincter dysfunction such as urinary incontinence, and left quadriceps femoral muscle hypotrophy. The patient could walk without crutches but this was very difficult when using her toes. Fifteen days after surgery the patient could walk with aid, both on her toes and heels, with slight ataxic disturbanc-

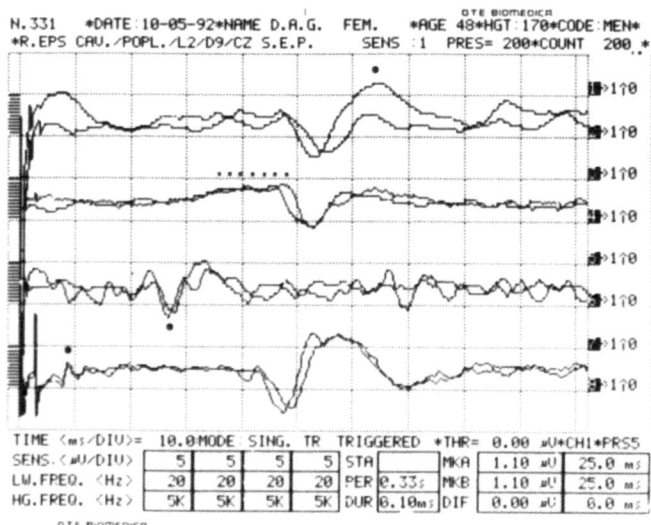

Fig. 94. Preoperative SEPs obtained by right superficial peroneal nerve stimulation at ankle level. Derivations: popliteal fossa, L2, T9, Cz'/Fpz'. Evoked responses are evident and clear at the popliteal and lumbar levels, having normal latency. A wide negative wave is, instead, observed at dorsal level. Cortical response has clearly increased latency: 64-65 ms.

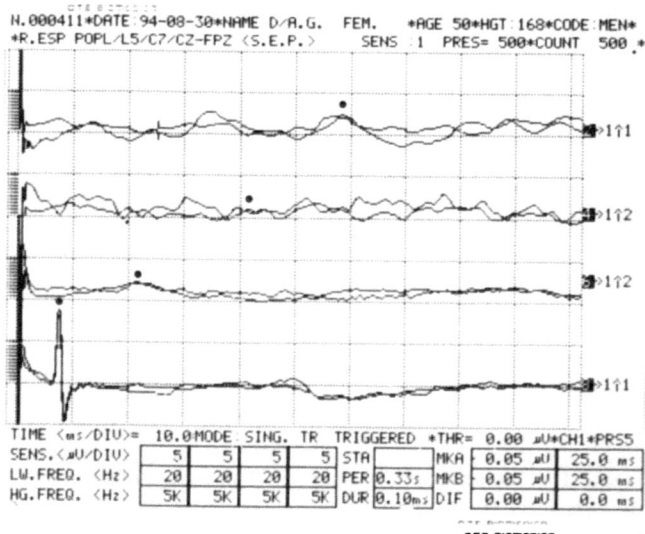

Fig. 95. Postoperative SEPs performed with the same stimulation procedures as for the preoperative. Derivations: popliteal fossa, L5, C7, Cz'/Fpz'. Evoked responses are normal at popliteal and lumbar levels. Cervical response shows a low voltage and mildly increased latency. The cortical response shows a latency of 56-58 ms, with a 7- to 8-ms reduction compared to the preoperative value.

es. Sensation was improved in the lower limbs, with slight deficit at distal level.

Preoperative SEPs showed a normal response at popliteal level, a clear absence of EPs at lumbar and cervical levels and a slowed conduction with an increased latency of cortical response: 53 ms (Fig. 96). Intraoperative SEPs showed a mild decrease in latency of the cervical and cortical responses following tumour removal (Fig. 97). A postoperative SEPs confirmed normalization of SEPs (Fig. 98).

Case No. 37:

A 64-year-old woman (1991). Left posterolateral meningioma in T11. For 10 years she had complained of pain frequently arising at the medial dorsal level which extended on both sides but more severe on the right, while on the left she felt warm paraesthesias. For 6 months this diffuse pain had extended to the entire lower right limb and towards the anterior surface of the left leg, accompanied by predominantly right spastic paraparesis, which required first an

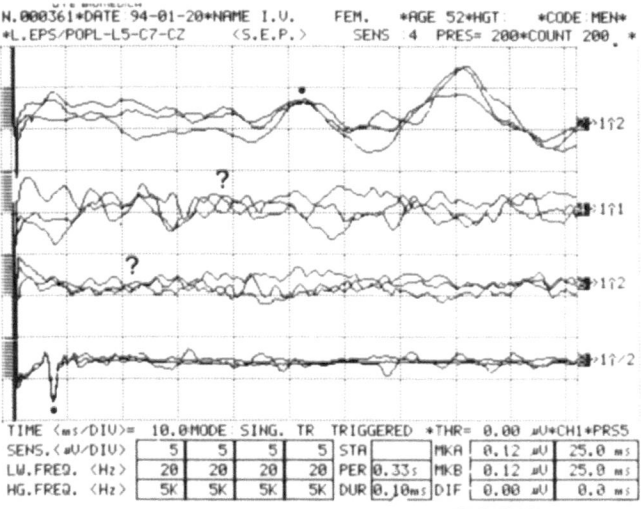

Fig. 96. Preoperative SEPs obtained by left superficial peroneal nerve stimulation at ankle level. Derivations: popiteal fossa, L5, C7, Cz'/Fpz'. Clear evoked response at popliteal level with normal latency, morphology and amplitude. Lumbar and cervical evoked response are not recognizable. Clear cortical evoked response with a slight increased latency: 53 ms.

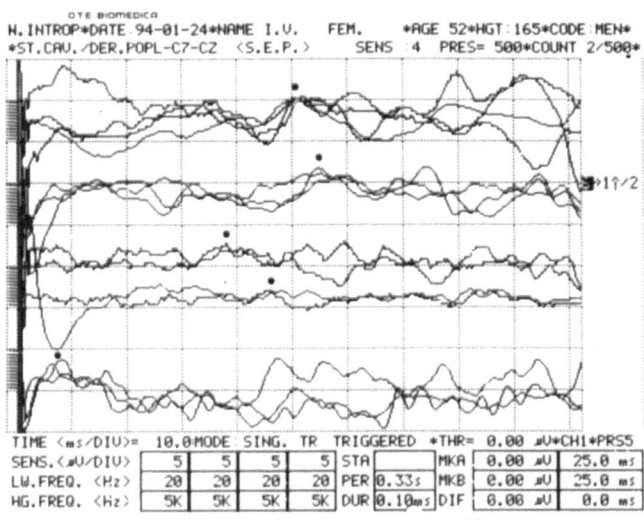

Fig. 97. Intraoperative SEPs obtained by left superficial peroneal nerve stimulation at ankle level. Derivations: popliteal fossa, C7, Cz'/Fpz'. *Lowest traces*, popliteal derivation at the fibula head level showing evoked responses with normal latency although presenting a low amplitude and irregular morphology. These abnormalities are frequently observed during intraoperative recordings, most probably due to the patient's position on the operating table. Surgery is performed with patient lying on one side with flexion of the lower limb towards the hip. *Two middle traces*, cervical derivation: *below* before, *above* after the dorsal meningioma was removed. There is a clear postoperative reduction of latency: 46 ms before tumour removal, 38 ms at the end of surgery. *Two upper traces*, cortical evoked response before and after surgery. A reduction in the cortical latency is also visible: 54-59 ms before and 50-51 ms after the removal of the meningioma.

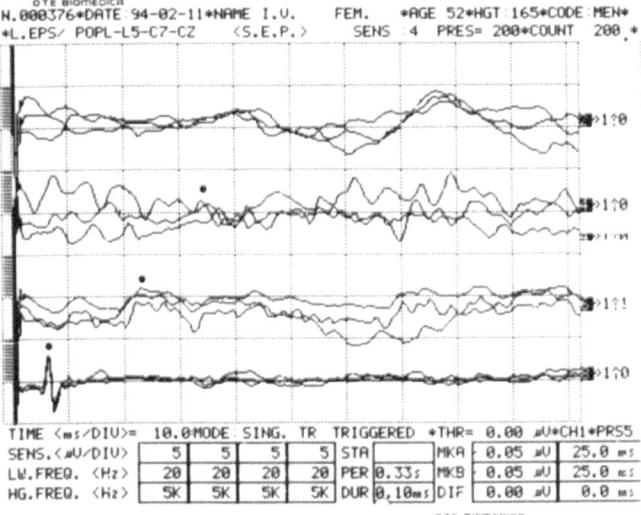

Fig. 98. Postoperative SEPs obtained 18 days after surgery. Same stimulation and derivation parameters as preoperative SEPs. Clear evoked responses at popliteal and lumbar levels with normal latency, morphology and amplitude. Cervical responses are clear and show a further decrease in latency in relation to intraoperative values: 40-43 ms.

aid on the right and then on both sides for walking. She complained of sphincter disturbances for 2 months, appearing first as incontinence then as severe retention which required a permanent catheter placement. Severe motor disturbances appeared for 20 days followed by almost complete plegia of right lower limb and severe paresis on the left, where only residual movements against gravity were seen. Complete motor inhibition of lower limbs and bilateral T10-T11 anaesthesia was reported after surgery, but a rapid and progressive regression of motor and sensory disturbances occurred. The patient was able to walk using crutches after less than 1 month; 4 months later she was able to walk without support, although she was slightly lame in the right leg. She recovered good sphincter control after 2 years; slight motor and sensory deficits were still present on the lower right limb.

Preoperative SEPs showed an almost complete conduction block at the lesional level (Fig. 99). The intraoperative SEPs revealed a recovery and improvement in conduction (Figs. 100, 101), and postoperative SEPs taken 2 years later were normal (Fig. 102). This picture corresponds exactly to the patient's improvement status. However, we consider this a particularly interesting case for another reason: intraoperative SEPs monitoring was not able to predict the motor and sensory inhibition observed after surgery and during the first postoperative days but confirmed instead a clear improvement in respect to the preoperative SEPs. We have discussed above some reports in the literature of false-positive/false-negative results (Ginsburg 1985; Kaplan 1986; Lesser 1986; Molaie 1986; Salzman 1986;

Chatrian 1988) and the relative considerations (Friedman 1987; Grundy 1988). We believe that our false-negative result confirms the observation from neurotraumatology of the maintance of SEPs in the case of a transitory functional medullary disturbance, and the reverse occurring in transverse anatomical lesions which cause a complete disappearance of evoked responses above lesion level. This phenomenon may be compared to neuroapraxis as observed in peripheral nerve injuries.

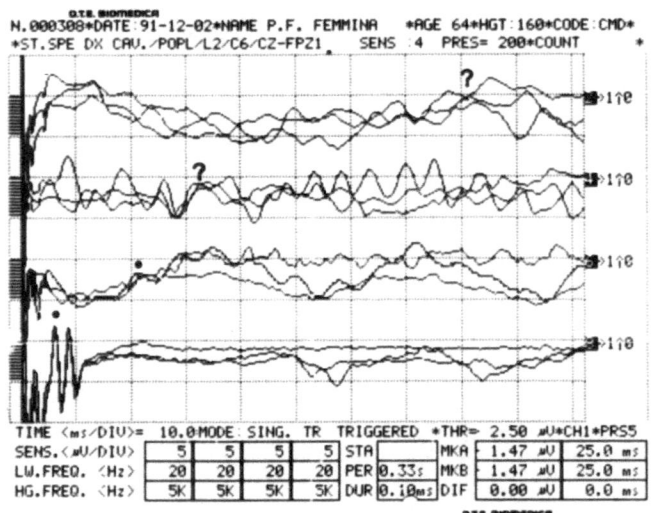

Fig. 99. Preoperative SEPs obtained by right superficial peroneal nerve stimulation at ankle level. Derivations: popliteal fossa, L2, C6, Cz'/Fpz'. Clear evoked responses at popliteal and lumbar levels with normal latency and amplitude, although some morphological abnormality is seen. Cervical responses are dubious, and those recorded from the cortex are substantially absent.

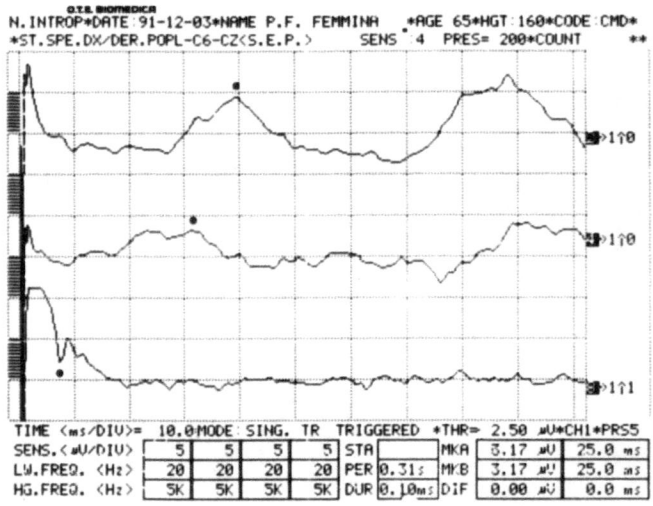

Fig. 100. Intraoperative SEP monitoring. Superficial peroneal nerve stimulation at right ankle level. Derivations: popliteal fossa, C6, Cz'/Fpz'. Evoked responses obtained during the opening of the dura mater. Medullary decompression improves responses, with normal latency even at cervical and cortical levels.

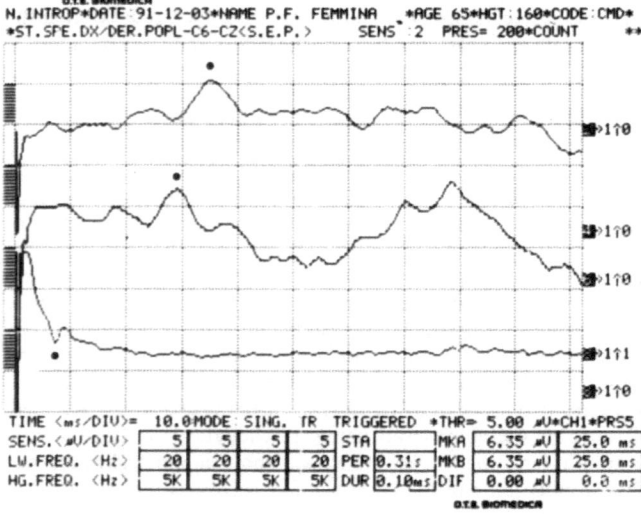

Fig. 101. Intraoperative SEP monitoring. The same parameters as in the previous figure. Responses obtained after the removal of the meningioma. Clear evoked responses both at peripheral and central levels. There is a clear reduction in both cervical and cortical latency of nearly 5 ms compared to those before removal of neoplasm

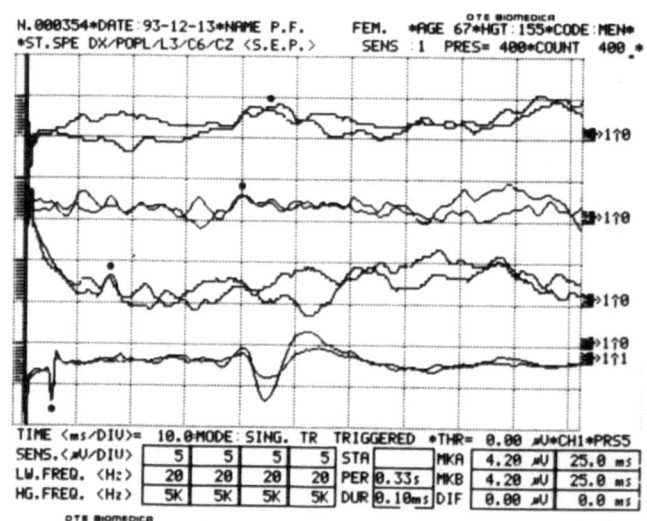

Fig. 102. Postoperative SEPs performed 2 years after surgery. The same parameters as preoperative SEPs. SEPs are normal at peripheral and central levels

Case No. 38:

A 55-year-old man (1994). Right posterolateral meningioma at T11 level. For 10 years the patient reported occasional back pain with a paraesthetic irradiation on the right towards the inguinal region. For 3 years worsening of back pain on the right paravertebral side with pain, paraesthesias and dysaesthesias on the inguinal region, the gluteus, lower limb and posterior surface of the right leg towards the foot and on the perineal region. Five months previously there was a painful lumbar block accompanied by paraesthesias spreading towards the middle and lower abdominal quadrants and ataxic signs rising in both lower limbs. Sphincter disturbances in the form of urinary incontinence and sexual disturbances such as priapism and nocturnal spontaneous ejaculations. After surgery the patient reported lumbar dysaesthesias extending towards the anterior surface of both lower limbs which disappeared completely within 7-10 days, resulting in total recovery.

Preoperative SEPs showed a substantial increase in central conduction time between L2 and C7, but with very clear responses from all sources (Fig. 103). Intraoperative SEP monitoring showed a reduction in latency of cortical responses by nearly 20 ms (Fig. 104). Postoperative SEPs check confirmed the reduction in central conduction time of nearly 4 ms with respect to preoperative values (Fig. 105).

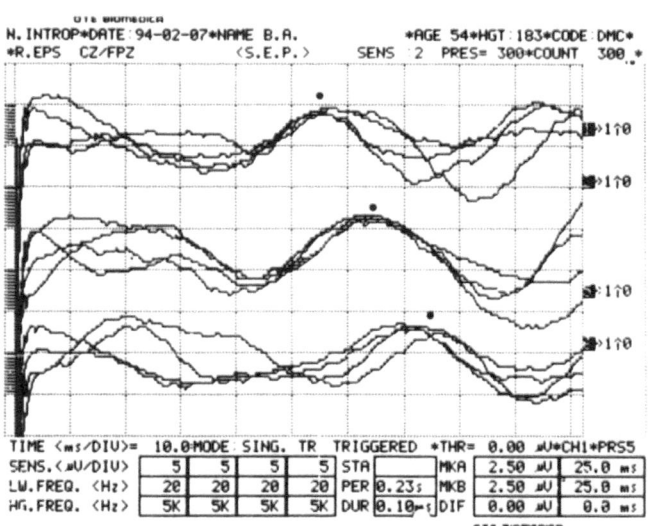

Fig. 104. Intraoperative SEPs monitoring. Superficial peroneal nerve stimulation at right ankle level. Cortical derivation. *From bottom to top,* the three groups each with four traces, at the beginning of surgery, the opening of dura mater and the removal of meningioma. A progressive reduction in cortical response latency from 75 ms to about 55 ms is visible.

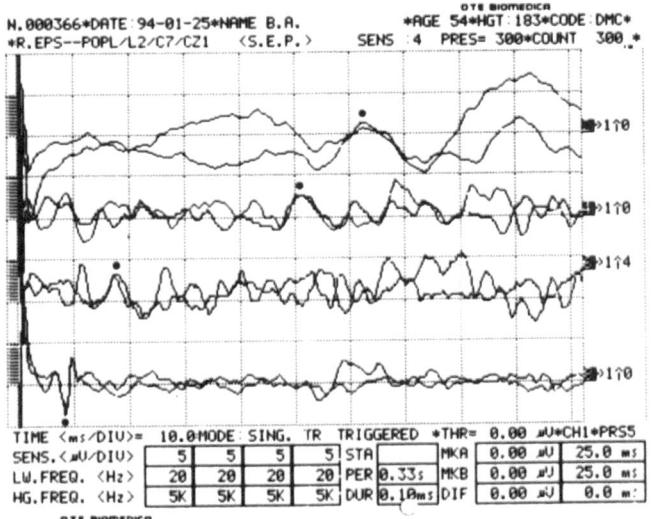

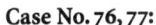

Fig. 103. Preoperative SEPs obtained by superficial peroneal nerve stimulation at right ankle level. Derivation: popliteal fossa, L2, C7, Cz'/Fpz'. Popliteal and lumbar responses are normal for latency, morphology and amplitude. Cervical and cortical evoked responses are evident with normal amplitude and morphology, but show an evident increase in latency (considering the patient's height, 183 cm).

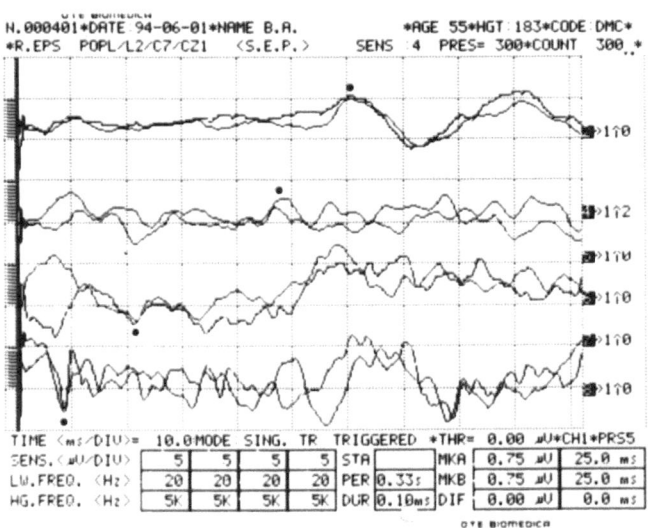

Fig. 105. Postoperative SEPs obtained 4 months after surgery. The same parameters as preoperative SEPs. The evoked responses are evident in all derivation sites and have normal morphology and amplitude. Latency of cervical and cortical responses seems to reach the limits in respect to normal.

Case No. 76, 77:

A 28-year-old woman (1988). Eight years previously she was affected by peripheral right facial nerve paresis, preceded by occasional headaches, with residual facial synkynetic movements and bilateral mimic spasm. Bilateral hypoacusis with tinnitus and occasional phosphenes. For 3 years difficulty in head and neck movements accompanied by paraesthesias along the entire upper left limb, then extending to the body and lower limbs, followed by a constriction

sensation at medial dorsal level. Progressive motor deficency of both lower limbs occurred later, allowing the patient to walk only for very short distances without crutches. Sphincter disturbances in the form of urinary incontinence. Clinical examination revealed left eyelid ptosis, left to right pupil anisochoria, spontaneous horizontal nystagmus, right 7th cranial nerve peripheral paresis, bilateral hypoacusia, left lateral positive Romberg test, slight upper left limb paresis and severe apastic paraparesis with Babinski sign and ataxia, deep and superficial hypoaesthesia of the upper left limb and distally at T6 level on both sides of the body. No skin signs suggesting von Recklinghausen's disease. The patient underwent five operations over 2 years resulting in the removal of 3 meningiomas and 14 neurinomas. First operation (16 Sept. 1988): a left ventrolateral meningioma and an intramedullary cystic neurinoma at C1- C2 level. Second operation (28 Sept. 1988): a left paramedian premedullary meningioma at T 7 level and a small subarachnoidal lamina calcification. Third operation (9 March 1989): ten caudal

neurinomas. Fourth operation (23 May 1990): three terminal cone neurinomas. Fifth operation (30 Jan. 1991): right frontal parietal endocranial meningioma. The patient gradually improved after these operations and showed recovery of sensory and motor disturbances in the upper left limb and improvement in disturbances in the lower limbs. She was able to walk without aid, but spastic-ataxic signs persisted. Sphincter disturbances recovered completely.

SEPs obtained before the two operations in September 1988 showed an almost complete conduction block at cervical level, fol-

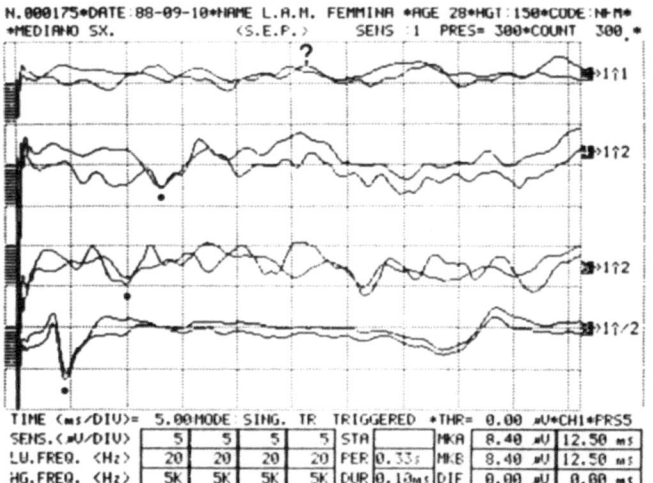

Fig. 106. SEPs obtained by left median nerve stimulation at wrist level. Derivations: elbow, Erb's point, C4, C4'/Fpz'. Peripheral and cervical evoked responses are evident and with normal latency, morphology and amplitude. No responses at cortical level.

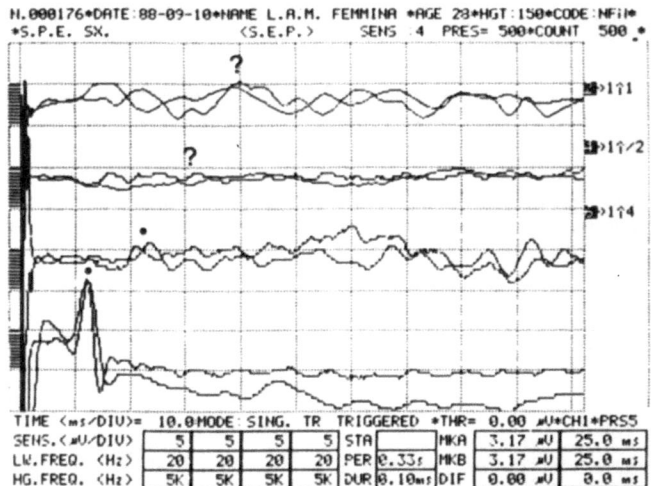

Fig. 107. SEPs obtained by superficial peroneal nerve stimulation at left ankle level. Derivations: popliteal fossa, L5, C7, Cz'/Fpz'. Evoked responses are evident and normal at popliteal level; those obtained at lumbar level appear to have an irregular morphology. No reliable evoked responses are revealed at cervical and cortical levels.

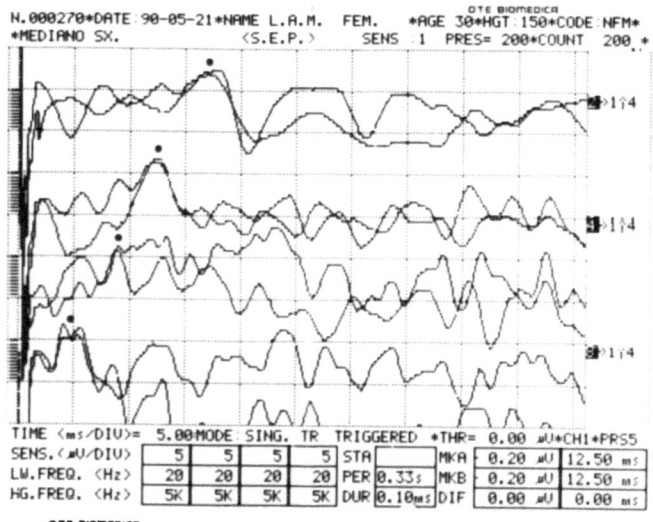

Fig. 108. SEPs obtained by left median nerve stimulation at wrist level. The same parameters as in the former examination (Fig. 106). The evoked responses, although presenting some morphological abnormality, are evident from all derivations and have normal latency and amplitude.

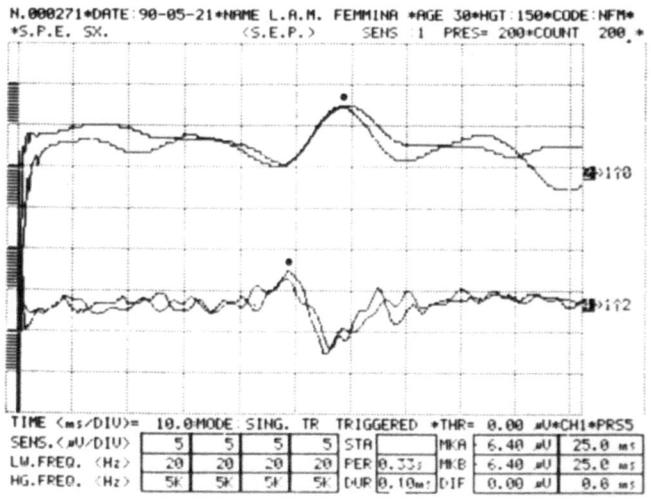

Fig. 109. Evoked cervical (C7) and cortical (Cz'/Fpz') responses obtained by left superficial peroneal nerve stimulation at ankle level. The responses are evident; however, latencies of 48 and 58 ms at the negative peak are increased, particularly if correlated with the patient's height, 150 cm.

lowing left median nerve stimulation (Fig. 106), and a similar block at lumbar level after left peroneal nerve stimulation (Fig. 107). SEPs checks in May 1990, however, showed complete normalization of EPs after left median nerve stimulation (Fig. 108) and recovery of somatosensory conduction after left peroneal nerve stimulation, with EPs both at cervical and cortical levels, but with increased latency (Fig. 109). Intraoperative MEPs on 23 May 1990, obtained by direct stimulation of a clearly compressed right L3 nerve root and recorded from right quadriceps femoral muscle after decompres-

sion, showed an excellent recovery of the motor conduction (Fig. 110). Postoperative SEPs control for the lower limb performed 10 days after the operation confirmed total normalization of somatosensory conduction (Fig. 111). The last postoperative SEPs check performed 15 days after right frontal-parietal meningioma removal was made for the upper and lower left limbs and showed EPs with normal latency, morphology and amplitude on all sources (Figs. 112, 113).

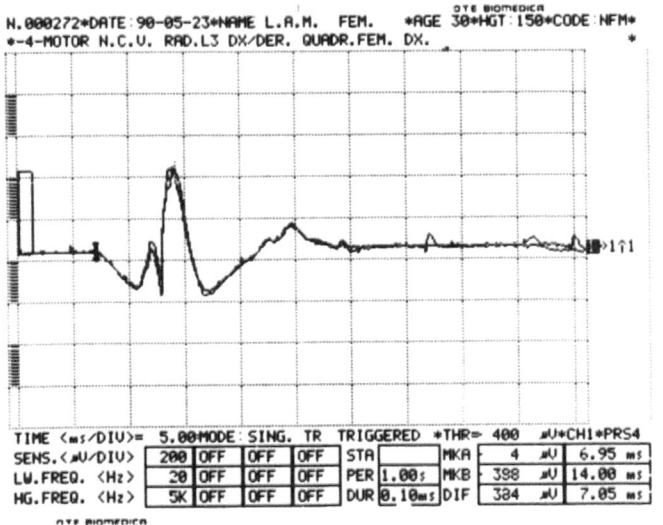

Fig. 110. Intraoperative MEPs obtained by direct radicular stimulation of L3 on the right (20 V, 0.1 ms) and with a coaxial needle electrode placed on quadriceps femoral muscle on the same side. The muscle responses obtained after decompression manoeuvres of the nerve root are well superimposed and have normal latency, morphology and amplitude.

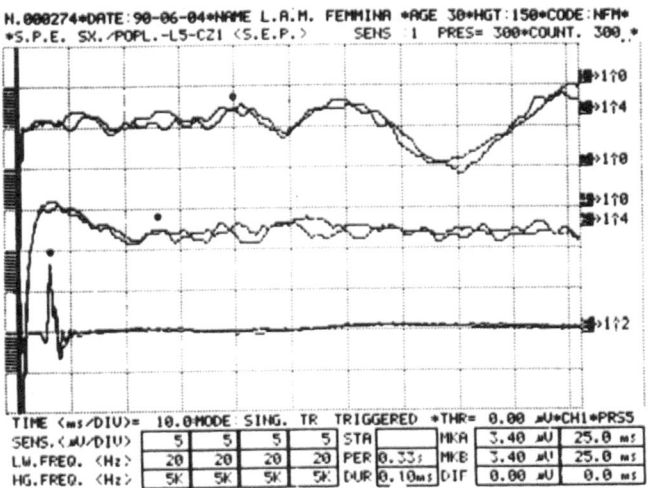

Fig. 111. Postoperative SEPs check obtained 10 days after the previous operation. Left superficial peroneal nerve stimulation at ankle level. Derivations: popliteal fossa, L5, Cz'/Fpz'. This examination shows clear evoked responses with normal amplitude, morphology and latency from all derivation sites. An evident reduction (18 ms) in cortical latency (40 ms) compared to preoperative SEPs (Fig. 109) is seen.

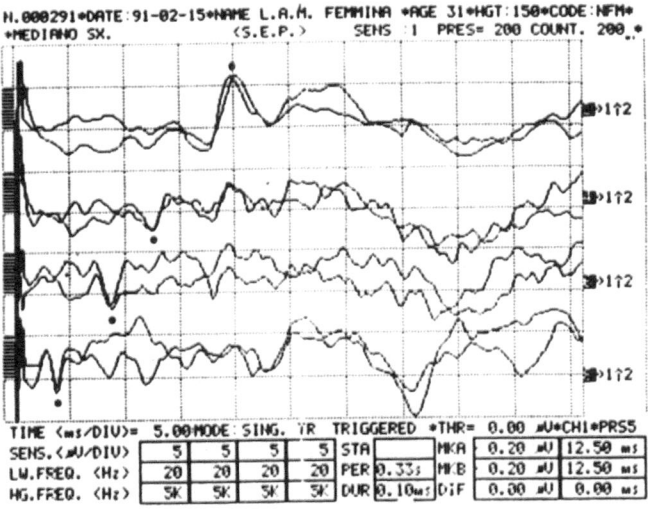

Fig. 112. Postoperative SEPs 15 days after the last operation for right frontal-parietal meningioma. Stimulation of left median nerve at wrist level. Derivations: elbow, Erb's point, C4, C4'/Fpz'. The evoked responses at various levels, peripheral and central, are perfectly normal

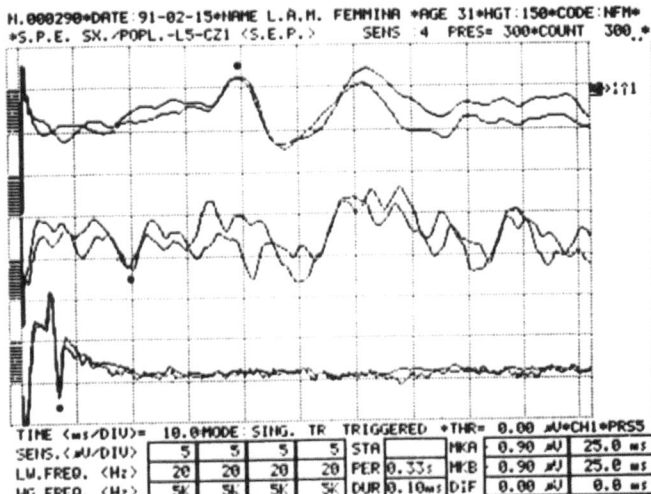

Fig. 113. The same as for Fig. 111. In this examination SEPs are obtained by stimulation of superficial peroneal nerve at left ankle level and derivations at popliteal, lumbar (L5) and cortical (Cz'/Fpz') levels. In addition to having normal latency, the responses show a greater amplitude and very good morphology, much more normal than those obtained 8 months earlier.

7.5 Results, Discussion, Conclusions

To evaluate the efficiency of SEPs as diagnostic and prognostic parameters we compared instrumental results with the clinical course of motor, sensory and sphincter disturbances. The average follow-up period was 12 months. Pre- and postoperative motor deficits were evaluated by Levy's scale: total preoperative score of the 11 patients was 15, while the postoperative score was 2 (Graph. 1). We therefore observed the clinical trend of the sensitive, radicular and cord deficiences and sphincter disturbances. Nine patients suffered from pain in radicular areas at the lesion level, and two of these patients still presented these symptoms after surgery. Hypoanaesthesia at lesion level, observed in three patients, had not changed after surgery. Preoperative cord pain and paraesthesias were present in ten patients and remained in three of these after surgery. Cord hypoanaesthesia was present in seven and persisted in three after surgery. Six patients were affected by ataxia before surgery, and two presented this symptom after surgery (Graph. 2). Sphincter disturbances were present in eight before surgery and only one after sur-

gery (Graph. 3). SEPs were divided into the five categories described above (see Sect. 7.4); the total preoperative score was 17 in seven patients, and a postoperative score of 5 in nine (Graph. 4). Table 15 summarizes the results.

The small number of patients and the lack of some pre- and/or postoperative SEPs evaluation tests do not allow us to draw substantial conclusions from these data. However, as mentioned above, few cases are reported in the literature of patients affected by spinal neoplasms undergoing SEPs evaluation, and very few affected by spinal meningiomas. This makes statistical comparisons impossible. Our SEPs quantification scale was based on Levy's scale but only in a structural way, as higher scores indicated severity of clinical and neurophysiological findings. No scoring was made for sensory deficits or sphincter disturbances due to lack of adequate methods; we limited our observations to the presence or absence of these. In spite of this, however, there is a clear relationship between the clinical picture and course of the disease on the one hand, and pre- and postoperative SEPs on the other.

This underlines the importance of this neurophysiological method in the field of neoplastic spinal compres-

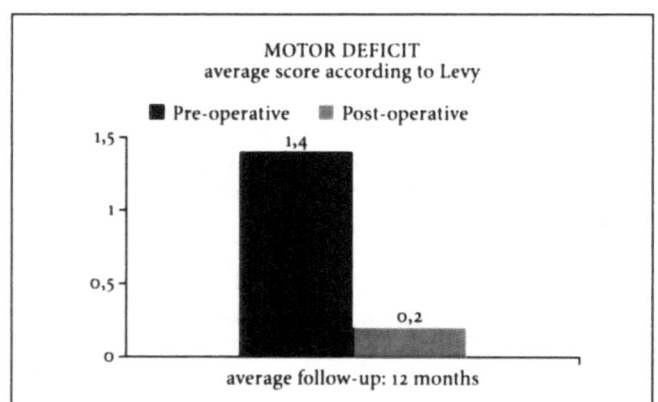

Graph 1

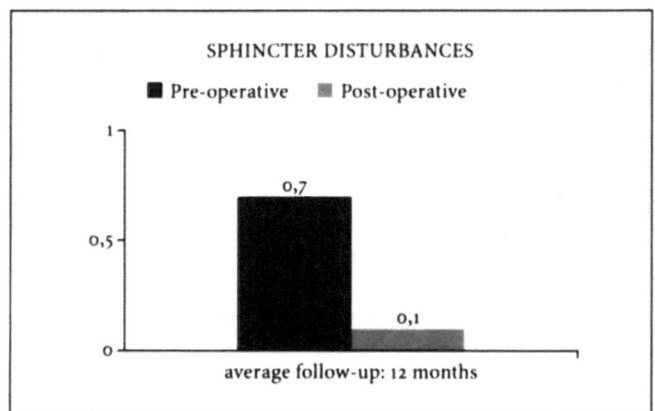

Graph 3

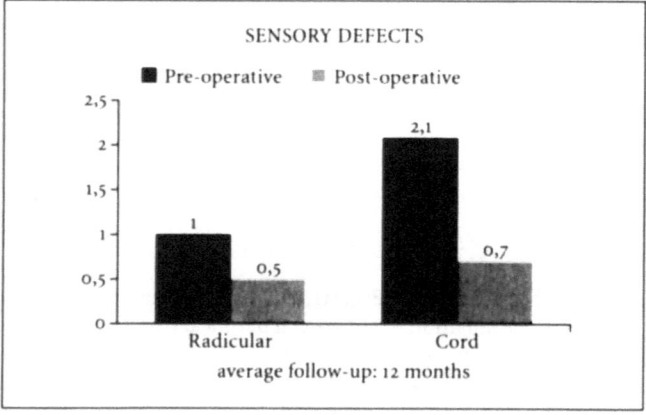

Graph 2

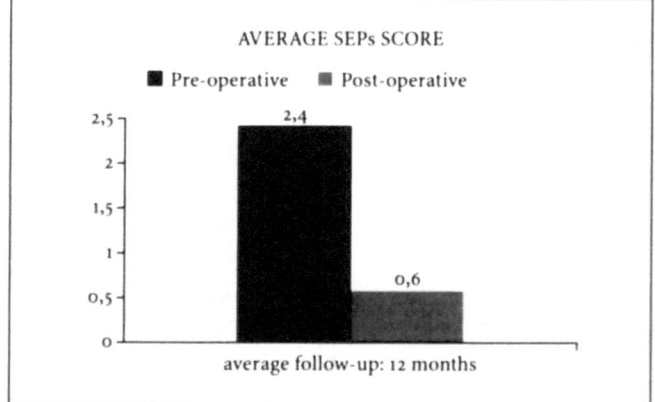

Graph 4

Table 15.

	Preoperative	Postoperative
Motor deficit (Levy's scale)	15 ($n=11$)	2 ($n=11$)
Radicular paraesthesias	9/11	2/11
Radicular hypoaesthesia	3/11	3/11
Cordonal paraesthesias	10/11	3/11
Cordonal hypoaesthesia	7/11	3/11
Cordonal ataxia	6/11	2/11
Sphincter disturbances	8/11	1/11
SEP score	17 ($n=7$)	5 ($n=9$)

sions, particularly for neoplasms with very slow development, as in the case of meningiomas. The sometimes occult and asymptomatic beginning of meningioma development can be revealed by SEPs and MEPs and it is therefore a valuable procedure for correct and early diagnosis. The simplicity and speed of these noninvasive procedures, together with low cost and absence of contraindications are also important features. In particular these procedures enable us to perform frequent checks on patients to determine the course of the disease and to verify the efficacy of specific therapeutic approaches.

8 Neuroradiology

A. Pansini - P. Conti - R. Conti - F. Lo Re

8.1 Bone Alterations from Compression of the Meningioma on the Vertebral Sac

Gaidolfi et al. (1991) emphasize the importance of standard radiological studies of the rachis and express their belief that primary or metastatic pathology may be responsible for the symptoms of myeloradicular disturbance. In some meningioma cases an X-ray of the rachis can provide precise information to help in determining the level and can also identify specific rachidian alterations that are secondary to the slow compressive action of a tumour and thus suggest the presence of a meningioma. In contrast

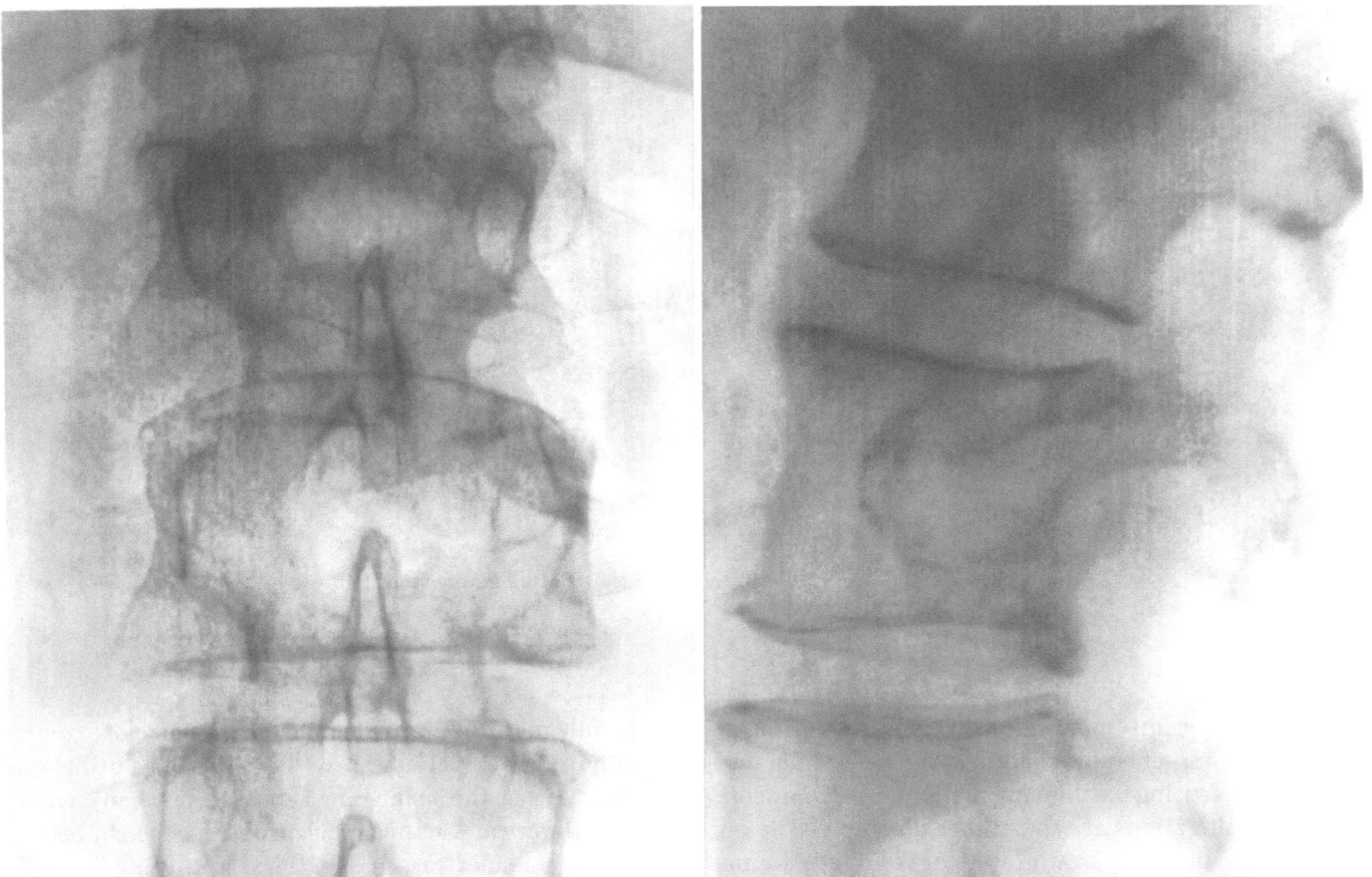

Fig. 114. In anteroposterior projection, narrowing of articular pedicle in L2 with enlargement of the spinal canal. In lateral projection, erosion of posterior surface of L2 body. The lamina of L2 appeared thinned

83

A. Pansini et al.
Spinal Meningiomas
© Springer-Verlag Italia 1996

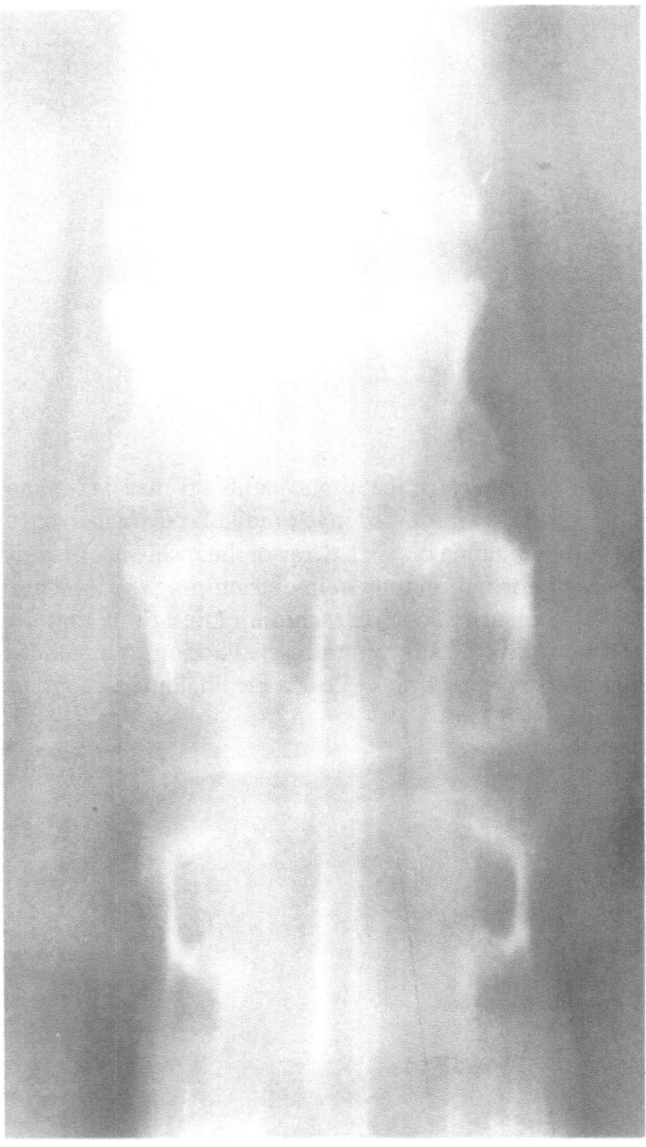

Fig. 115. Anteroposterior stratigraphy. Bone modifications of the pedicles are clear. Great excavation of the vertebral body of L2 on the left

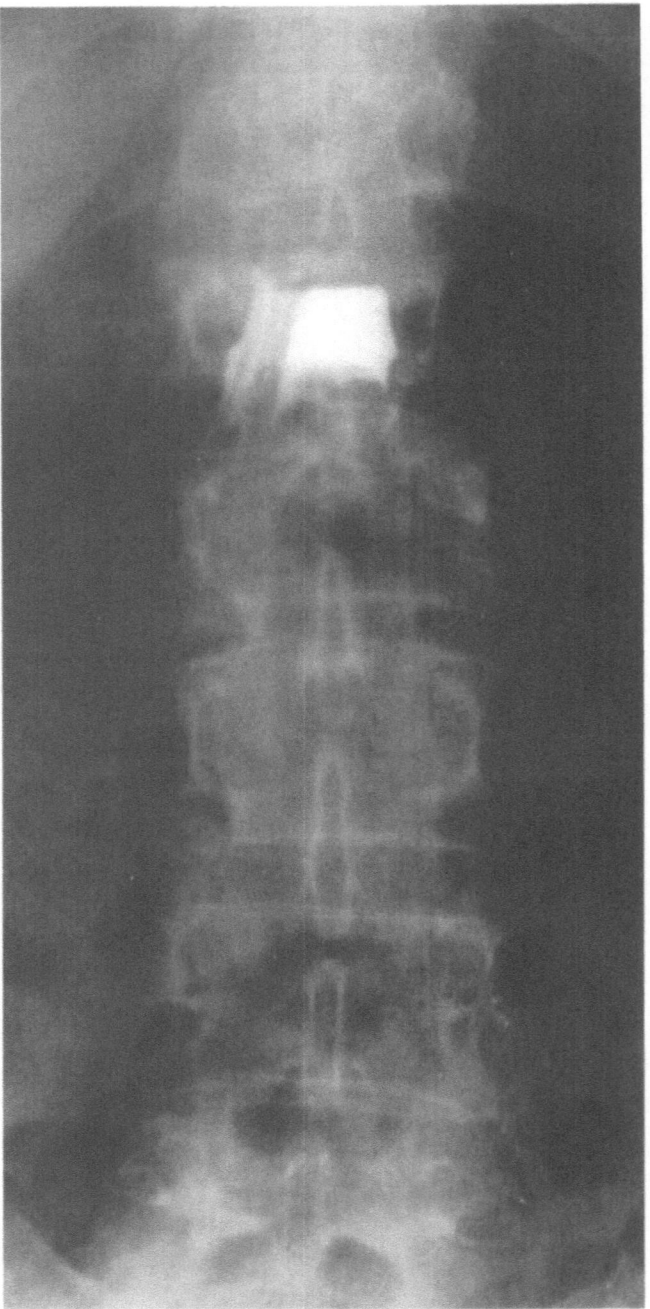

Fig. 116. Myelography: total block in L1

to other neoplasms, meningiomas (due to their dural attachment) are generally adjacent to the walls of the vertebral canal, causing the thinning of the internal bone cortex. These alterations are sometimes directly visible on plain X-ray and on a stratigraphy or indirectly found because the normal measurements of the interpeduncular distance (Lindgren 1952; Decker 1968) identify the metamere where the compression lies. The salient features are caused by erosion of the pedicles, laminae and posterior somatic walls (scalopping). The latter appears more fre-

quently in extradural forms that develop in close contact with the vertebral bodies. The alterations in a pedicle are evident when the meningioma enlarges, or when it erodes the intravertebral foramen wall on one side thereby becoming intra- and extrarachidian (Figs. 114-117).

Case No. 69: Meningothelial Meningioma
A 56-year-old woman (1978). Left intra- and extradural meningioma, with extrarachidian extension in a posterolateral site in L1-L3. *Clinical Course.* 18 years. At the age of 38 years the patient was

affected by pain with pluriradicular pattern, first in the lower third of the thigh and then spreading progressively to the anteromedian surface medially to the leg. The painful radicular symptoms associated with lumbago occurred at intervals over the years. The pain became constant only 9 months before hospitalization and more intense with radicular irradiation to both sides. Loss of strength in the left lower limb with difficulty in walking and paraesthesia to the feet. Sphincter disturbance in the form of retention of urine.

Neurological Examination. Flaccid paraplegia affecting the left (Levy grade III). Pronounced hypertrophy in the lower third of the femoral quadricep. Hypoaesthesia from L1 on the left to L2 on the right. Hyperaesthesia at both feet.

X-Ray of Upper Lumbar Tract. Anteroposterior narrowing of articular pedicle in L2 and L3 on the left, presenting a widening of the rachidian canal. A lateral projection showed erosion in a semilunar shape, as an excavation of L2. The lamina of L2 appeared thinned and intervertebral foramen widened (Fig. 114-115).

Myelography (performed suboccipitally). Partial dome-shaped block in L1. Slight lateral flow on the right. The medullary corridor appears displaced on the right (Fig. 116).

Surgical Treatment. The laminae appeared thinned and the articular mass of L2 eroded on the left. The lesion infiltrated and surrounded the dura, compressing the caudal roots and the medullary cone which was displaced to the right. The upper pole of the neoplasm was intradural. Its consistency was dense, lumpy and the size of a mandarine. The major part of the tumour on the left extended outwards from the rachis through the intravertebral foramens of L1 and L2. Fragmented removal completely freeing the caudal fascia. The tumour was pushing the dura against the posterior excavation of the vertebral body L2 (Fig. 117).

Results. Progressive recovery of flex extension of legs after 1 year, persistence of deficit in left foot. Walking was possible with support. Sphincter disturbances regressed.

In anteroposterior projections when erosion of the peduncle is more pronounced on one side the upper spinal processes of the adjacent vertebral body lose their outlines, presenting a calcified thickening, particularly when the meningioma grows beyond the intravertebral foramen. This is seen better on stratigraphy (Fig. 115) as a hyperdense peripheral area. In these forms the alteration of the pedicle may be associated with enlargement of the intravertebral foramen, an increase in the interpeduncular distance or the thinning of one or two laminae (Fig. 114).

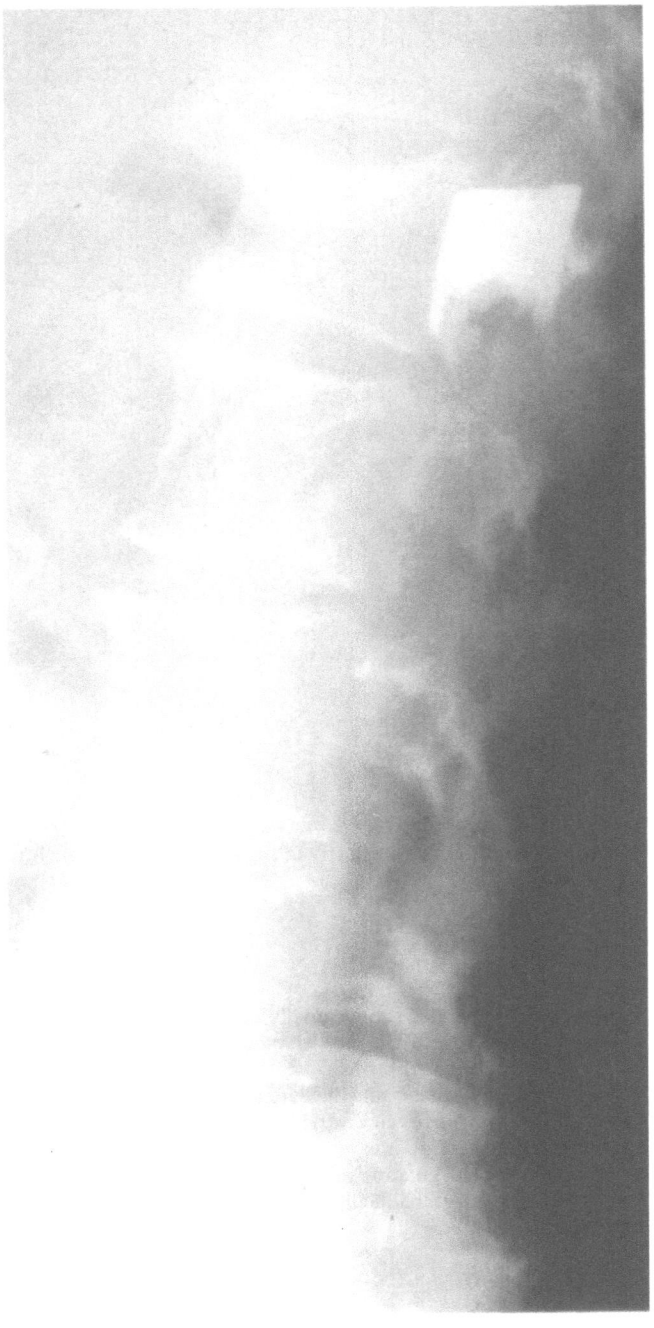

Fig. 116. Myelography: dome-shaped block in L1

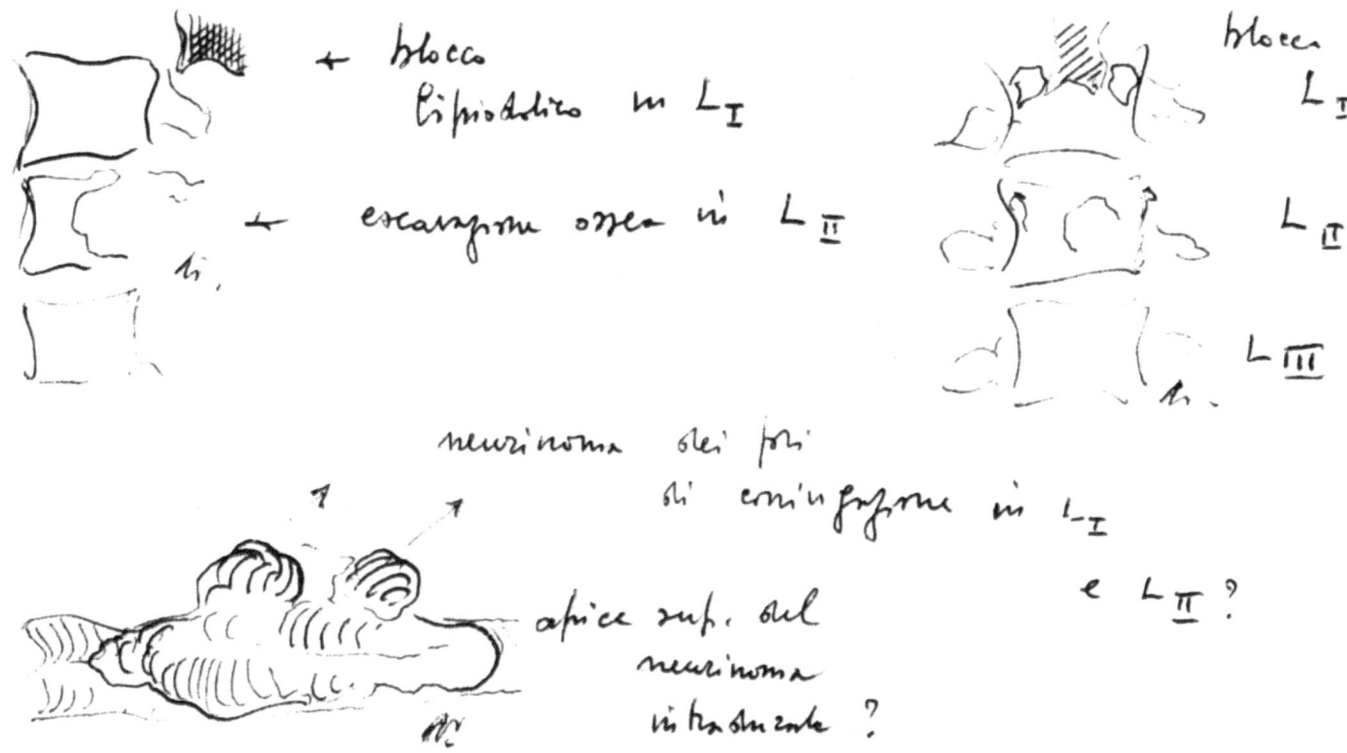

Fig. 117. Schematic reconstruction of case 69. During the operation the large compression suggested a partly intra- and extradural neurinoma extending beyond the intravertebral foramen of L1-L2

8.1.1 Modification of a Single Pedicle

The modification of a pedicle causes a minimum thinning in lateral meningiomas which are very close to the meningeal funnel near the two nerve roots (Figs. 118, 119).

Case No. 107: Meningothelial Meningioma with Psammomatous Expression

A 57-year-old woman (1978). Left posterolateral intradural-extramedullary meningioma in D7
Medical History. Surgery for the removal of a fibroid at age 40 years.
Clinical Course. Initial sensation of instability and weakness in the two lower limbs on the left with slight motor claudication. Distal paraesthesias such as tingling sensations to the lower limbs on the right. In another hospital multiple sclerosis was suspected. Paraparesis on the left for 6 months leading to the impossibility of walking. Hypoaesthesia at D7 level on the right. Sphincter disturbances.
X-Ray. Signs of osteoporosis affecting medial dorsal tract with diffused arthrosis. Calcifications on discs in D6-D7. Slight scoliosis with lateral tendency to ankylosis of various vertebral bodies which appeared malformed and spindle-like.

Myelography (performed suboccipitally). The block in D6-D7 located the lesion on the left. The arch-shaped image defined a roundish filling defect (Fig. 118).
Surgical Treatment. On incising the dura a posterolateral tumour the size of an almond was seen on the left. It was removed from the arachnoid adherent structures and the spinal roots above and below the compression. Coagulation of the base of attachment (Fig. 119).
Results. Walking was still difficult after 10 days. Clinical recovery after 2 months.

When the tumour extends forwards and posteriorly to the denticulate ligament compression of the meningeal sheath occurs at the level of invasion and its point introduction into the intravertebral foramen causing resorption phenomenon of the cortex. Erosion affecting a pedicle ipsilaterally to the compression was found in 41 posterolateral meningioma cases, and only 2 were found in the cervical tract and 14 at thoracic level. Alterations in one peduncle seem rare only in dorsal locations, although bone alterations appear variable.

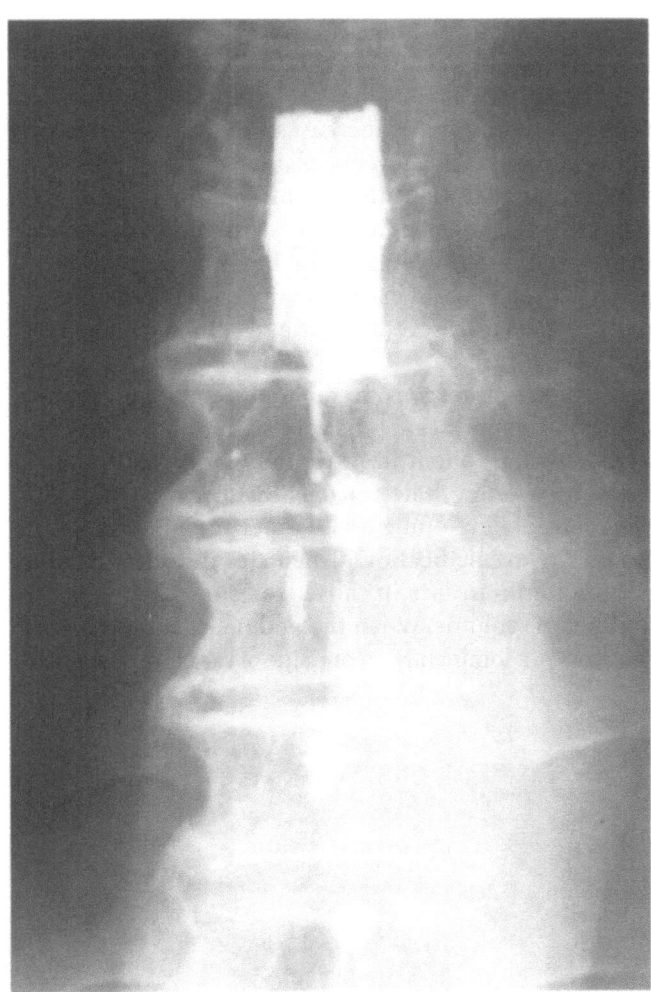 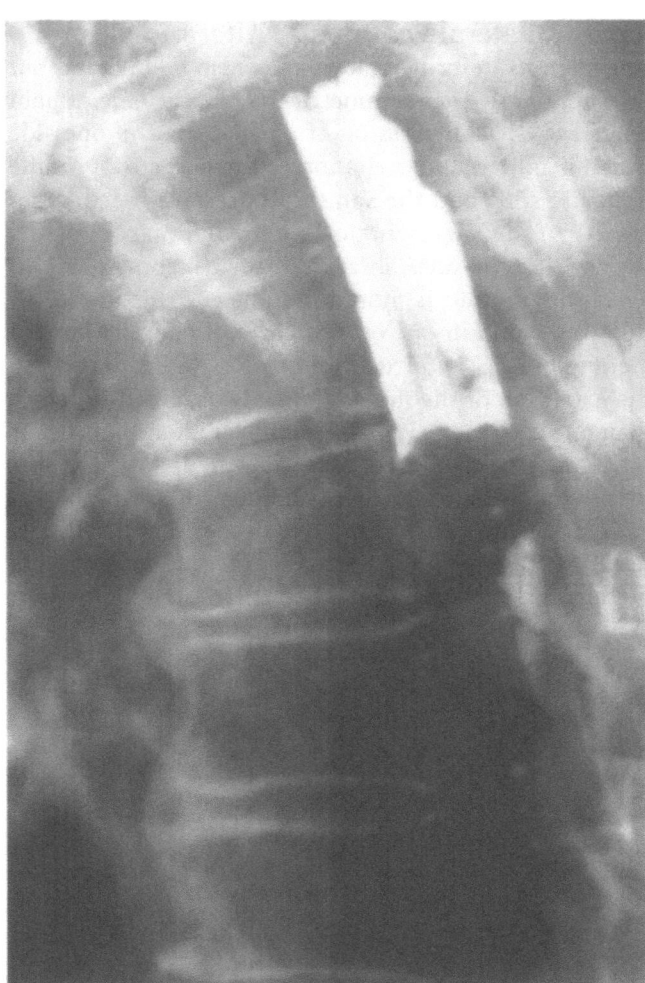

Fig. 118. Suboccipital myelography. Block in D7 producing a linear dome-shaped feature and slight flow along the medial line which defines a roundish-shaped filling defect on the left

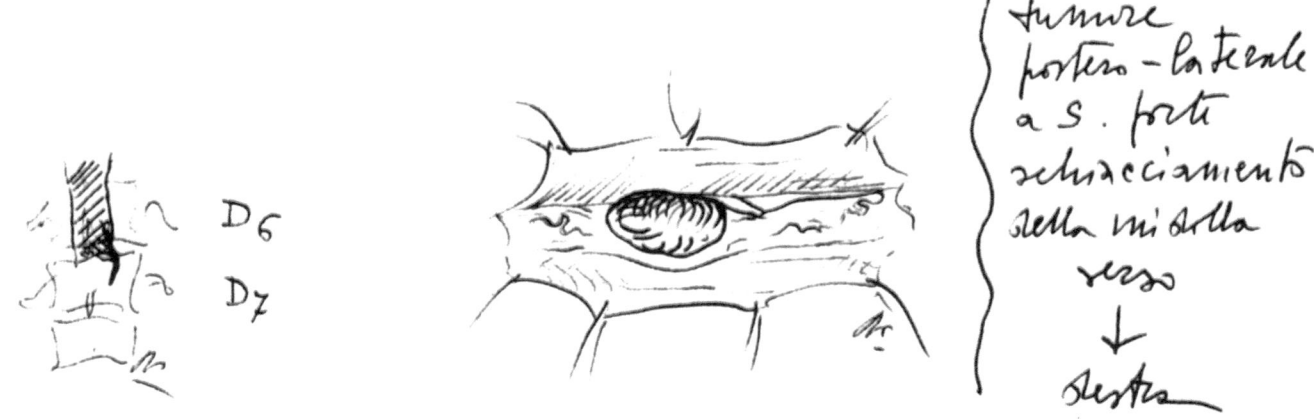

Fig. 119. Diagram of case 107. The left posterolateral tumour reduces the thickness of the pedicle in D7 (see Fig. 118)

8.1.2 Bilateral Peduncular Alterations

The features described above may also be bilateral but they are hardly ever symmetrical. As in the case of pain related to the compression of a nerve root on one side which is followed by irritation of the nerve root on the opposite side, and the same compressive mechanism results in the narrowing of the medial margin of the peduncle on two sides, always more evident on the side on which the tumour is more pronounced. This modification was found in one of four cases of laterally located meningiomas. The process of erosion, in proportion to the extention of the meningioma, is observed on more than one metamere. When peduncular alterations occur on numerous vertebrae X-rays show the same characteristics found in intramedullary tumours and correspond in extension to the maximum width of the rachidian lumen resulting from the interpeduncular measurements transversally on various levels. When there is a reduction in height together with a reduction in thickness of the laminae one finds an alteration in the interpeduncular spac-es, predominantly on lateral projections. These characteristics suggest a pathological condition of intramedullary formation such as that seen in glioma cases when the medullary volume increases not only transversally but also in length as a myelitic plial-form enlargement. The peduncular alterations that occur in syringomyelia (Fig. 120) are very similar, as in rare cases of intra- and extradural arachnoidal cysts, on the basis of a dysembryogenetic nature and in exceptionally rare cases of scarred cysts formed over several years as a result of a traumatic event (Fig. 121).

These features are only an indication of how the slow process of compression can cause alterations that are normally more frequent in intramedullary glial tumours, without excluding, however, the rare form of meningioma with central development and other premedullary locations. The decalcification of pedicles in intramedullary meningiomas occurs in those tracts of the spinal cord with major volume. When the peduncles undergo modification, predominantly on one side of numerous vertebrae,

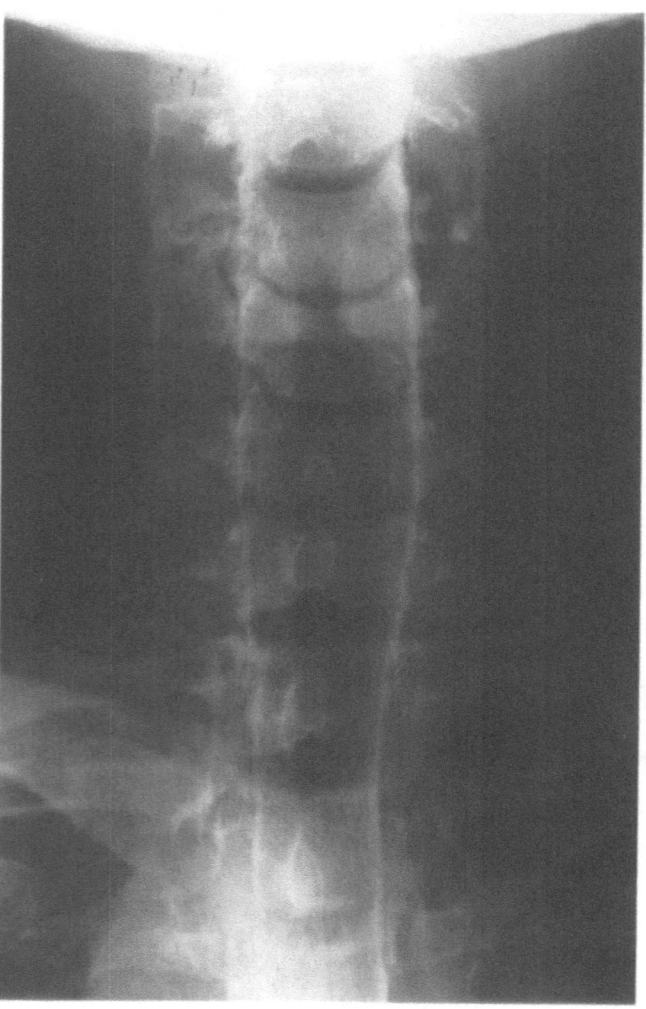

Fig. 120. Thinning of pedicles in syringomyelia on myelography

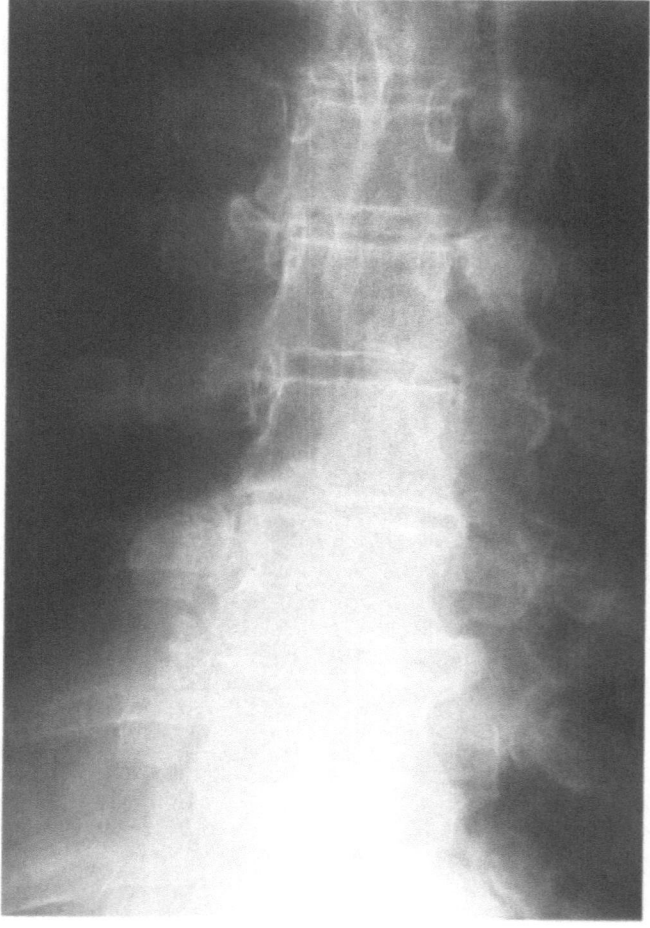

Fig. 121. Thinning of pedicles in a case of an arachnoid cyst

the enlargement of the spinal cord is greater on the same side.

As we begin to view the upper metameres and gradually work our way to observing those below the alterations become less visible and the interpeduncular distance gradually becomes normal. If one could draw an imaginary line vertically along the erosion of the pedicles, for example along the various metameres on both sides of the cervical tract, the radiographic reading would be facilitated in defining the increased volume of the cord and the extent of the spinal canal's enlargement. Apart from these rare intramedullary forms, usually only one pedicle is modified in intradural and juxtamedullary meningiomas. A minimal thinning of the medial and lower margin of a pedicle indicates the level of the meningioma's upper pole, while the same modification at the pedicle's upper margin of the vertebra below on the same side corresponds to the lower pole of the compression. Erosion on X-ray is also indicated by the alterations in the enlarged subarachnoidal space at the upper and lower pole level of the meningioma. The asymmetry of the pedicle depends on the kind of compression: on one side there is direct compression from the meningioma while on the other the compression is caused by displacement of the cord pushed against the meningeal sac resulting in dilatation of the subarachnoidal space above and below the tumour.

With extradural meningiomas the alterations are limited to the locations of the tumour and the extent of modification depends on its length. Every degenerative modification of the cord nature worsens the existing compression of the myeloradicular structures on the side of the tumour. Therefore meningiomas, with their slow development, often affect older patients suffering from arthrosis, vertebral stenosis and segmental scoliosis. In one of our patients affected by arthrosis below the meningioma site in D8-D9 we suspected a second tumour on the right, which was later excluded by CT. It was merely a lateral hypostosis in stenotic hourglass arthrosis in D10-D11 (see case 57, Chap. 6). Scoliosis affecting the rotation of one or more vertebral bodies can obstruct the radiological evaluation of the rachis, making it difficult to identify the initial structure alterations of the pedicle or to evaluate the interpeduncular spaces. The morphological alterations described above interfere with the vertebral column by modifying the physiological curvature (Figs. 122-124).

Case No. 97: Transitional Meningioma

A 71-year-old woman (1980). Anterior intradural-extramedullary meningioma in D11.
Medical History. Operated for ovarian cysts.
Clinical Course. 1 year. Ingravescent lumbago irradiating to the right lower limb, then spreading to the left. Progressive motor deficit.
Neurological Examination. Spastic paraparesis. Babinski sign and clonus on the left. Occasional ataxia while walking. Hypoaesthesia from D12 more pronunced on the left. Sphincter disturbances in the form of retention.

Rachicentesis. 6.8 g protein per thousand.
X-Ray of Dorsolumbar Tract of Rachis. Right convex scoliosis affecting rotation of vertebral bodies and a reduction in their height at D10 (Fig. 122).

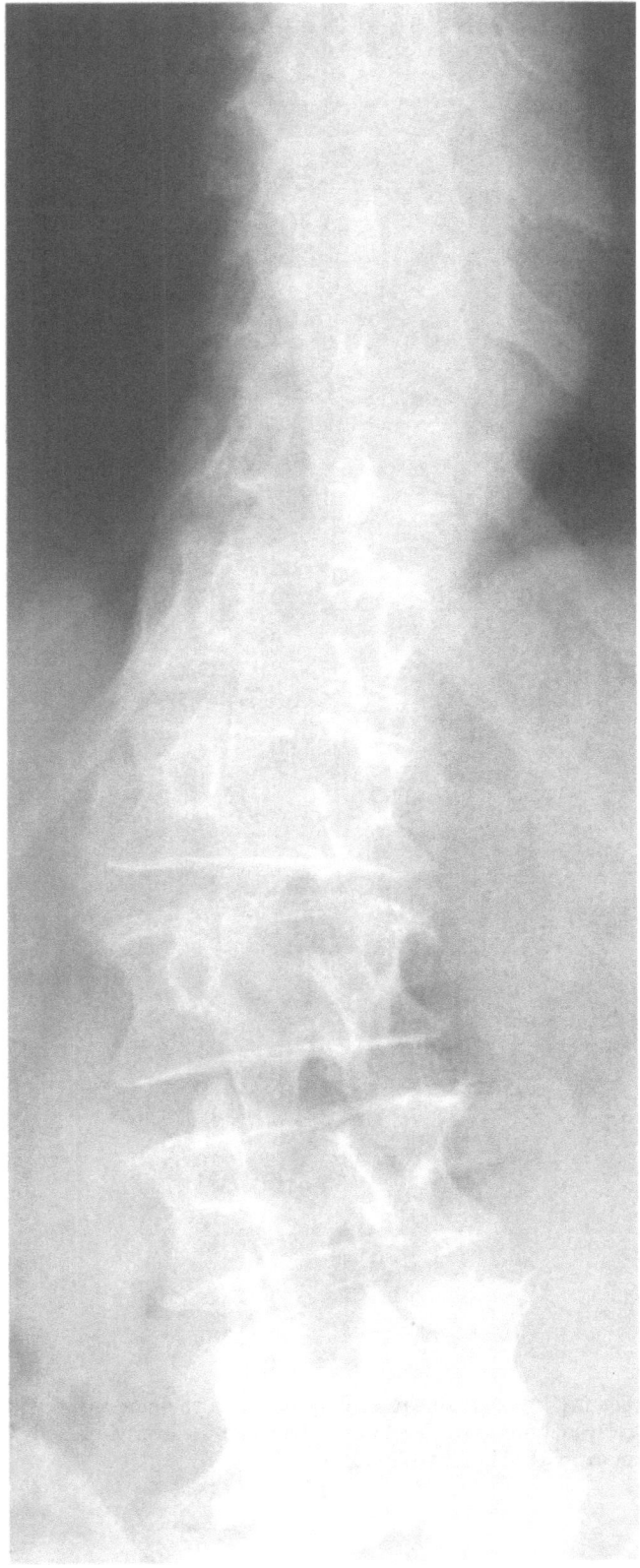

Fig. 122. X-ray of dorsolumbar rachis. Right-convex scoliosis

Myelography (performed suboccipitally). Block in D10-D11 producing a dome-shaped image (Fig. 123).

Surgical Treatment. Opening the dura the cord appeared pushed backwards and presented a very thin surface-layer blood supply. Once the arachnoid was opened a tumour was seen on both sides. It appeared a reddish-wine colour and in a premedullary site. The posterior columns appeared atrophic. Incision of the capsule on one side and fragmented removal was performed together with the calcified base of attachment (Fig. 124).

Results. After 1 week regression of sphincter and sensory disturbances. After 20 days gradual recovery of motility took place on the right. One month later, walking was possible with support.

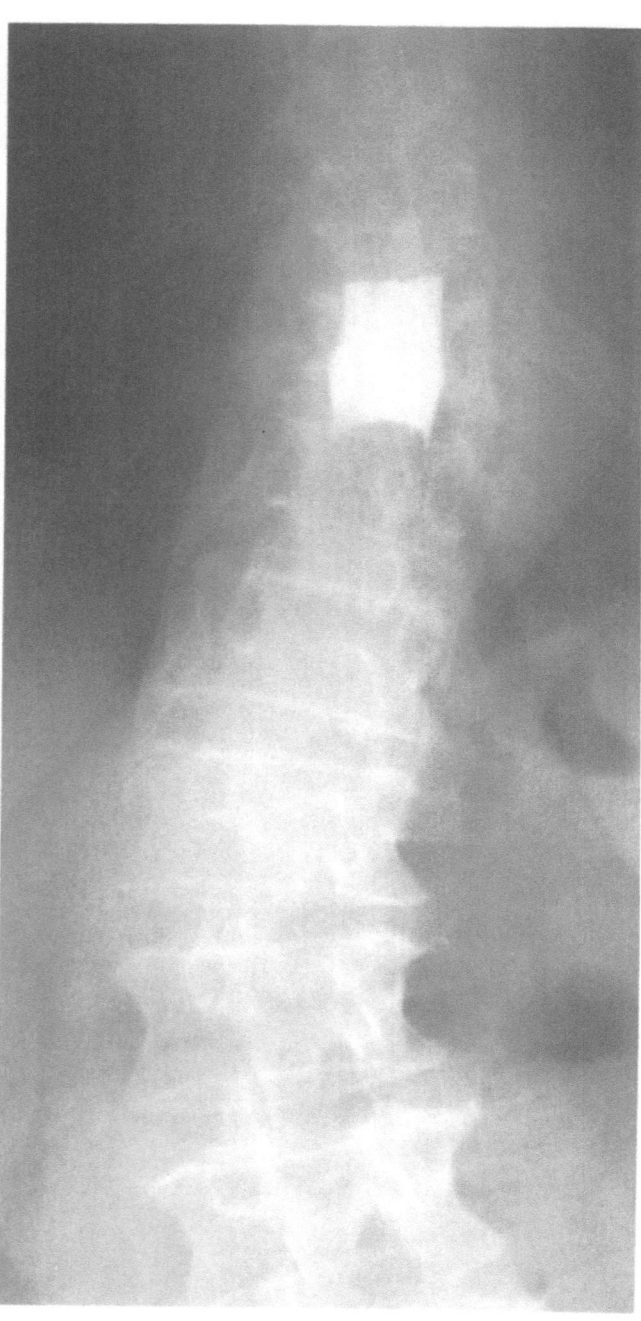

Fig. 123. Myelography. Total block producing a dome-shape, with clear margins at D11 level where the malformed vertebral body is more marked in the scoliotic fulcrum

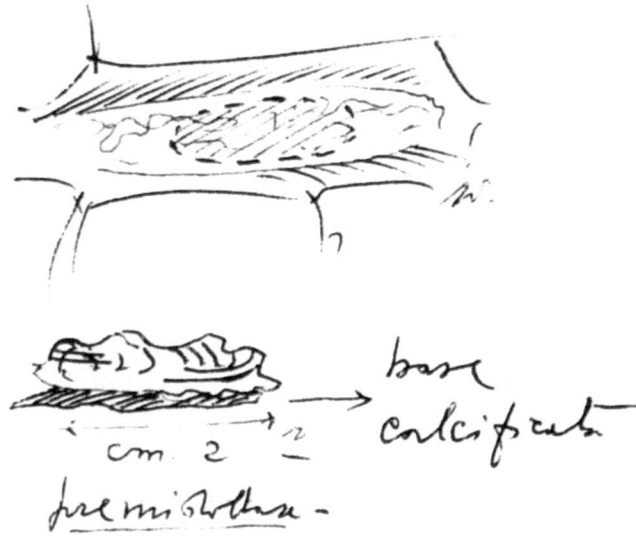

Fig. 124. Diagram of operating field with reference to the calcified base of the premedullary dura

8.1.3 Morphological Alterations in the Vertebral Body

This suggests posterior wall scalopping of one or more vertebral bodies which is very clear on lateral projections. This shell-shaped recess is found on the posterior somatic wall and during surgery corresponding to the ventral potrusion of the tumour. This feature, more frequent in lumbar tumours, is found not only in meningiomas but also in neurinomas (Fig. 125), ependymomas of the cauda, teratomas and dysembryogenetic arachnoidal cysts. Not only do the excavated vertebral bodies show an alteration in their thickness but also usually the laminae.

The differential radiological diagnosis of these three oncotypes is difficult especially when the posterior wall of the vertebral bodies appears very regular (Fig. 125) showing a dense or schlerotic border. In giant ependymomas of the cauda, ependymoblastomas and rare forms of angioblastic meningiomas the bone erosion presents an osteo-

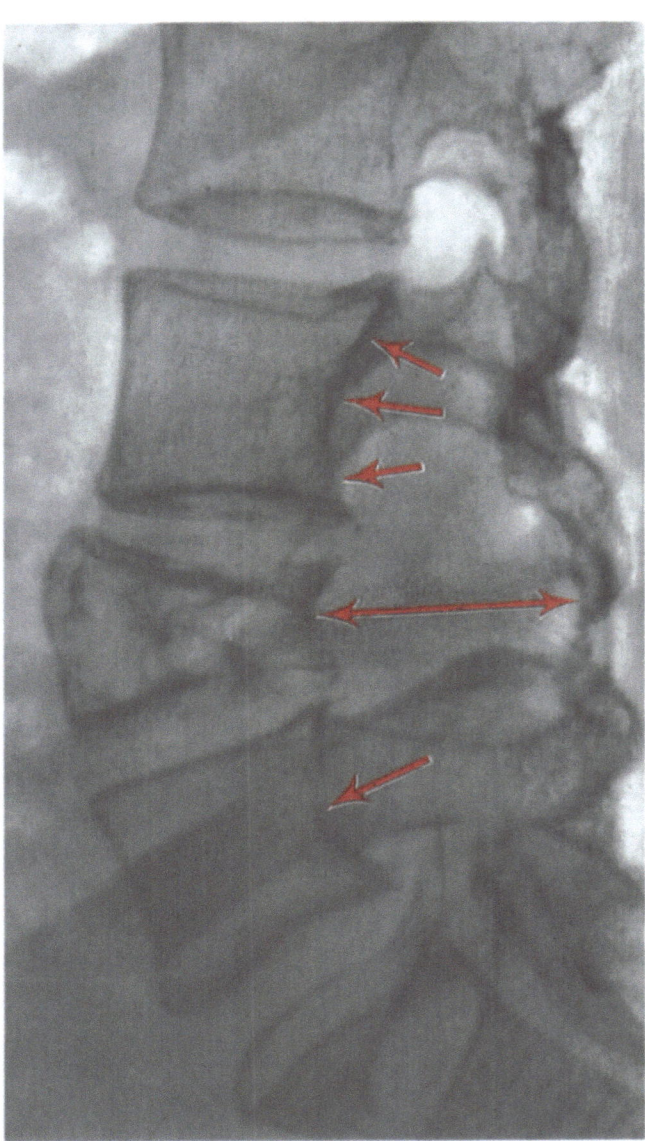

Fig. 125. Erosion of many vertebral bodies in a case of spinal neurinoma

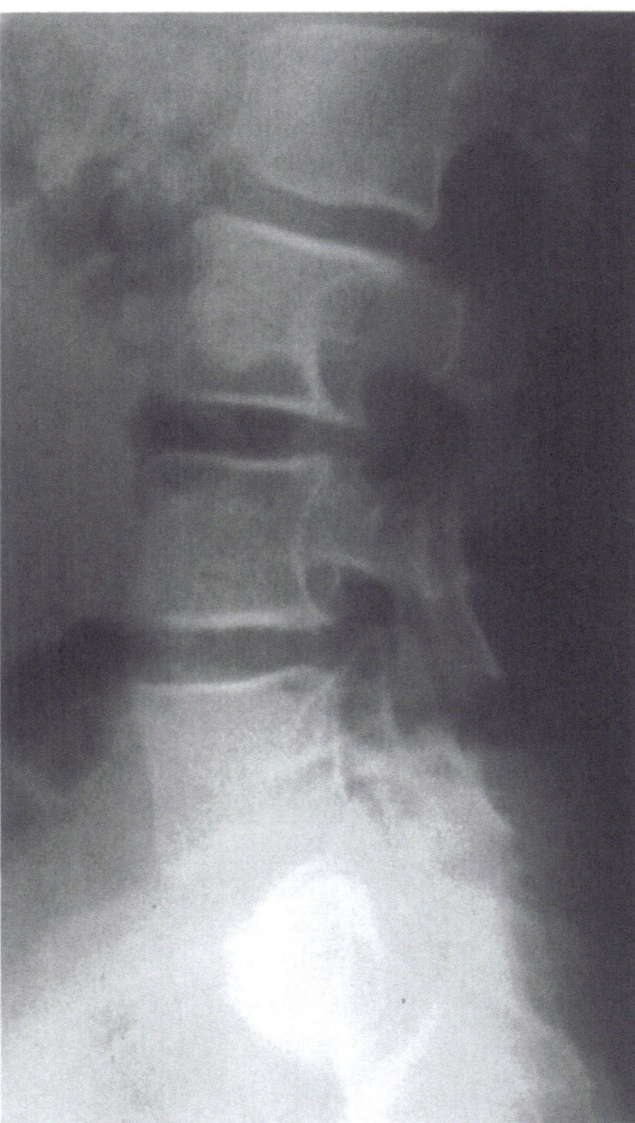

Fig. 126. Pathological fracture of L4 in a case of ependymoblastoma

lithic and irregular nature occupying the ventrolateral wall of the rachis canal, intravertebral foramen and one or two sides of the peduncle. In an ependymoblastoma case we observed the fracture of a vertebral body (Figs. 126, 127) but never in our rare meningioma cases. In meningiomas we have sometimes found that the infiltration of tumoral tissue on the bone walls is homologous to the osteogenetic processes in cranioencephalic meningiomas: "at osteolitic area level the neoplasm infiltration penetrates gradually" (Cushing 1938). Sometimes the scalopping of the posterior walls of numerous vertebrae indicate the exact vertical extent of the expansive process and its volume. Alterations in one or more vertebral bodies have been found by Decker (1968) even in osteosarcoma cases. When a meningioma greatly modifies the morphological structure of a vertebra the histological examination usually shows signs of immaturity (Figs. 128-130). In a few cases we have noted on plain X-ray examination that a vertebra located in a different area to that in which a meningioma has developed retains its normal morphological features but presents vertical striae similar to the vertebral angioma ones (Fig. 131).

Case No. 44: Transitional Meningioma

A 69-year-old woman (1973). Right posterolateral intradural-extramedullary meningioma in D6-D7.

Clinical Course. 2 years. Pain initially located at mediodorsal tract but 8 months before hospitalization it irradiated in a hemigirdle to the right into the submammary region. Progressive loss of strength in lower limbs to the right. Ataxia made walking impossible 15 days prior to hospital admission. Retention of urine.

Neurological Examination. Rigid and kyphotic dorsal rachis. Right monoplegia; some slight contralateral flex-extension movements. Contracture and left Babinski sign. Hypoaesthesia from D7 to the left.

X-Ray of Dorsal Tract. Slight convex scoliosis on the left. In D7 the vertebral body presented vertical striae of an angiomatous type (Fig. 131).

Myelography (performed suboccipitally). Partial block in D6-D7, with dome-shaped image.

Surgical Treatment. On incising the dura a neoplasm the size of an almond was seen posterolaterally on the right. The meningioma invaded the internal surface of the dura and adhered to the sensory roots of D7.

Results. Complete recovery after 3 months.

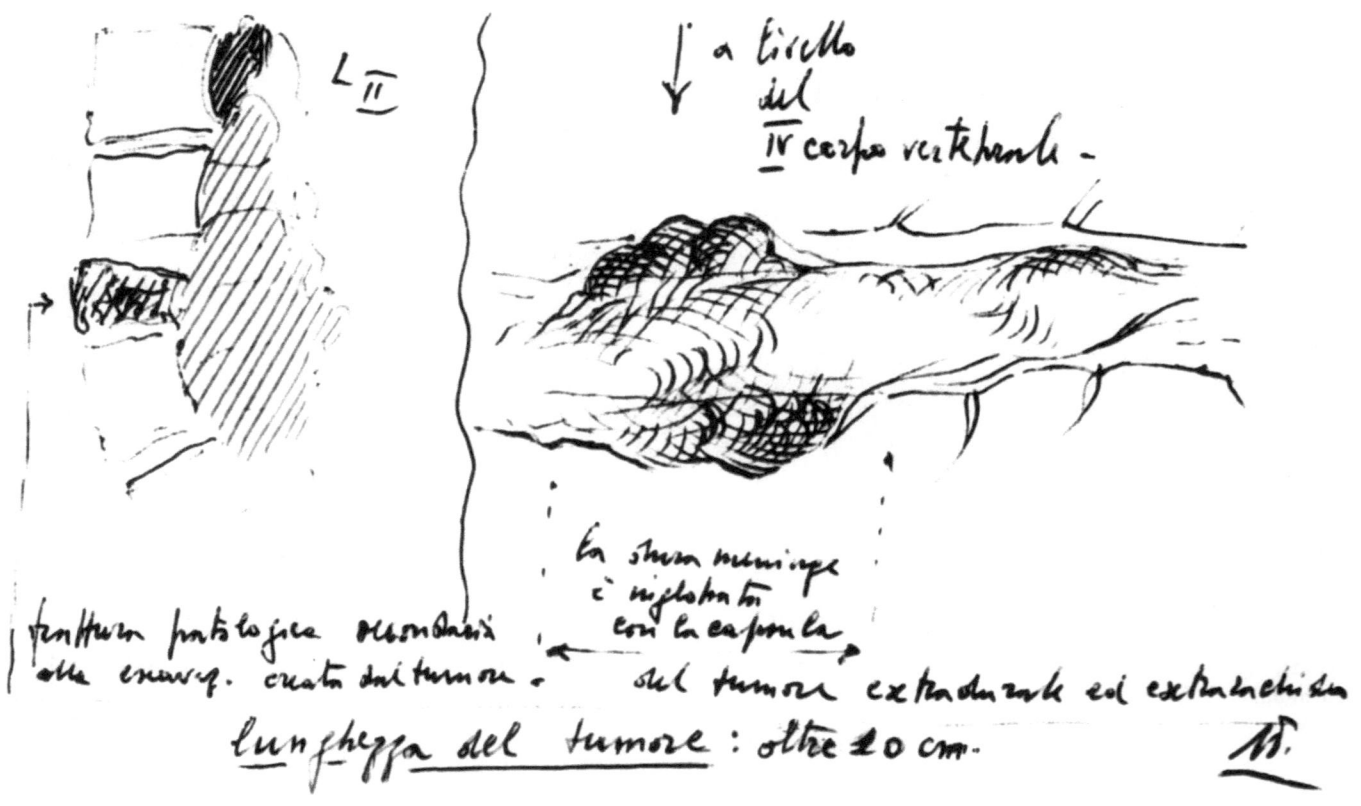

Fig. 127. Drawing of the case of ependymoblastoma of the cauda equina

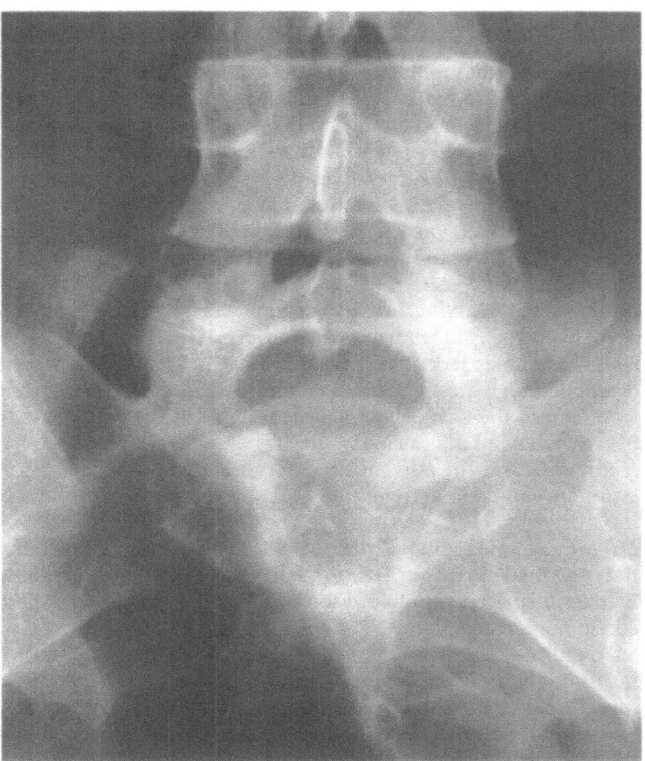
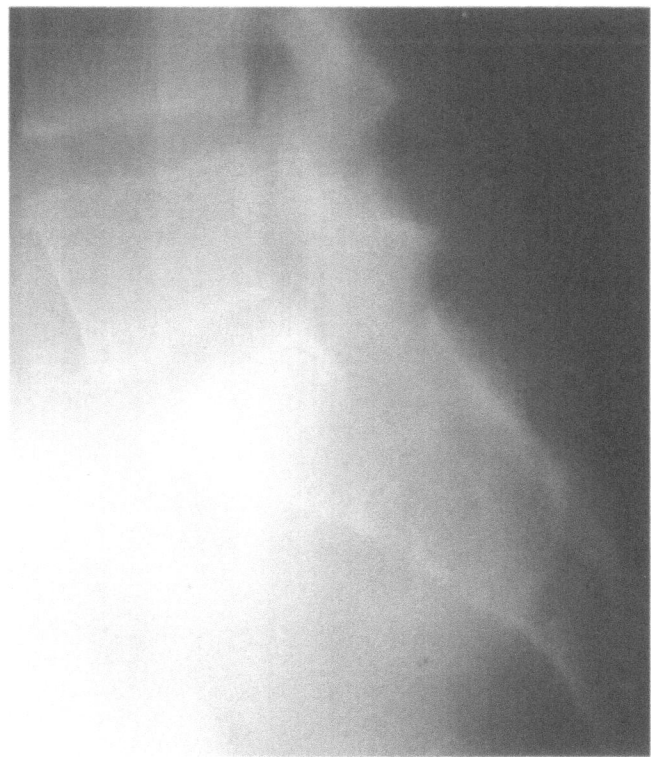

Fig. 128. Large destroyed area in the sacral wall with excavation of the vertebral body anteroposteriorly in S1 and laterally

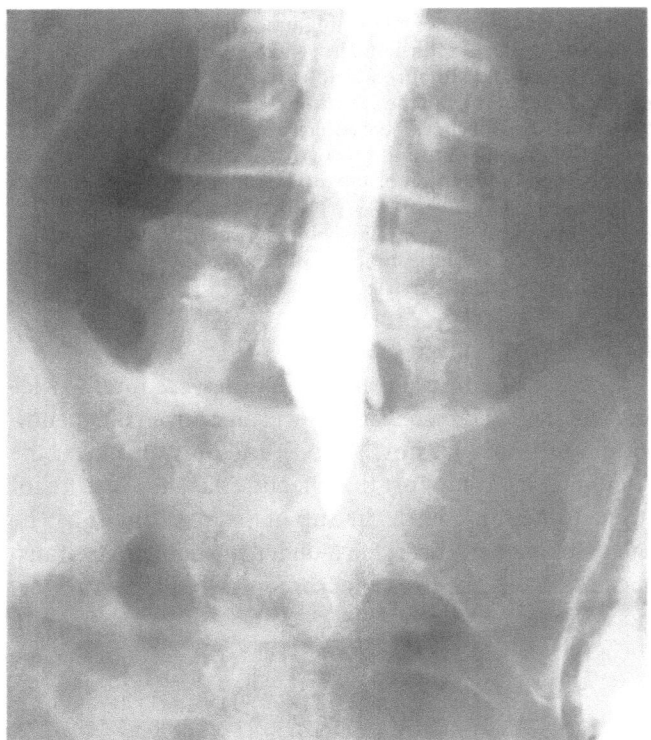

Fig. 129. Radicolography shows a shadow and the amputation of the meningeal sac and roots on the right near the destroyed sacral bone

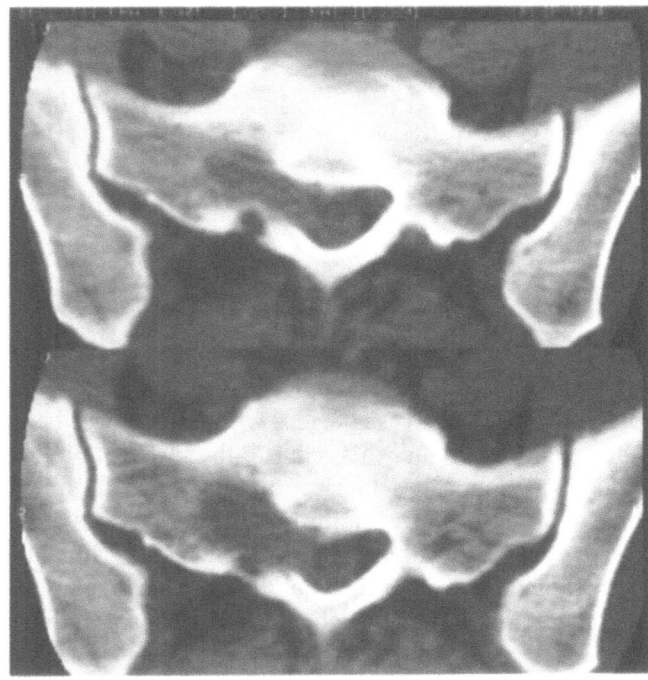

Fig. 130. CT scan: erosion of the sacral bone

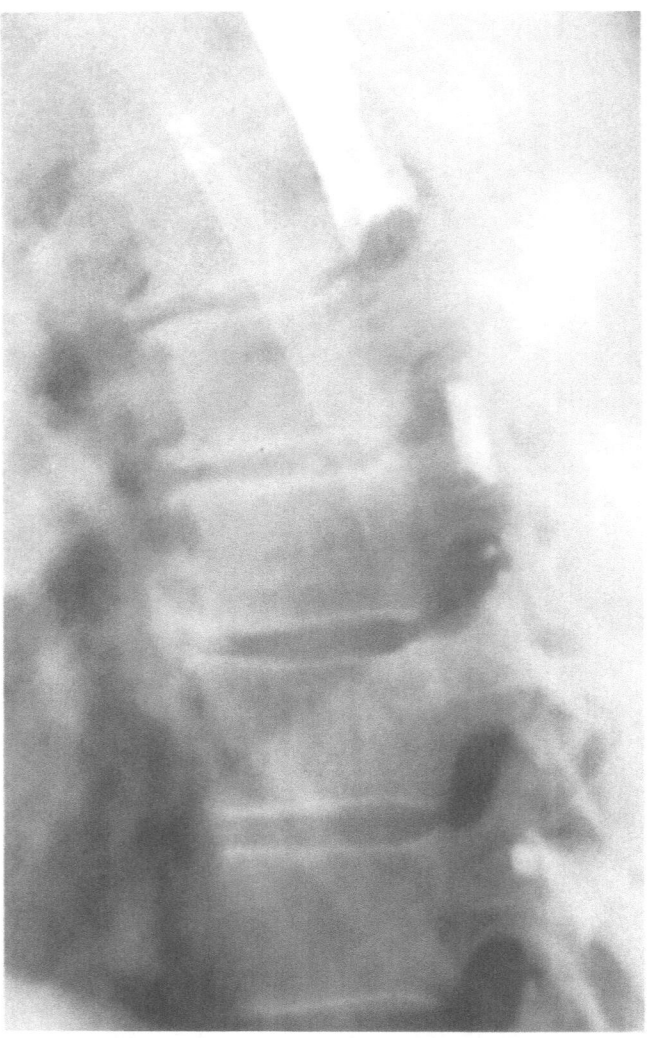

Fig. 131. Suboccipital myelography. Block producing a dome-shaped image in D6-D7. The vertebral body of D9 appears striated as an angiomatous vertebra

Case Nos. 83, 84: Psammomatous Meningioma in Two Sites

A 48-year-old woman (1992). Left posterolateral meningioma in D9-D10 and right premedullary meningioma in D11.

Clinical Course. 10 years. Occasional feeling of "heaviness" in lower limbs on the right with painful paraesthesias along the posterior surface of the right thigh and leg (another hospital suspected disc herniation in L5-S1, and surgery was performed). Dorsolumbar pain then appeared irradiating in girdle-like manner in the suprapubical and inguinal regions on the right. Paraesthesias ascending from the sole of the feet to the right. The patient suffered from motor claudication for 2 years.

Neurological Examination. Hypertonia to right lower limb and slight hypotrophy of left femoral quadricep. Hyperreflexia of patellas. Flaccid ankle jerk. Bilateral Babinski sign. Spastic. Paraparetic deambulation with slight ataxia. Painful and tactile hypoaesthesia from D10 to the right. Hypopallaesthesia from the iliac crests to the right. Retention of urine.

X-Ray of Dorsal Tract. In anteroposterior area, calcified density in D10 between right articulation and spinous process obliquely towards right.

Myelography (via lumbar puncture). Densified contrast medium near the medial tract in D11: oval-shaped filling defect on right. Evident displacement of cord towards left. In D10 the medullary corridor appeared on the right due to block on the left, producing an irregular outline. The iodine contrast medium showed a neoplasm in D11 on the right and a block above on the left (Figs. 132-133).

Myelo-CT. The two compressions were well-defined; the larger was located in D9-D10. In the very clear medial sagittal reconstruction the cord appeared pushed forwards by the posterior compression. The smaller compression below pushed the medullary corridor backwards because of the premedullary compression (Figs. 134-135).

MRI of Dorsal Tract. In D10-D11 extramedullary expansive process 3 cm long in posterolateral site on the left. With gadolinium the two compressions in an extramedullary site were greatly enhanced (Figs. 136-139).

Surgical Treatment. Splitting of the dura and coagulation within its depth of the arachnoidal meningioma's invasion of the internal surface of the dura on the left. The sensory root of D10 covered the tumour as a band. Total removal by fragmentation after having removed the roots from the adherent arachnoidal process. Coagulation of the base of attachment (which was partly calcified). The cord was gently reclined until the second, premedullary, meningioma was revealed on the right of the dura. Removal by fragmentation (Figs. 140-144).

Results. Improvement in motility with regression of sensory disturbances in 1 week. After 1.5 months walking was normal but a minimal degree of ataxia persisted.

The typical vertebral angioma feature appears more precisely on CT (see case no. 100) without, however, being able to define whether this is due to the simple modification of a spongiosa vacularization or to a true modification of a malformative nature. In some cases only MRI can reveal areas of adipose transformation (Fig. 136) in the bone spongiosa of a vertebral body. It must be remembered that these images occur frequently as occasional findings.

Areas of adipose transformation were found twice in rachidian metameres, at some distance from the meningioma site (see case nos. 44, 100), and only once near the tumour level. We report these features as there are histological phenomena in the intrinsic component of the meningiomatous tissue which undergo a lipomatous transformation, visible even macroscopically in the surgical field.

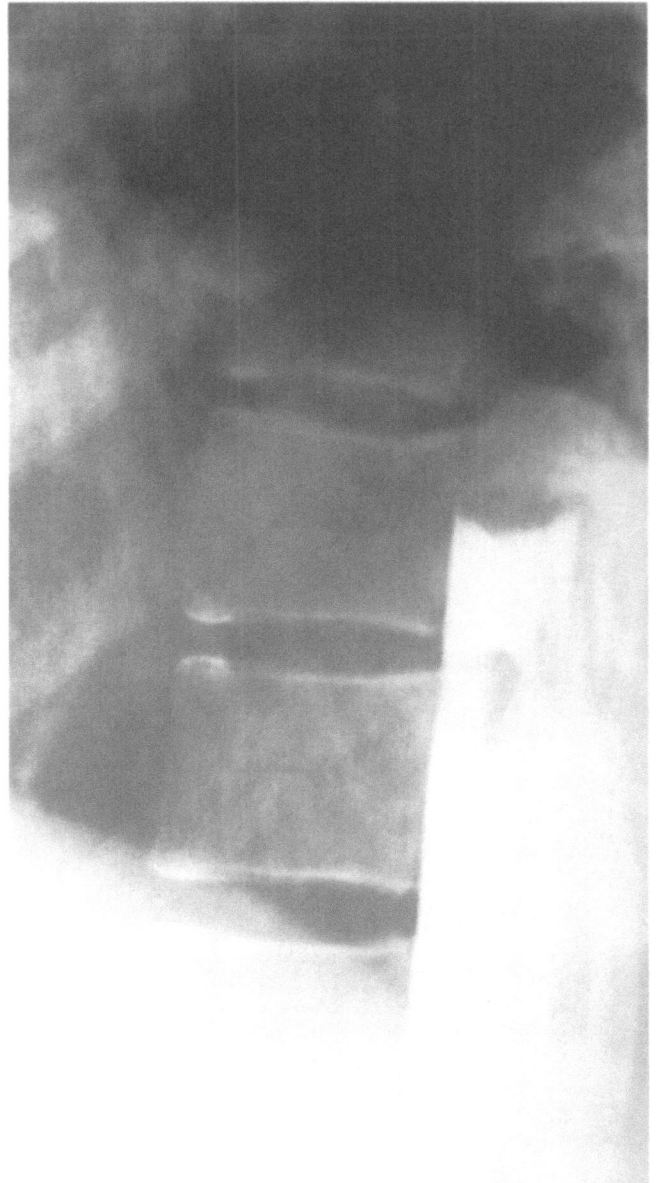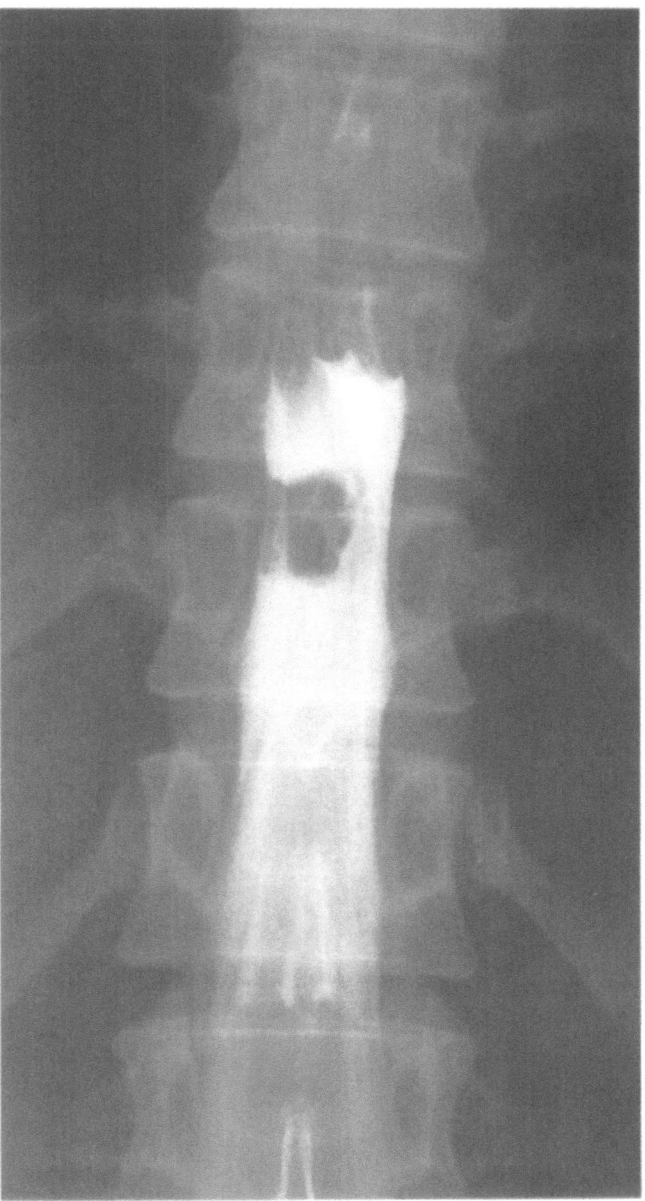

Fig. 132. Myelography via lumbar puncture. In a lateral projection a roundish-shaped filling defect shows the enlarged anterior subarachnoidal space at the upper half of the vertebral body of D11 up to the space D11-D12. The cord appears thinned and displaced towards the back. The contrast medium passes this level and comes to a total block behind the vertebral body of D10. Anteroposteriorly the filling defect produces an image which occupies the canal almost completely at D10-D11 level and is slightly greater on the right. Above this level the subarachnoidal space appears dilated on the left. The cord appears S shaped due to displacement towards the left in D11 and towards the right in D10

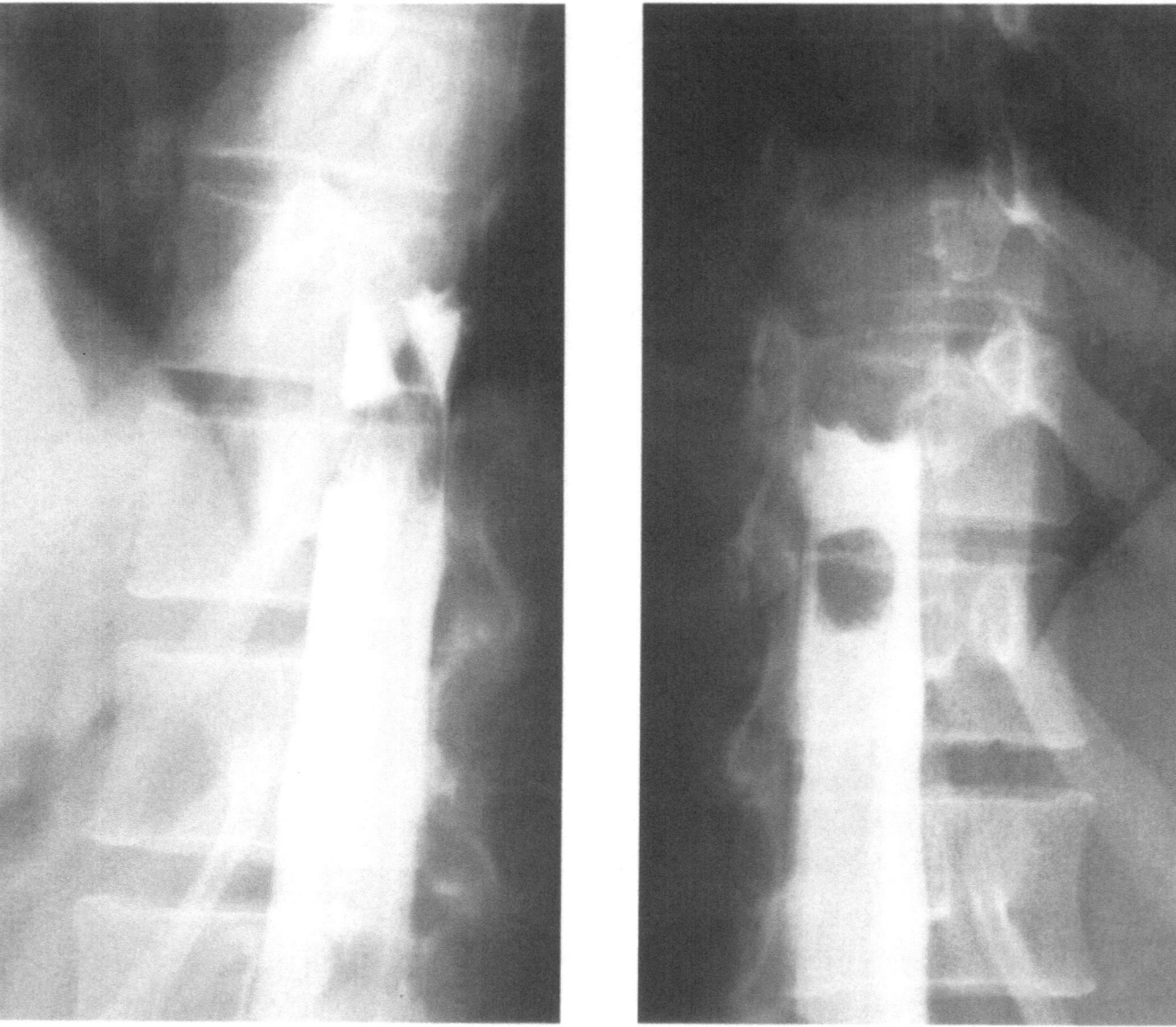

Fig. 133. The two oblique projections, left and right, confirm a double lesion: the smaller one in D11 and predominantly anterior on the right, and the larger one in D9-D10 on the left

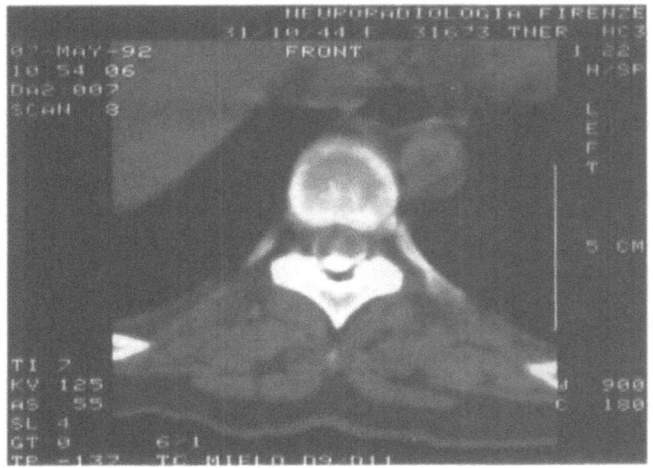
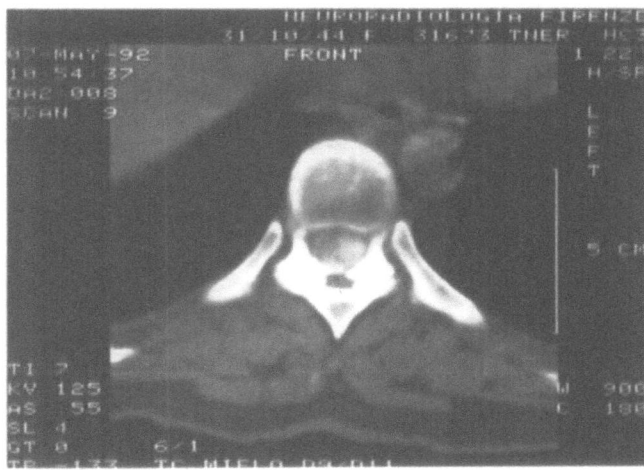
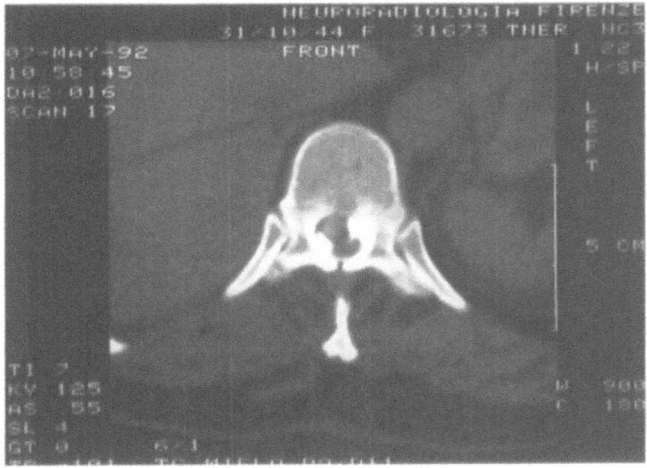

Fig. 134. Myelo-CT. In the sections made at the myelographic filling defects level the lesion is seen in an upper area and extending from D9-D10, occupying the left half of the canal with contralateral displacements of the cord. In the lower sections the totally anterior right lesion appears surrounded by the contrast medium and is seen clearly displaced towards the back of the cord

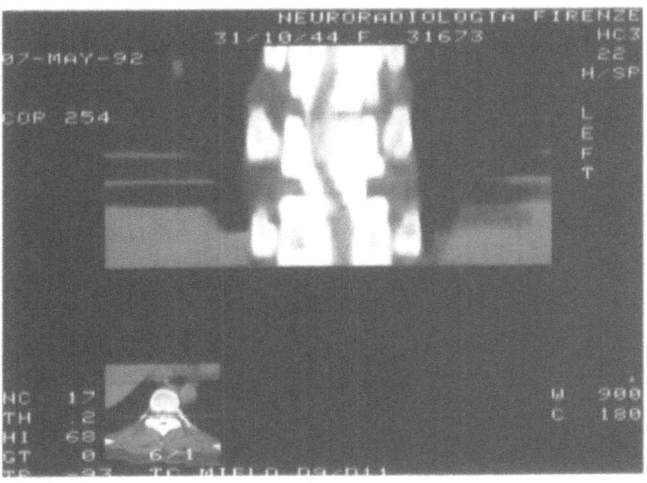
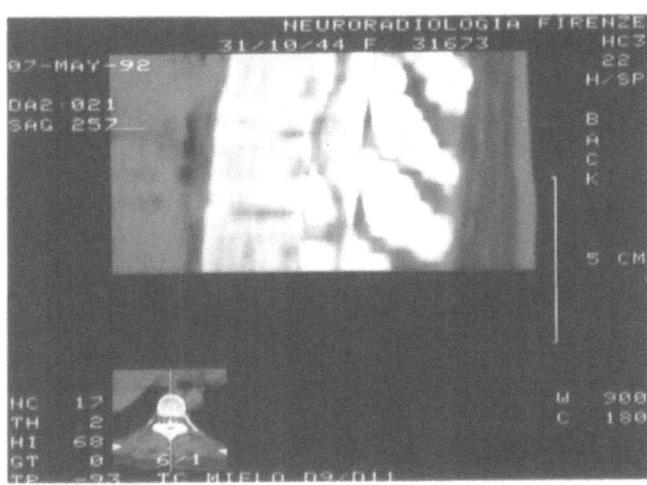

Fig. 135. CT reconstructions. The S-shaped cord with the two lesions is clearly seen

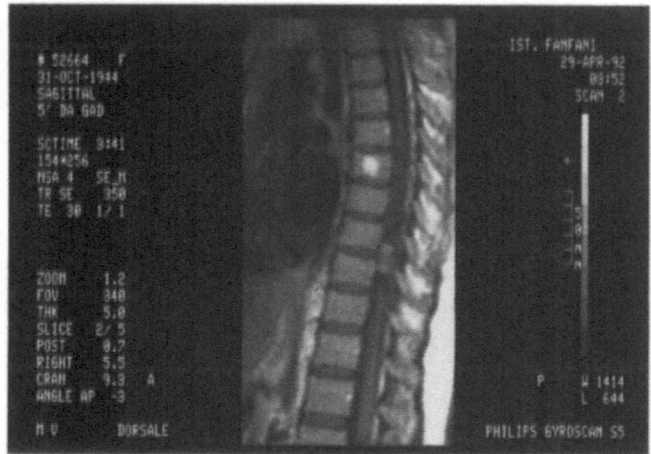

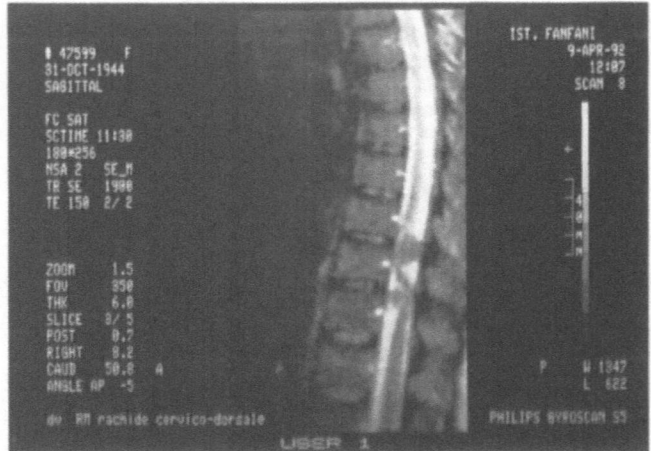

Fig. 136. MRI. Sagittal projections (Figs. 136, 138) and direct coronal projections (Fig. 139) SE T1 (TR 350 ms and TE 30 ms) and sagittal T2 (Fig. 137; TR 1900 ms and TE 150 ms). MRI directly identifies the two lesions which have a slightly isodense signal compared to the cord in the following sequence (SE T1) and isointense in T2. The tract of the cord between the two neoformations appears flattened and confirmed by its S shape. A small lipomatous vertebral area is visible in the vertebral body of D7

Fig. 137. MRI: sagittal projection

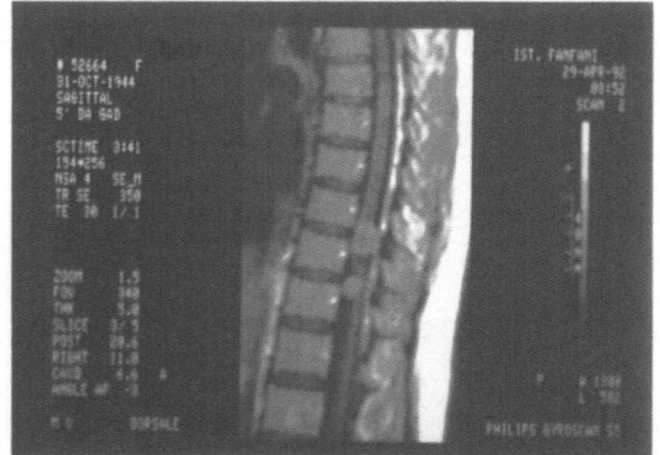

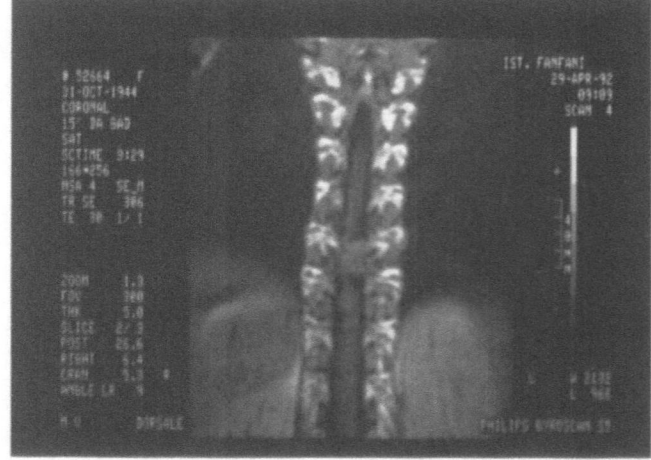

Fig. 138. MRI: sagittal projection

Fig. 139. MRI: coronal projection

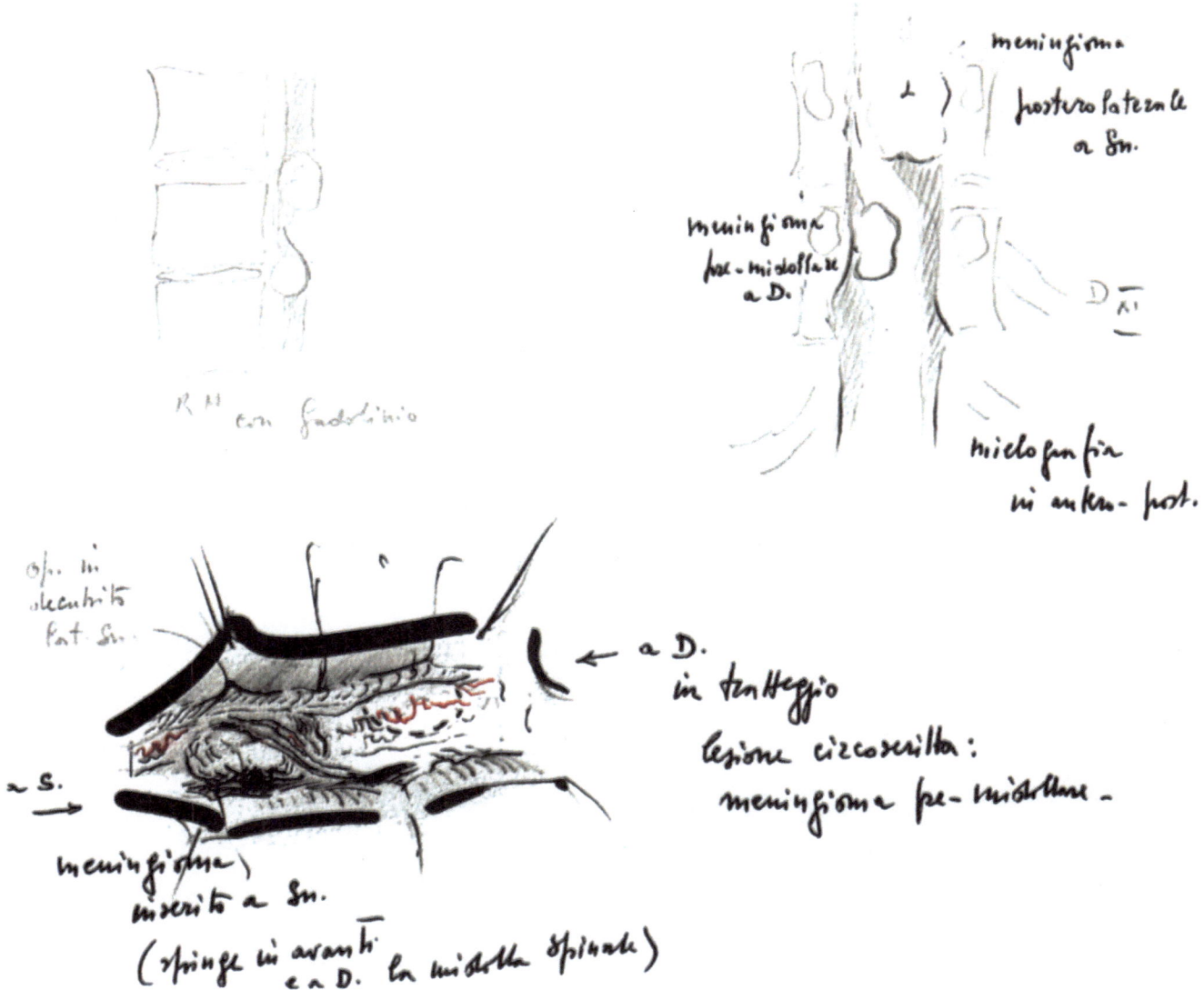

Fig. 140. Diagram of operating field. The splitting of the dura: the left posterolateral meningioma pushes the cord forwards; the right premedullary lesion is outlined

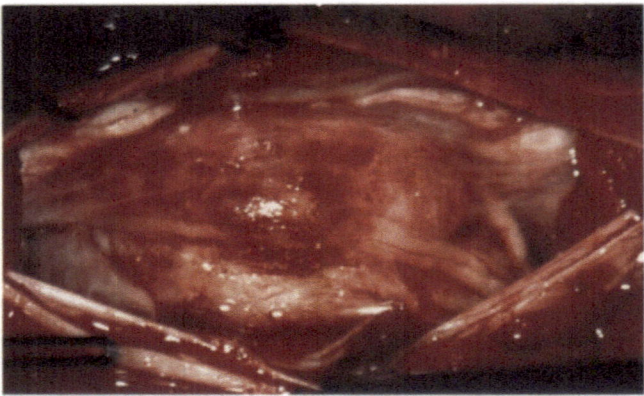

Fig. 141. The operating field with neighbouring meningioma and dura. In this case the splitting of the dura is performed on the left. The tumour is subarachnoidal and adheres to the radicular bundle of D10 and is pushed upwards

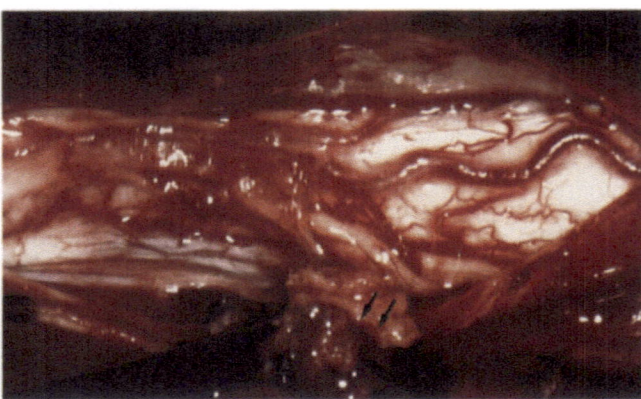

Fig. 142. The removal of the last part of the tumour inserted in the leptomeninges of the dura (*arrow*). The cord is compressed contra-laterally on the right and is partly turned (see Fig. 143)

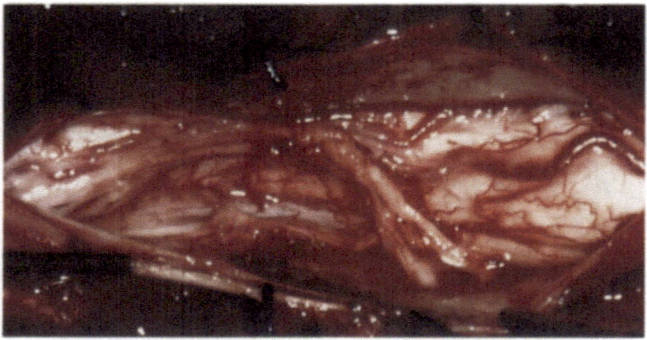

Fig. 143. The operating field with the total removal of the neoplasm. Above the shadow left by the removed meningioma the medullary arterial circulation is dilated and at the same time there are whitish ischaemic areas near an evident protrusion at another pre-medullary meningioma in D11 on the right (see Fig. 144)

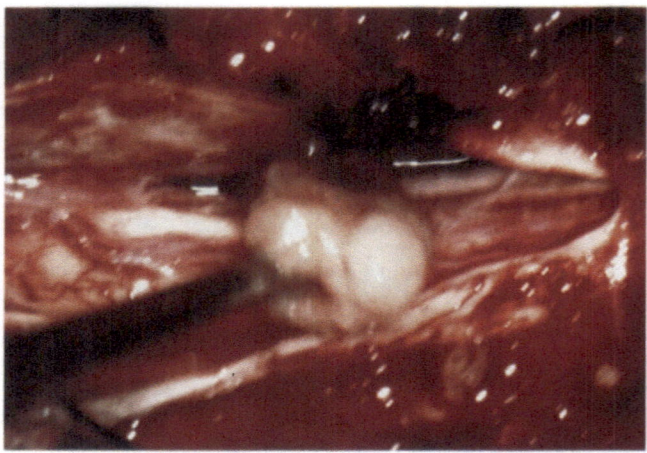

Fig. 144. The totally premedullary meningioma has already been arranged in toto towards the exterior

8.2 Calcifying Features of a Meningioma

The reported frequency of calcifications in meningiomas varies considerably depending on the author (from 1% to 33%). The presence of calcifications detected by X-ray examinations does not always resolve the nature of the calcifications, although those found inside the rachidian canal are almost certainly due to compression. Irregular and scattered calcifications have been described in dermoids and epidermoids by List (1941), Lombardi and Passerini (1964) and Rath et al. (1967). The diagnosis of the nature of a meningioma is reached when the tumour is globally calcified. Not every author would agree that this is a particularly rare condition. *Levy et al. (1982)* report one case in 97 meningiomas, Camp (1938) 4.6%; and Culver et al. (1949) 5 of 15, 33%. Pagni (1989) evaluated other authors'

reports and collected a total of 599 meningiomas, with the addition of two personal cases, reaching an incidence of 3.5%. Most authors seemed to consider the incidence as 1%-2%.

The calcifications described in the literature without the characteristics of an entirely psammomatous meningioma refer to emangioblastoma cases (Cecchini and Gozzini 1984). According to Nittner (1976), calcifications are present in teratomas, ependymomas and neurinomas. There have also been cases of calcifications at arachnoidal level (Herren 1939; Slager 1960). The entirely calcified intrarachidian meningioma seen on X-ray is exceptional, as in the case of intercranial meningiomas. Spinal ones appear as a high-density mass within the rachidian lumen and the image shows almost the entire volume of the tumour. In a stratigraphy the image is not always homogenous, as the central area sometimes seems more compact than the peripheral area where the borders appear less well defined due to a less densely calcified area (Figs. 145, 146). Regarding the calcified aspect of the possible compressive formation in an intrarachidian site we note the rare forms of osteochondroma at thoracic level. These cases can be considered on a neuroradiological differential diagnosis plane as they always refer to post-traumatic lesions which appear after several years, often due to a fall affecting the sacrum or heels (Fig. 147).

Another differential diagnosis case between meningiomas and osteochondromas is represented for the osteochondroma by the evident superimposition of the calcified intrarachidian component with the transversal pattern of most of the disc. The continuity of the disc calcifications with the intrarachidian subligamentous component is clearly visible on CT of the bone as sometimes a cartilaginous rupture of the anulus fibrosus is clearly seen (Fig. 148). MRI facilitates a differential diagnosis in these rare cases as it identifies the rupture and the reaction above and below the point at which the chondroma is seen across the posterior longitudinal ligament (Fig. 149). There are also meningiomas that appear as a homogene-

ous calcareous mass (Pear and Boyd 1974). A more accurate incidence of these pathological features can be obtained by observing the number of meningiomas studied on CT. It is more sensitive than direct X-ray or stratigraphy due to the use of contrast medium and axial scans which eliminate overlapping. When the calcifications on an X-ray are minute and scattered it is difficult to determine whether they lie deep in the meningioma or whether it involves expansive processes of a different nature.

In our series of 432 primary spinal tumours we found complete calcification of the meningioma only twice (cases 66, 38). In 18 cases we have identified direct radiographic features such as small congenital anomalies: three cases of synostosis in C2-C3 (body and laminae), one of which affected only the laminae with meningioma below in D1-D2, D2-D3, D10-D11 (cases 53, 59, 100).

Case No. 100: Transitional Meningioma
A 73-year-old woman (1988). Right ventrolateral intradural-extramedullary meningioma in D2-D3.
Medical History. Right hemiparesis of an unknown nature 20 years before hospital admission.

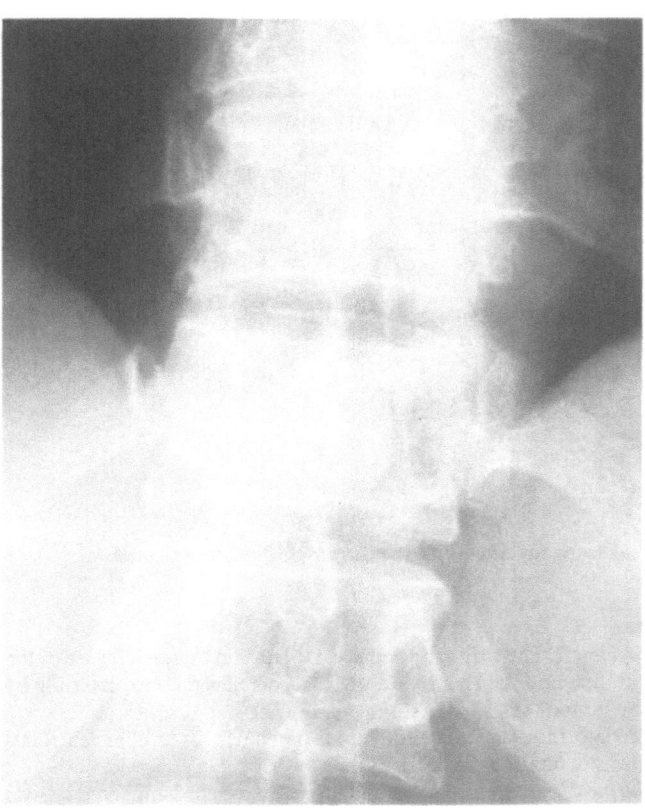

Fig. 145. X-ray of dorsal rachis with stratigraphy. In an anteroposterior projection, left-convex scoliosis. A roundish calcified type of structure is seen at the vertebral body of D11. The medial side of the right articular facet in D11 appears eroded. The transverse diameter of the rachis is wider

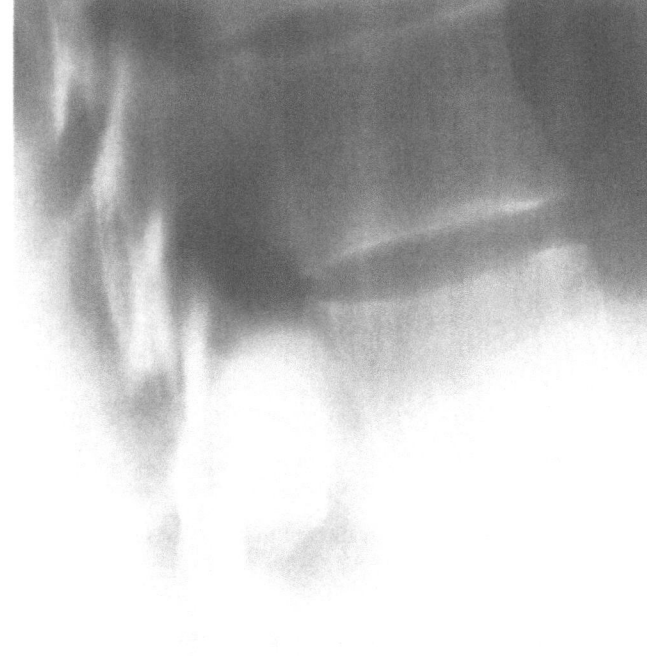

Fig. 146. The lesion in lateral projection appears inside the vertebral canal

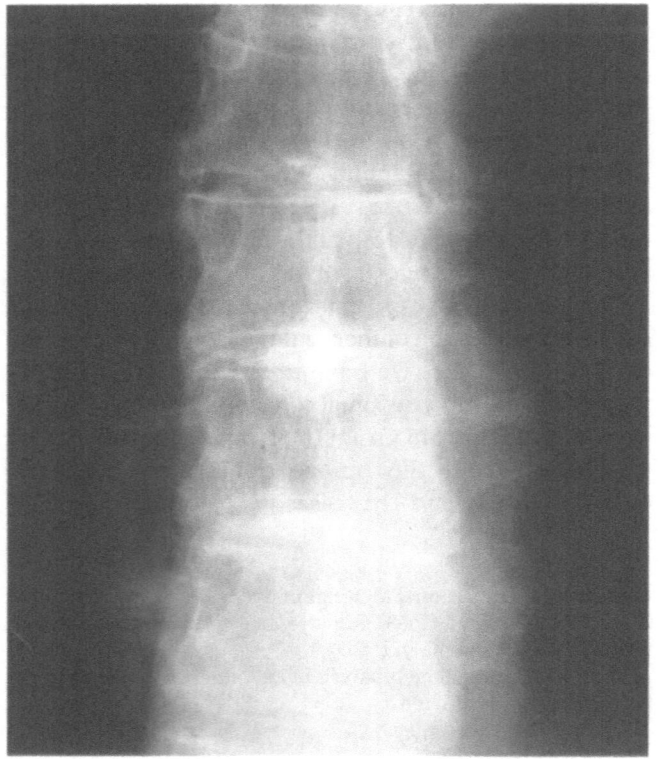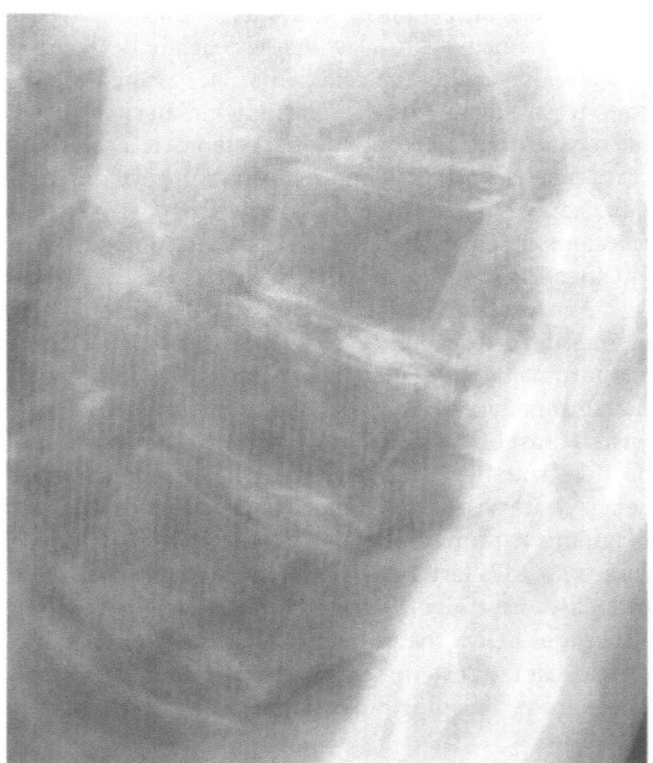

Fig. 147. Chondroma on plain x-ray films

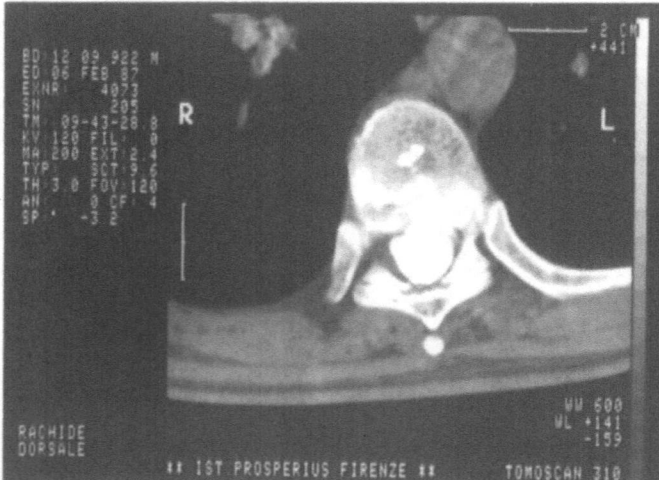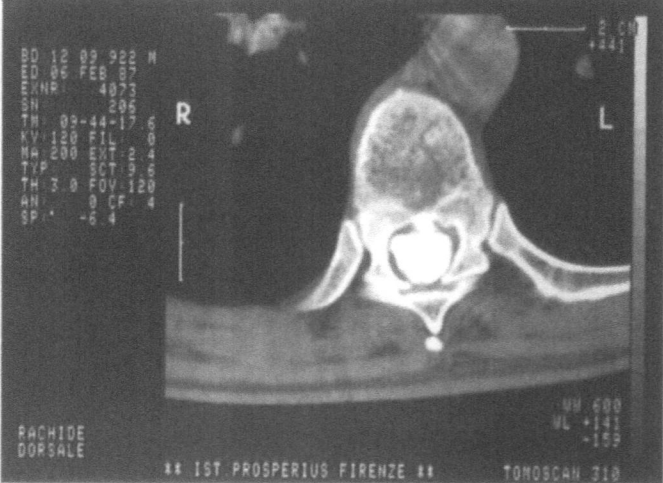

Fig. 148. The posterior calcification of the disc is visualized on the two dorsal scans together with the intrarachidian chondroma

Clinical Course. 1 year. Cold sensation type of paraesthesias, at both lower limbs followed by motor claudication to the right; 6 months later the patient complained of band-like constriction sensation at abdomen, with difficulty in walking.

Neurological Examination. Spastic paraparesis with right Babinski sign. Hypoaesthesia from D9, distally pronounced. Sphincter disturbances in the form of incontinence.

X-Ray of Cervical Rachis. Synostosis C2-C3 (Fig. 150).

X-Ray of Dorsal Rachis. Scoliosis on medial tract. Angioma of vertebral body in D11.

Myelography. Partial block in D2 producing a dome-shaped filling defect.

Myelo-CT. The scans showed great dilatation on the left side of the sub-arachnoidal space, and the cord displaced controlaterally by the tumour (Figs. 151-152).

MRI. Intradural-extramedullary lesion at D2-D3 level in ventrolateral site on the right (Fig. 153).

Surgical Treatment. On opening the dura the cord appeared curved posteriorly with a reduction in the surface-layer blood supply. Exploring the right showed the neoplasm with its anterolateral invasion on the right. Removal of the arachnoidal adherent structure. Incision of tumourous capsule and excision by fragmentation. Coagulation of base of attachment.

Results. Postoperative motor inhibition to lower right limb accompanied by cord paraesthesias to the right. From the third day clear recovery of the motility on the right. After 10 days walking exercises and after 6 months the patient achieved clinical recovery and normal walking.

Case No. 59: Meningothelial Meningioma
A 63-year-old man (1985). Left posterolateral and anterior intradural-extramedullary meningioma in D1-D2.
Medical History. Diabetes.
Clinical Course. 7 months. Dorsal pain followed by motor deficit of left lower limb after 3 months, with an impediment in walking. The patient complained of a band-like constriction sensation in the upper dorsal area. Three months prior to hospitalization the same symptoms appeared on the right with an ingravescent nature leading to paraplegia.
Neurological Examination. Flaccid paraplegia. Equinism of right foot. Diffused flaccidity of muscular masses. Left Babinski sign. Hypoaesthesia from D4 which became anaesthesia distally. Sphincter disturbances in the form of retention.
Rachicentesis. 0.70 g protein per thousand.
X-Ray of Cervical and Dorsal Rachis. Slight scoliosis. Synostosis C2-C3 (Fig. 154). Thinning of peduncle of D3 on the right.
Myelography (via lumbar puncture). Almost total block in D1-D2. Slight lateral flow defining neoplasm on the right. Ample dilatation of subarachnoidal and sublesional space posteriorly and laterally (Fig. 155).
MRI. Tumour in D1-D2 with narrowing visible of cord above and below.
Surgical Treatment. Tumour well incapsulated and of pinkish colour compressing the cord towards the right. Freeing the arachnoid from adherent structures and observing the invasion on the internal dural surface corresponding to the dural funnel of D2 on the left. Removal of adhering process and removal of neoplasm en bloc. Severe atrophy of the cord which, however, retained a considerably dilatated surface-layer circulation (Figs. 156, 157).
Results. A few hours after regaining consciousness, the patient was affected by Jacksonian convulsions at brachial-facial muscles on the left which occurred with prolonged hypotension. The patient was taken to the intensive care unit where he died due to loss of metabolic equilibrium.

There were small dysmorphia regarding the hypoplastic and upward arch of L5 associated with the asymmetry of the metemere laminae above, with a megalamina on one. Schistasis of L5-S1 with mega-apophysis above in a mengioma case in D1-D2. Spondylosis and spondylolisthesis in L4-L5 in a meningioma case in D9. One of our patients with a lesion in D11; synostosis of the laminae of C2-C3, with a vertebral angiomatous aspect visualized on CT. Another patient, aged 64 years presented a meningioma in C4-C5 associated with some small laminae dysmorphias in the dorsal tract accompanied by a diffused medialization of the articular interlines due to congenital stenosis in L1-L3. This patient suffered from congenital luxation of the hip (Figs. 158, 159).

Case No. 49: Meningothelial Meningioma
A 64-year-old woman (1977). Left posterolateral extradural meningioma in C4, C5 enveloping the roots C5-C7.
Medical History. Congenital luxation of the hip bilaterally. Operated on at age 25 and 48 years.
Clinical Course. 5 years. Impediment in walking, worsening and cervical pain. One year before hospitalization lack of strength in the

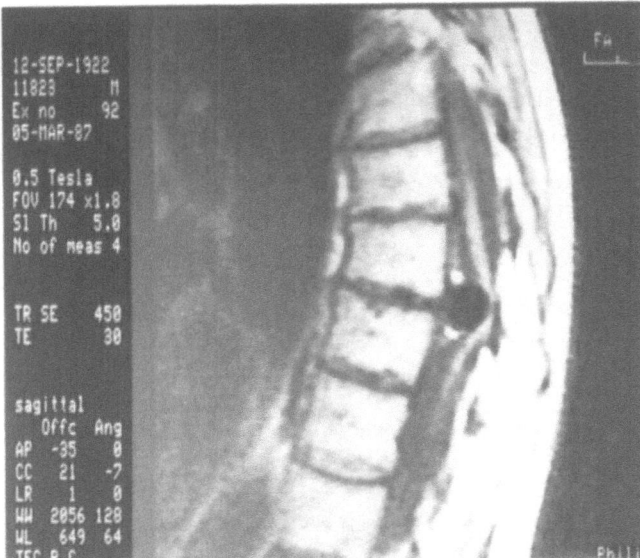

Fig. 149. MRI. Sagittal projection T1 (TR 450, TE 30 ms). Large roundish-shaped area without signal, compared to the high calcium content at the intersomatic space D8-D9. Two small areas with high signal are seen at the upper and lower poles of the tumour with the thickening of the posterior longitudinal ligament

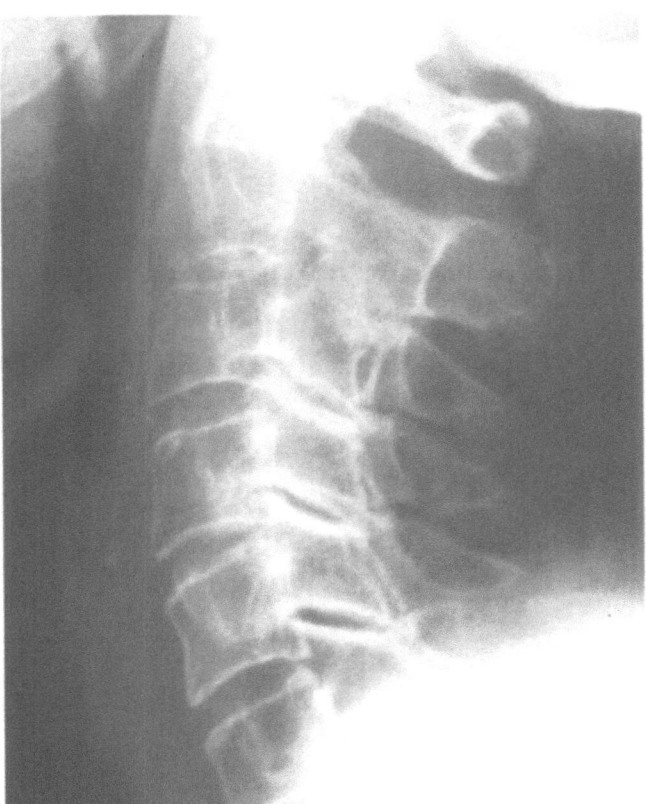

Fig. 150. Plain X-ray of cervical rachis in lateral projection. Sinostosis of the laminae of C2-C3

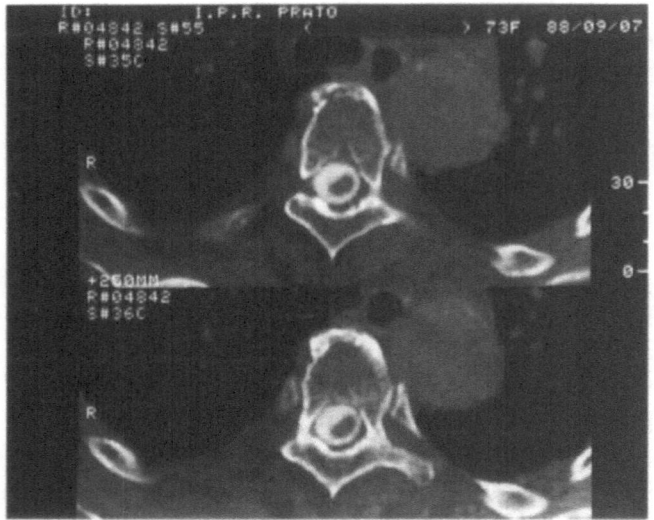 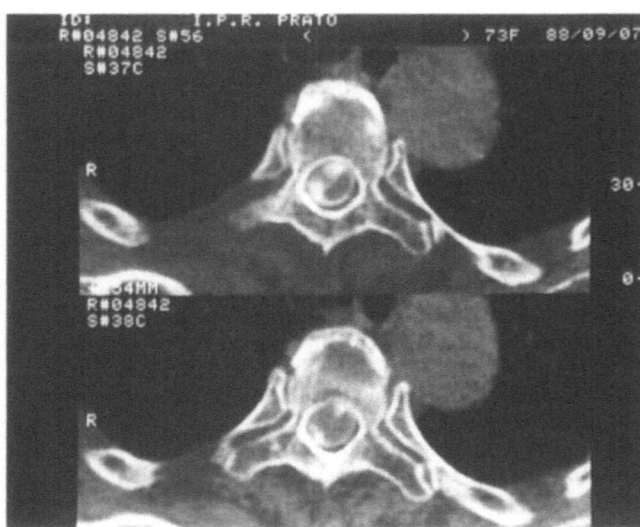

Fig. 151. Myelo-CT performed after the myelography via lumbar puncture which shows a dome-shaped block in D2. The scans show great dilatation on the left side of the subarachnoidal space and the cord is displaced contralaterally by the tumour

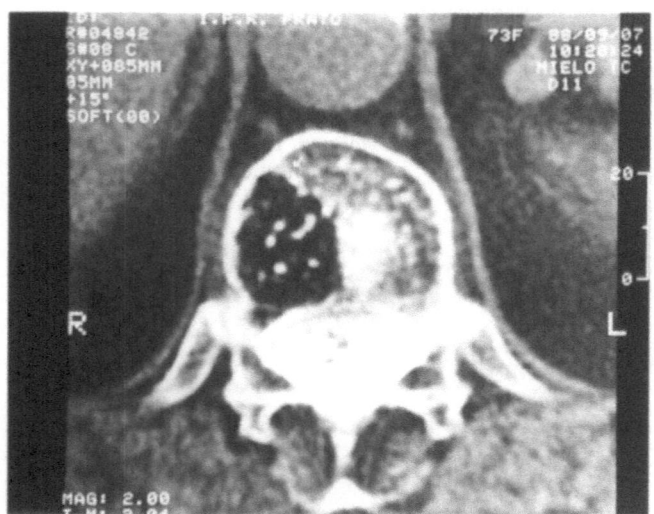 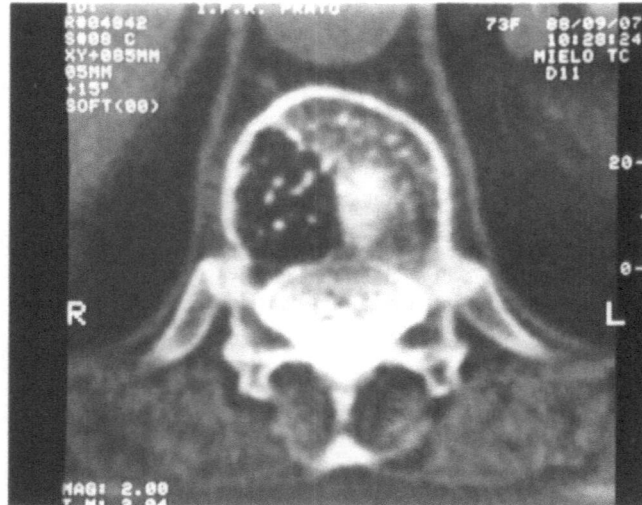

Fig. 152. Scans relating to the same case documenting angiomatosis of the right hemisome

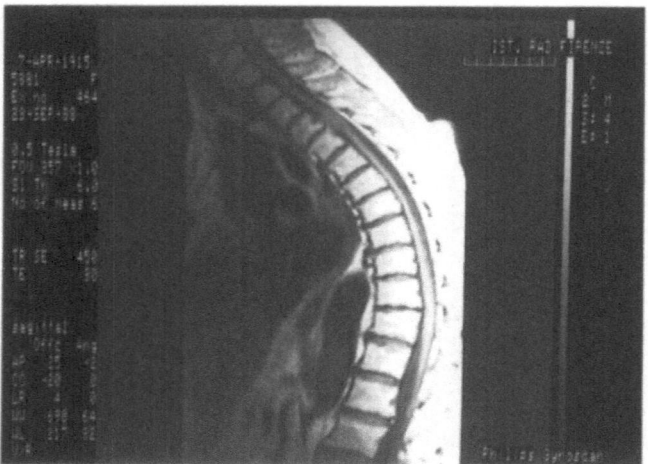 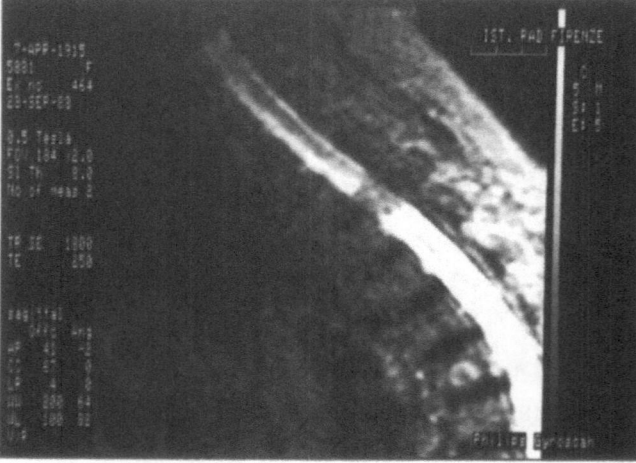

Fig. 153. MRI of dorsal rachis. Sagittal projection SE T1 (TR 450 ms and TE 30 ms) and T2 (TR 1800 ms TE 250 ms) direct test. An oval shaped neoformation with regular margins in D2-D3 with intense signals as for the posteriorly displaced cord

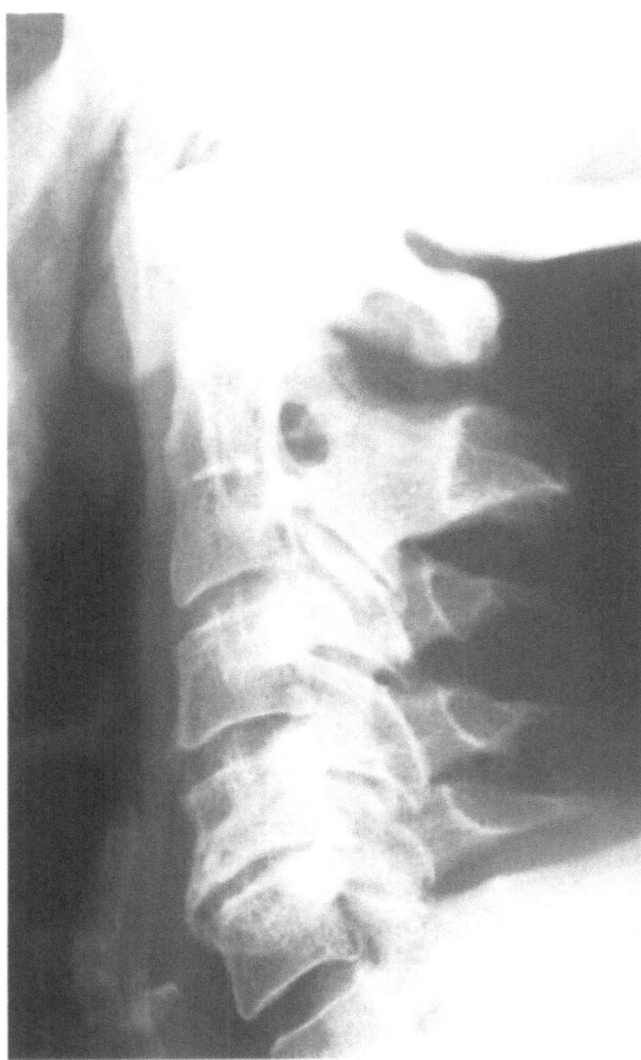

Fig. 154. Myelography via lumbar puncture. Almost total block in D1-D2 on the left. A very slight flow of contrast medium passes the block and surrounds the oval-shaped lesion, defining also its upper pole. The subarachnoidal space appears widened on the left

hands and later in the lower limbs, with rapidly ingravescent characteristics leading to severe paraparesis.

Neurological Examination. Severe paresis of both hands to the left and unable to clench a fist. Hypotrophy of the first interosseous bilaterally. Good reflexes except for the right deltoid. Severe spastic paraparesis to the right (Levy grade 3). Hypoaesthesia from C6. Sphincter disturbances in the form of retention.

Rachicentesis. 0.42 g protein per thousand.

X-Ray of Cervical Rachis. Discoarthrosis with posterior esostosis in C5-C6 and C6-C7.

X-Ray of Lumbosacral Rachis. Left convex scoliosis with rotation of vertebral bodies. Dysmorphia of posterior arch with upturned laminae. The articular interlines in L2-L4 were medialized.

Myelography (performed suboccipitally). Transitory block in C3-C4: the iodine contrast medium partly passed this level on the left with block in C4-C5 (Fig. 158).

Surgical Treatment. The meningioma occupied an extradural site adhering to the posterior and lateral surface of the dura on the left. The roots of C5-C7 were enveloped by the tumour. Total microscopic removal after foramenoctomy. The neoplasm invaded the

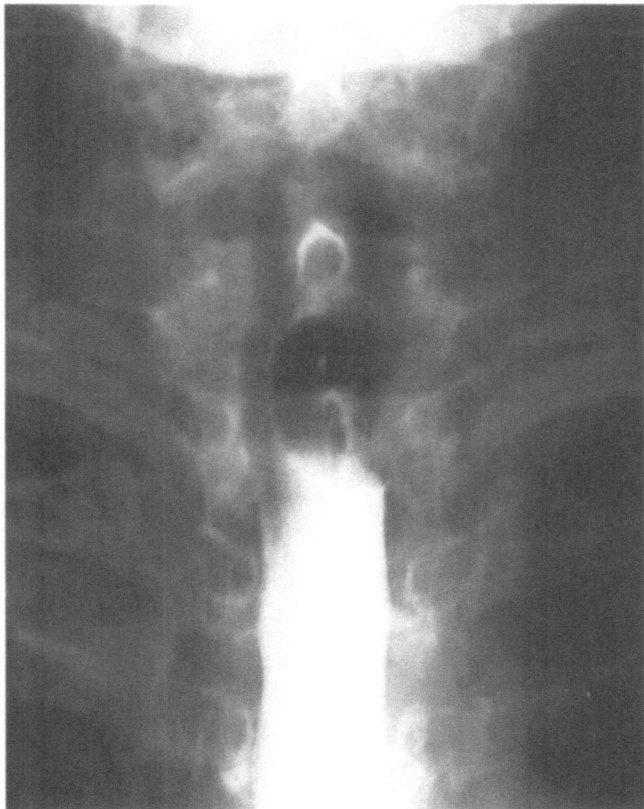

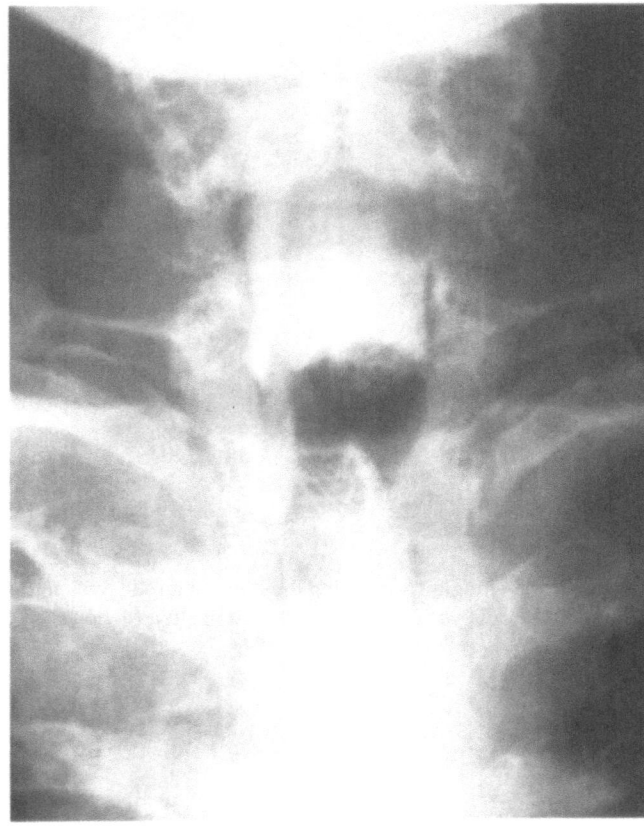

Fig. 155. Myelography: almost total block in D1-D2

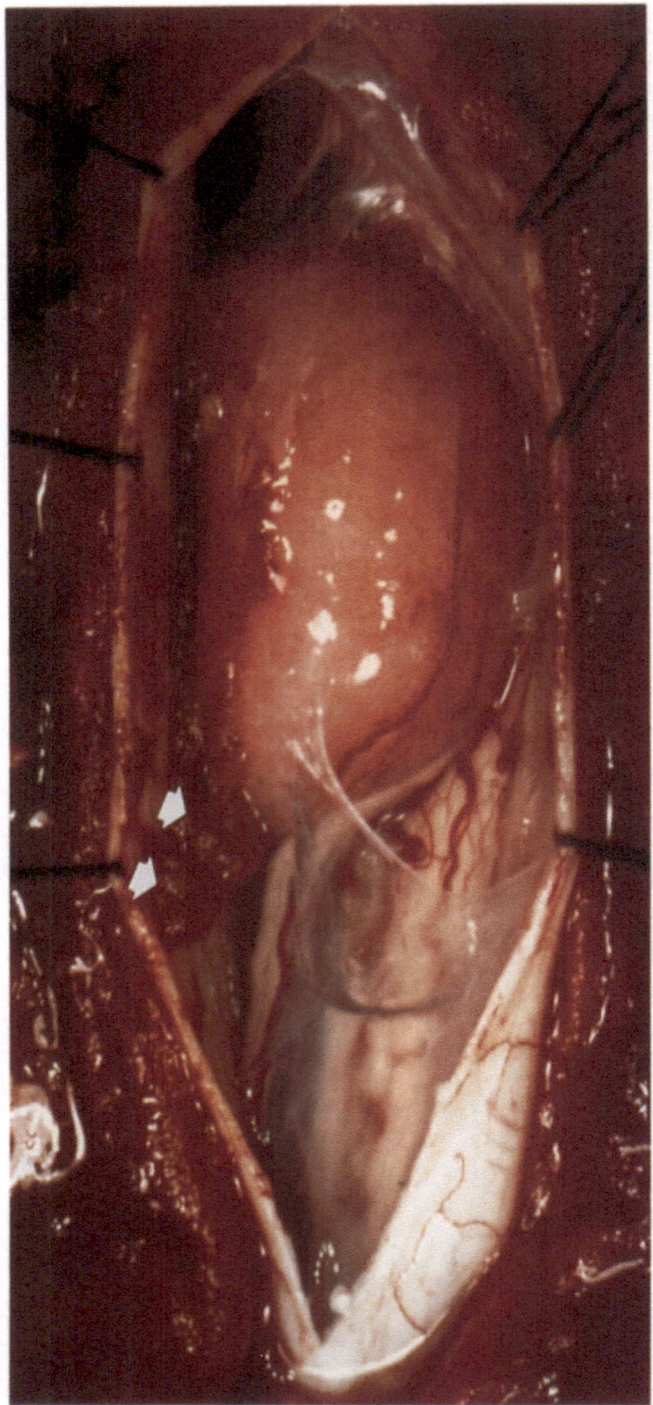

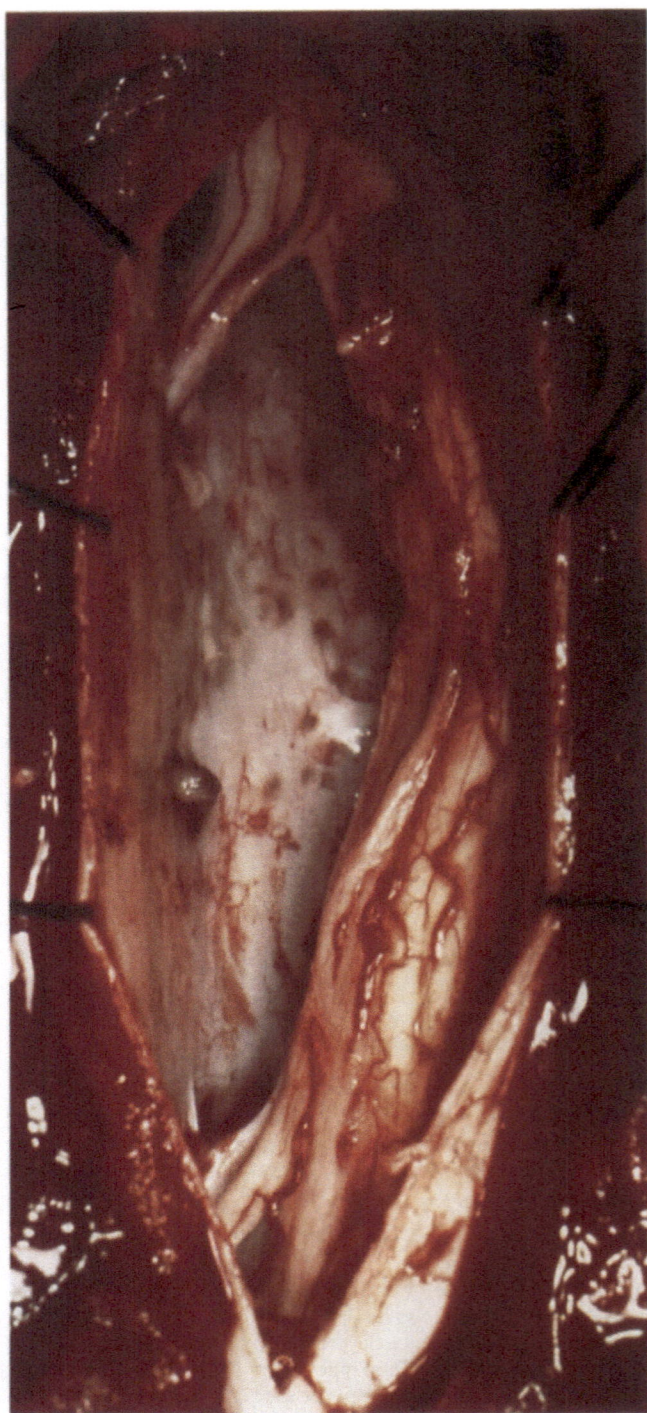

Fig. 156. The meningioma invading the internal dural layer on the left envelops a root with angiectatic vascularization (*arrow*)

Fig. 157. The greatly displaced cord which maintains a good surface layer circulation. The internal ventral surface layer of the dura shows an increased capillary bed

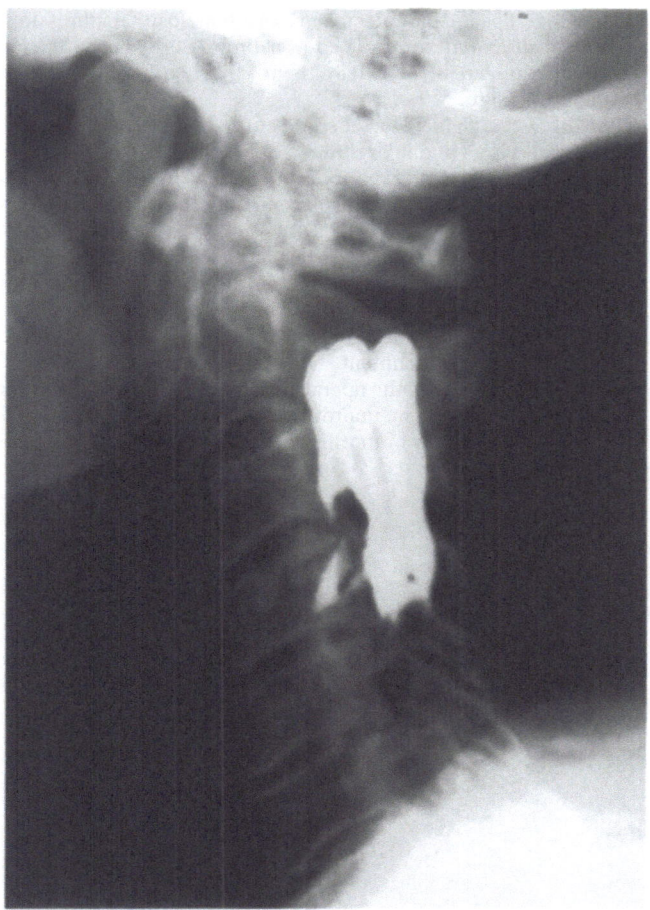
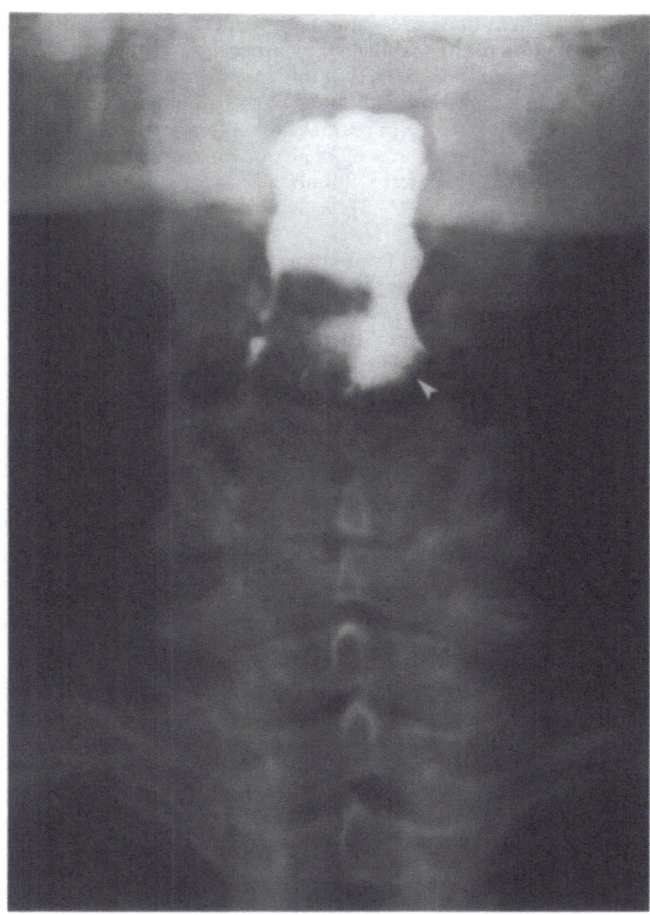

Fig. 158. Suboccipital myelography. Transitory block in C3-C4. A small amount of contrast medium passes the block on the left, filling the left radicular pocket (*arrow*), and comes to a complete block in C4-C5 producing a negative image of the cord displaced towards the right

anterior and lateral epidural space near the roots (Fig. 159).

Results. Gradual recovery of motility leading to walking without support for about 5 years. Following this the patient complained of paraesthesias in the form of a tingling sensation and cramp-like pains to the feet and legs to the right. Simultaneously the patient presented a deteriorating lack of strength in the lower limbs and hypoaesthesia in the left hand. During the following 2 years the patient developed paraesthesias and loss of strength even in the upper right limb. In the following months violent attacks of cervical pain and a further deterioration of paraparesis leading to incapability of standing upright and walking.

Neurological Examination. (1986) The patient was admitted to hospital for a second time 9 years after the operation. Lack of strength in the hands with severe hypotrophy of the interosseous, thenar and hypothenar eminence. Spastic paraparesis; only slight flexion of the thigh and the leg on the right side was possible (Levy grade 3). Hypoaesthesia from D7. Sphincter disturbances in the form of retention.

Rachicentesis. 0.98 g protein per thousand.

Myelography (via lumbar puncture). Block at half the height of the vertebral body of C7.

CT. In C4-C6 (at level of previous laminectomy) vast hypodense area behind the vertebral bodies from a calcified residue. Surgical instructions for another operation which was not performed, due to the patient's severe cardiac insufficiency. In addition to the dysmorphia described above, malformations of the meningeal sheaths of a meningocele nature reached the first sacral metameres with par-

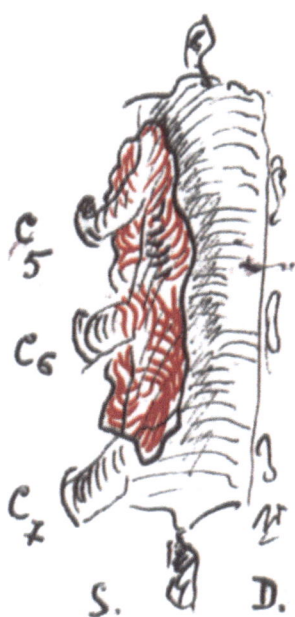

Fig. 159. Postoperative plan with details of the extradural meningioma's location enveloping C5-C7

ticularly evident bone excavations. In the lateral projections the ventral portion of the malformed meningeal sac corresponded to the bone excavation in S1. MRI in this case identified a meningioma in D9. In connection with other bone pathologies previously noted by Cushing (1938) in cranial meningiomas we observed a meningioma in D8-D9 in a 67-year-old woman suffering from Paget's disease on the lower left limb.

Case No. 119: Transitional Psammomatous Meningioma

A 72-year-old woman (1972). Intradural-extramedullary meningioma in D6-D7.

Medical History. Paget's on the left femur (Fig. 160)

Clinical Course. 20 years. For some time the patient had complained of weakness in the right lower limb. For 8 months there was a further lack of strength with contracture in flexing the lower limbs and the beginning of paraesthesias in the lower thoracic and abdominal regions. Spastic paraplegia developed on hospital admission.

Neurological Examination. The lower limbs were kept in flexion and abduction, unable to extend them actively or passively. Bilateral Babinski sign.

X-Ray of Dorsal Spine. Dorsal spine curved due to arthrosis and anterior ankylosis of one or more vertebral bodies.

Myelography (performed suboccipitally). Block in D6-D7 with lateral flow on the left. Evident displacement of the medullary corridor towards the left (Fig. 161).

Surgical Treatment. The cord was displaced towards the left. Below the arachnoid and adhering to the dura on the right there was haemorrhagic tumoural tissue of a reddish-wine colour (Figs. 162, 163). Incision of the tumoural surface, debulking and total removal. Coagulation of the attachment.

Results. A few days after the operation slight flexation of the lower limbs persisted but with an improvement in sensation. After 2 weeks first signs of a recovery of motility of the lower limbs.

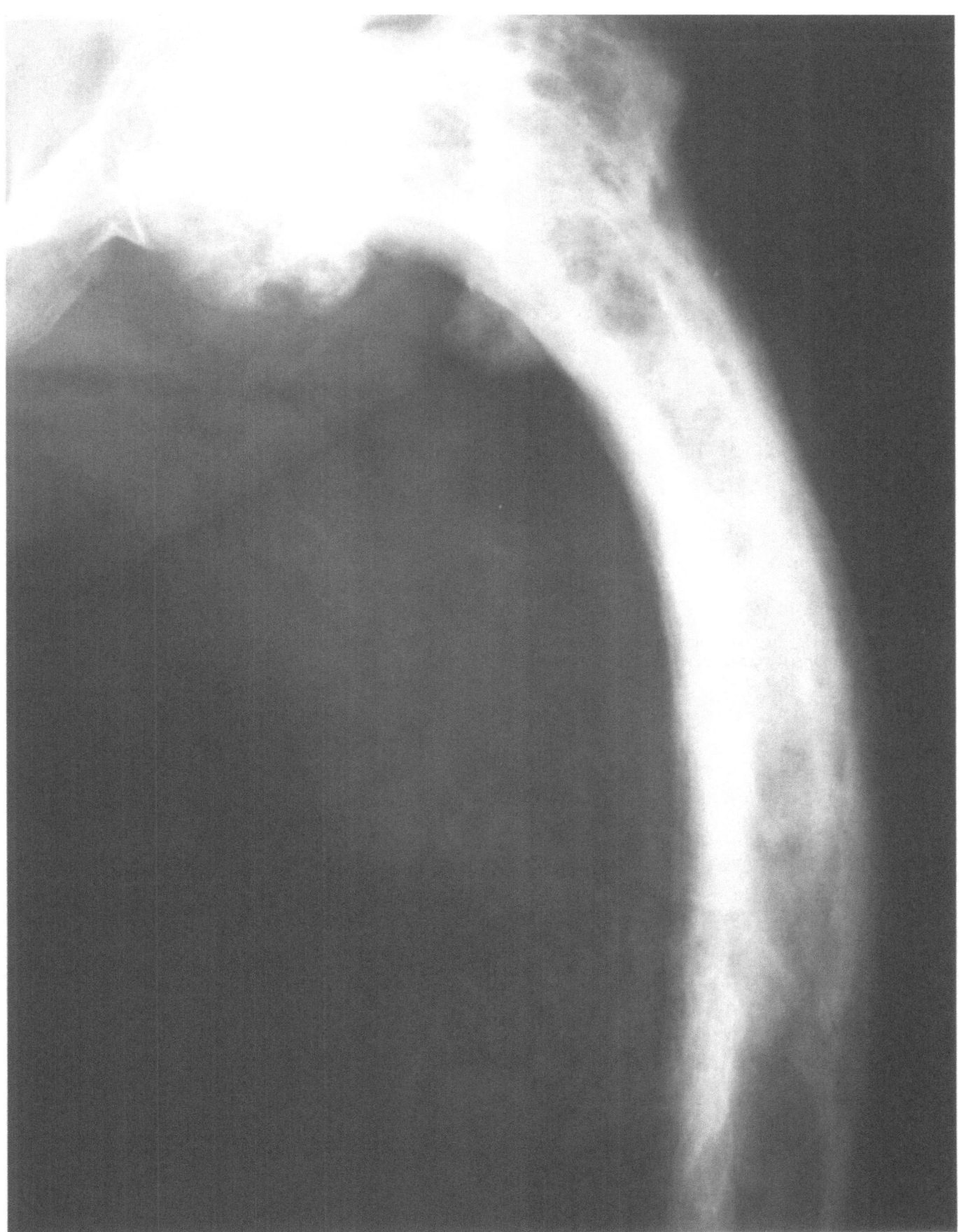

Fig. 160. Paget's disease of the left femur

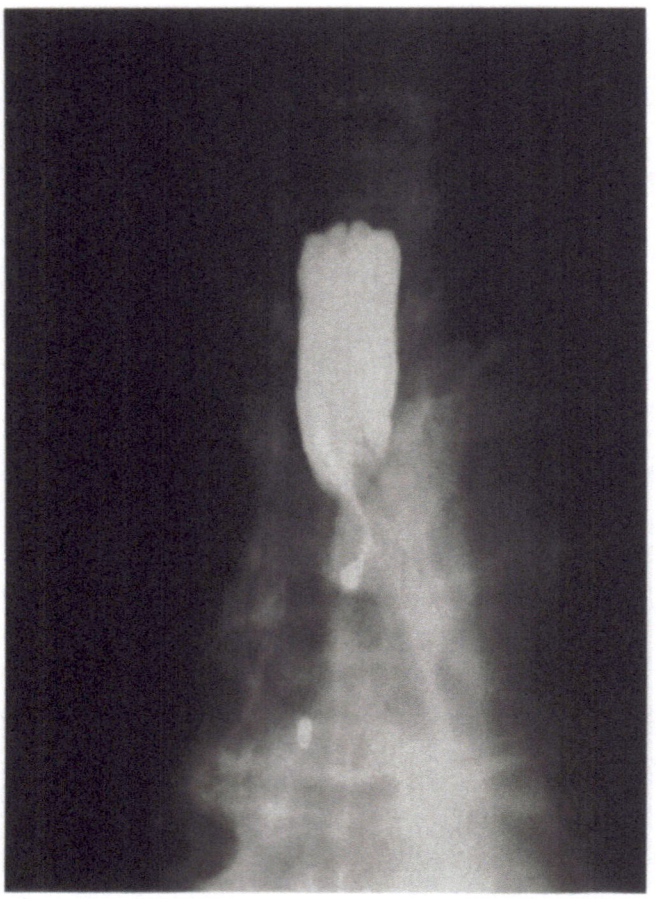

Fig. 161. Suboccipital myelography. Anteroposteriorly, block in D6-D7 on the right defining the expansive lesion displacing the cord to the left

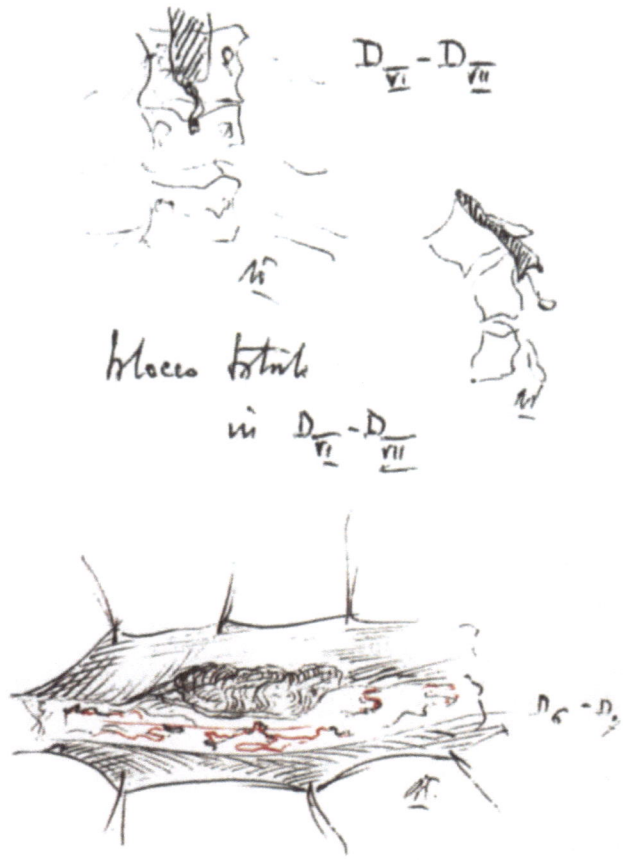

Fig. 162. Scheme of the myelography and the operating field

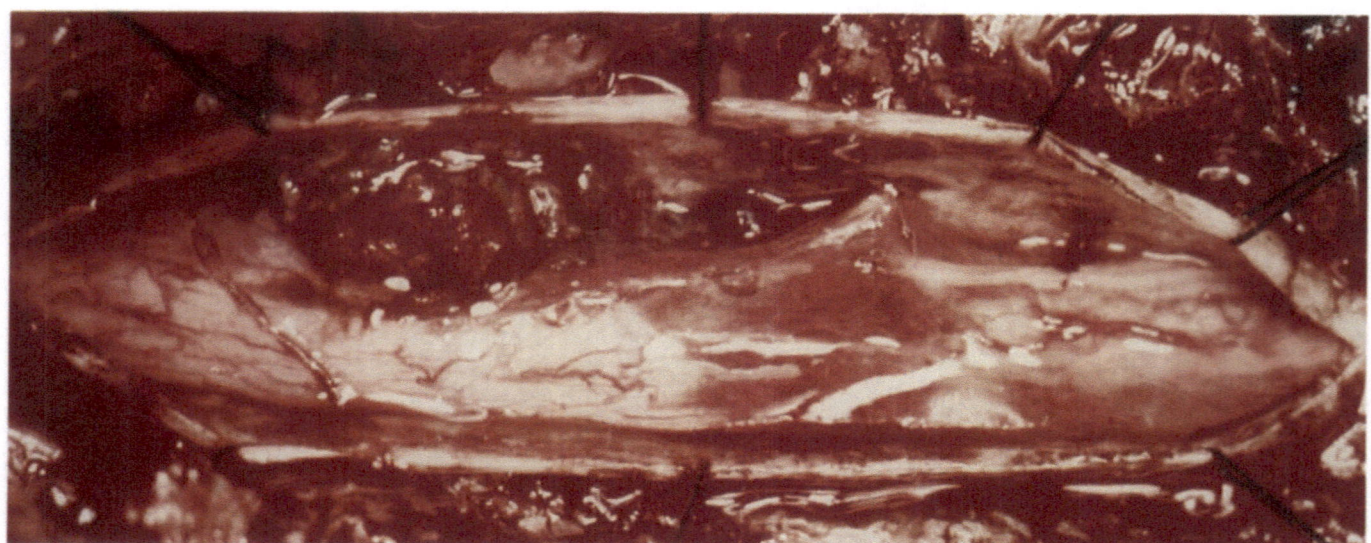

Fig. 163. The tumour, below the arachnoid, displaces the spinal cord laterally

8.3 Neuroradiological Diagnostic Examinations

Continuous progress in the neuroradiological field has provided us today with instruments such as CT and MRI which enable us to identify every form of endorachidian pathology. They not only supply us with images, through which we can identify various features of tumour compressions but also increase our field of vision thereby making it possible to visualize the tissue adjacent to the site where the lesion has formed. Although we are thankful for the outstanding results that we can achieve with modern diagnostic methods in meningiomas, we still rely on myelographic results which continue to be extremely valuable. For this reason we compare the various methods used for a complete preoperative examination.

8.3.1 Myelography

In 98% of cases myelography assists in the diagnosis of the tumour site, its relationship with the meningeal sheath, cord displacement and alterations in the subarachnoidal space. For many years the myelographic examination was performed suboccipitally with lipiodol (Sicard 1922) and was the only diagnostic aid for identifying the level of the compression, offering a valuable means of determining the nature of endorachidian neoplasms. In cases with very small tumours it is sometimes necessary to adjust the patient's position if satisfactory results are not achieved by slowing the flow of the iodine contrast medium along the subarachnoidal space.

Every total or partial block produces an image which corresponds to the upper pole of the tumour but when the iodine contrast medium flow stops, producing a dome-shaped image, this does not mean that the problem of a differential diagnosis between a meningioma and a neurinoma has been resolved (Figs. 164, 165). An iodine contrast medium produces an irregular block more often in meningioma cases. Another favourable feature in diagnosing a meningioma is the image of the dural sac showing as a straight line because of the attachment of the tumour to that side.

Case No. 56: Transitional Meningioma
A 75-year-old woman (1987). Right posterolateral intradural-extramedullary meningioma in D7-D8.
Medical History. Diabetes.
Clinical Course. 3 years. Initial acute motor deficit manifested by sudden weakness of the lower limbs. Fracture of the left femur. The patient recovered walking ability 4 months before hospitalization. Slight motor claudication accompanied by paraesthesias at right lower limb.
Neurological Examination. Presence of a dyschromic birthmark at the right thigh level. Spastic paraparesis with right monoplegia and Babinski sign. Hypoaesthesia from L1 to the left.
X-Ray of Dorsal Tract of Rachis. Kyphosis with dorsolumbar scoliosis.
Myelography (via lumbar puncture). Block in D7-D8 producing

oval-shaped filling defect. The cord appeared displaced forwards and to the left.
Myelo-CT. Confirmation of the location of the tumour. Clear view of the right posterolateral attachment of the tumour.
Surgical Treatment. Opening of the dura showed a roundish subarachnoidal neoplasm which pushed the cord forwards. Freeing of the arachnoid and removal en bloc of the tumour with coagulation at the base of attachment.
Results. The flexion contracture of lower limbs disappeared, and the gradual improvement in voluntary motility led to walking within 1 month. Slight ataxia persisted.

The medical literature does not report the difficulty connected with myelography in defining upper locations in C1 or the occipito-atlanoid forms of meningiomas in the great occipital fossa. In one of our patients suffering from spondyloarthrosis in C5-C6 we were not able to identify the tumour location in C1-C2 with a myelogram and therefore misinterpreted the clinical syndrome, diagnosing a compression from myelopathy in dicouncusarthrosis. In another case the complete block for meningioma in C1-C2 showed a characteristic dome-shaped image which occupied the entire premedullary region (Figs. 166, 167).

Case No. 114: Meningolithial Meningioma
A 70-year-old woman (1971). Ventrolateral to the right, intradural-extramedullary meningioma in C1-C2.
Clinical Course. 1 year.
Neurological Examination. Motor deficiency hemisyndrome on the right with spasticity and bilateral Babinski sign. Painful hypoaesthesia in C3 on the right.
Rachicentesis. 0.72 g per thousand.
Myelography (performed suboccipitally). Total block in C1-C2 with dome-shaped image which appeared widened and a slight sideways flow to the left (Fig. 166).
Surgical Treatment. On opening the dura the cord and lower portion of the bulbar were seen pushed posteriorly to the left by a well-defined neoplasm the size of a cherry and of hard consistency. The surface layer of the cord had an ischaemic appearance. Opening of the arachnoid. Incision of the capsule on one side after sensory radectomy of C2 and the gradual removal of the tumour by fragmentation. The invasion was entirely ventral (Fig. 167).
Results. Recovery of the voluntary motility at right hemisome in 2 days. After 1 week walking was possible with support. After 3 months clinical recovery.

The use of hydrosoluble iodine medium via lumbar puncture facilitates the flow to pass the dorsolumbar passage and reach the upper cervical metameres level. The nature of the tumour is diagnosed by a clear definition of the compression and the neural structures close by. This hydrosoluble method, which sends the liquid along the radicular funnels, shows the filling of the subarachnoidal space on one side (even if slight), the medullary corridor (which is less contrasted) and the tumour block at the same time. The various myelographic images inside the dural sac in extramedullary compression cases depend on various factors. The most important are the volume

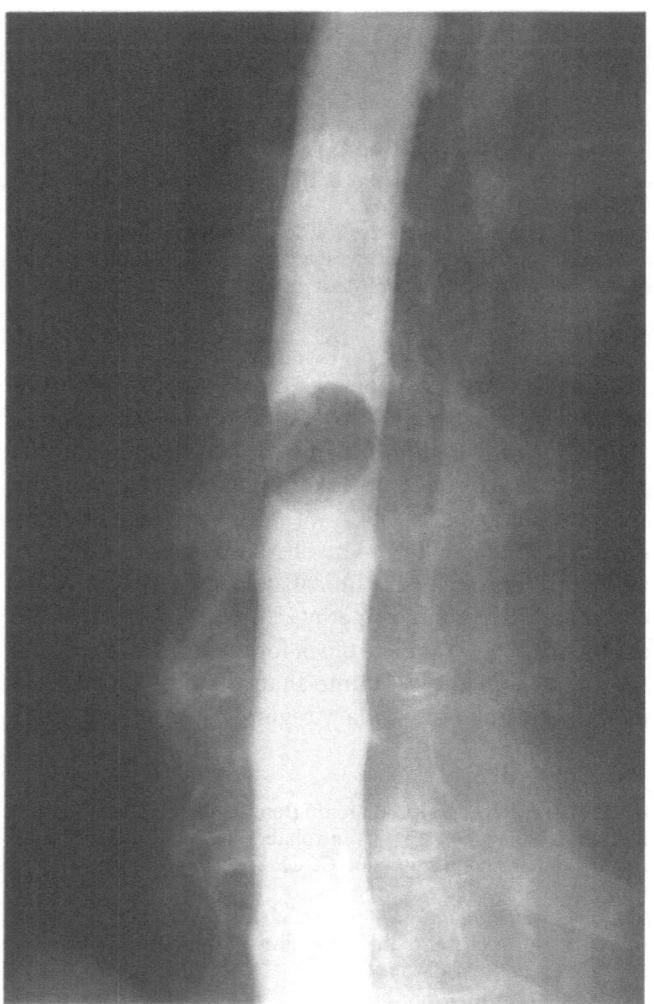
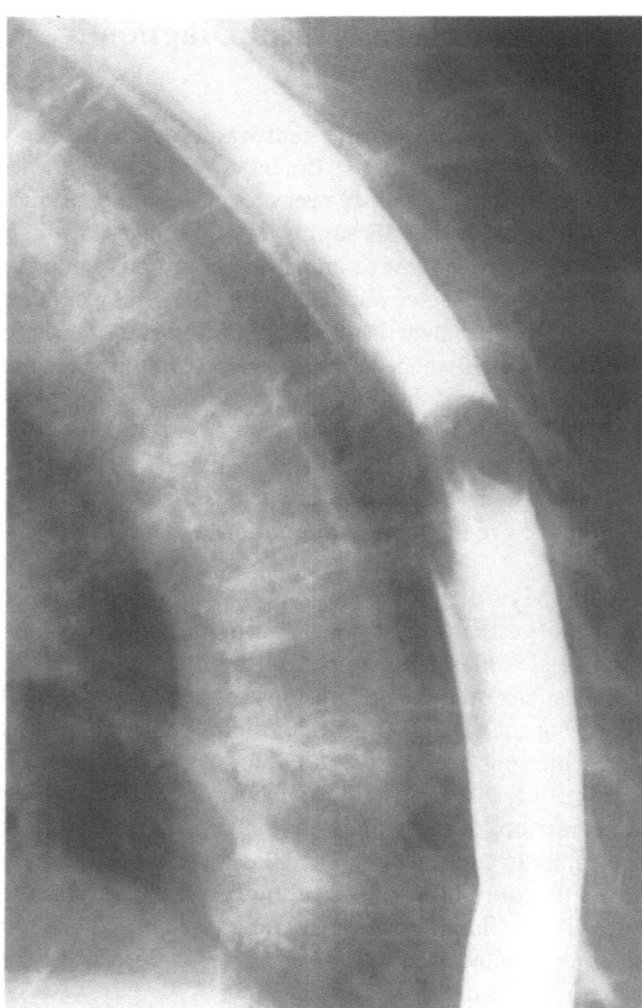

Fig. 164. Myelography via lumbar puncture. Oval-shaped filling defect in D7-D8 atypical for meningiomas. The arachnoidal space appears widened anteroposteriorly on the right, also laterally and posteriorly

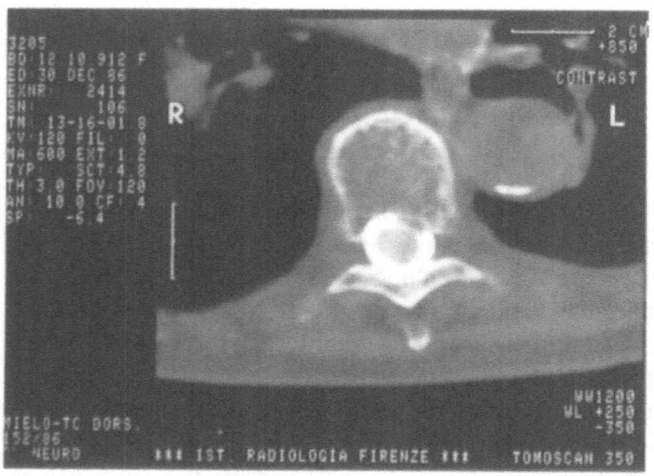
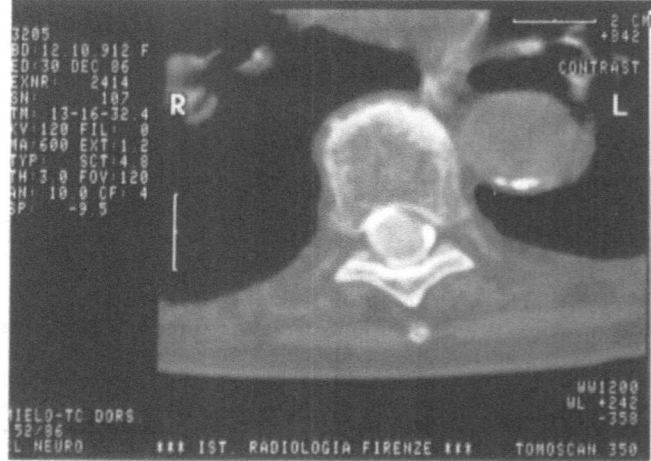

Fig. 165. Myelo-CT. Two sections at D7-D8 level show an expansive round lesion occupying a great part of the rachidian lumen and three-quarters surrounded by contrast medium. The cord is pushed forwards and to the left

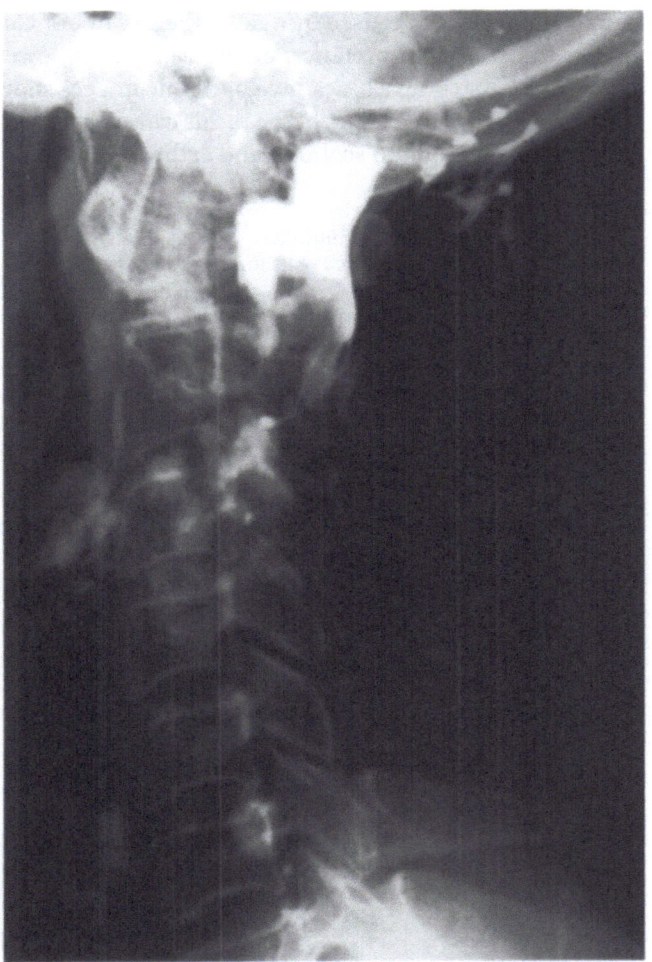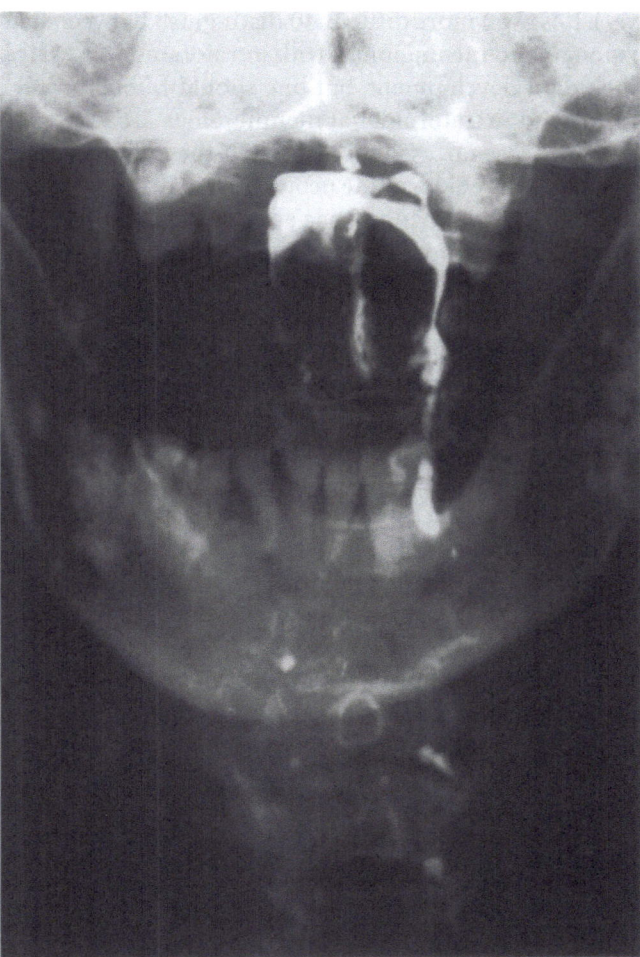

Fig. 166. Myelography performed suboccipitally. Total block in C1-C2 producing an irregular feature in a lateral projection. Anteroposteriorly the contrast medium thickens producing a dome-shape with a slight left lateral flow. The image shows a widening of the transversal diameter of the rachidian canal

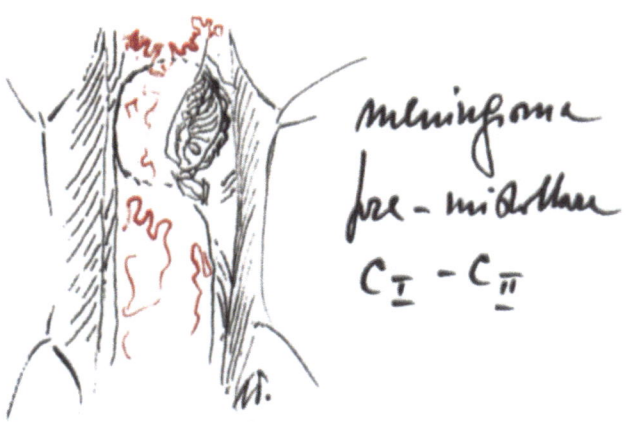

Fig. 167. Scheme of the operating field: the tumour is premedullary

of the neoplasms, the microscopic characteristics of the whole in the presence of a more or less linear capsule and the possible reactive adherent processes of the peritumourous leptomeninges. Usually the iodine medium blocks producing dome-shaped images identifying either a meningioma or a neurinoma. However, a clear dome shape suggests more probably a neurinoma of a cystic nature with smooth surface.

In the diagnosis of a meningioma the iodine medium often produces an irregular image, very similar to that of the neurinoma but with a less uniform surface. If the block on one side is oblique and near an intravertebral foramen the image shows the neurinomatous nature of the compression, but this does not exclude the type of meningioma which has an intradural attachment adjacent to the radicular funnel (see case no. 47, Figs. 173-

177). It is even more difficult to distinguish between neurinomas and meningiomas with intraforamen and extrarachidian development, but one should remember that intra- and extraforamenal meningiomas are extremely rare (see case no. 45, Fig. 183-187). If the iodine medium flows along the sides of the neoplasm and defines it entirely it is probably a meningioma attached to a sensory nerve root. A myelogram may prove unsatisfactory when the tumour is in a premedullary site.

The first types of iodine medium used in myelographic practice for intrarachidian pathologies were liposoluble (Torotrast and Lipiodol); these were followed by ionic hydrosoluble ones (Conray, Methiodal, Dimer-X, Uromiro). These have now given way to nonionic types (Iopamidol). The latter, due to their low viscosity and neurotoxicity, produce satisfactory images in the diagnosis of level and nature.

Lumbar punctures allow us to examine the entire iodine passage along the subarachnoidal space of the entire rachis and therefore in some cases to identify even two locations or more. The range of possibilities offered is very important because the clinical picture of a compression in an upper site caused by a rather large tumour can hinder the exact interpretation of clinical signs in lower sites. Before reaching a block myelographic images show the possibly narrowed edges of the rachis caused by osteoporosis developing into scoliosis and arthrosis.

Case No. 36: Transitional Meningioma

An 82-year-old woman (1984). Posterior, intradural-extramedullary meningioma in D5-D6.
Clinical Course. 7 months. Ingravescent weakness sensation at lower limbs to the left.
Neurological Examination. Severe spastic paraparesis with clonus at the patellar and foot bilaterally. Bilateral Babinski sign. Hyperaesthesia on D4 and hypoaesthesia from D5 distally. Hypopallaesthesia from the iliac crests. Sphincter disturbances in the form of retention.
Rachicentesis. 1.50 g per thousand.
X-Ray of Dorsal Rachis. Very evident osteoporosis with reduction in height in D11 and D12 and segmental kyphosis.
Myelography (via lumbar puncture). The contrast medium contracted at D11-D12 where the reduction in height of the vertebral bodies occurred. Then total block in D5-D6 (Fig. 168).
Surgical Treatment. On opening the dura, the cord was seen to be pushed forwards by a neoplasm invading the internal part of the dura (Fig. 169). Gradual removal by fragmentation. The cord was reduced

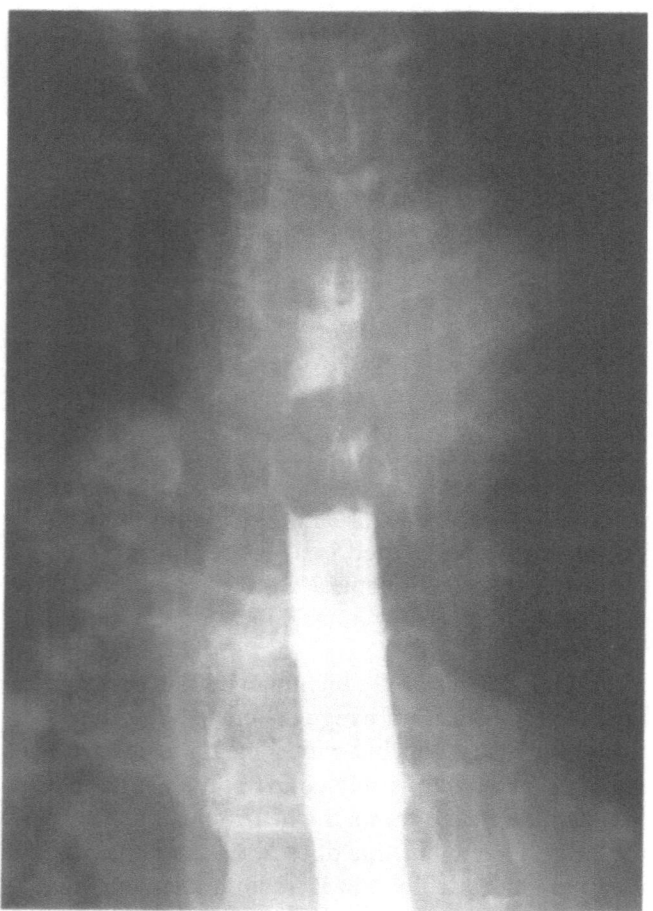
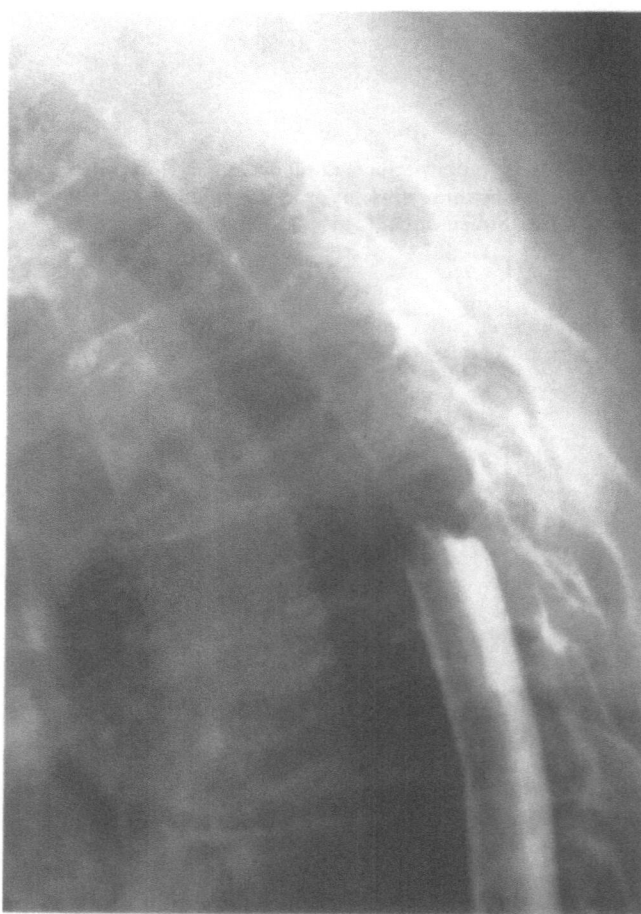

Fig. 168. Myelography via lumbar puncture. Transitory block defining an oval-shaped filling defect in D5-D6 which is slightly irregular in the lower tract. Laterally the subarachnoidal space is wider posteriorly

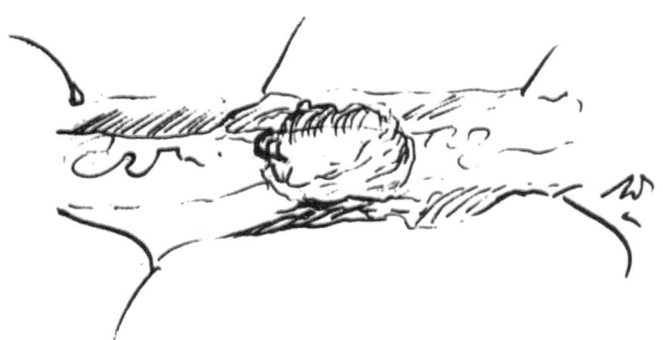

Fig. 169. Diagram showing the meningioma and its inscertion base on the inner surface of the dura

in volume and appeared ischaemic.

Results. Gradual improvement of motility. Two months later the patient was walking normally. Disappearance of sphincter disturbances. Five years later the patient complained of a persisting distal hypopallaesthesia.

Iopamidol, apart from continuing along the entire extent of the meningioma, diffuses near the lateral recesses and frequently demonstrates the exact relationship between the meningioma and the subarachnoidal space. To define the relationship between a meningioma and the nearby structures it is indispensible to carry out, in addition to anteroposterior projections, lateral and oblique projections with patients in a supine decuputis position to determine the exact location of the tumour, particularly in ventral and posterior sites. Iopamidol defines the lower pole of a tumour when the image is blocked at irregular intervals along a horizontal plane, which is sufficient in making a probable diagnosis of meningioma (Figs. 170-172).

Case No. 90: Transitional Meningioma

A 57-year-old woman (1989). Posterolateral intradural-extramedullary meningioma in C7-D1.

Clinical Course. 8 years. Recurrent back pain in cervicodorsal region irradiating to medial surface of the left arm. Four months before hospitalization paraesthesias of a burning nature at right lower limb with weakness felt at the knee.

Neurological Examination. Flexion response of the fingers of the right limb. Spastic paraparesis to the right. Bilateral Babinski sign; tactile, thermal and painful hypoaesthesia at D1-D2. Hypopallaesthesia from D7-D8 which became anaesthesia distally. Sphincter disturbances in the form of retention.

Rachicentesis. 0.26 g per thousand.

X-ray of Cervicodorsal Rachis. Slight asymmetry of pedicles in C7-D1 (left to right).

Myelography (via lumbar puncture). Block at lower border of D1 level (Fig. 170).

Myelo-CT. Oval neoformation with defined intradural-extramedullary borders in C7-D1 which caused the displacement of the cord towards right side (Fig. 171).

MRI. Lesion measuring maximally 2 cm in diameter posteriorly and located laterally on the left. Displacement of the cord forwards and to the right. The MRI showed sensitivity to the cord in T2 (Fig. 172).

Surgical Treatment. Meningioma invading the internal dural surface on the left adhering to the cord which was reduced in volume.

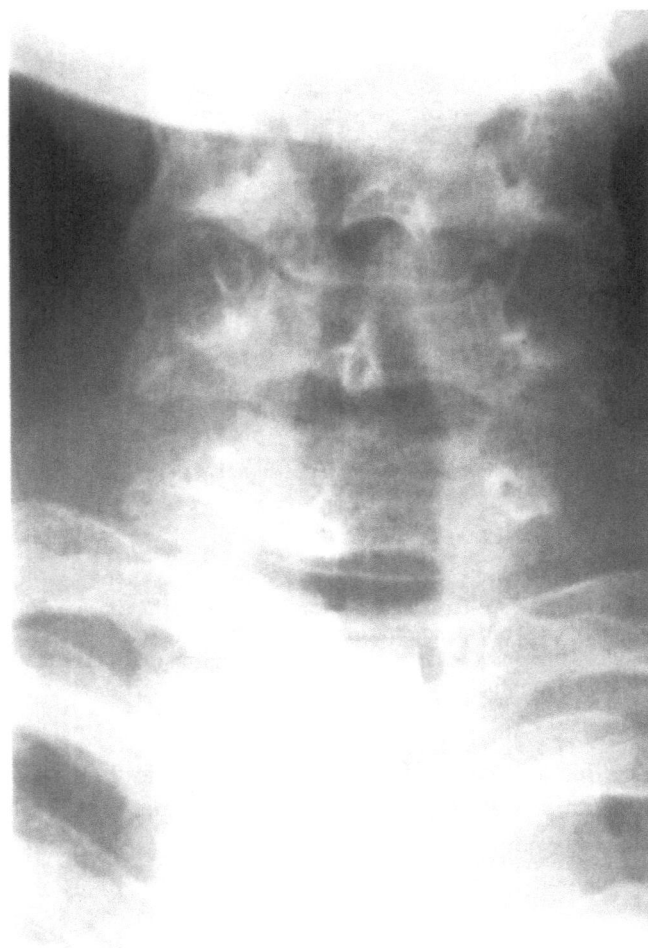

Fig. 170. Myelography via lumbar puncture. Anteroposterior block producing an irregular image of the pedicle's upper margin on the right side and complete stop below the pedicle on the left side at C7-D1

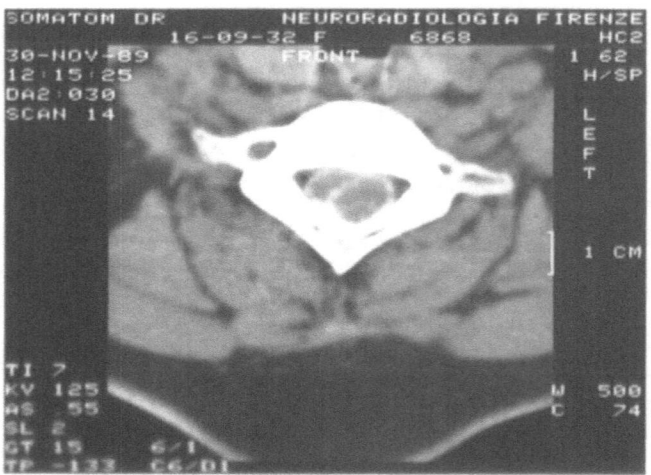 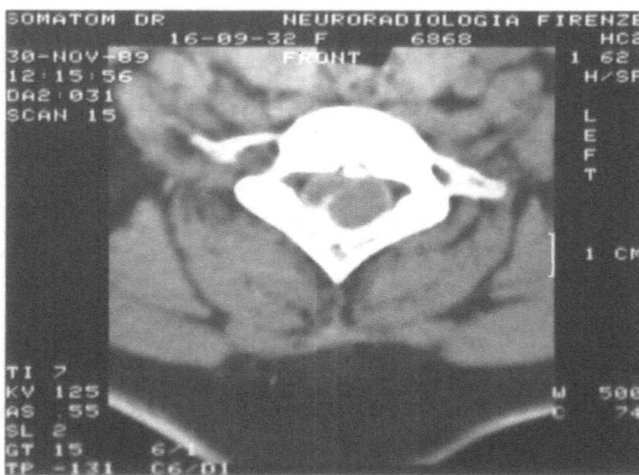

Fig. 171. Myelo-CT. In the two images the homogeneously dense meningioma is visible in toto at the cord which is pushed ventrally and to the right

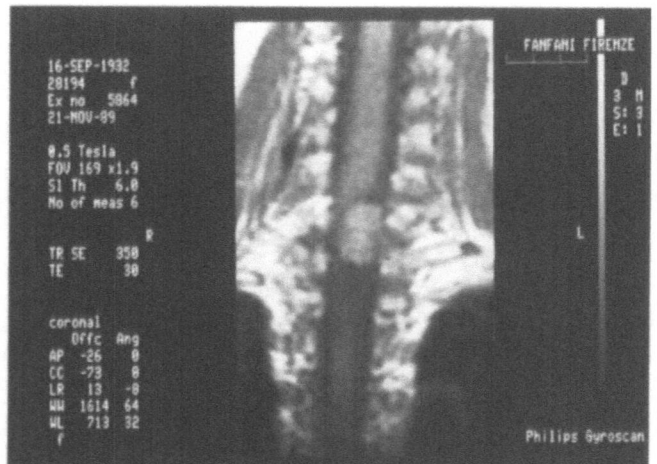 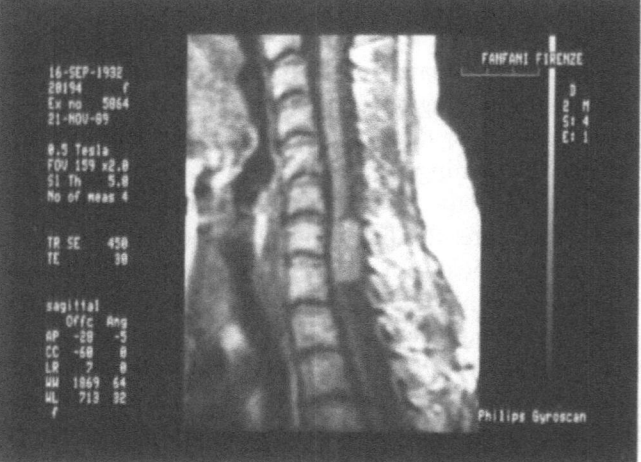

Fig. 172. MRI. Spin-echo sequence T1 (TR 450 ms; TE 30 ms), sagittal and coronal planes. The meningioma at C7-D1 has an irregular ovaloid feature with homogeneously isodense signal at the spinal cord which seems displaced forwards and to the right

Ischaemic surface-layer vascularization. Freeing the arachnoidal adherent structures and excision of the tumour by fragmentation. *Results.* After 5 days walking returned almost normal. Clinical recovery after 3 months.

Between cervical and dorsal levels the iodine medium can prove less uniform, unlike for the entire dorsal tract. When the upper pole of the block is strictly concave it is easier to observe the corridor which has not been filled with the iodine medium and to identify the degree of cord displacement caused by the tumour. Sometimes the iodine medium is linear, without flowing laterally along the subarachnoidal space. This image suggests the invasion of a meningioma.

8.3.2 Computed Tomography

Direct CT scans, thanks to the axial projections, identify bone alterations which are not always recognizable by direct radiography but are correlated with the presence of a meningioma. The principal ones are:

- Modification of one or more pedicles
- Increase in space between pedicles
- Possible increase in anteroposterior distance of rachidian diameter
- Simple and defined modification of the vertebral body's posterior wall cortex at the level of the tumour
- Narrowing or modification of a lamina on the side of the tumour formation
- Presence of intrarachidian calcifications
- Possible discoarthrotic associations such as potrusions inside the canal
- Alterations in the bone spongiosa at the site of the meningioma or in metameres at some distance from the site of the tumour
- Simple vertebral anomalies (schistasis, anomalies of the laminae or of the articular masses including the articulate interline of one side, sinostosis of two adjacent vertebral bodies or of the laminae, alterations in toto of a spinous process and spondylolisthesis).

Three-dimensional reconstructions and very close scans make possible very precise images of every type of bone alteration (Figs. 173-177).

Case No. 47: Transitional Osseous Meningioma
A 60-year-old woman (1989). Left anteroposterior, intradural-extramedullary meningioma in D4-D5.
Clinical Course. 7 months. Paraesthesias, hot and cold sensations, and sometimes electric shocks initially to the left lower limb, then affecting the right limb. Two months prior to hospitalization contracture of the lower limbs occurred with progressive difficulty in walking.
Neurological Examination. Spastic paraparesis, mainly left (Levy grade 0). Hyperaesthesia on D4 on the left. Hypoaesthesis from D5. Sphincter disturbances in the form of retention.
Rachicentesis. 0.2 g protein per thousand.
X-Ray of Dorsal Tract. The pedicle of D5 was narrowed.
Myelography (via lumbar puncture). Transitory block in D5 with widening of the arachnoidal space on the left. A minimal portion of the contrast medium passed the block and defined the right outline and upper pole of the lesion (Fig. 173).
CT. Lesion occupying a large part of the vertebral canal at D4-D5 level, substantially hyperdense with the presence of medial calcifications. The cord above and below the compression seemed displaced towards the right. Reconstructed images showed the calcified component in positive diagnosis for meningiomas (Figs 174-175).
Myelo-CT. The canal was almost completely occupied by a calcified solid mass on D4-D5. The cord was displaced towards the right (Fig. 176.a-176.b).

MRI. Neoplasm in left anterolateral site. Hyperdense area of lesion (Fig. 177).
Surgical Treatment. On opening the dura, the cord appeared atrophic with poor surface-layer vascularization, displaced towards the right. The almond-sized meningioma invaded the dura below the root and had premedullary development. Total excision after removing arachnoidal adherent structures and coagulation of the base of attachment.
Results. In the following 10 days paretic-ataxic gait. After 1 month normal walking which continued 1 year later.

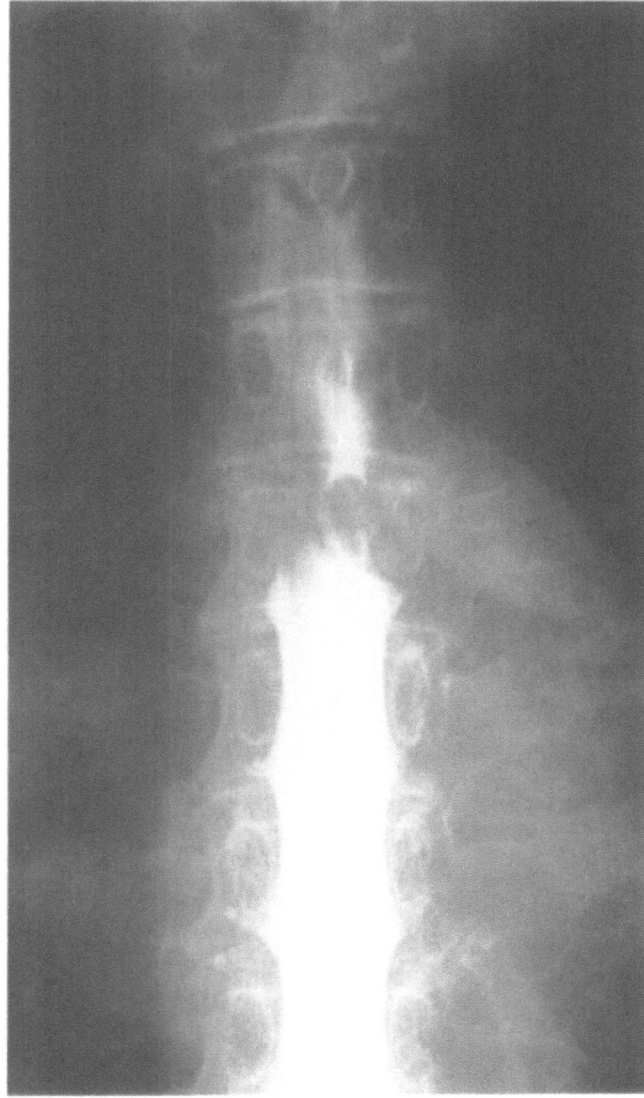

Fig. 173. Myelography via lumbar puncture. Transitory block in D5 widening of the subarachnoidal space on the left. A small amount of contrast medium passes the block and defines the right outline and upper pole of the lesion

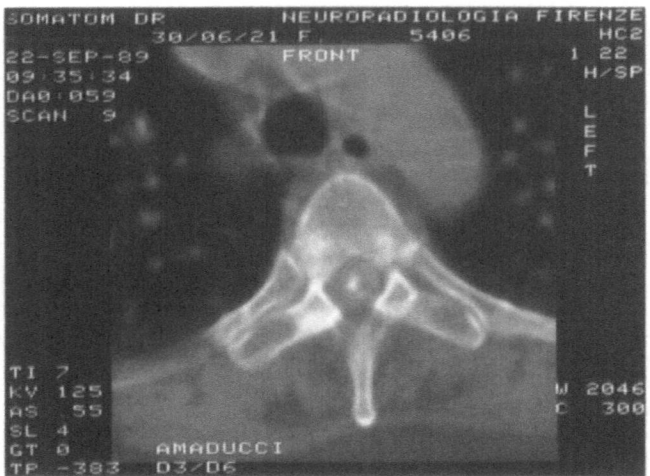

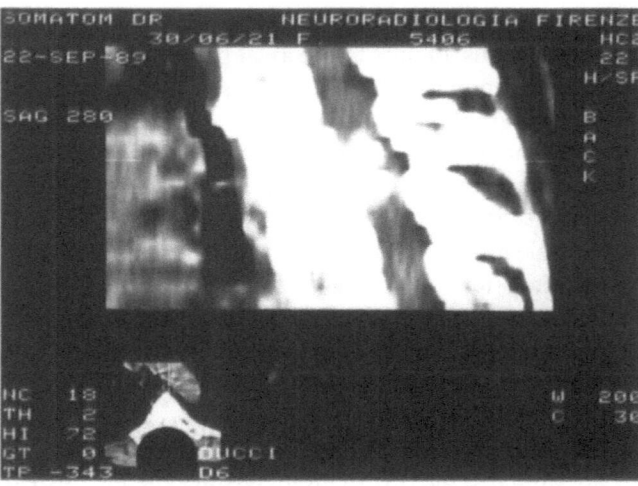

Fig. 174. Plain CT. The roundish-shaped tumourous lesion inside the canal is hyperdense at the periphery and extends towards the left

Fig. 175. The calcified area of the tumour is seen better in the sagittal reconstruction of its vertical extension

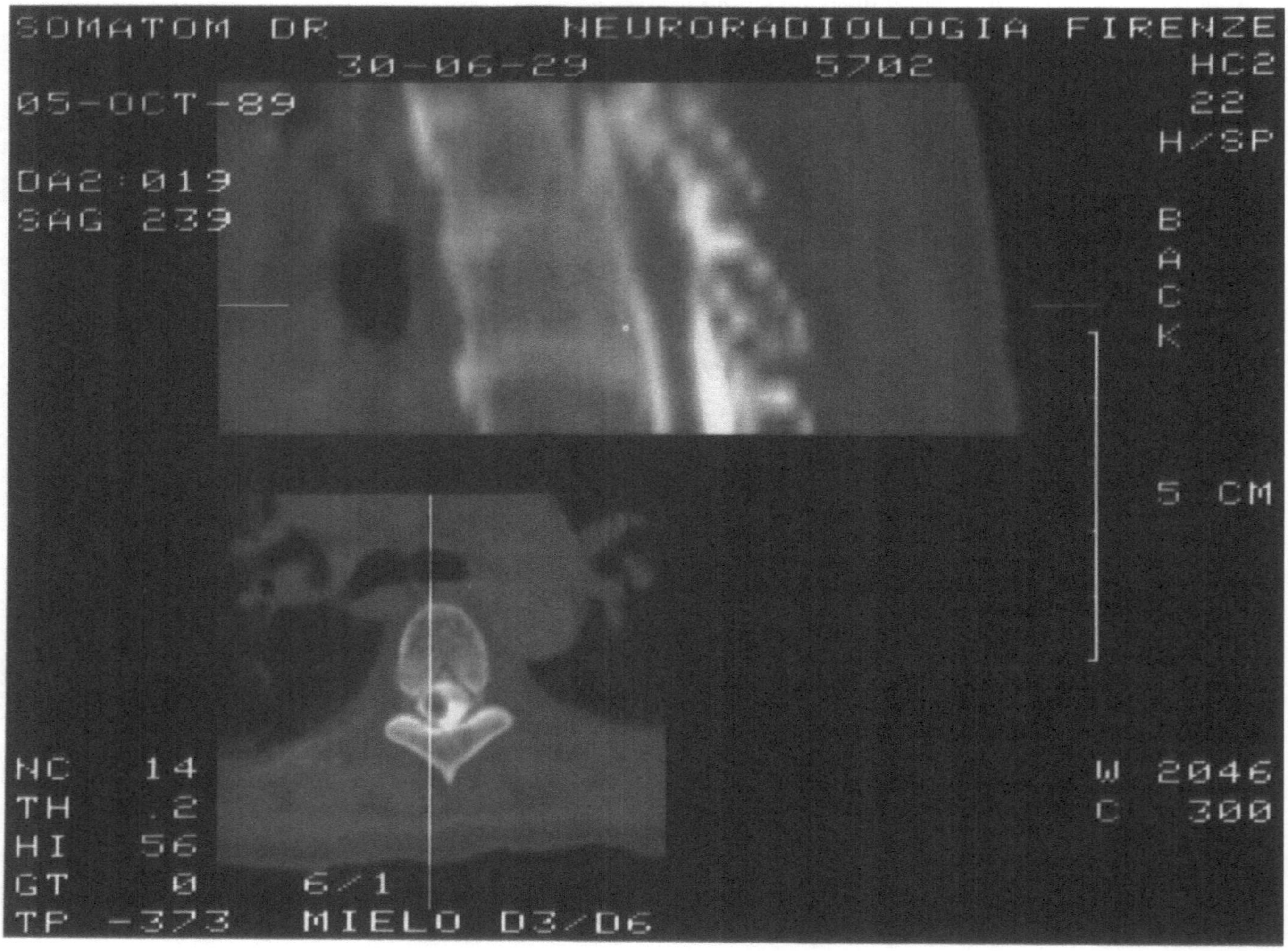

Fig. 176.a. Myelo-CT reconstruction. In a right paramedian sagittal scan, the canal is enlarged transversally at the compression level. The relationship between tumour and dilatation of the subarachnoidal space above and below is very precise

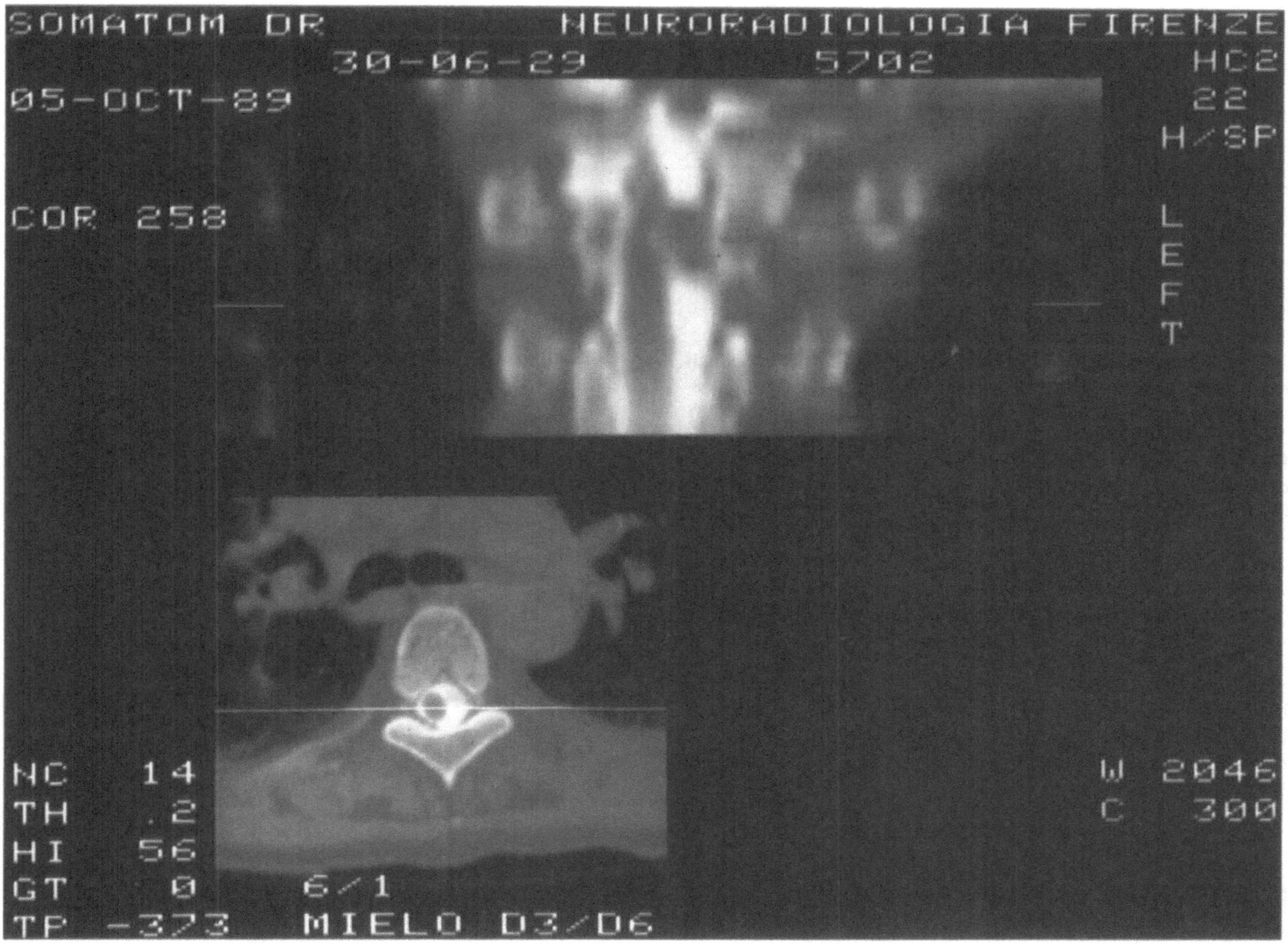

Fig. 176. b. Myelo-CT reconstruction in coronal scan

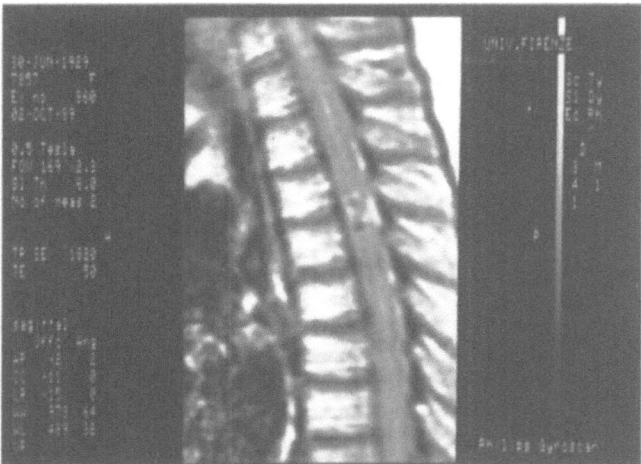

Fig. 177. MRI. DP sequence (TR 1800 and TE 50) median sagittal plane. The lesion in toto is less evident but the two calcified areas show the areas without a signal

8.3.3 Myelo-Computed Tomography

Myelographic images become complete and highly revealing when associated with CT scans because the axial scans are capable of exploring the entire tract in which the tumour is located. Myelo-CT scans are indispensable in defining the preoperative radiological anatomy of the tumour in its exact juxtamedullary site inside the dura mater. This type of examination is extremely useful in the rare cases in which the meningioma is both intra- and extrarachidian through an intravertebral foramen. Both CT and MRI directly define the entire volume of the tumour, while myelography and myelo-CT show the relationships between tumour, leptomeninges and cord.

Case No. 42: Meningothelial Meningioma
A 64-year-old woman (1989). Intravertebral foramen, extradural meningioma in D9-D10 on the right.
Medical History. Haemangioendothelioma on the right foot. Surgery performed for an intercostal glomus tumour at 55 years; sacral lip-

oma at 60 years and right underarm lipoma at 62 years. Two years before hospitalization in another hospital, percutaneous, cervical cordotomy on the left for pain on lower right limb.

Clinical Course. 4 years. Widespread pain on dorsal rachis without specific pattern. Subsequent painful episodes with pain distribution from the mediodorsal tract anteriorly to upper right abdomen presenting as a suspect colocystic calculus. The patient was advised to wear a plaster corset. Impediment in walking over the previous few months.

Neurological Examination. Spastic paraparesis. Foot clonus. Bilateral Babinski sign. Difficulty in evaluating the sensibility due to past cordotomy; however, painful hypoaesthesias felt from D8, distally pronounced with slight hyperaesthesia on the two dermatones above.

X-Ray of Dorsal Tract. Diffuse osteoporosis, right convex scoliosis in upper tract. Articular masses were narrowed on the right in D8-D9 and D9-D10; schistasis in L4-L5 and excavation of the sacrum.

Myelography (via lumbar puncture). No block. Ample vision of D9-D10 due to epidural compression (Fig. 178) Lower, in L5-S1, large sac of a pseudomeningocele type (from previous surgery for discus haernia with complications due to a fluid fistula; Fig. 179).

MRI. Large neoformation which occupied the paravertebral douche on the right and the intravertebral foramen in D9. The cord appeared reduced in volume (Figs. 180, 181).

Surgical Treatment. Lateral right laminectomy to reach the enlarged intravertebral foramen. The neoplasm, apparently in continuity with the root, had developed towards the thoracic cavity. Intradural exploration showed a normal root up to the dural entry zone but confused with the extradural component of the meningioma. Partial removal and preganglion radicotomy.

Results. Walking with support after 1 month. Complete recovery at 5 year check-up.

To judge the conditions of meningioma formation we can obtain precise anatomical-radiological information for a topographic diagnosis. If CT shows suspect calcifications within the structure of the meningioma which are not evident on X-ray or stratigraphy, the myelo-CT can identify every form of cord displacement and malformation. The width of the subarachnoidal space depends on the volume and location of the meningioma. The images of ascending myelography correspond perfectly to the axial scans of a myelo-CT, but an iodine image can more clearly show the narrowing of the radicular funnels and the perimedullary subarachnoidal space on the opposite side of the tumour.

Case No. 58: Transitional Meningioma
A 76-year-old woman (1987). Right posterolateral intradural-extramedullary meningioma in D2-D3.
Clinical Course. 1 year. Weakness at lower limbs to the right with par-

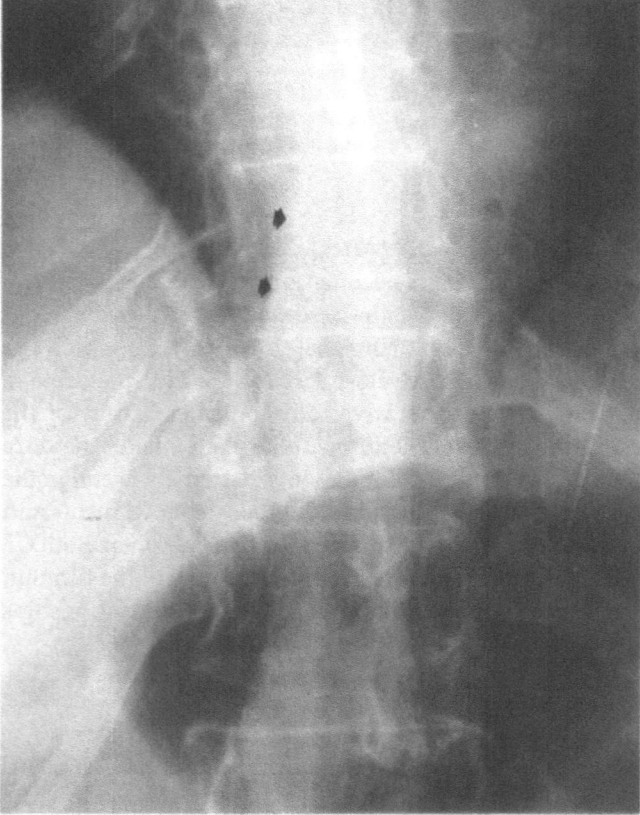

Fig. 178. Myelography: extradural compression *(arrows)*

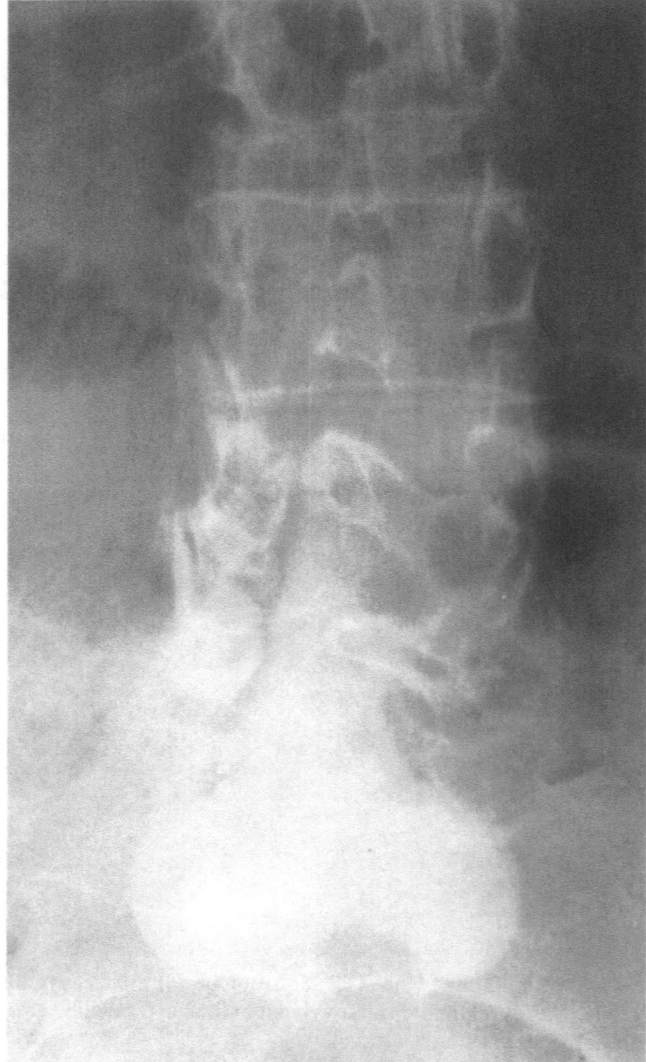

Fig. 179. Pseudomeningocele in L5-S1

aesthesias such as tingling sensations. The symptoms grew worse until walking became impossible.

Neurological Examination. Spastic paraplegia with clonus at the patella. Tactile and thermal pain hypoaesthesia from D4. Pallaesthesia from the iliac crests. Constriction felt at upper thorax.

Rachicentesis. 0.68 g per thousand.

X-Ray of Cervicodorsal Rachis. Kyphoscoliosis.

Myelography (via lumbar puncture). Transitory block at D2-D3 level with slight lateral flow only on the left revealing the upper pole of a tumour (Fig. 182).

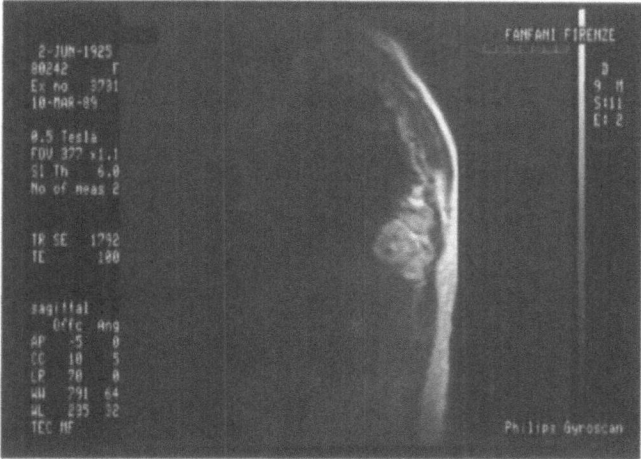

Fig. 180. MRI: right sagittal paramedian scan

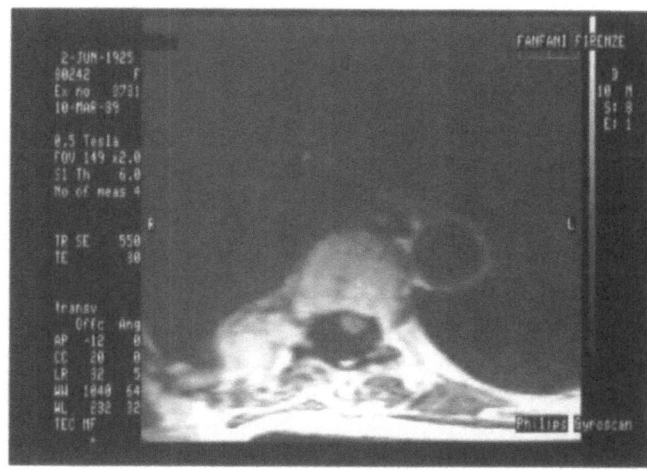

Fig. 181. MRI: the tumour occupies the right paravertebral region

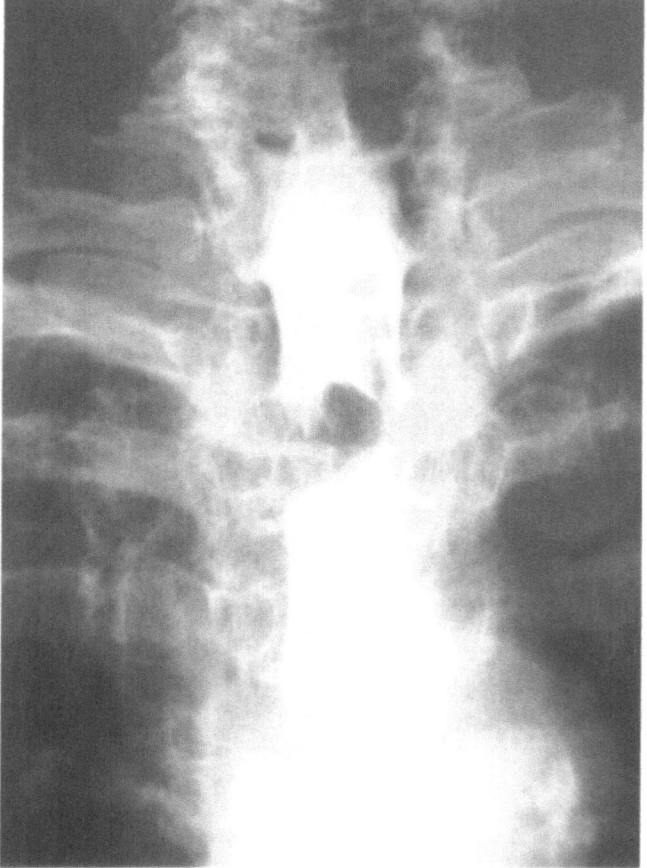

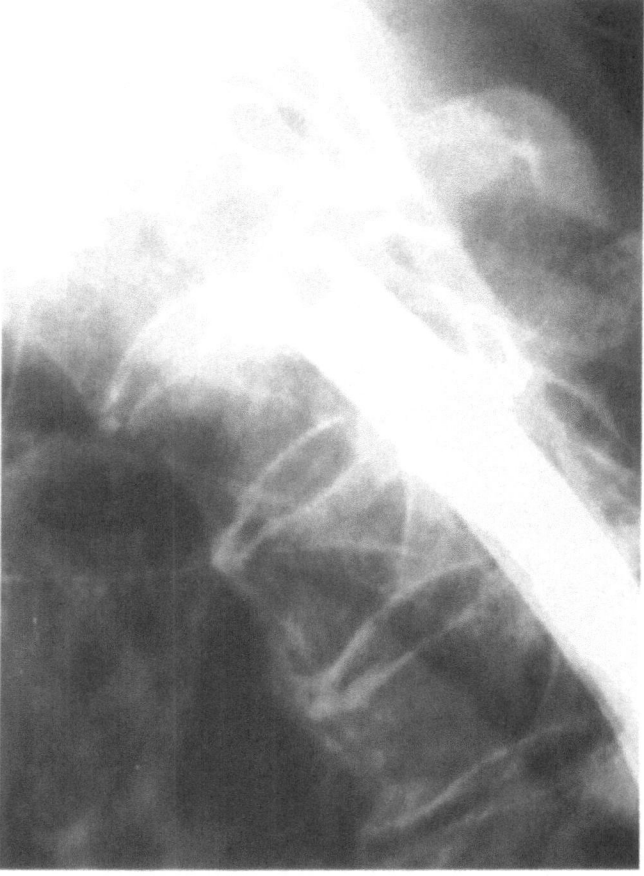

Fig. 182. Myelography via lumbar puncture. Transitory block in D2-D3 on the right. The contrast medium flows into the subarachnoidal space which is enlarged on the right and surrounds an oval-shaped area. The cord is displaced towards the left. Laterally the total block defines a concave area with dilatated subarachnoidal space posteriorly. Slight flow in the dural funnel of the root which is displaced towards the exterior

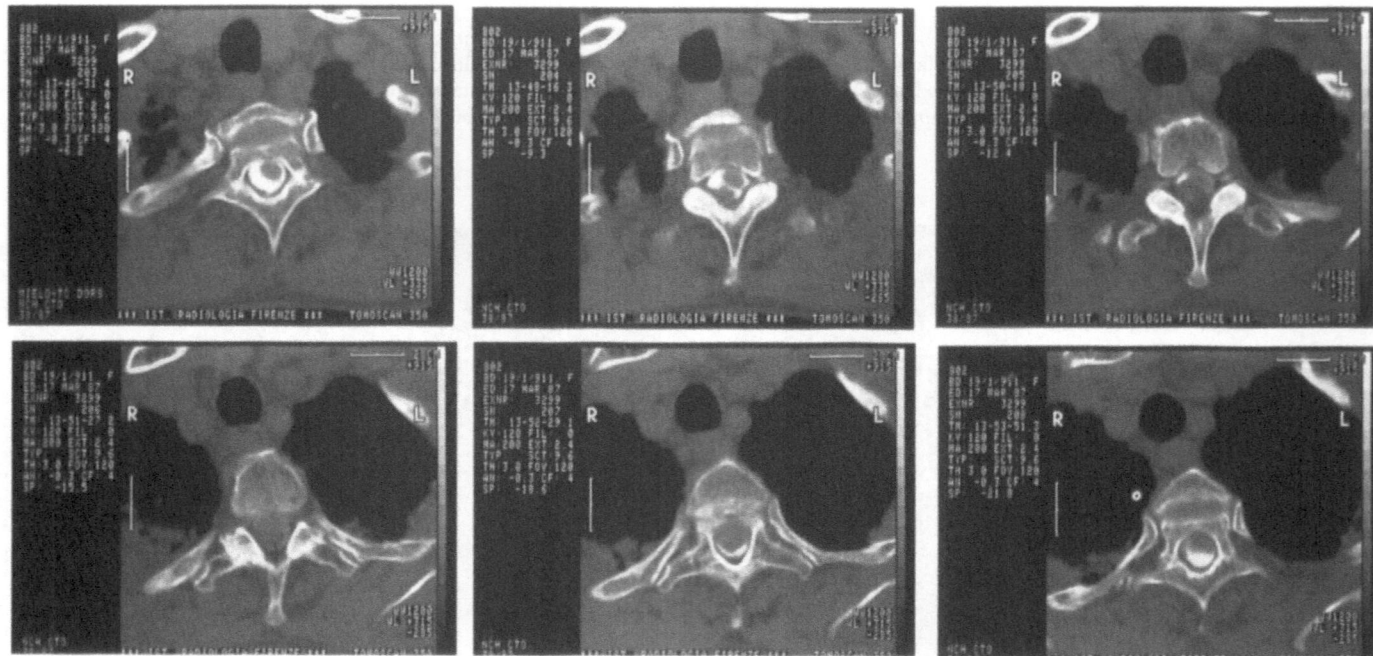

Fig. 183. The tumour is located posterolaterally on the right

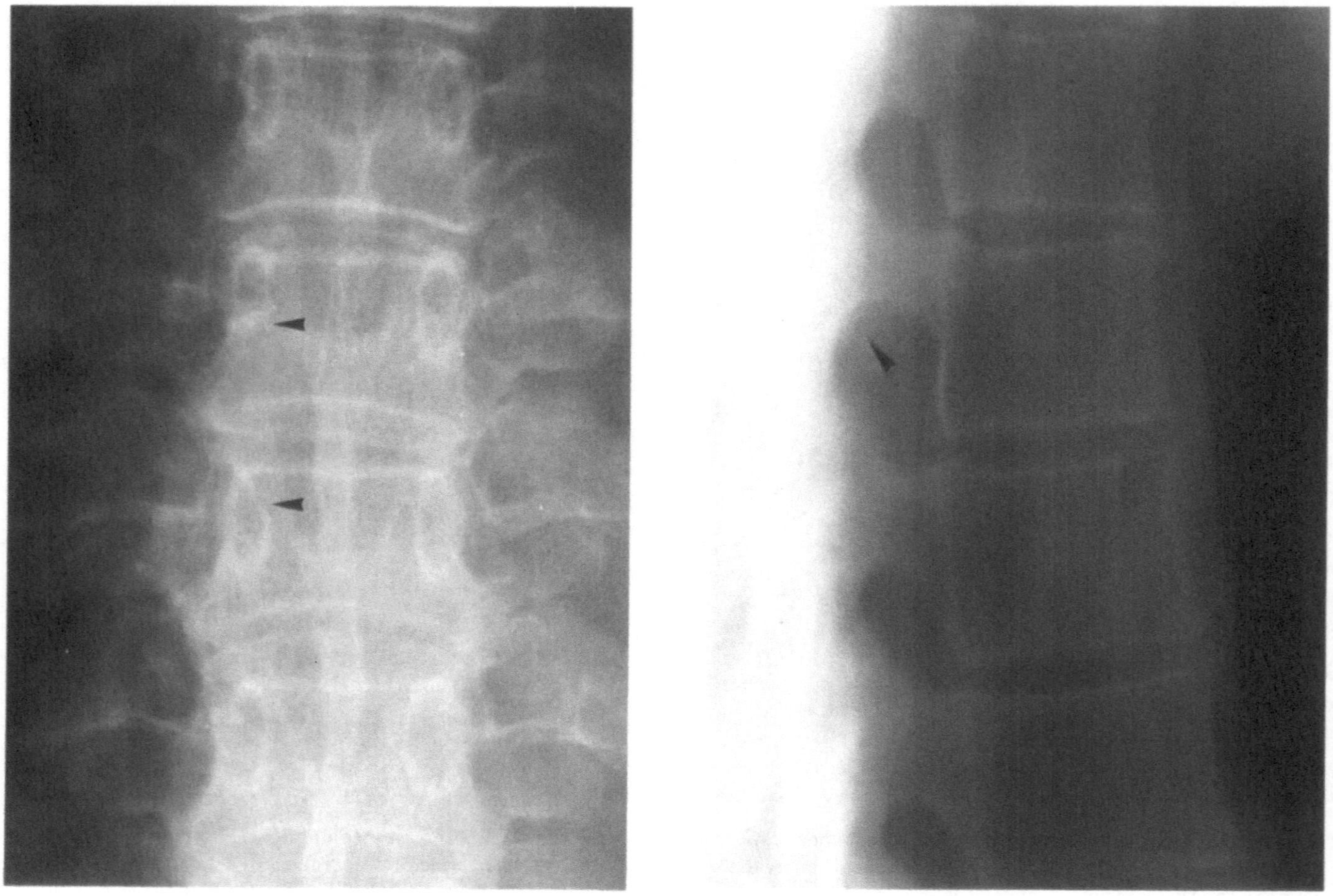

Fig. 184. The articular facets in D5-D6 on the right were thinned. The intervertebral foramen in D6-D7 is enlarged *(arrows)*

Myelo CT. In D2-D3 the expansive intradural lesion was located posterolaterally on the right. The corridor, corresponding to the cord displaced to the right, was clearly seen (Fig. 183).
MRI. Confirmation of findings in previous examinations.
Surgical Treatment. Curved paramedian incision on the right of the dura. The cord appeared pushed forwards by a calcified tumour. Total excision of neoplasm and base of attachment. The surface-layer vascularization presented very fine vessels with signs of ischaemia especially at the posterior columns.
Results. After 10 days walking with bilateral support. After 3 months walking with only one support. Seven months later the patient's condition persisted.

A suspect decalcification of a pedicle with an enlarged intravertebral foramen as shown in X-ray sometimes finds confirmation in a myelo-CT which identifies the reduction in subarachnoidal space exactly medial to the level of bone modification. In these cases the meningioma which occupies the epidural space is principally extradural and intraforamenal.

Case No. 45: Meningothelial Meningioma

A 59-year-old woman (1987). Right posterolateral intradural-extra-medullary meningioma in D5-D7.
Clinical Course. 2 years. Pain at right hemithorax at intervals then becoming continuous. In a few months a band-like constriction was felt at the right hemithorax with hot and cold paraesthesias of the legs. Progressive impediment in walking to the lower right limb.
Neurological Examination. Spastic-ataxic paraparesis to the right (Levy grade 2). Thermal-pain and superficial tactile hypoaesthesias from D6-D8 on the left. Hypopallaesthesia from last ribs. Sphincter disturbances in the form of incontinence.
Rachicentesis. 0.98 g per thousand.
X-Ray of Dorsal Rachis. Left-convex scoliosis. The articular facets in D5, D6, D7 and D8 on the right were thinned. The intervertebral foramen in D6-D7 were enlarged (Fig. 184).
Myelography (via lumbar puncture). Block anteroposteriorly in D6, D7. The contrast medium passed D7, flowing sideways on the left (Fig. 185). Lateral and oblique block at lower pole of meningioma and concavity towards the upper areas producing an irregular image.
Myelo-CT. Axial and sagittal scans reconstruction of the compression showed extradural location and isodense for two-thirds of the rachidian lumen. The cord, which was reduced in volume and pushed towards the left, passed the enlarged intervertebral foramen in D6-D7 (Figs. 186, 187).
Surgical Treatment. Extradural neoplasm which if moved laterally occupied the intravertebral foramen, thereby becoming extrarachidian. The tumour enveloped the root of D7 which had increased in volume (Fig. 188).
Results. Neurological examination appeared normal after 7 months. Paraesthesias at intervals at the left thigh. After 5 years the patient was operated on in another hospital for recurrent lesion. Histological examination showed an angioblastic meningioma.

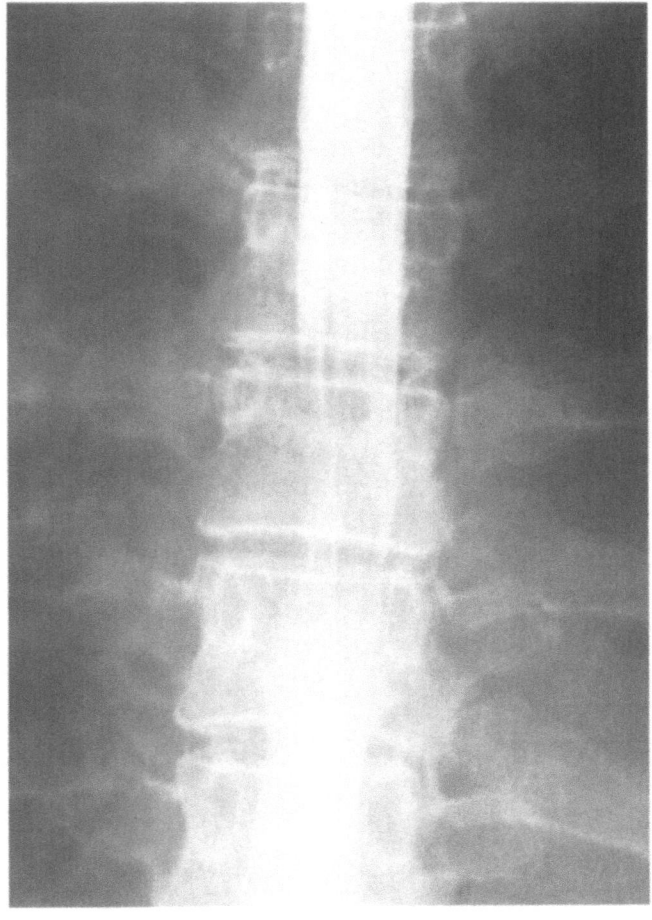

Fig. 185. The contrast medium flows on the left side

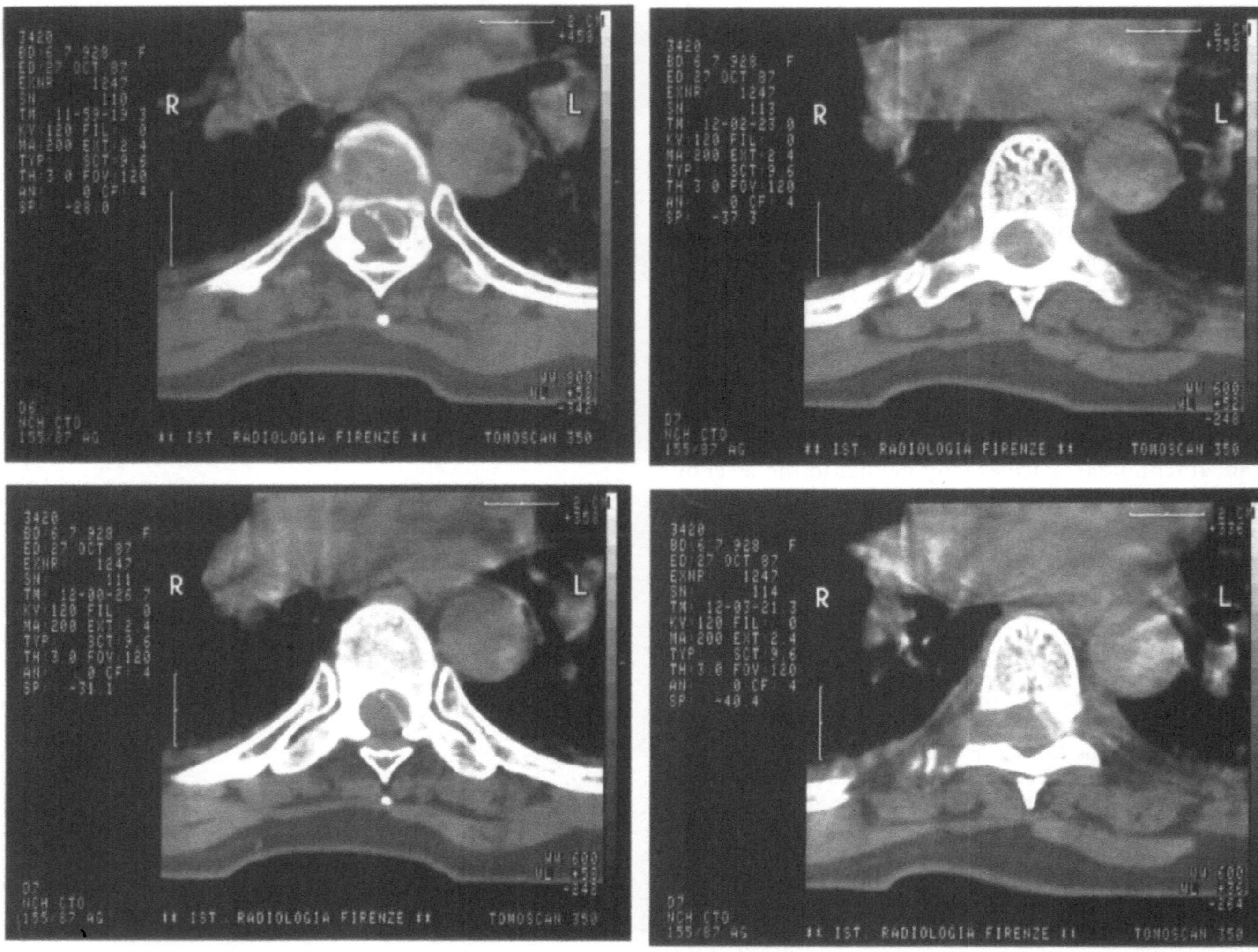

Fig. 186. Myelo. CT: spinal cord is reduced in volume and pushed towards the left side

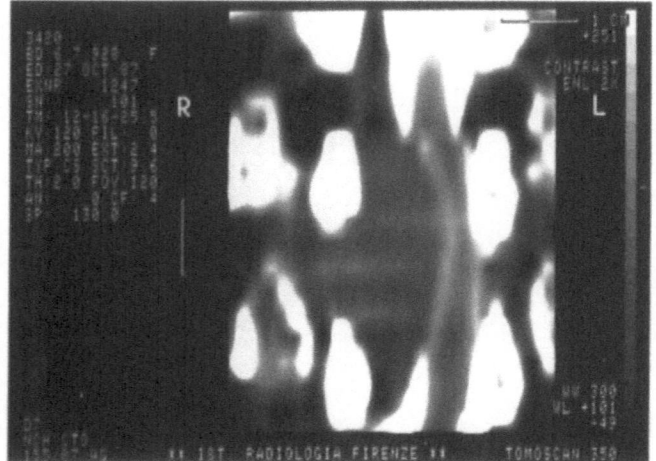

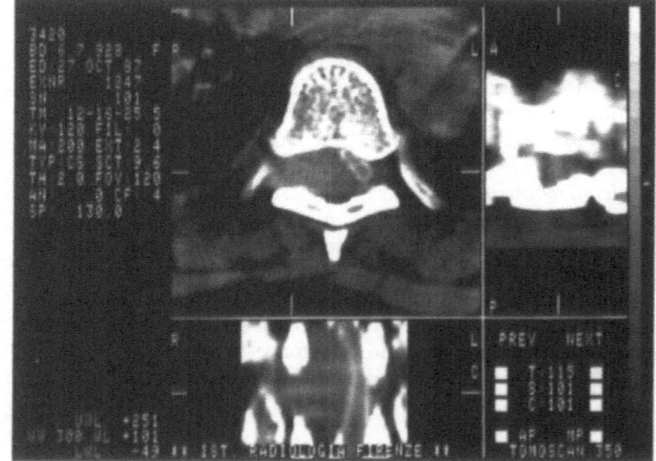

Fig. 187. The tumour occupied the right two-third of the spinal canal

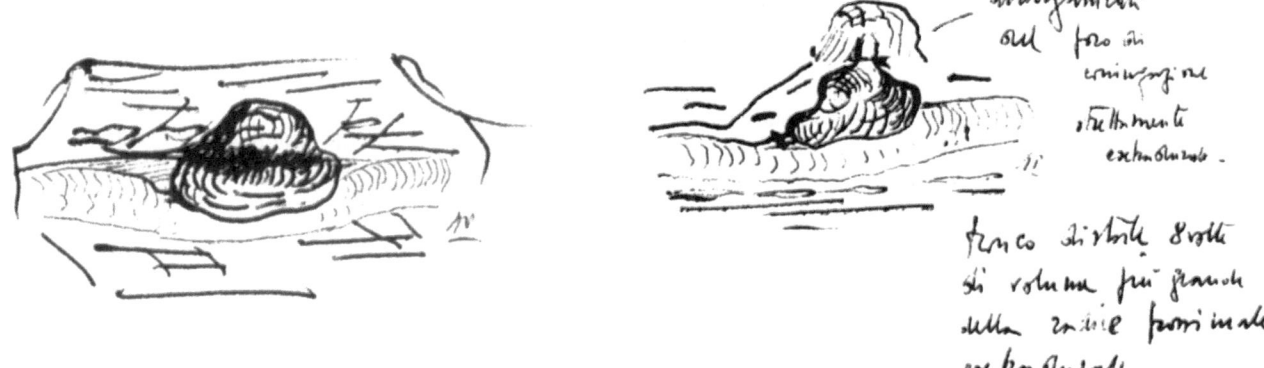

Fig. 188. Drawing of the operating field

In this case the diagnosis of tumourous compression, originally made by myelography as being extradural and intraforamenal, was subsequently confirmed by myelo-CT which also supplied the exact extension of the lesion. These techniques provide results which complement one another and for this reason neither can be excluded. The diagnostic results depend on a global evaluation of the various features. The principal features of the images lead us to an anatomic-radiological finding based on the nerve structures above and below the meningioma and on alterations in the subarachnoidal space. With myelo-CT the meningioma attachment can retrace the site of the previously identified calcifications and supply other elements of the morphological characteristics of the tumour. Reconstruction in various planes reveals the topography of the variations affecting the nerve structures above and below the meningioma and show the tumour's extention (Figs. 189-194).

Case No. 99: Transitional Meningioma

A 79-year-old man (1989). Left ventrolateral intradural-extramedullary meningioma in D4.

Clinical Course. 5 years. Intermittent back pain, for 6 months irradiating band-like to the left mammary region. Burning paraesthesias distally to feet and legs with impediment of voluntary movements. For 5 months walking had been extremely difficult.

Neurological Examination. Spastic paraparesis to the left. Foot clonus and left Babinski sign. Hypoaesthesia from D6, distally pronounced.

X-Ray of Dorsal Rachis. Scoliosis of cervicodorsal passage. Obvious narrowing of articular facets of D4 and D5 on the right.

Myelography (via lumbar puncture). Transitory block anteroposteriorly in D4-D5. Very little contrast medium defined the upper pole of the tumour. In lateral projection the dilatation of arachnoidal space above and below the compression in the ventral part. Myelographic examination perfectly defined the right ventrolateral position of the meningioma (Figs. 189-190).

Myelo-CT. Intradural-extramedullary neoformation of an oval shape in left anterolateral site which displaced the cord contralaterally (Figs. 191-192-193-194).

Surgical Treatment. On opening the dura, the cord appeared to cover the tumour but showed major displacement towards the right. Opening of the subarachnoidal space facilitated the view of the reddish-wine coloured neoplasm. Incision of the capsule and removal by fragmentation. Coagulation of the base of attachment.

Results. Improvement in paraparesis until normal walking achieved. After 4 years (age 83 years) walking was possible, step by step, of a pseudobulbar type.

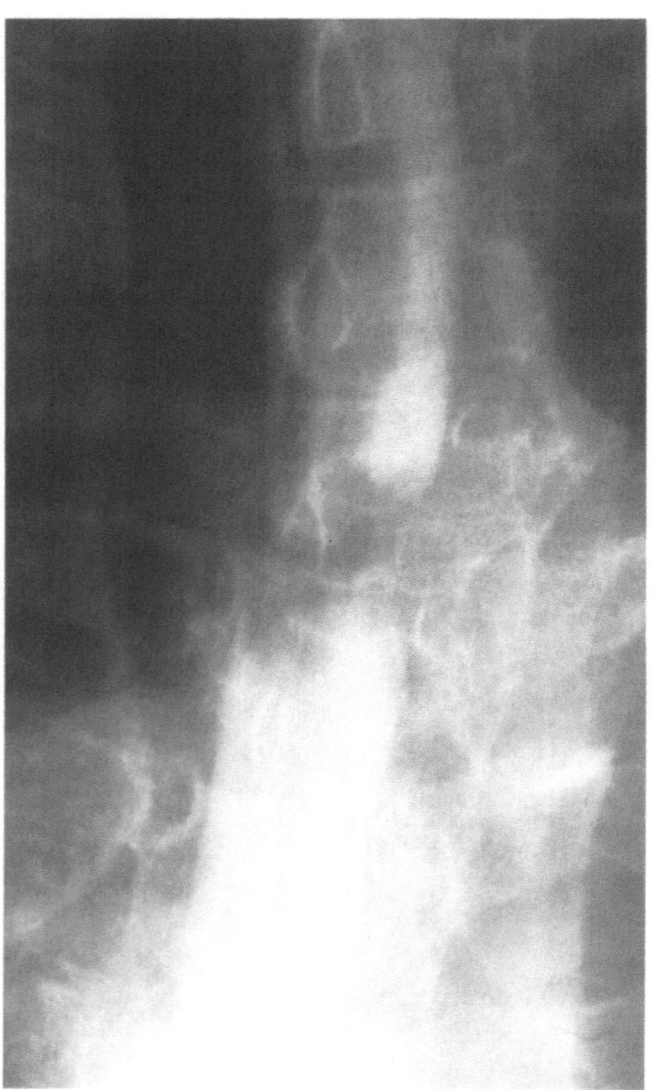

Fig. 189. Myelography via lumbar puncture. Enlargement of the subarachnoidal space on the left. Transitory block in D4-D5 defining the outline of an oval-shaped intradural mass

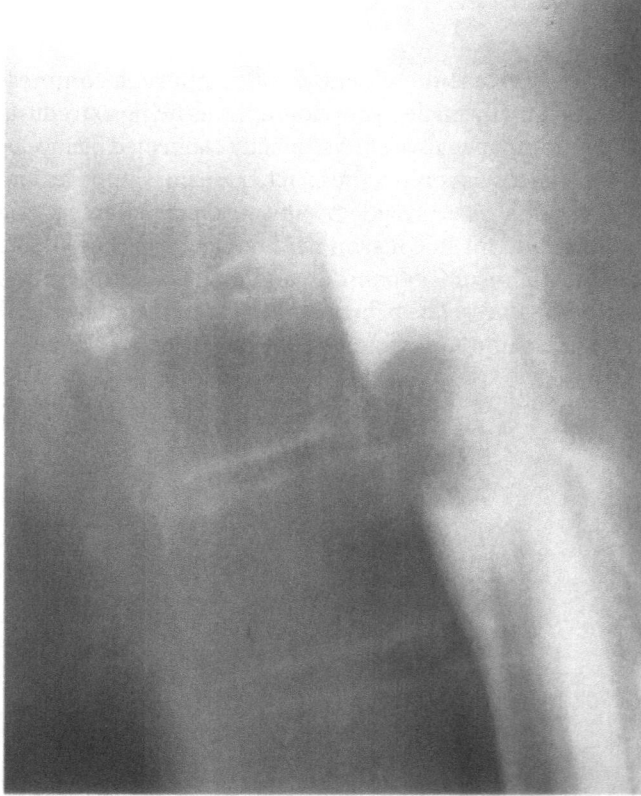

Fig. 190. Lateral stratigraphy shows a negative image of the oval-shaped expansive process which enlarges the subarachnoidal space above and below the cord, pushing it sideways and towards the back

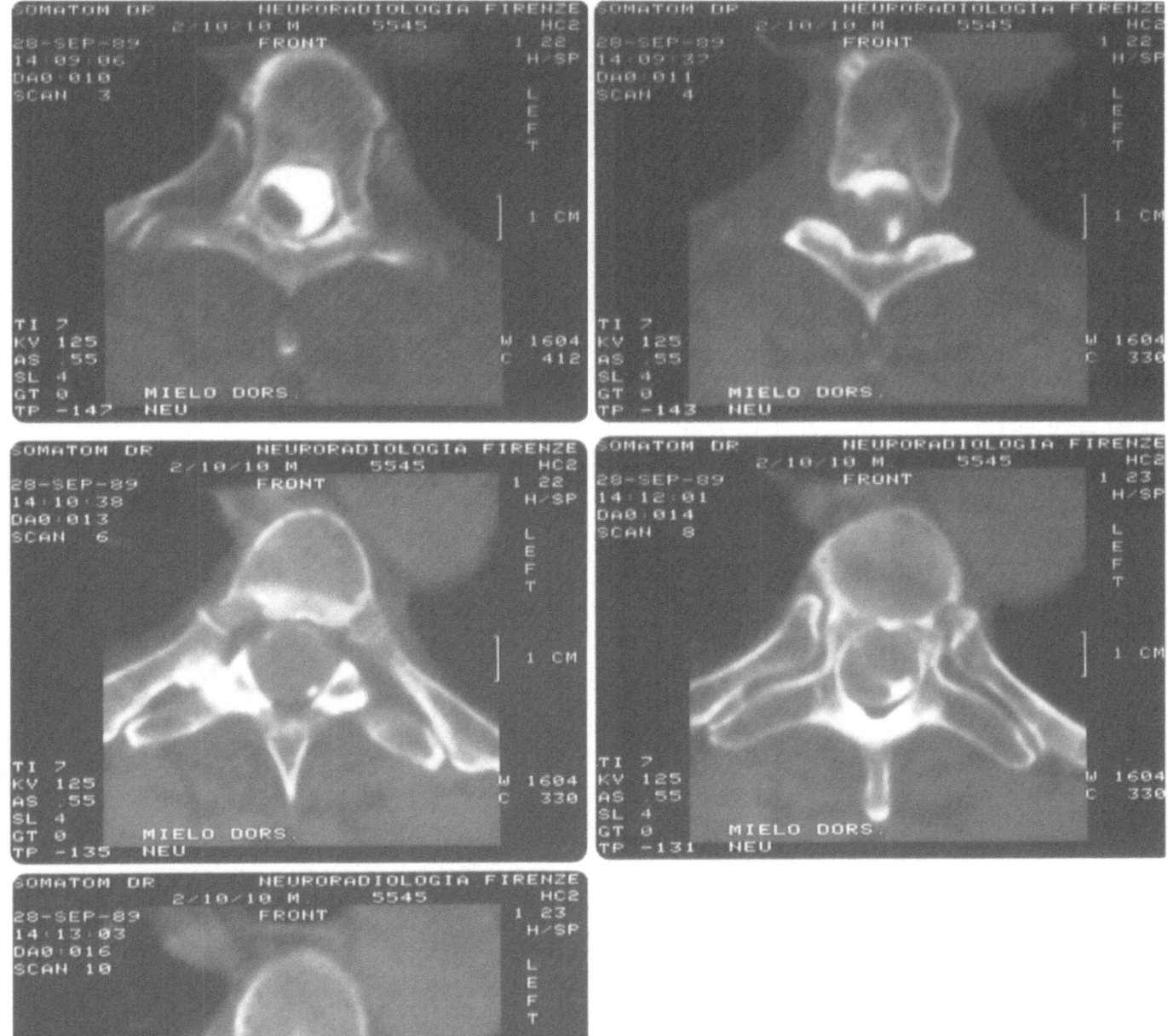

Fig. 191. Myelo-CT. Confirmation of the left anterolateral widening of the subarachnoidal space. In central sections the expansive process which deforms and displaces the cord to the posterolateral right side is plainly seen. In the last axial scan the reappearance of the dilatation of the subarachnoidal space below the lesion

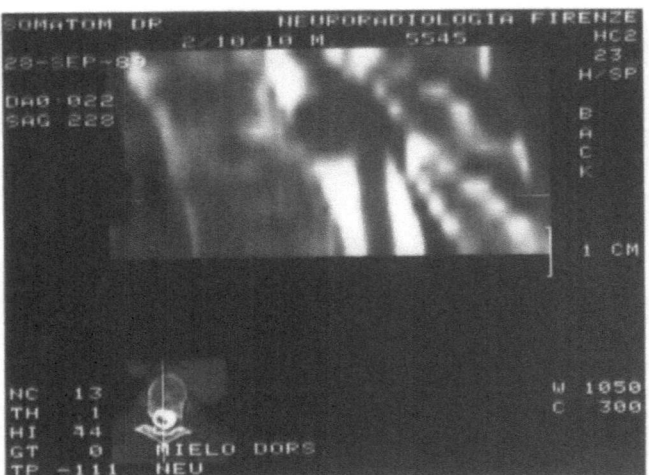
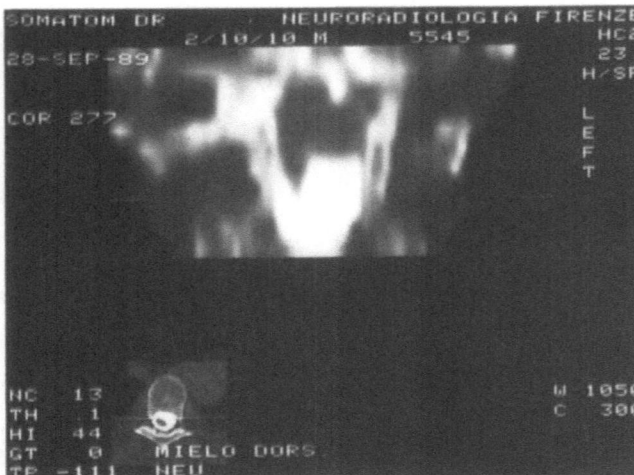

Fig. 192. Electronic reconstruction on a sagittal and coronal plane corresponds perfectly to the myelography and provides additional detail of the cord displacement on the right and to the rear

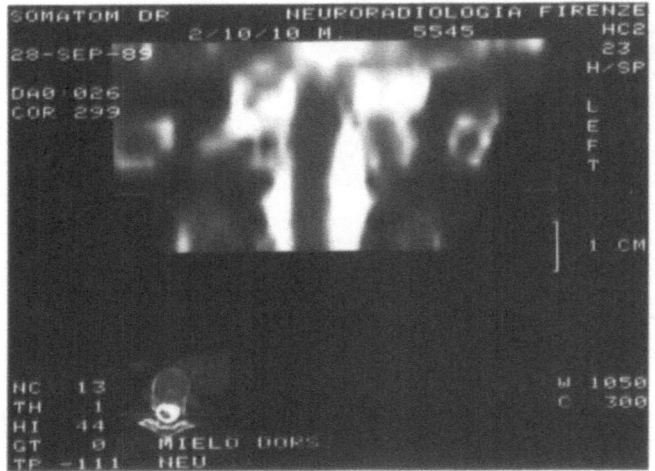
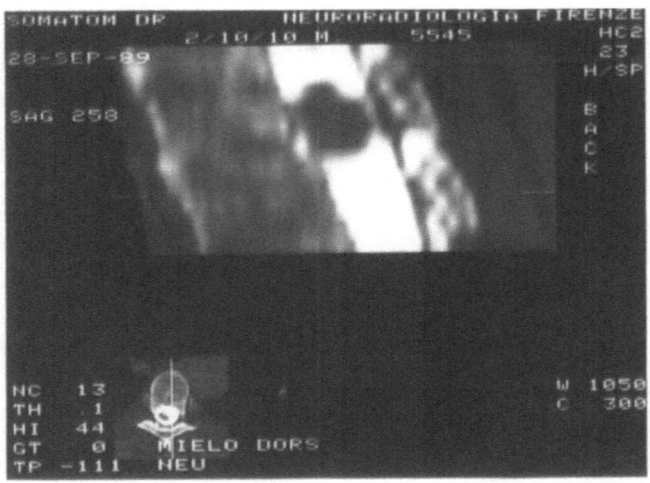

Fig. 193. Myelo-CT: coronal reconstruction

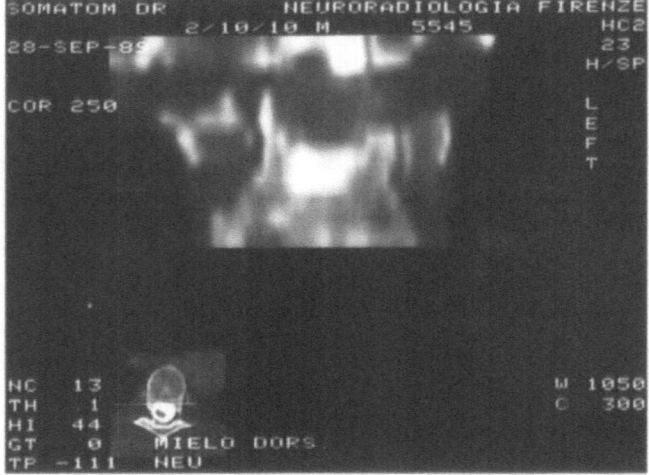
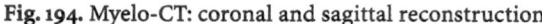
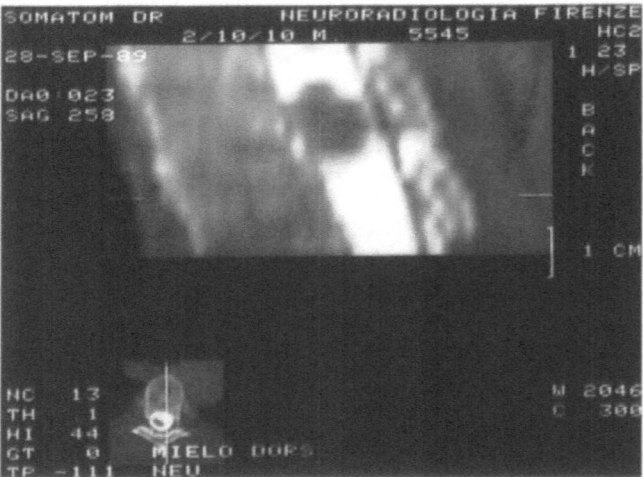

Fig. 194. Myelo-CT: coronal and sagittal reconstruction

8.3.4 Magnetic Resonance Imaging

MRI produces without a doubt the most valuable information in all compressive myeloradicular pathologies. In addition to being noninvasive, it allows a panoramic study on multiple planes (axial, sagittal, coronal) and can detect even the smallest lesion. MRI is superior to all other examinations and is crucial in detecting the nature of tumours when the attachment base is narrowed along the entire length of the tumour. These aspects of narrowing disappears except on the upper and lower poles of the meningioma because the dura mater returns to its normal thickness in the tract where the attachment ends.

Case No. 29: Transitional Meningioma
A 63-year-old woman (1987). Left ventrolateral intradural-extramedullary meningioma in D5-D6.
Medical History. Surgery to remove a fibroid.
Clinical Course. 15 years. Intermittent back pain. For 2 years motor impediment to the left and slight motor claudication. Band-like constriction at medial dorsal tract level and hot and cold paraesthesias at lower limbs.
Neurological Examination. Spastic paraparesis to the left. Bilateral Babinski sign. Superficial tactile and pain hypoaesthesia from D6. The oscillating sensibility felt less by the iliac crests. Sphincter disturbances in the form of retention.
Rachicentesis. 0.73 g protein per thousand.
X-Ray of Dorsal Spine. Scoliosis.
Plain CT. Neoplasm occupying left anterolateral portion in D6. The cord appeared displaced backwards and to the right. Along the posterolateral wall of the vertebral body of D6; area of irregularly shaped calcifications (Figs. 195-197).
MRI. In D5-D6 intradural-extramedullary neoformation measuring maximally 3 cm in diameter. The neoplasm invaded the left anterior side, and its maximum width occupied the rachidian canal almost entirely. After having administered the contrast medium there was fairly a good enhancement of the neoplasm (Fig. 198).
Surgical Treatment. Hypervascularization of the laminae and venous haemorrhages along the epidural space. The cord was displaced backwards and reduced in volume. By freeing the arachnoid the reddish-wine coloured neoplastic tissues appeared on the left. Fragmented removal of the tumour. A portion of the dural invasion was calcified near the 6th dorsal root on the left. Coagulation of the base of attachment and removal of contralateral adherent processes (Fig. 199).
Results. Within 15 days the patient began to walk. Clinical recovery after 1 month.

In addition to defining the characteristics of a compression, MRI is able to throw light on possible degenerative lipoid, intratumourous phenomena with or without fatty deposits deep in the vertebral body at the level of the tumour site or at various vertebral points. Another element that can be seen only indirectly with a myelogram but is clearly visible with MRI is the concomitant modification of the medullary vascularization for its entire length above and below the meningioma.

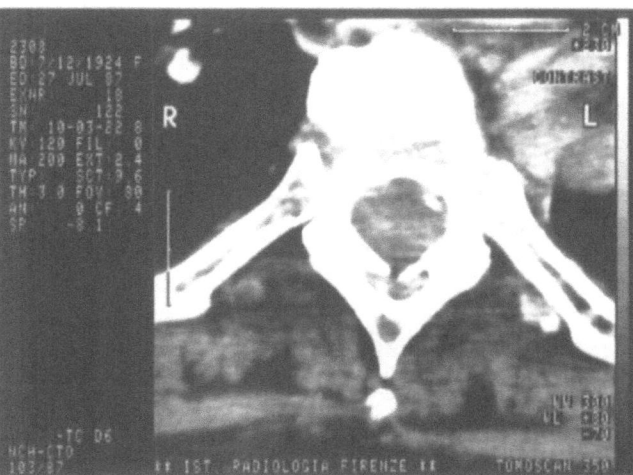

Fig. 195. The meningioma occupies the left anterolateral portion of the spinal canal in D6

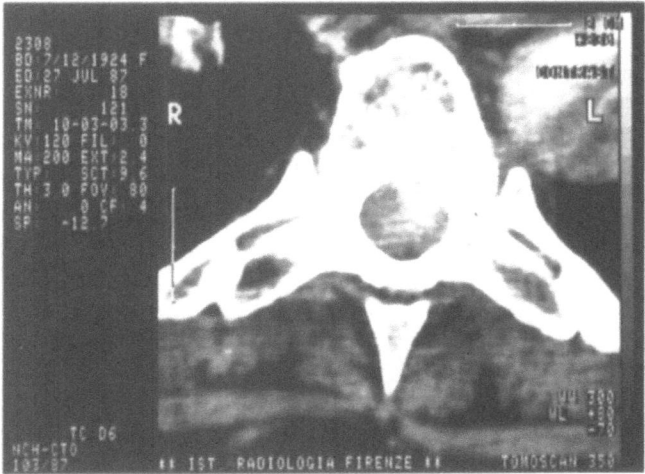

Fig. 196. A lower section

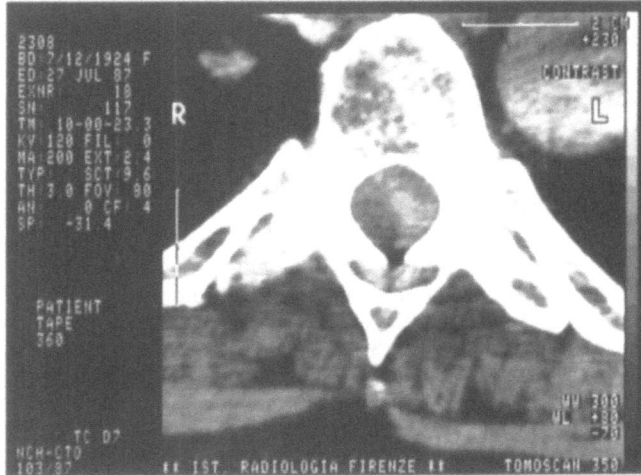

Fig. 197. Calcification of the tumour

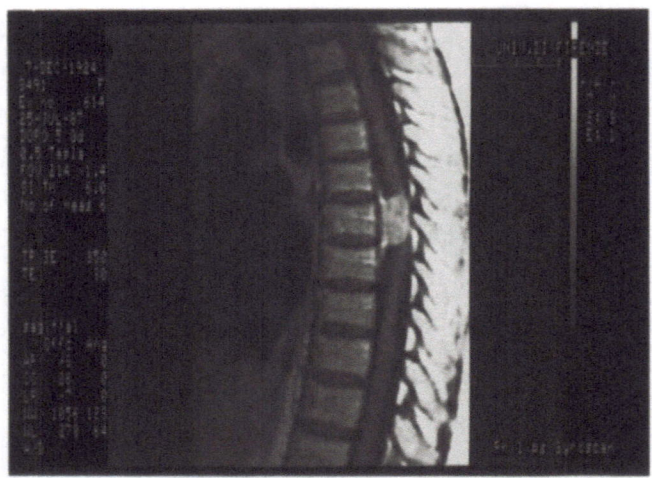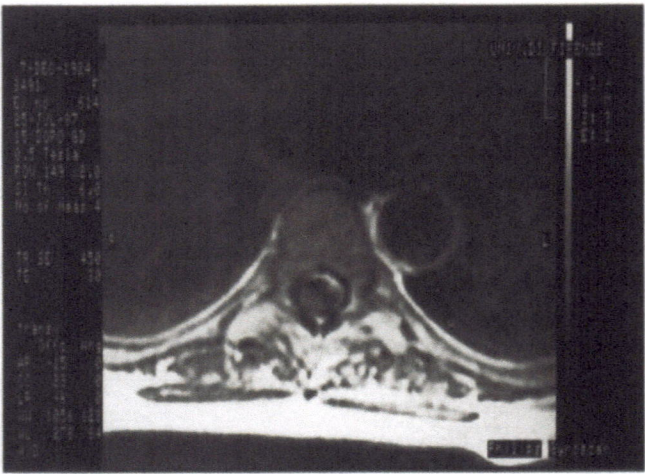

Fig. 198. MRI. Sagittal and axial projections T1 (TR 350, TE 30 ms) after injecting the paramagnetic contrast medium: nonhomogeneous feature of the tumour with a "mouse-tail" insertion near to the upper and lower poles. This feature is important for the diagnosis of the diagnosis of the nature of the tumour

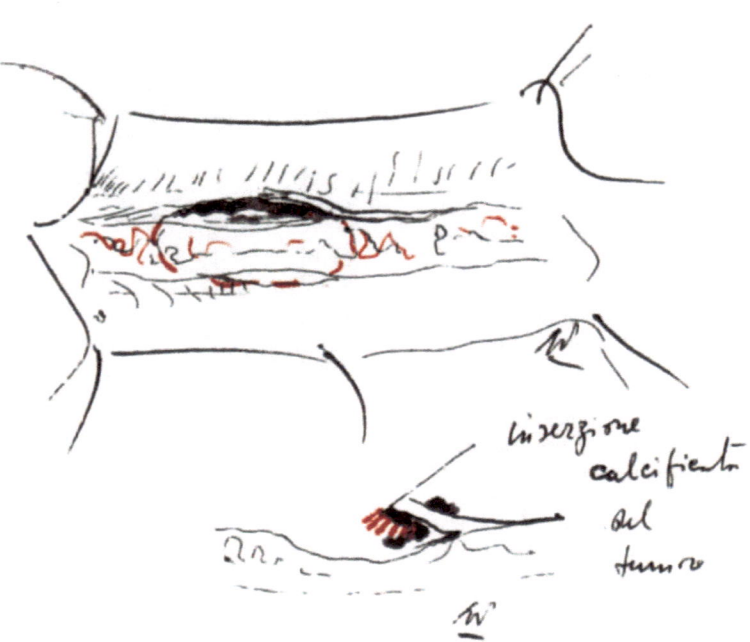

Fig. 199. Picture of the operating field

Case No. 70: Transitional Meningioma

An 81-year-old woman (1993). Right posterolateral intradural-extramedullary meningioma in D10.

Clinical Course. 10 years. Sense of constriction on lower thorax on the right with intermittent pain in umbilical region, pronounced when standing upright or at night. Hot and cold paraesthesias to lower limbs. Impediment in walking for 1 year.

Neurological Examination. Spastic paraparesis. Bilateral Babinski sign. Lack of medial and lower abdominal reflex. Superficial tactile and painful hypoaesthesia from D10, pronounced from D12 towards the left. Hypopallaesthesia to the left below 12th rib.

X-Ray of Dorsal Rachis. Left convex scoliosis.

MRI. In D10 the vertebral canal was occupied by a roundish formation measuring a little under 2 cm in diameter. It had a well-defined outline, was homogeneous and showed sensitivity to the cord in early sequences with an increase in protonic density signal. The neoplasm displaced the cord upwards and to the right (Figs. 200, 201).

Surgical Treatment. A reddish-wine coloured tumour occupying the right posterolateral region. The cord appeared reduced in volume and a root extended over the surface of the tumour reaching the dural funnel on the left. Removal by fragmentation while debulking the tumour; a partial repletion of the surface layers blood vessels occurred in the direct vicinity of the neoplasm. The partly calcified attachment of the meningioma was near the dural funnel of the tenth root.

Results. In the following 10 days walking was still difficult for the right lower limb. Clinical recovery 1 month later.

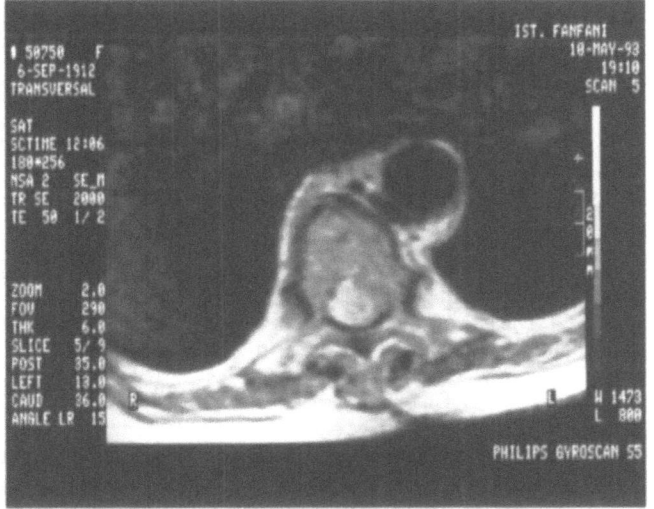

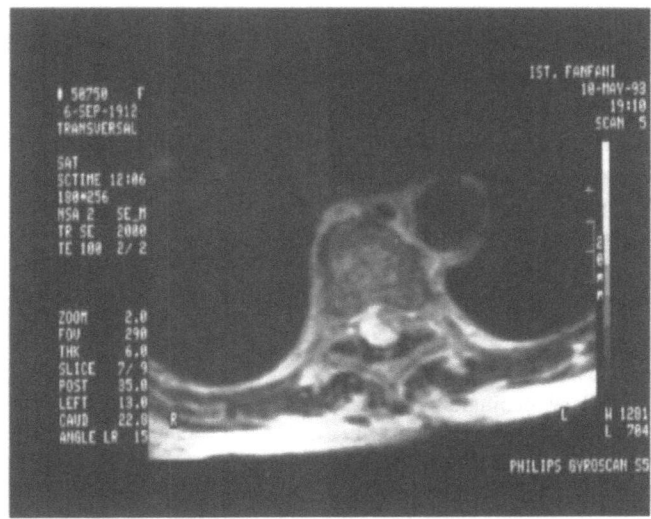

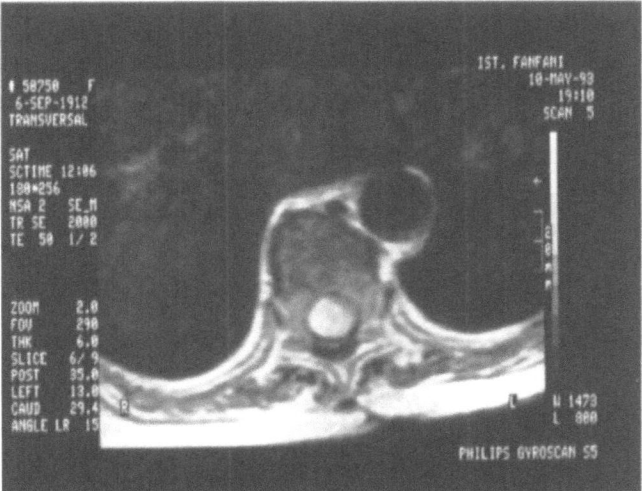

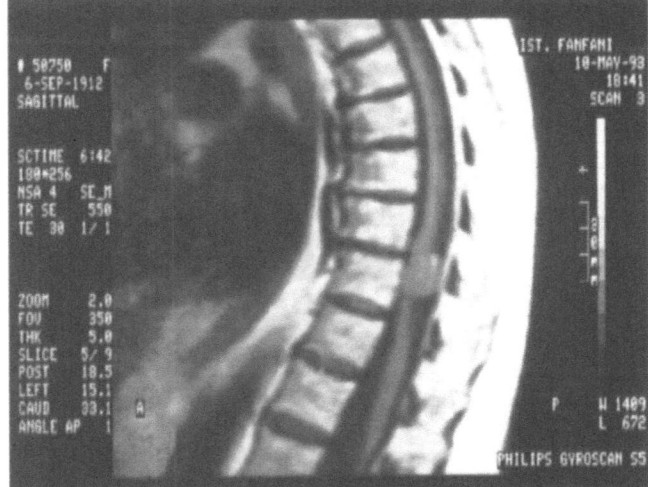

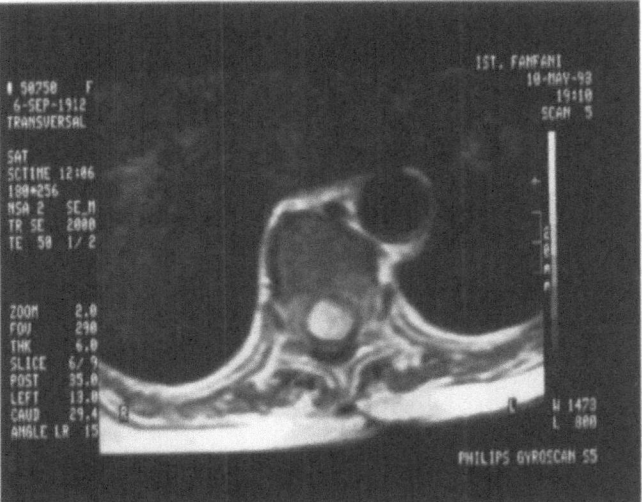

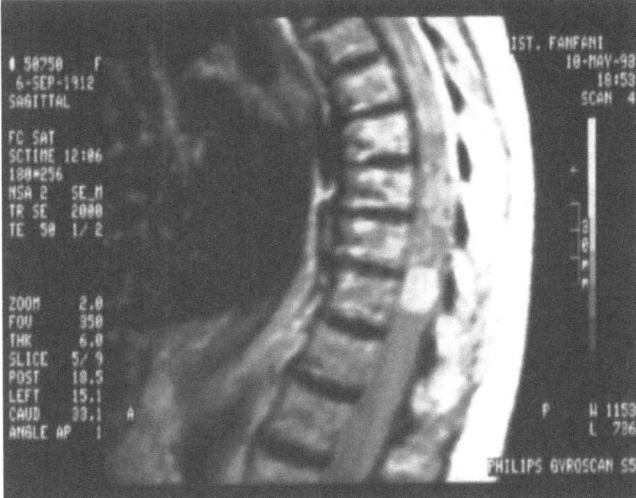

Fig. 200. MRI. Axial projection DP and T2 (TR 2000 and TE 50, 100 ms). Sagittal projection T1 (TR 550 and TE 30) and DP (TR 2000 and TE 50). The expansive intradural process in D9-D10, isodense to the cord in the T1 sequence and hyperintense in the protonic density and T2 in right posterolateral location

Fig. 201. MRI. The sagittal sequence (DP) shows dilatation of the medullary vascularization above the lesion

MRI can detect intramedullary ischaemia in meningioma cases with intense perifocal oedema. Every clinical tool can give positive results regarding the extension of a tumour in meningiomas with intra- and extrarachidian development, even if their nature remains uncertain. Frequently the diagnosis of location reached only by MRI is not sufficient and a myelo-CT even today plays an essential role in obtaining preoperative elements which are particularly useful.

Case No. 52: Fibroblastic Meningioma

A 63-year-old woman (1987). Right ventrolateral intradural-extramedullary meningioma in D1-D2.

Clinical Course. 20 years. Long-standing dorsal pain with transitory fastidious irradiation on the right. One year before hospitalization paraesthesias to the lower limb with loss of strength. After a few months the same symptoms appeared on the left.

Neurological Examination. Spastic paraparesis to the right. Bilateral Babinski sign. Hypopallaesthesia distally to right malleolus. Sphincter disturbances in the form of imperious micturation.

X-Ray of Dorsal Rachis. Dorsal left convex kyphosis-scoliosis from D1 to D5-D6 (Fig. 202).

Plain MRI. In D2-D3 the compression occupied the vertebral canal particularly on the right. It was difficult to verify whether the lesion was intra- or extradural (Fig. 203)

MRI with Gadolinium. Expansive, oval-shaped structure with diameter measuring maximally 2 cm and occupying the rachidian canal on right anteroposteriorly. The cord of a thread-like appearance presentd a mark and was displaced towards the left (Fig. 204).

Myelo-CT. The site of the meningioma was more clearly in a right anterolateral position. The cord was displaced posteriorly (Fig. 205).

Surgical Treatment. On opening the dura the cord appeared curved backwards with a very narrow surface-layer vascularization. After opening the arachnoid a slight reclination of the cord on the right was essential to remove the neoplasm, pushing it against the dural wall.

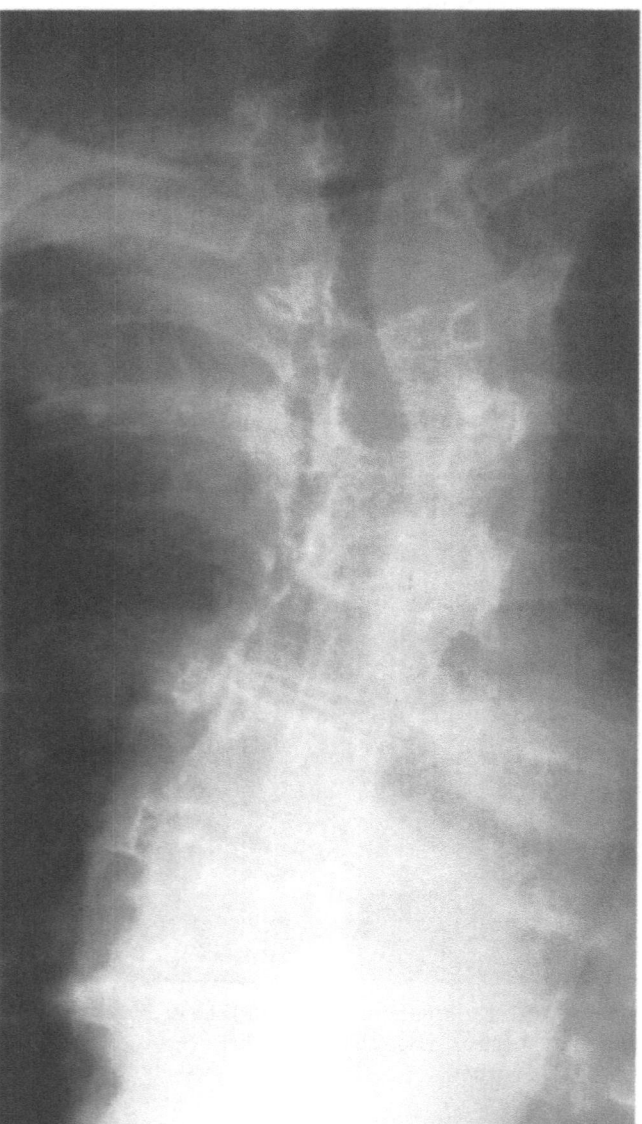

Fig. 202. Dorsal kyphoscoliosis

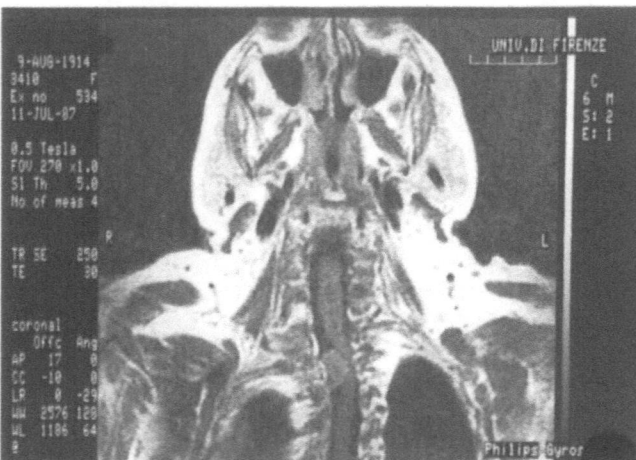

Fig. 203. MRI. SE T1 sequence (TR 350 and TE 30) on coronal and sagittal planes and after injection of contrast medium into a vein. The tumour, at a right anterolateral location, assumes little contrast medium. The cord is compressed and displaced towards the left

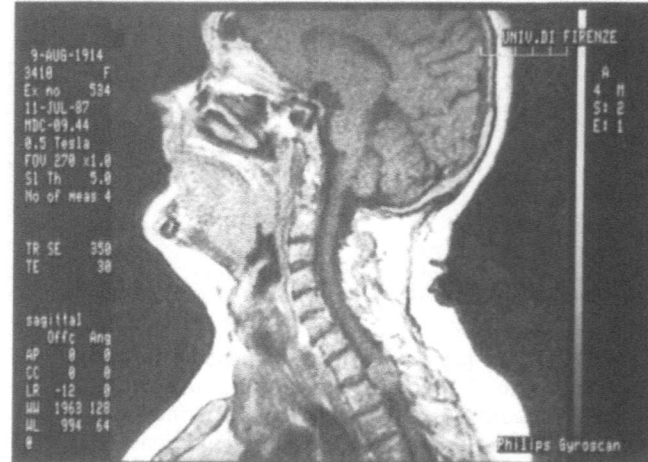

Fig. 204. MRI sagittal section

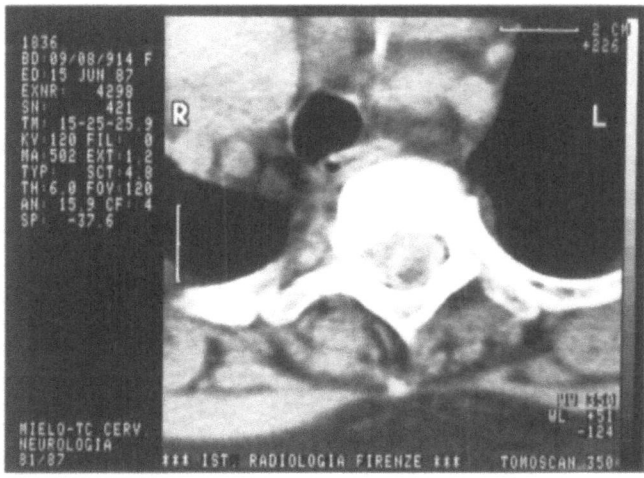

Fig. 205. Myelo-CT. An expansive intradural lesion in D1-D2 is of the same density as the cord. The contrast medium thickens on the right below the lesion

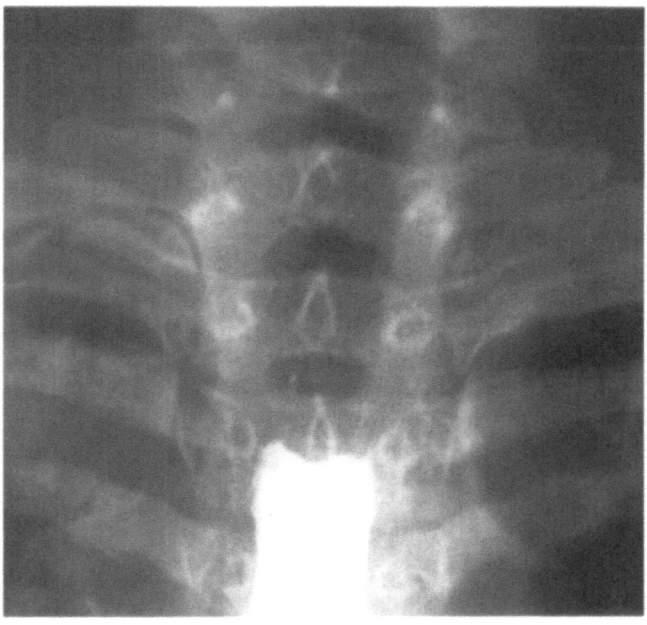

Results. Postoperative motor inhibition persisted after 1 month. Bronchopneumonia complications and transfer to intense care unit.

A number of investigations must be carried out depending on the specifics of the individual case without preconcptions idea that only CT and MRI offer methods capable of reaching a diagnosis and exact localization (Figs. 206-210).

Case No. 46: Transitional Osseous Meningioma
A 36-year-old woman (1990). Posterior intradural-extramedullary meningioma in D2-D3.
Medical History. Acute anterior poliomyelitis at a young age.
Clinical Course. 3 months. Progressive difficulty in walking and motor claudication to the right. The patient had to use bilateral support. Burning paraesthesias to lower limbs.
Neurological Examination. Dyschromic cutaneous birthmark on the left lower abdomen. Spastic-ataxic paraparesis. Bilateral foot clonus and Babinski sign. Hypoaesthesia from D4.
Rachicentesis. 0.55 g protein per thousand.
Myelography (via lumbar puncture). Block in D2-D3 with slightly dome-shaped filling defect. In lateral projections the iodine column gradually narrowed from the back to the front, thus revealing the posterior site of the tumour (Fig. 206).
Myelo-CT. In D2-D3 widespread calcifications within the dural sac. In the reconstructions the lesion was in a posterior site; an elongated form with calcified densities. The posterior subarachnoidal space was wider below the lower pole of the tumour (Figs. 207-208).
MRI. In close relation to the posterior wall of the rachidian canal there were small round expansive formations clearly defined and measuring about 1 cm in diameter which compressed and displaced the cord forwards marking the posterior profile. The signal of this formation appeared homogeneous in the various sequences and sensitive to the cord (Fig. 209).

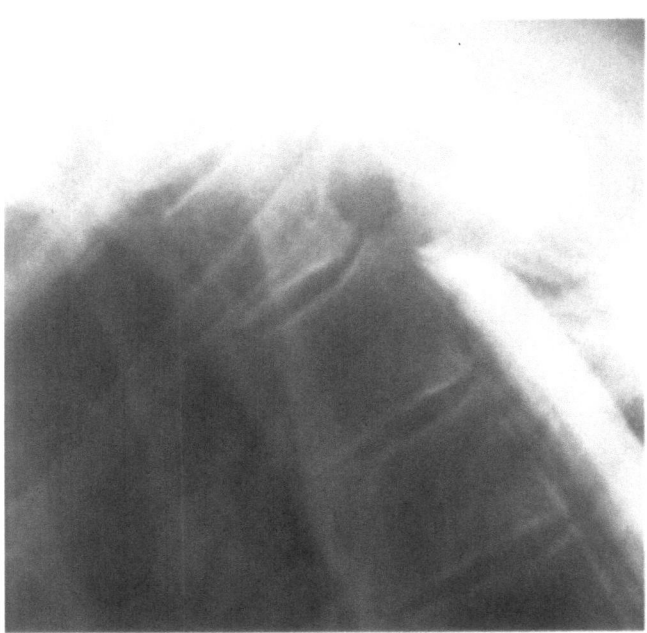

Fig. 206. Myelography via lumbar puncture. Total block at the D2-D3 level. Laterally the column thins as it moves forwards defining the lower posterior tract of the neoplasm

Surgical Treatment. The dura was taut, nonpulsating, of hard consistency and calcified. A curved incision was made below the most resistant dural point which led to the lower pole of the meningioma. The incision was continued upwards revealing the tumour in toto. It was removed together with its attachment (Fig. 210).
Results. Gradual reduction in hypertonia to lower limbs with spontaneous motility.

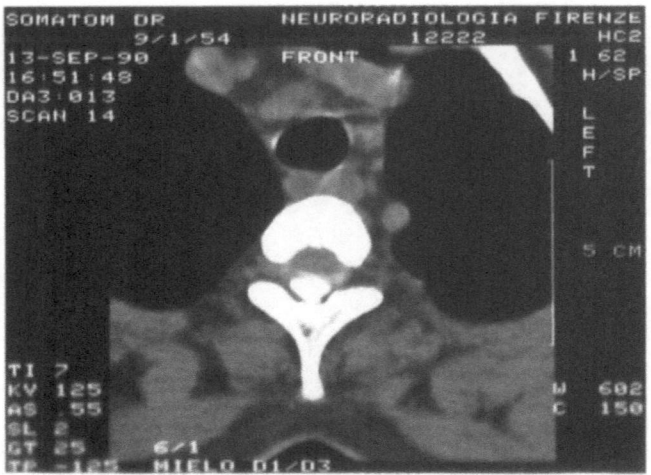

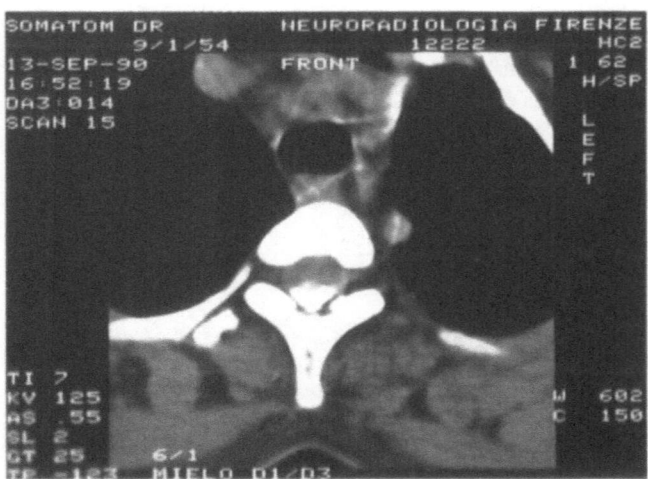

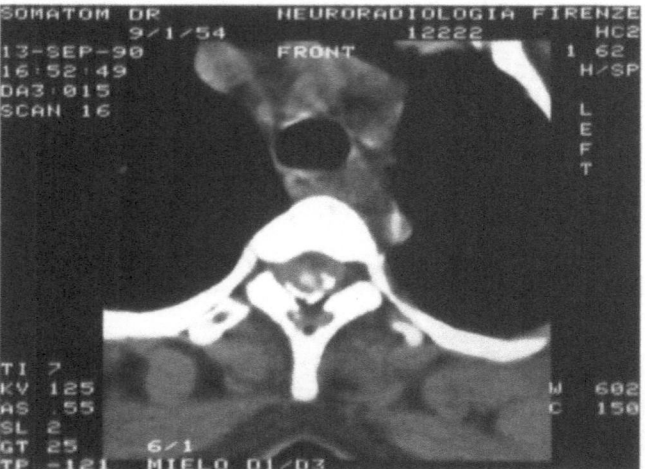

Fig. 207. Myelo-CT. Contiguous axial scans, 2 mm thick. Small calcifications are present in the intersomatic area of D2-D3 in the posterior part of the dural sac. Total block. The vertebral canal in D2 is completely occupied by a homogeneous tissue with a similar density to the cord

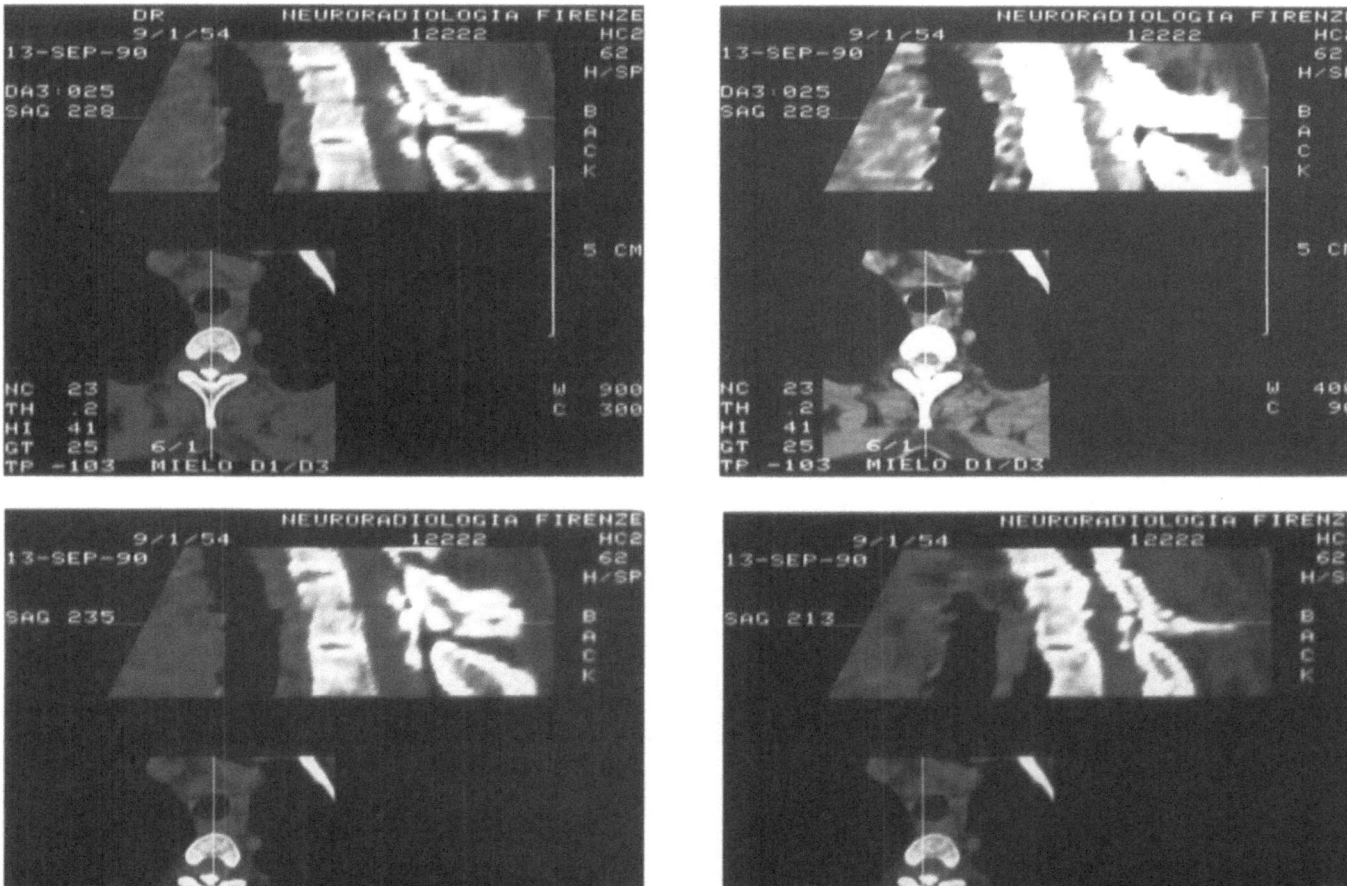

Fig. 208. Electronic reconstruction on the sagittal plane. The calcifications identified as the irregular areas are more evident

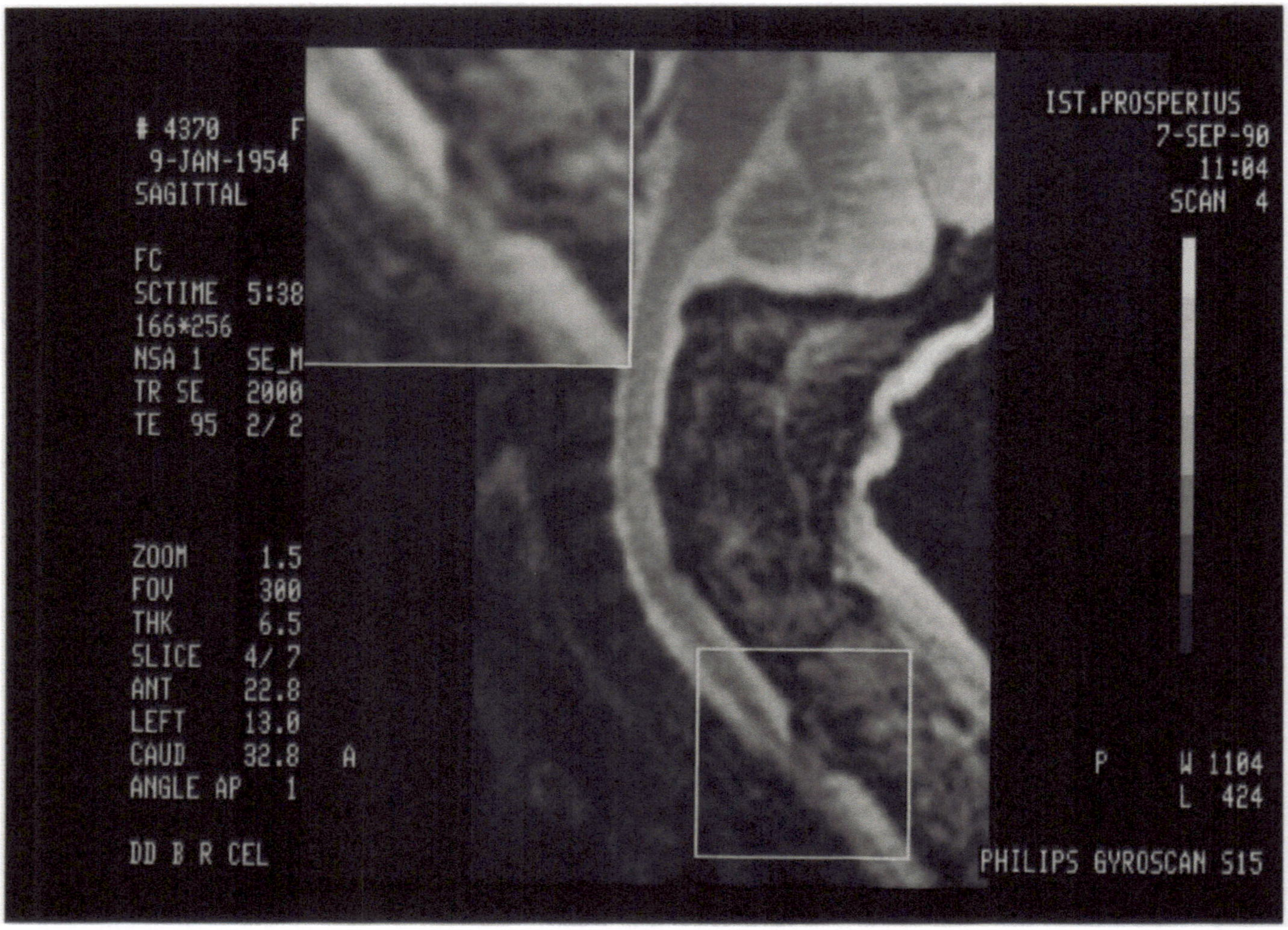

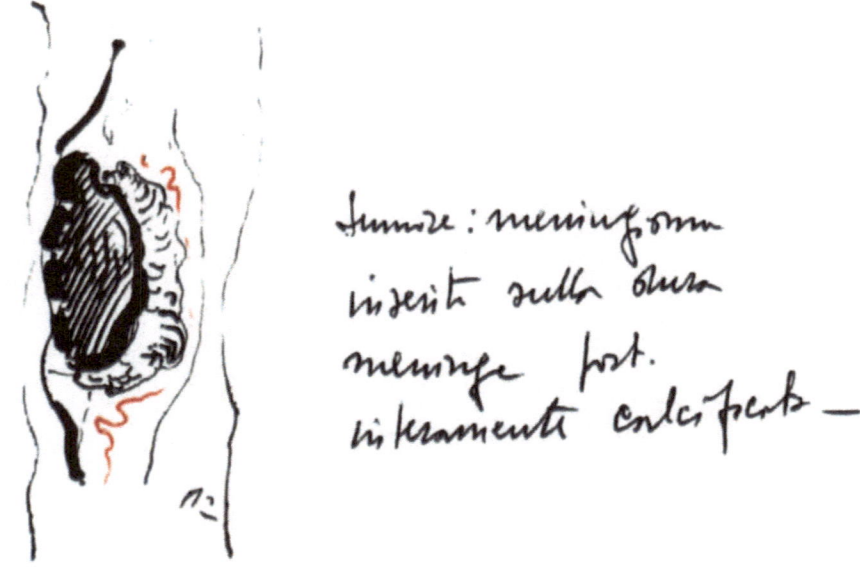

Fig. 209. MRI. Sagittal projections T2 (TR 2000 and TE 95). An expansive ovaloid formation in D2-D3 with compression of the ventrally displaced cord

Fig. 210. Drawing of the operating field. The tumour is completely calcified

In some cases, even when myelography performed via lumbar puncture supplies the positive image for a compression with a suspected meningioma, on the basis of a lumpy irregularity in the anteroposterior total block we are convinced that other neuroradiological investigations are able to supply details for defining the relationship between a tumour and the neural structures (Figs. 211-215).

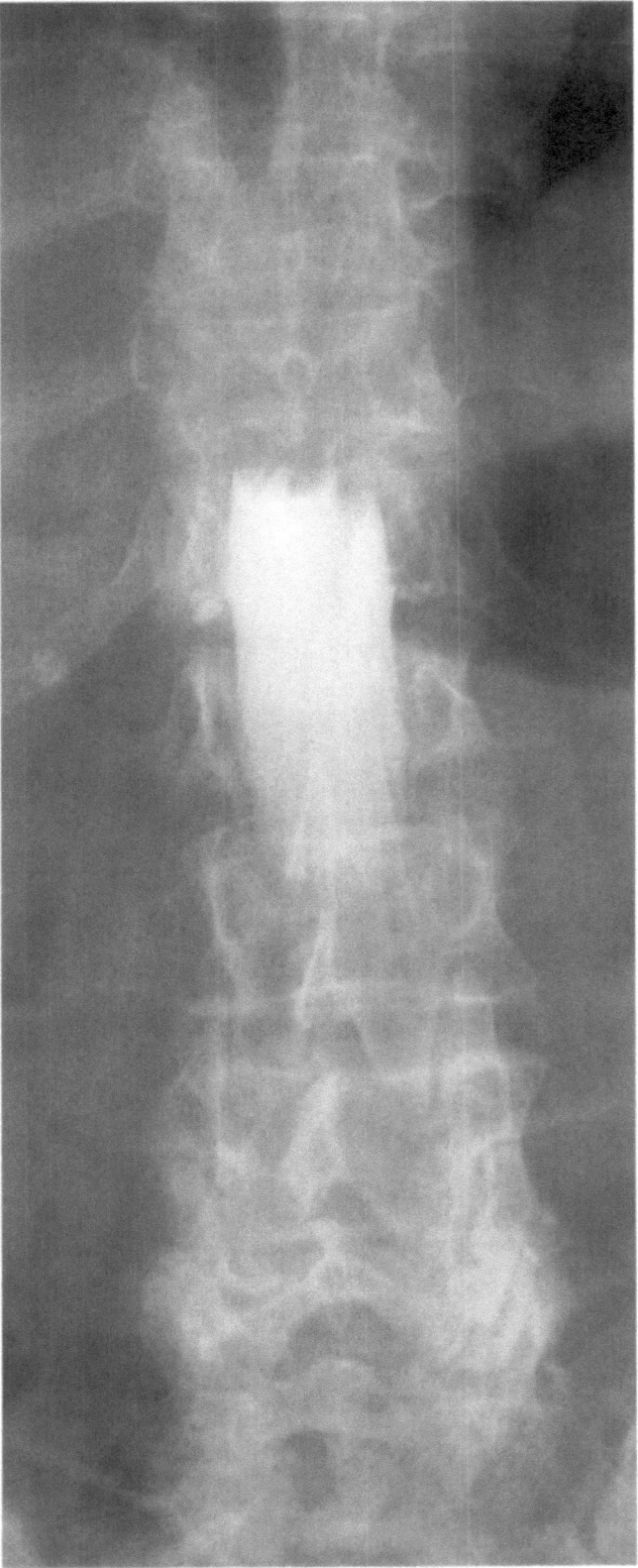

Fig. 211. Myelography via lumbar puncture. Anteroposteriorly, total block in D11-D12. Double concavity upwards. The medullary corridor is displaced to the left. The block is more linear in the lateral projection (see Fig. 212)

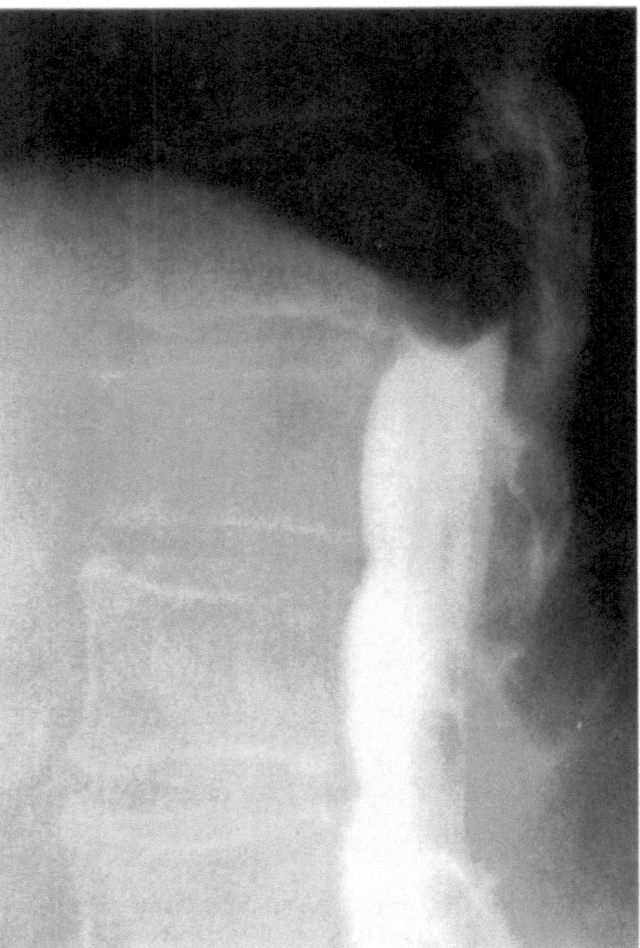

Fig. 212. Lateral view

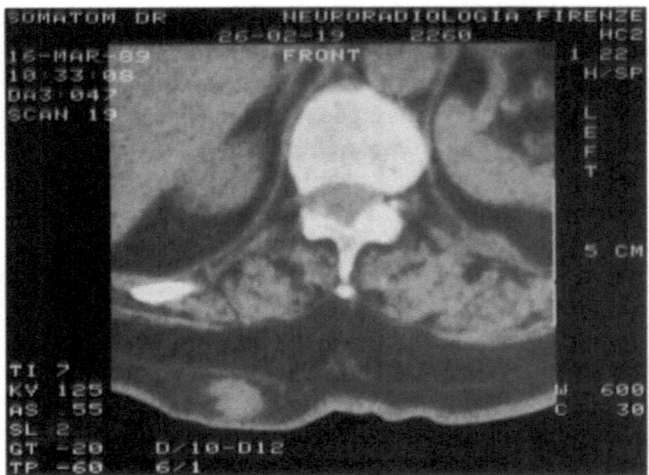

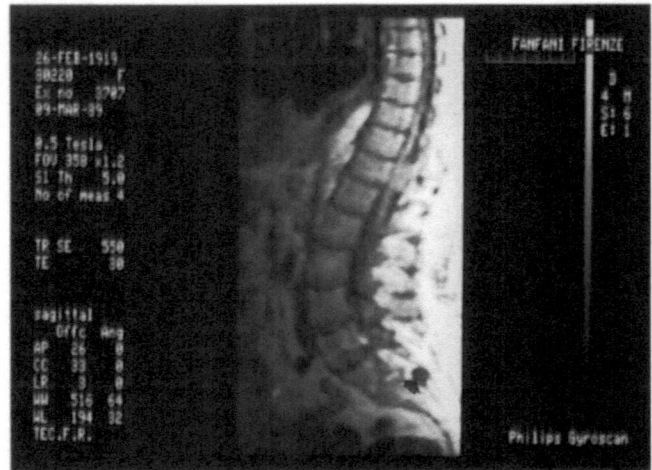

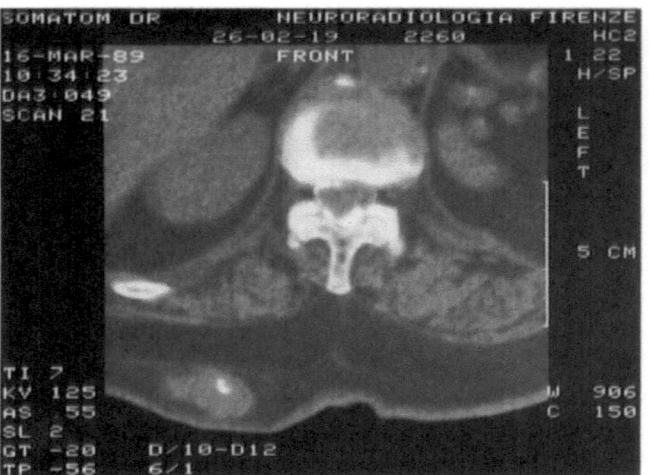

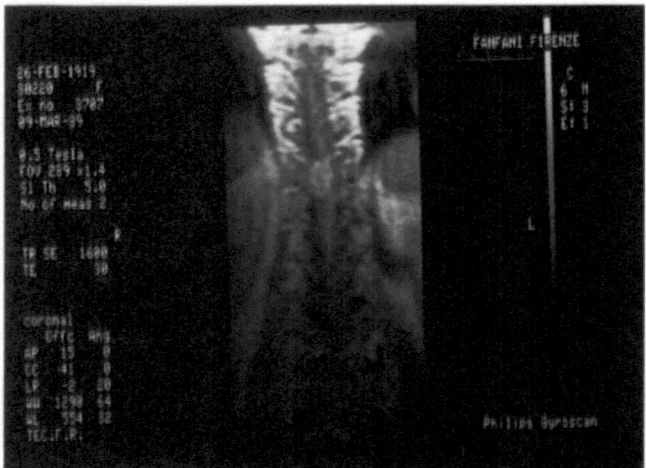

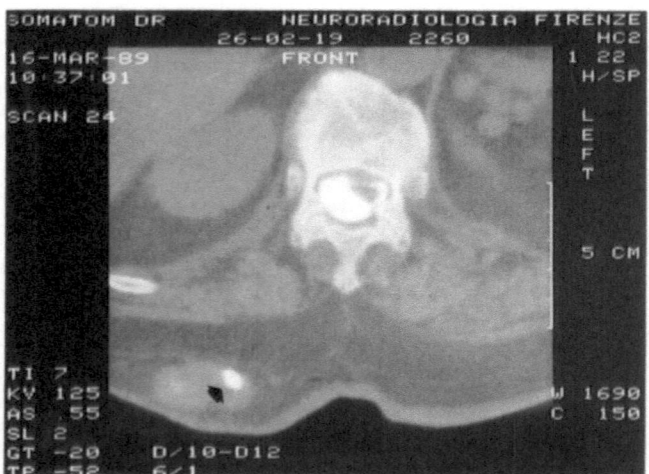

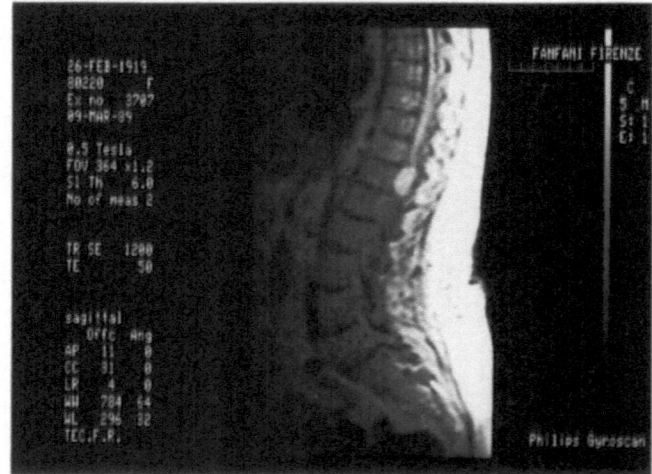

Fig. 213. Myelo-CT (2 mm contiguous scans). Sections in D10-D11. *Above*, the vertebral canal is occupied by a lesion whose density appears similar to that of the cord. The central section shows only a small part of the right posterolateral subarachnoidal space. *Below*, the subarachnoidal space is dilated against the displacement of the cord towards the left. Collateral findings in the three sections include an ovaloid lesion subcutaneously to the right and a nonhomogeneous structure due to a hyperdense calcified type area (arrow)

Fig. 214. MRI. Sagittal and coronal projections. Spin-echo sequence T1 (TR 550 ms, TE 30 ms) and DP (TR 1200 and TE 50 ms) direct test. An ovaloid lesion extending along the height of the vertebral body of D11, located on the right side of the vertebral canal, which displaces the cord contralaterally forwards and to the left. This expansive process is of an isointense nature with the cord in a T1 sequence but appears unevenly hyperintense in DP due to the presence of internal hypointense areas, probably small calcifications. Sacral level presents a linear roundish-shaped arachnoidal cyst

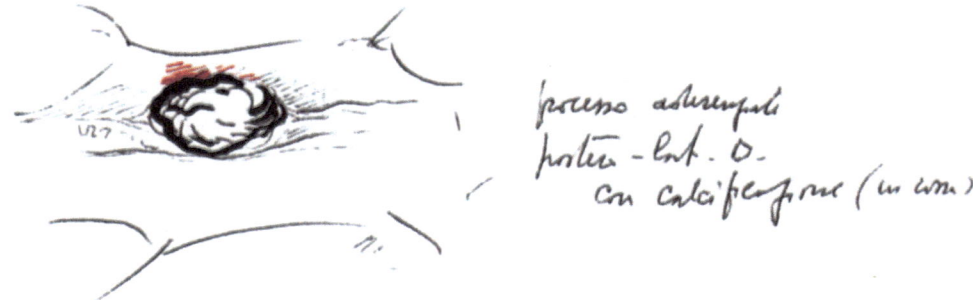

Fig. 215. The calcified part of the tumour is shown red

Case No. 95: Fibroblastic Meningioma
An 89-year-old woman (1989). Right posterolateral intradural-extramedullary meningioma in D12.
Clinical Course. 10 years. Intermittent pain in the lumbodorsal passage. Three years before hospitalization the patient complained of heaviness to the lower limbs with motor claudication. Burning paraesthesias to lower limbs. One month before admission to hospital the patient suffered deterioration of the motor deficit leading almost to paraplegia.
Neurological Examination. Severe paraparesis to the right. Hypotrophy of femoral quadricep to the left. Flaccid patellas and lack of ankle jerk. Right Babinski sign. Band of hyperaesthesia in D10-D11 and hypoaesthesia below. Sphincter disturbances in the form of incontinence.
Rachicentesis. 3.75 g protein per thousand.
X-Ray of Dorsolumbar Rachis. Scoliosis on dorsolumbar passage. Disappearance of articular facets at D11 on the right. Very slight retrolisthesis in D11-D12.
MRI. In D12 oval formation measuring maximally 2.5 cm in diameter which occupied the canal almost entirely and displaced the fascia of the cauda towards the left (Fig. 214).
Myelography (via lumbar puncture). Total block in D11-D12 with well-defined lower pole of the neoplasm, irregular in shape and multilobed (Figs. 211-212).
Myelo-CT. Visualization of neoplasm in D11-D12. Widening of subarachnoidal space below the block. The cord appeared displaced towards left (Fig. 213).
Surgical Treatment. On opening the dura the tumour appeared compact and was covered by the arachnoid and was invaded on the right posterolateral internal surface. Calcifications on the dural side of the attachment. The cord was completely displaced ventrally and towards the left. After removal by total fragmentation, removal of perimedullary adherent structures and straightening of the cord (Fig. 215).
Results. Gradual recovery of walking but persisting ataxic gait. After the patient had been sent home, and 3 weeks from surgery, she was readmitted for cephalalgia syndrome and operated on for a chronic sublesional haematoma. Complete recovery in 1 month. Patient considered clinically cured; neurologically negative during a check-up after 6 years. (This was the oldest meningioma patient in the present series.)

We consider MRI essential in identifying the exact dimensions of a tumour and the features of dilatation in the subarachnoidal space above and below the neoplasm.

However, when the meningioma almost entirely occupies the rachidian lumen and is of premedullary development, but its exact location is undefined, myelography proves very useful. This is because the indirect images produced for locating tumours present various angles of the corridor at the displacement produced by the meningioma and allow us to define its exact location and dimensions. Although the axial scans produced by MRI are extremely valuable, a myelogram offers a more detailed study of the subarachnoidal space. This is very useful in evaluating the width of the laminectomy which varies from case to case especially when the meningioma is premedullary (Figs. 216-218).

Case No. 40: Fibroblastic Meningioma
A 74-year-old male (1988). Intradural-extramedullary-premedullary meningioma in D2.
Clinical Course. 2 months. Diminution in the subjective sensitivity of the skin of the abdomen. Severe motor difficulty for 1 month at right lower limb and frequent attacks of motor claudication leading to paraplegia.
Neurological Examination. Spastic paraplegia and equinism at the feet. Bilateral Babinski sign. Hypoaesthesia from D2-D3, distally pronounced. Pallaesthetic anaesthesia from the iliac crests. Sphincter disturbances in the form of retention.
X-Ray of Dorsal Rachis. Arthrosis.
Myelography (via lumbar puncture). Almost total block in D2. Slight diffusion and flow of iodine medium along both sides (Fig. 216).
MRI. Extramedullary neoformation with clear outline located anteriorly to cord in D2 (Fig. 217).
Surgical Treatment. On opening the dura the cord appeared normal in volume but the surface-layer vascularization was thinned. The neoplasm was strictly anterior and was observed only after the dentate ligament had been cut. Removal by fragmentation and gentle reclining of the tumour to right and to the left of the cord. The incision was paramedian and made to the right of the motor root of D1 (Fig. 218).
Results. Twenty-four hours after surgery slight reaction to right femoral quadricep under stimulus. One month later some spontaneous movements of toes and incomplete flexion of voluntary movements. A check-up after 6 years showed the persistence of severe spastic paraparesis.

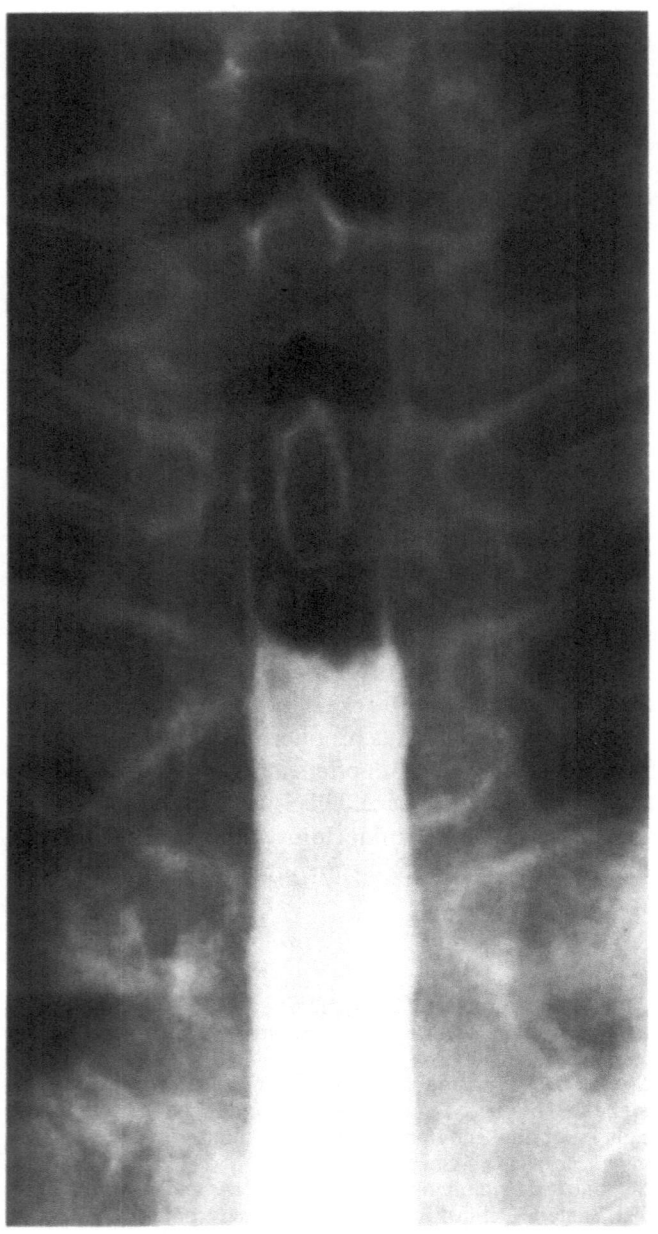

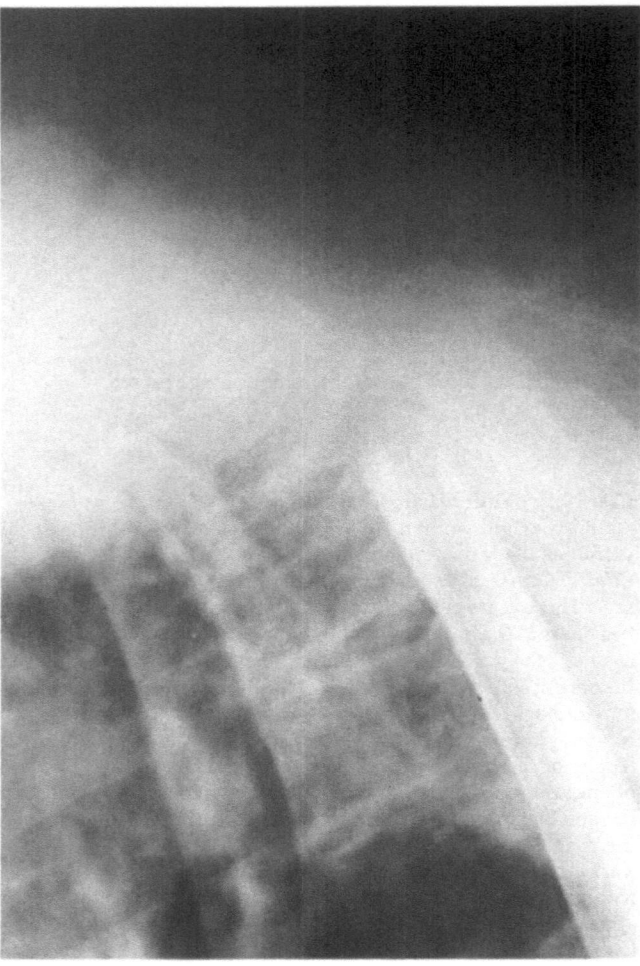

Fig. 216. Myelography via lumbar puncture. Anteroposteriorly, total block in D2 producing a dome-shaped aspect in an upward direction. Laterally, a detailed myelographic description of the subarachnoidal space with evident posterior rounding of the medullary corridor

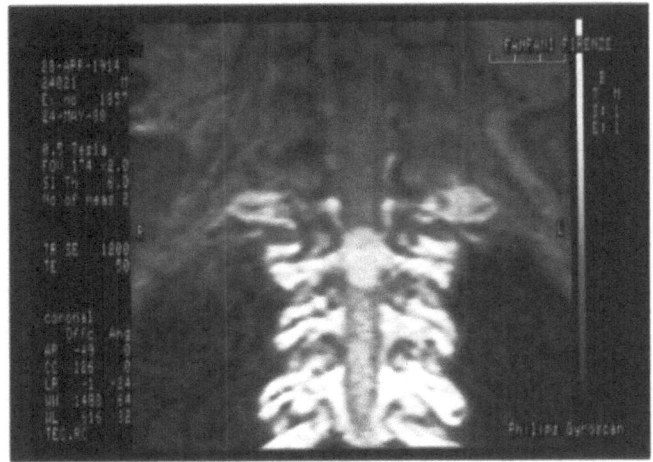

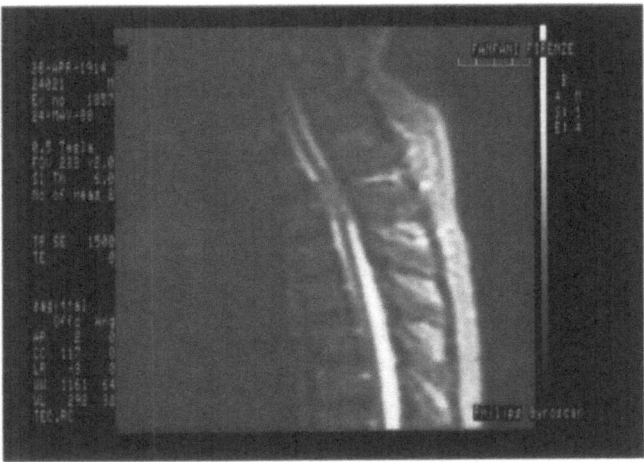

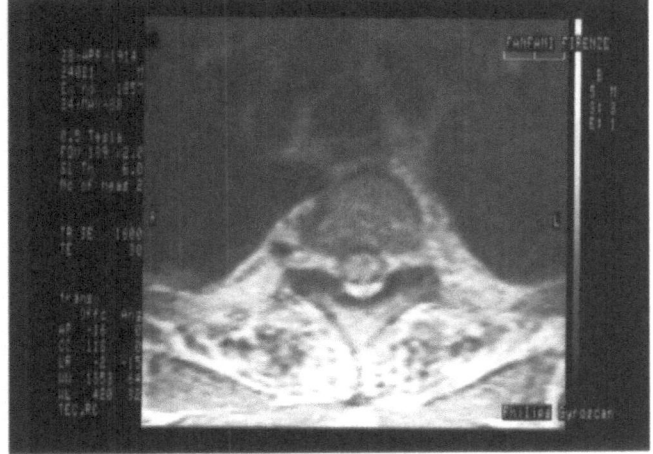

Fig. 217. A-C. MRI. Anterolateral location of extramedullary tumour in D2

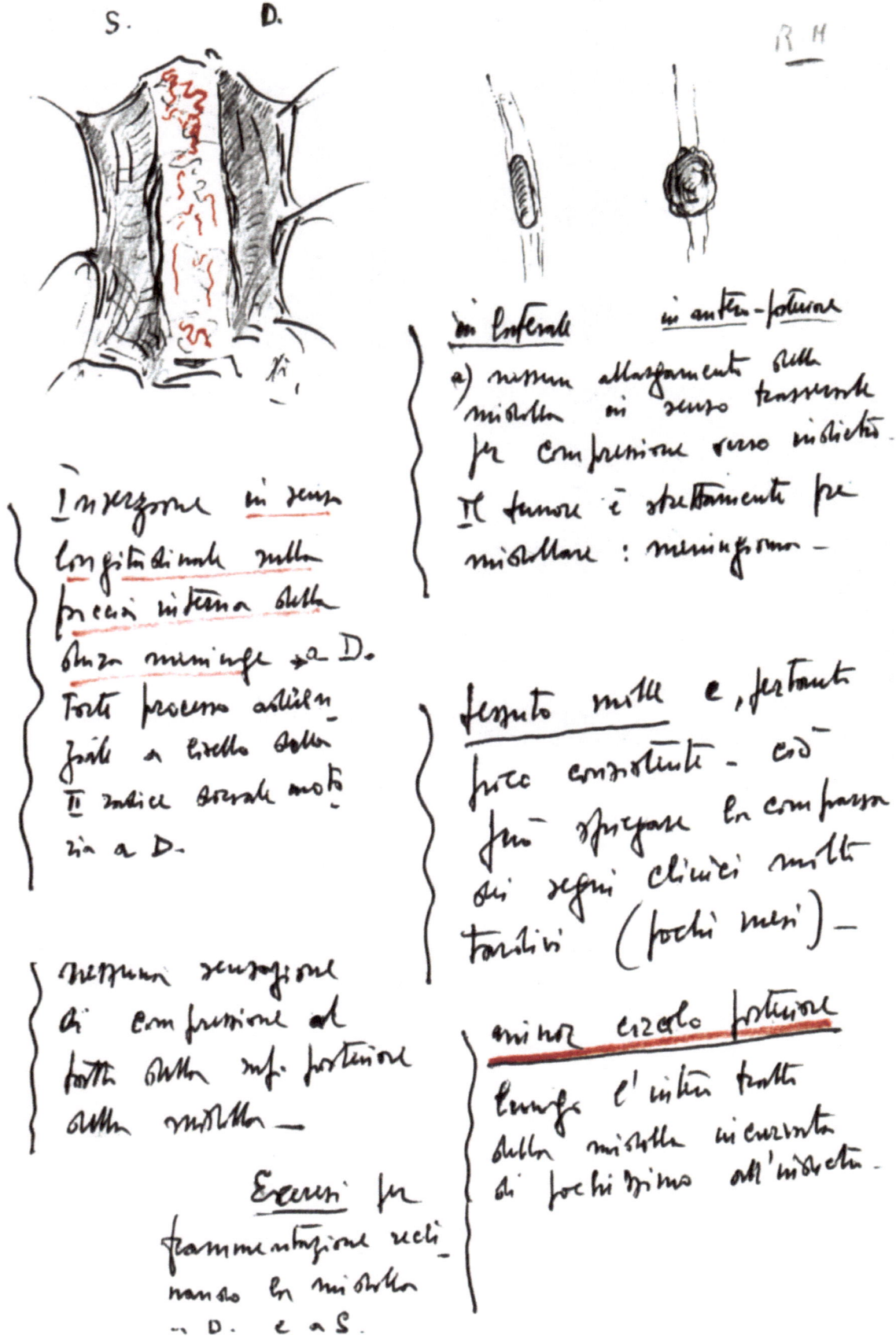

Fig. 218. Fragmentation of the tumour was possible after reclining the cord on both sides. In contrast to other premedullary processes this case did not present important signs of transversal enlargement

8.3.5 Angiography

Djindjian (1970) demonstrated with medullary angiography the way in which vascular neoplasms with intra- and extrarachidian development fill. Vertebral angiography for cervical locations can supply clear images of the vascularization of some meningiomas. The examination consists of injecting a contrast medium into the subclavian artery and has been practised for many years, but today the approach is by an indirect route (through catheterization) which has proved helpful even in relapse cases years after the first operation (Figs. 219-222).

Case No. 123: Psammomatous Meningioma
A 76-year-old woman (1987). Right posterolateral intradural-extramedullary meningioma in C2-C6.
Clinical Course. 6 months.
Medical History. Underwent surgery at 37 years for cervical neoplasm leading to monoparesis at right upper limb. Ingravescent weakness to lower limbs with impossibility of walking.
Neurological Examination. Spastic tetraparesis to the right. Flaccid monoparesis at right upper limb. Tactile and painful hypoaesthesia from D4 and hypopallaesthesia from the iliac crests.
X-Ray of Cervical Rachis. Results from a laminectomy C4-C7.
MRI. Expansive lesion extending from C5 to C6-C7 (approx. 5 cm), spindle-shaped and with clear outlines. The cord was displaced to the left and showed sensitivity.
Femoral Angiography. Injection into the subclavian artery on the left and thyreocervical on the left and relative right artery. In the area corresponding to the laminectomy performed previously on the right a slight intrarachidian blush was seen, with its upper pole at C4 and spreading further down for 4 cm.
Surgical Treatment. On opening the dura the tumour invaded the posterolateral internal surface layer on the right compressing the cord contralaterally. The cord had been flattened. Longitudinal incision of the tumourous capsula and removal by fragmentation. Removal of adherent structures along the lateral surface of the cord.
Results. Respiratory insufficiency immediately after surgery resulted in death after 20 days.

This case shows an irregular pathological cycle, predominantly extrarachidian, developing from a relapsed meningioma after 39 years. At the time of surgery the extensive healing process can explain the modification of all the vascularization including the cervical paravertebral. A selective medullary angiography is not part of the diagnostic routine; however, we believe that it can be a particularly valuable technique in the diagnosis of special cases, above all for intra- and extrarachidian forms, particularly those in dorsal sites. It is helpful to identify at a preoperative stage which blood vessels may be excluded without creating insufficiency in the medullary vascularization. When the meningioma is very lateralized angiography is used to visualize the lumen of the vertebral arteries to indicate narrowing in the extension of the tumour. The use of neurosurgical techniques in a preoperative stage should lead to surgery which takes into account the close morphological relationship between the lesion and the nearby structures.

8.4 Conclusions

Since our first use of MRI in the diagnosis of medullary compressions and particularly in intrarachidian neoplasms, we have attempted to define the connections between the results of the histological examination and the alterations visualized by MRI. However, even today we have not been able to identify all the features relating to histological types. Nevertheless we are sure that the spectroscopic examination of MRI provide contingent criteria for a clear differentiation. A MRI, as noted above, can visualize the dural site of a meningioma and with the images of T2 we are more frequently able to identify their hyperdensity. This simple examination, or one using gadolinium, can be used to accurately define all morphological details of intrarachidian neoplasms. This is not to belittle the value of other examinations such as CT and myelo-CT. In its own way each is helpful in defining a tumour and the adjacent structures. These investigations used together are useful but one generaly proves particularly appropriate in any individual case.

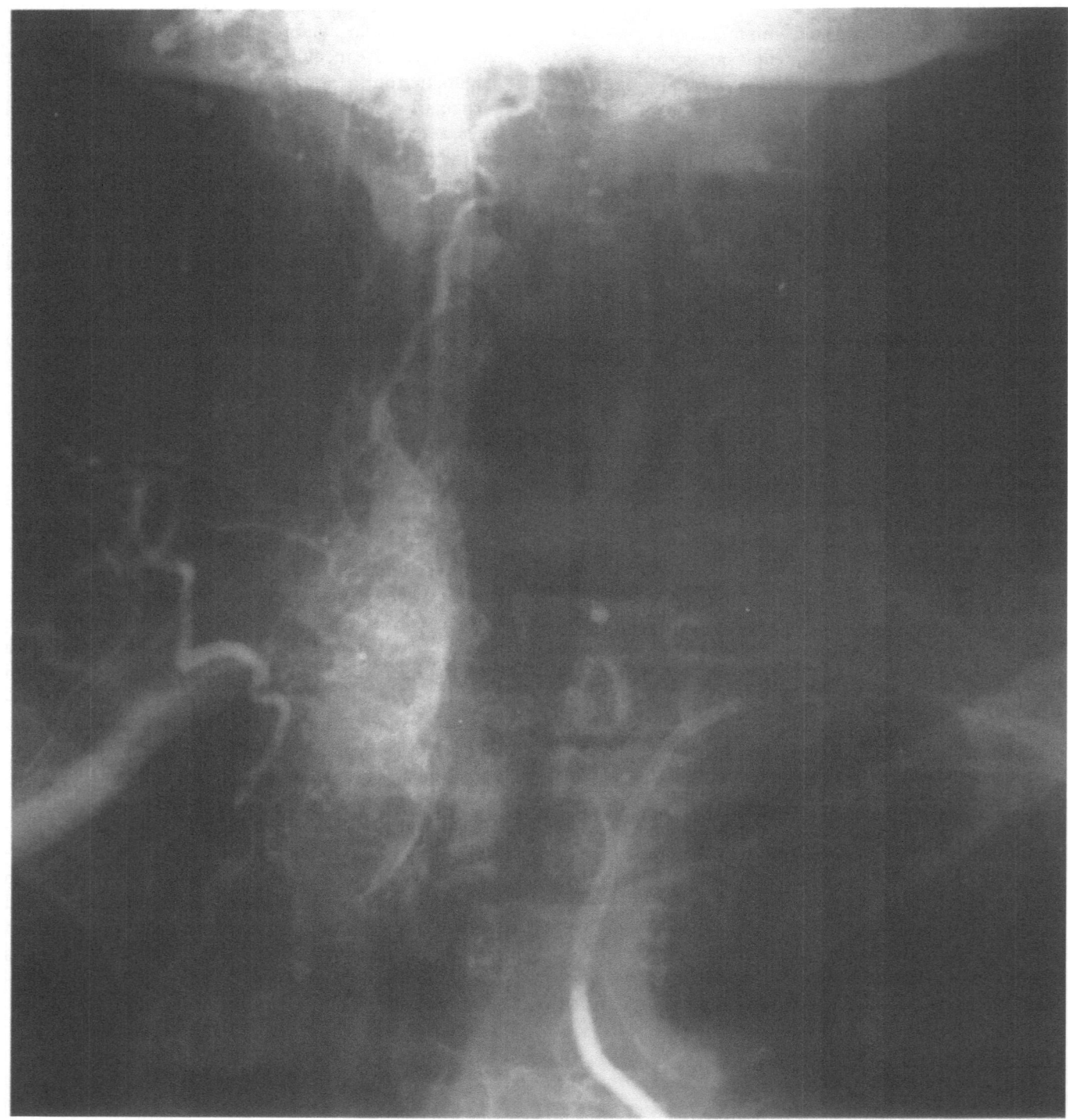

Fig. 219. Angiography, through left brachium via subclavian injection of the thyreocervical artery and the anonymous artery. Blush inside the lesion which is injected via the arterial structures of the right. No vascular supply from the left

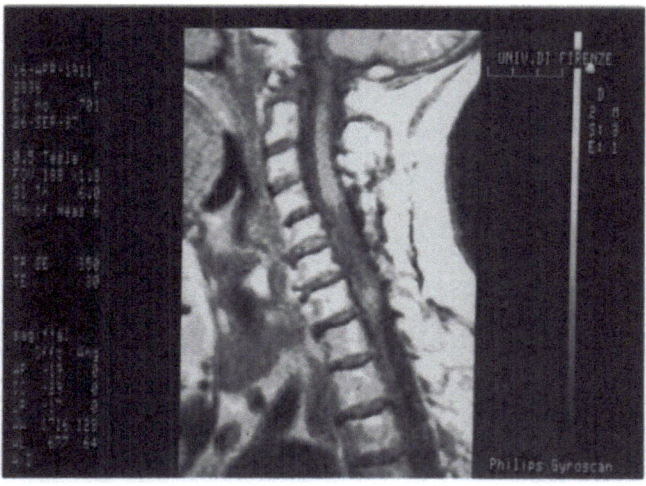

Fig. 220. Plain cervical MRI. Median sagittal projection. Spin-echo sequence T1 (TR 350; TE 30 ms). Results of cervical laminectomy from C3-C6. A large roughly ovaloid lesion with regular margins is present from C4 to C7 which shows itself to be homogeneously low to magnetic resonance

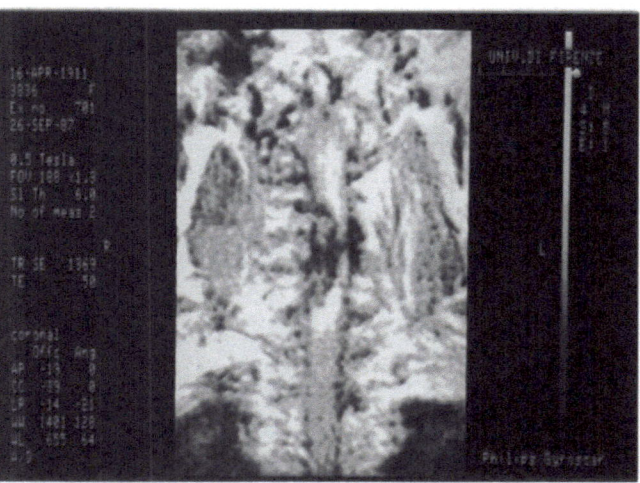

Fig. 221. Spin-echo sequence DP (TR 1369; TE 30 ms). Coronal projection. The expansive process even in this sequence shows low intensity signal and is located predominantly on the right, compressing and displacing the cord towards the left. The cord shows a diffused hyperintensity signal indicating an oedematous reaction

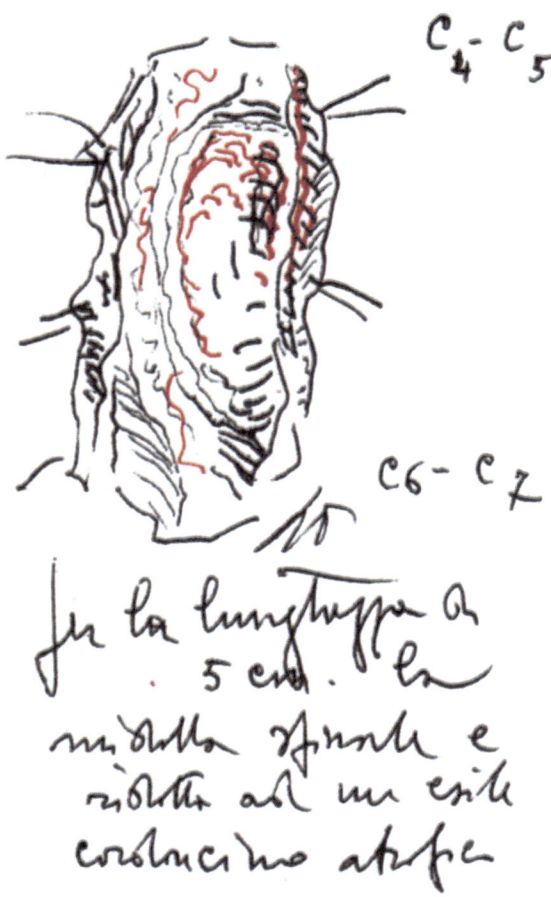

Fig. 222. The displacement of the cord is greatly increased and the surface layer shows signs of ischaemia

9 Surgical Techniques

A. Pansini

9.1 Microscopic Features and Variations in the Relationship with the Spinal Dura and Leptomeningeal and Myeloradicular Structures

Before describing variations in microsurgical techniques for the treatment of spinal meningiomas we review the most characteristic microscopic features of a meningioma and variations in its relationship to the dura mater, the leptomeninges and the cord.

Meningiomas generally reach 1.2 cm in size and are located on a single vertebral body, or they sometimes occupy an intradural site between two or more vertebral bodies. Tumours are frequently only a few centimetres long but there are some particularly large forms, as noted by Sawa (1993), which can reach the posterior occipital fossa through the foramen magnum. Here the tumour extends beyond the posterior arch and for this topographical extension must be considered exceptional. Our series deals only with meningiomas originating from the first vertebral body in C1. There are also extremely small meningiomas, as small as lentils, deep within the dura and often associated with von Recklinghausen's disease. The surface layer of meningiomas varies from case to case, for example the invasions can be in various parts of the internal or dural wall or occupying the entire meningeal layers with intra- end extradural development.

Meningiomas are generally roundish in shape in the forms in which the attachment is well defined. Others can be oval-shaped when the base of attachment is larger, and with or without a compact calcifying component in the form of a bony lamalla adherent to the internal dural wall. When the calcified portion occupies the base of the tumour, the passage of neoplastic tissues is clearly visible from the attachment point, and the tissues become less consistent with a smooth or irregular surface layer. However, in every form there is a more uniform and a less dense superficial layer in relation to the underlying friable and haemorrhagic tissue. During the operation, in an appropriate site, it is always useful to conserve this peripheral layer to avoid the tumour bleeding before it is removed from the meningeal plane.

In addition to the meningiomas with en plaque characteristics, there are also meningiomas in which the densely calcified base has the shape of a bony spur that is surrounded by the soft part of the tumour. The blood vessel layer of the meningeal sac near the attachment of the tumour and along the opposite part of the invasion presents irregular chain formations due to major dilatation of the arterial vascularization. This pronounced dilatation of the dural vascularization is still present on the internal side of the dura when the tumour has been removed. This feature is manifest more in anterior and posterior meningiomas. In the latter, major arterial participation in the external surface layer of the dura mater can reveal the extent of the base of invasion, which is rigid to the touch and thicker, allowing the possibility to decide how to proceed in opening the dura in relation to the volume and site of the meningioma. A major transversal development often produces a malformation of the entire posterior and lateral walls of the dura, varying in length according to the extension of the tumour.

9.2 Neighbouring Relationships with the Leptomeninges

A meningioma is frequently enveloped by the arachnoidal membrane which undergoes characteristic and variable displacement depending on the site and dimension of the meningioma and its adherent structures which develop between a meningioma and the leptomeninges. The alterations in the subarachnoidal space were identified

A. Pansini et al.
Spinal Meningiomas
© Springer-Verlag Italia 1996

for many years by using heavy iodine media long before the advent of CT and MRI. In the operating microscope, meningiomas with a lateral formation cause cord displacement towards the opposite side and the arachnoid moves further away from the medullary surface layer, like a curtain, immediately above and below the tumour. A varying morphological relationship between a lateral meningioma and the dentate ligament is formed; if the ligament is hidden by the tumour the meningioma develops in front of and behind the ligament. In these cases the dentate ligament appears as a sulcus on the surface layer of the meningioma. As the meningioma progressively occupies the central part of the rachidian lumen, the subarachnoidal space enlarges above the compression and the arachnoid moves still further away from the medullary surface.

In every form with partial or total block of the fluid the pulsations transmitted by the cord stop, and by simply puncturing the arachnoid to reduce the increased pressure of the fluid the pulsations reappear. We usually puncture the arachnoid above the meningioma because the myelitic vascularization is already affected at the time the operation takes place and a simple rachicentesis performed via lumbar puncture below the compression facilitates the diminution of nerve conduction (Garcin 1959).

The relationship to the nerve roots is also variable. In well-defined and lateral tumours the motor nerve root is pushed forwards against the dura mater while the posterior root appears stretched and elongated because the short distance between the medullary surface and the intravertebral foramen increases due to the tumour developing towards the back. This is caused by the force of the meningioma, so producing greater displacement of the cord in the opposite direction.

In most meningioma cases the arachnoid envelops the tumour as a veil along its surface, but some cases of tumours with the same attachment on the internal side of the dura mater remain totally extra-arachnoidal. These meningiomas sometimes have intra- and extrameningeal development. In these the densely calcified mass increases the compressive action and causes neighbouring bone alterations as described above (see case no. 66). Inside the dura mater adherent structures can be found between the arachnoid and the surface layer of the meningioma. Every type of adherent structure between the dura and the arachnoid is formed by a reactive and avascular tissue which is easily removed before opening the leptomeninges.

9.3 Position of the Patient

Patients with meningiomas of the cervical tract are usually placed in a sitting position without flexing the head, particularly in premedullary compression cases. In all forms of compressions the sitting position can be associated with a light, upward traction working up to the top of the head. With the electric table system any rear positioning of the patient on the operating table can be used during surgery to rectify any possible variation in pressure values. For all compressions below D3-D4 and for those in the lumbar tract we use the lateral decupitus position because having the patient positioned on the slightly rotating table that moves backwards and forwards allows a better view of the two lateral sides of the cord and of the relationship between meningioma and nearby structures.

Case No. 16: Transitional Meningioma
A 61-year-old woman (1966). Lateroventral intradural-extramedullary meningioma in D12-L1.
Clinical Course. 6 months. Back pain on dorsal tract when coughing. Subsequent transitory attacks of lumbago. Fifteen days before hospitalization the patient complained of acute and violent attacks of pain in lumbar area with irradiation to the anterolateral side of the thigh to the left.
Neurological Examination. Paraparesis to the left. Deficitary deambulation. Areflexia of patellas with pleuriradicular hypoaesthesia affecting L3-L4 and L5, on the left and on L4 on the right.
Rachicentesis. 7.20 g protein per thousand.
X-Ray of Lumbar Tract. Spondylolisthesis L5-S1.
Myelography (performed suboccipitally). Total block laterally and anteroposteriorly; the image was not clear enough to define the nature of the compression.
Surgical Treatment. Conus terminale of the cord was pushed posteriorly on the right. Dilatation of posterior spinal artery vascularization. On opening the arachnoid some roots adhered to the surface of the capsule. The lesion invaded on the left anterolateral internal surface of the dura (Fig. 223).
Results. Rapid and complete recovery after an initial motor inhibition of left lower limb. Results of neurological examination were negative after 3 years.

We do not exclude the ventral decupitus position used in many neurosurgical schools; however, we would like to add that in our long experience with over 900 medullary compressions, including both primary and secondary lesions, we have never encountered a case with deterioration of the venous stasis. For every operation preoperative fluoroscopy is used to define the borders exactly above and below the area where the laminectomy is be performed.

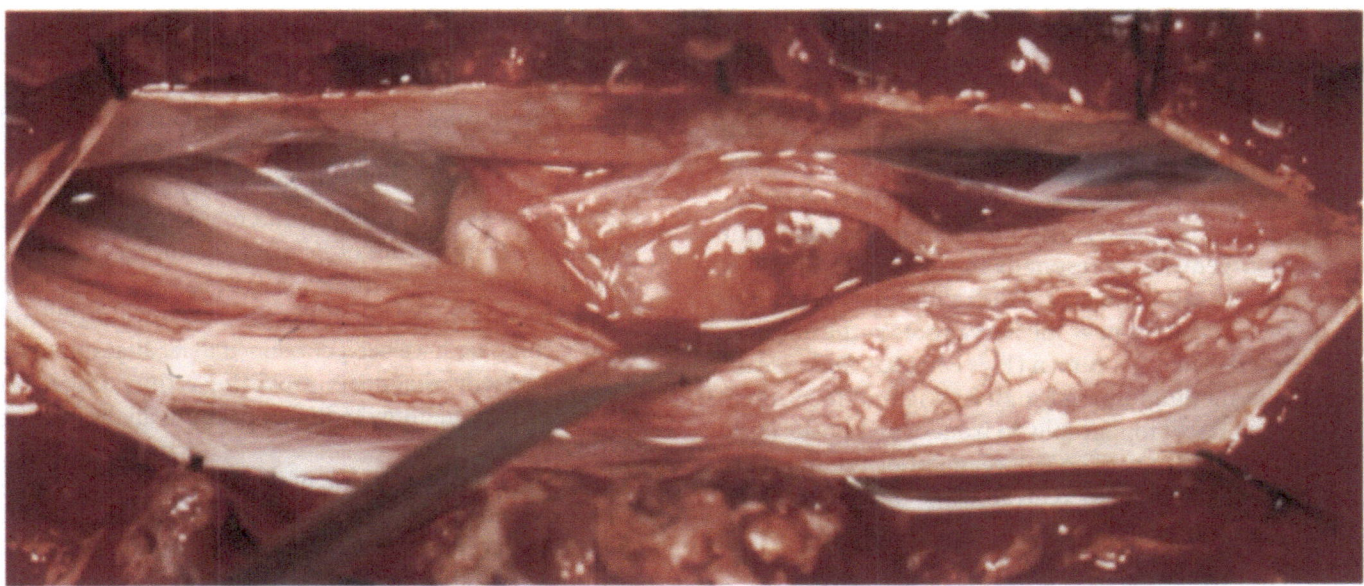

Fig. 223. Meningioma in left ventrolateral site. The adherent structure with a caudal root displaces posteriorly. Removal without radicotomy, sparing the radicular arterial circulation

9.4 Laminectomy, Lamina-Arthrectomy with Foraminotomy

Excision of the laminae requires just as much time as does excision of other forms of spinal compressions. In meningioma cases it is important to recall a number of factors once the length of the incision has been decided upon on the basis of the tumour's location and length. The laminectomy should be a few centimetres longer than the length of the lesion, and larger on the side on which the meningioma has principally developed. The lamina's narrow blood vessels should be daubbed with wax as the blood pressure would obstruct coagulation. Once the laminae have been removed, tactile resistance of the dural plane shows the tumour location when it is in a posterior or posterolateral region. In the preoperative definition of the site by CT, myelo-CT or MRI, the vertical extension of the meningioma and its transverse width are all factors in deciding whether to practice a simple laminectomy or a lamino-arthrectomy.

A much wider opening on one side and the excision of the articular mass is always practiced when the laterally located meningioma is advanced ventrally to the cord, or when it becomes partially extrarachidian. In these cases the level articulation at the opposite side is considered to avoid rachidian insufficiency particularly in patients over 70 years of age and with kyphosis, segmental scoliosis or osteoporosis. Once the osteotomy has been performed at the base of the spinous processes, the laminae are thinned until their total removal is achieved using a rongeur with thin points. This is kept along the surface of the laminal plane without fragmenting the laminae in their depth and avoiding microtraumas at the underlying dural plane in compressions such as a meningioma, where arterial vascularization variations of the neural structures frequently occur. If haemorrhages occur in the epidural plexus during surgery, it is preferable to control them by placing thin layers of haemostatic gelatine sponge between the dural plane and the bone walls rather than continuously coagulating, as this hinders venous drainage. The same procedure is followed in the case of slight venous haemorrhages during excision, when the relaxation of the meningeal sac occurs.

Some authors (Eggert et al. 1983) prefer the microsurgical technique as they consider the lamina approach more valuable in the excision of one or more hemilaminae and when it is necessary for the entire spinous processes and the contralateral hemiarches. They also state, however, that it may be advantageous to remove the articular process of one side together with the pedicle. The extension of laminectomy requires careful preoperative evaluation of the morphological characteristics of the meningioma, its site and volume. These are all features visible in the preoperative diagnostic images. A large bone aperture is preferable in all cases in which the cord is substantially malformed and flattened for freeing the tumour without traumatizing the cord and without bleeding. We accept the concept of leaving the hemiarches which can impede the protrusion of the cord at the operture of the dura mater in the case of a premedullary tumour. On the basis of experience acquired over time we have modified our surgical methods to suit each case in the incision of the spinal dura.

9.5 Deformations of the Spinal Dura as Seen in the Operative Microscope

These are found along the posterior plane where the tumour lies in the posterolateral dural tract or on the anterior area. In posteriorly located meningiomas the dural enlargement corresponds to the area of invasion, and in the posterolateral sites the malformation is limited to the spinal dura near the nerve roots at the entrance of the intravertebral foramen (Figs. 224, 225 and case no. 79). If the meningioma is small in a lateral location, it assumes a bilobal topography in front of and posterior to the dentate ligament. The enlargement of the dural sac remains well defined. In ventral forms the length of the dura is sometimes displaced and forms a shell shape against the posterior vertebral plane (see X-ray of vertebral bodies adjacent to the tumour, Sect. 8.1.3). Compared to other primary intrarachidian tumours the meningioma has particular characteristics, one of the most important

being its meningeal invasion. Sometimes the meningioma, with the base of its attachment to the spinal dura, can be of a subarachnoidal development, and sometimes, having the same dural attachment, it is extra-arachnoidal (Fig. 275).

We have stressed above the importance of neuro-radiological diagnosis. This is not to maintain that these techniques enjoy a kind of priority over others, but they do add significantly to the overall range of information upon which to make the diagnosis. CT, myelo-CT and X-ray techniques have been developed to facilitate accurate and very specific diagnosis, providing refined images of topographical "anatomy" which must be available during all phases of surgery.

Another characteristic of meningiomas is the evident displacement of the cord and nerve roots then cause. This may vary depending on the volume of the lesion, its position and the way in which the tumour adheres to the leptomeninges. In meningiomas with a posterior development (Fig. 226) the invasion along the internal part of the dura can be either symmetrical or longer on one side in a paramedian position.

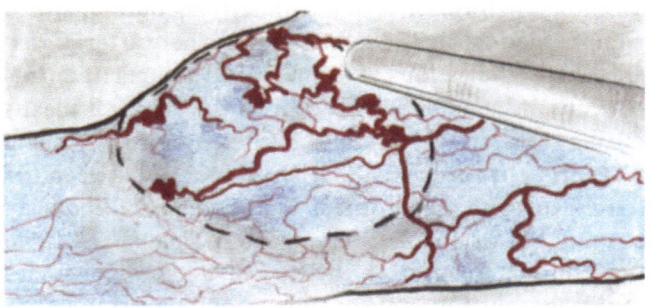

Fig. 224. Diagram of the dural enlargement near an intravertebral foramen in a right posterolateral meningioma case (see case no. 79). *Outlined,* the hypervascularized part of the dura. The circulation of the external dural layer is sinuous, irregular and below the tumour invasion (see Fig. 227)

Case No. 2: Transitional Meningioma

A 48-year-old woman (1965). Posterior intradural-extramedullary meningioma in C4-C5.
Medical History. Surgery for the removal of a fibroid at age 43 years.
Clinical Course. 1 year. Cervicobrachial pain with paraesthesias at the anteromedian side of the forearm with loss of strength in the whole limb. In the previous months ingravescent weakness in all limbs with distal paraesthesias to lower limbs.
Neurological Examination. Reduced movements of the head, particularly on flex extensions. Hypotrophy and hypotonia of muscles on the left scapula-humerus region. Flexation attitude on fingers of left hand. Paraparesis with hyperreflexia of upper limbs. Spastic paraplegia with clonus of the patellar on the left and polyphasia of Achilles tendon. Bilateral hyperaesthesia on C4-C5 and hypoaesthesia on C7 on the left. Tactile and painful hypoaesthesia from D4 to D7.
Rachicentesis. 1.88 g protein per thousand.

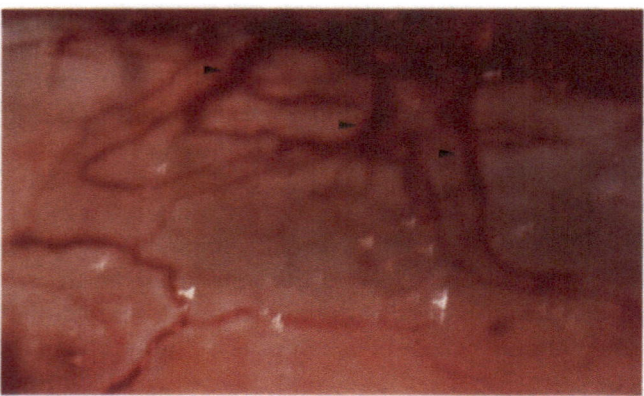

Fig. 225. Photograph from the operating microscope showing dilatation of the arterial circulation of the dura at the invasion below the meningioma (*arrows*)

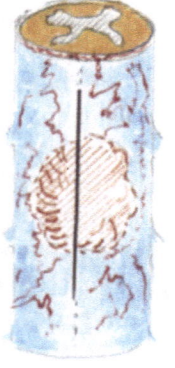
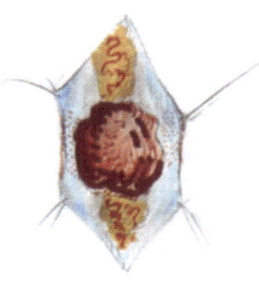

Fig. 226. Median longitudinal incision of the dura, with the attachment of the meningioma inserted to the internal posterior surface. Bilateral, symmetrical development

Myelography (performed suboccipitally). Total lateral block in C4-C5, confirmed anteroposteriorly, where the iodine column appeared irregular in central tract and with slight lateral flow (Fig. 227).

Surgical Treatment. Median incision of dura immediately showed the tumour adhering to posterior surface of the dura. The cord was displaced forwards. Sensory roots C5-C6 adhered to the surface of the meningioma. The arterial vascularization was dilatated above the neoplasm. Due to persistence of pronounced oedema at the cord in C6-C7 (after excision) the dura was not sutured. The dura was covered by a lamina of amnion (Figs. 228-230).

Results. Partial recovery of motility as early as the tenth day. After 1 month some flexion movements at lower limbs. After 6 months total recovery, which continued 2 years later (Fig. 231-233). Apart from the invasion area, the dura recovered a completely normal appearance, and for this reason there may have been an infiltration within its layer at the level of the meningioma (see Sect. 9.6).

Case No. 8: Transitional Meningioma

A 57-year-old woman (1964). Posterior intradural-extramedullary meningioma in D5-D6.

Clinical Course. 5 months. Distal paraesthesias to lower limbs with an ascending feature. Sense of constriction, band-like at subumbilical area, and gradual motor weakness to lower limbs to the left.

Neurological Examination. Small cutaneous angiomas scattered at the trunk and abdomen. Spastic paraparesis to the left. Hyperreflexia at patella and left foot clonus. Bilateral Babinski sign. Superficial tactile and painful hypoaesthesia from D12, distally pronounced.

Rachicentesis. 2.24 g protein per thousand.

Myelography (via lumbar puncture). Block in D5-D6 with slightly dome-shaped filling defect.

Surgical Treatment. Rich vascularization of muscular plane laminae. On opening the dura, immediate view of a posteriorly located neoplasm. The cord's surface-layer circulation appeared very dilatated and posterior columns were of a yellowish colour. Opening of the arachnoid above and below the meningioma and excision together with the surface of the dural invasion. The removed meningioma left a shell-shaped mark on the cord. No dural plastic; joining points and covering with gelatine lamina.

Results. From the very first days a gradual recovery of motor impairment. After 1 year slight hyperreflexia persisted but walking was possible without support. Complete recovery was reported after neurological examination 5 years later.

Sometimes the dural surface becomes very thin and the bluish red colour of the tumour can be seen. In meningiomas in a posterior position the alterations in the sur-

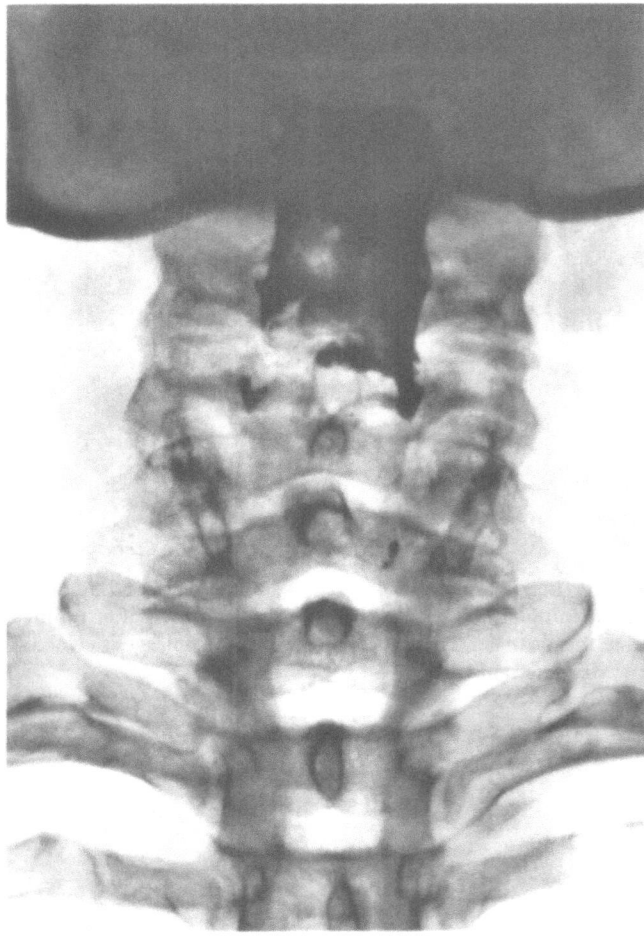

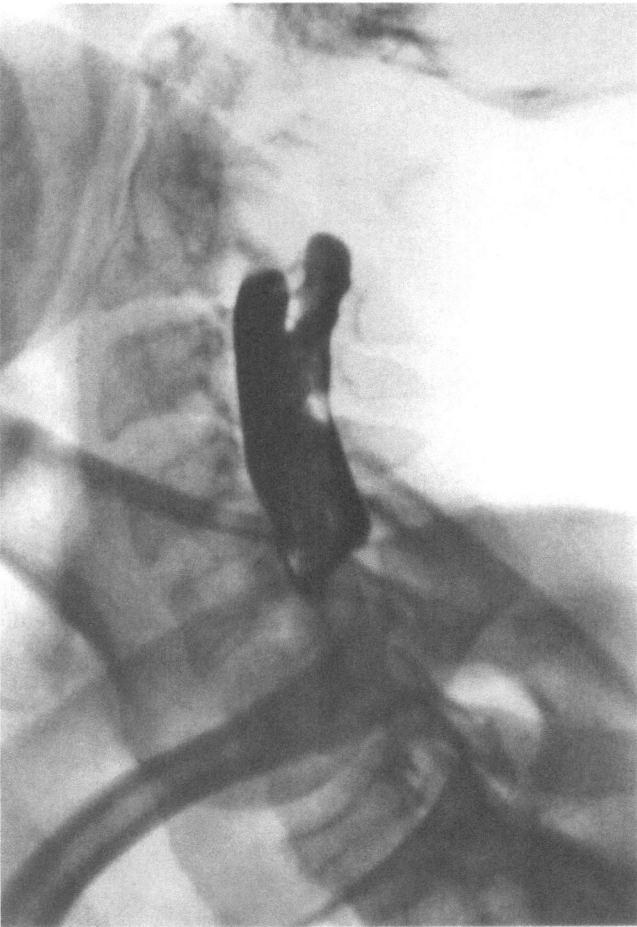

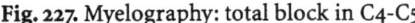

Fig. 227. Myelography: total block in C4-C5

face-layer circulation of the spinal cord are rendered visible by an increased vascular network which is continually dilatated through the meningeal layer with the neoplastic tissue (see case no. 2, Figs. 227-230). We use methods to open and incise the dural plane to reduce the haem-

orrhage as much as possible and to avoid further damage to the circulation of the tract where the tumour has already altered vascular supply of the neural structure, particularly to those myelomeres where the arterial supply network is already physiologically less rich.

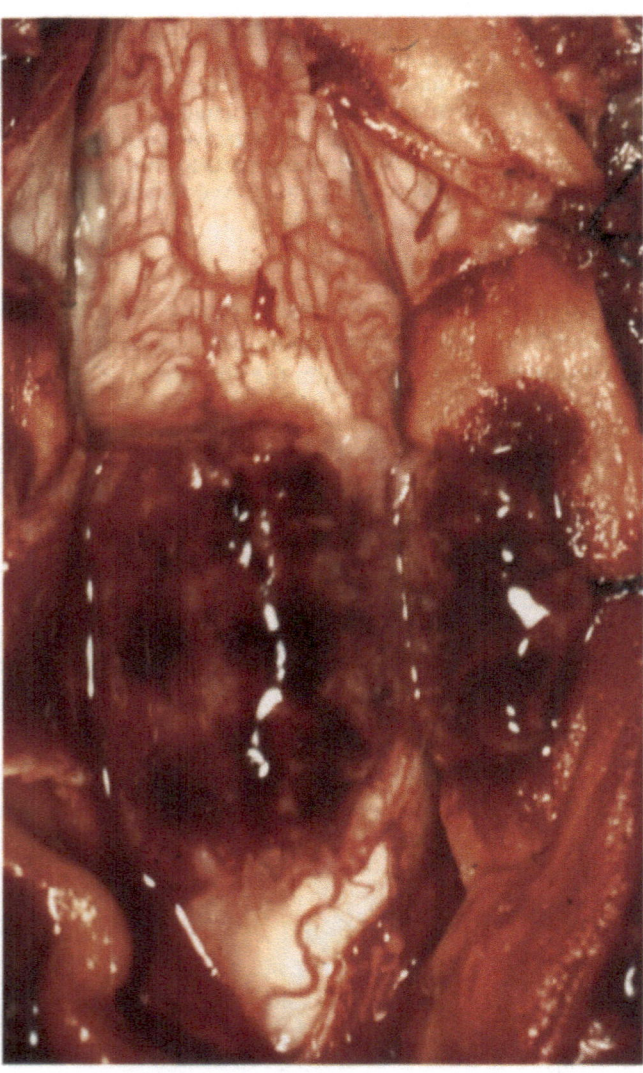

Fig. 228. On opening the dura the meningioma, which is definitely posterior, has a symmetrical development on both sides and infiltrates the dura, pushed to the right

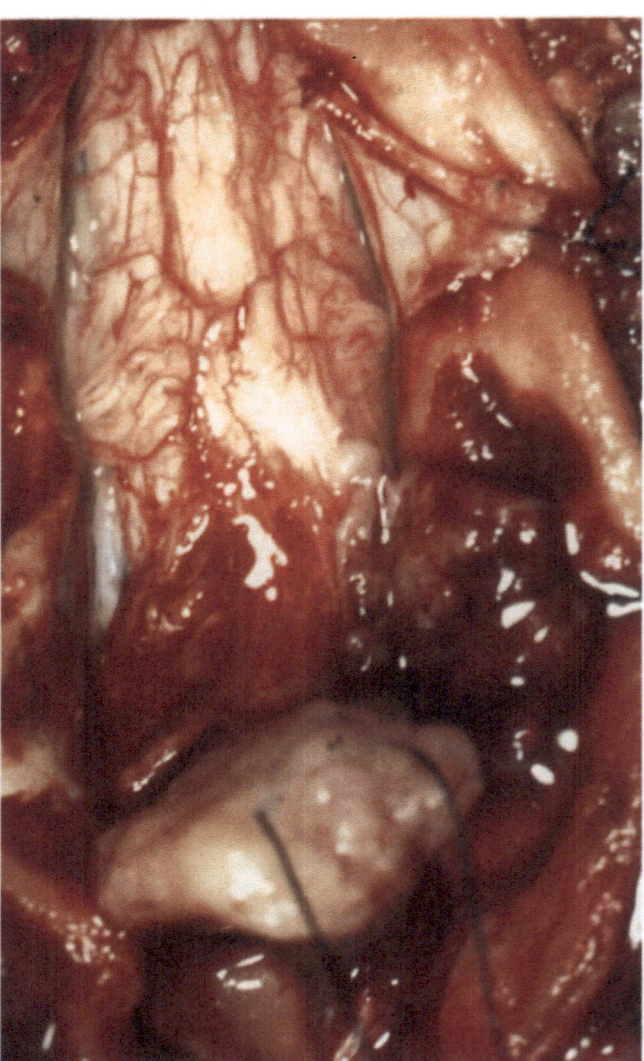

Fig. 229. In this case the whole area of dural infiltration is removed. The meningioma is pushed posteriorly and down after removal from the pia mater. The posterior compression enlarges the medullary diameter above

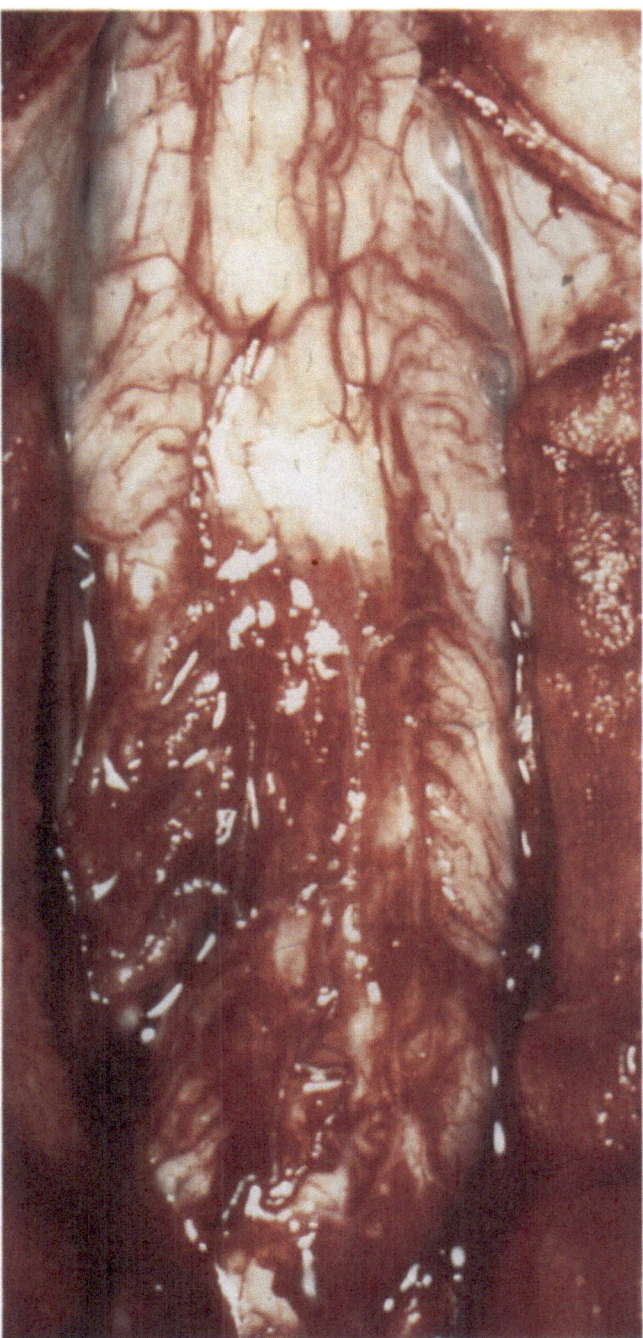

Fig. 230. Complete removal together with both sides of the dura; persistence of arterial dilatation of the surface layer circulation of the cord. In this case the ischaemic aspect is located above the meningioma

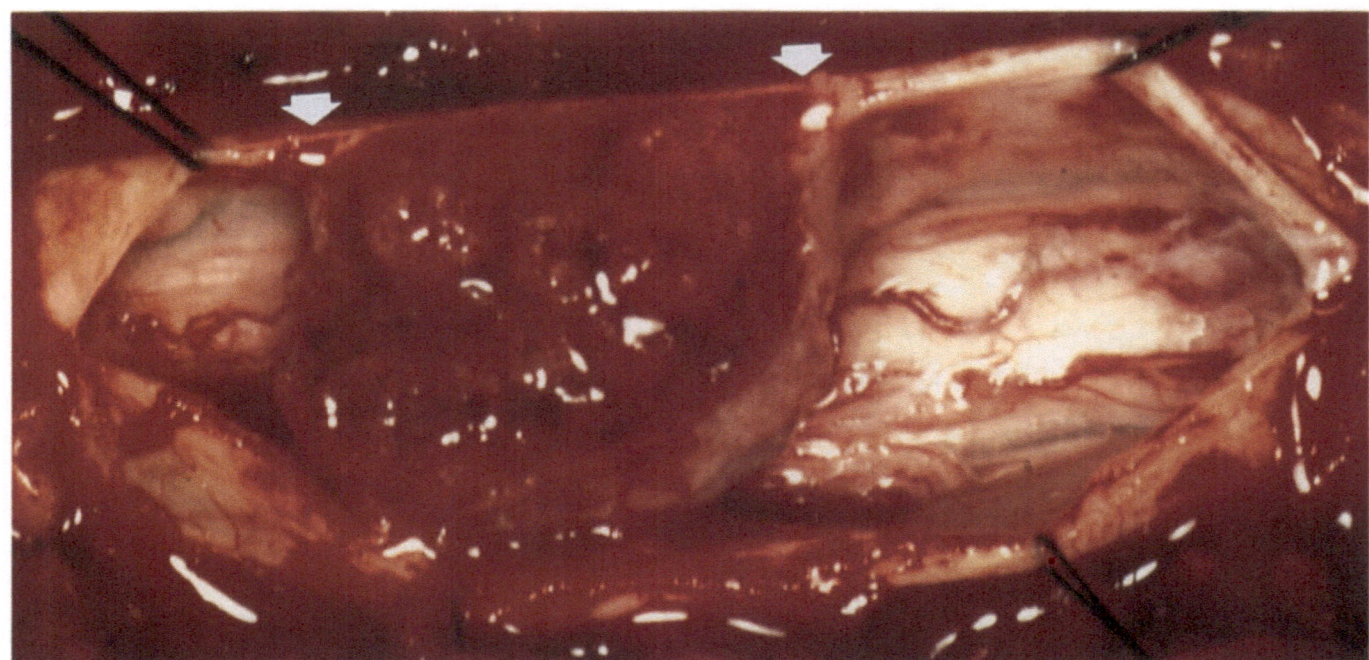

Fig. 231. The thinning and infiltration of the dura along the entire attachment of the meningioma (*arrow*). The dura above and below the invasion regains its normal thickness. This feature corresponds exactly to the MRI scans, with a "mouse tail" appearance of the dura

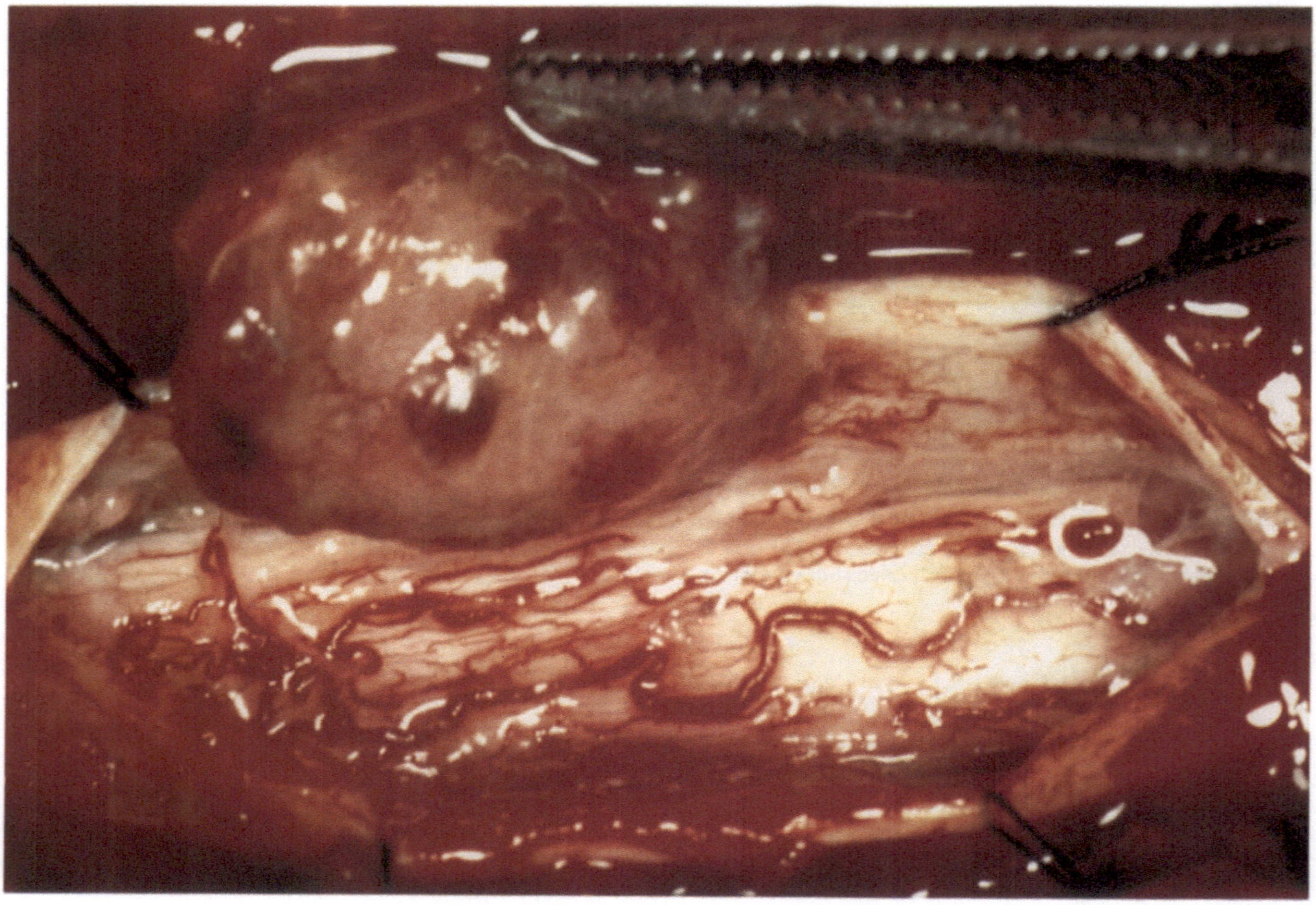

Fig. 232. It is possible to tilt the meningioma gradually, maintaining the entire surface layer of the cord

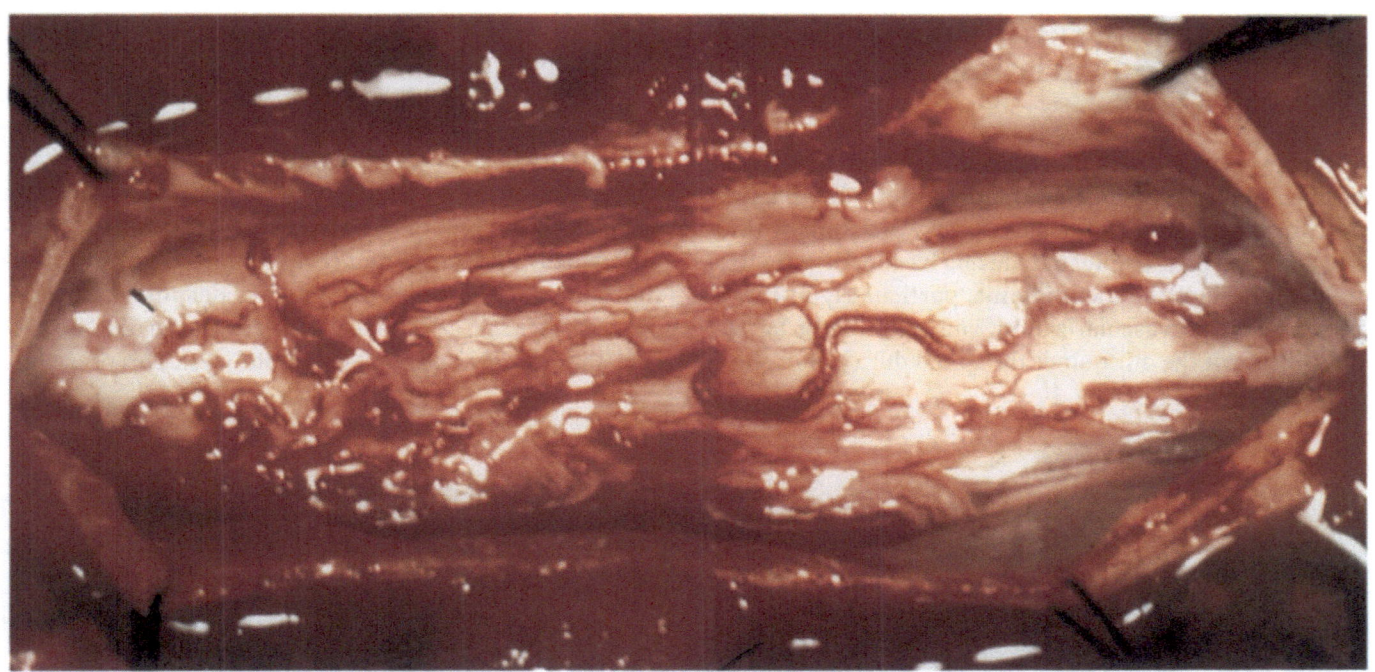

Fig. 233. Photograph of the operating field after cutting both sides of the dura at the dural invasion

9.6 Microsurgical Splitting of the Dura and Variations in Dural Incisions

For many years we have practiced the normal techniques of dural incision by cutting the dura along the medial line. In the past 5 years we have used a variation of this which we believe is helpful in reducing haemorrhage in the freeing phase of the meningioma, particularly in cases presenting hypervascularization. This technique is based on splitting of the dura, since the spinal dura is morpho-logically formed by two overlaying strata near the occipi-to-atlantoid.

There are two points to consider when using this technique. The first is suggested by the particular differen-tiation to which the spinal dura is subject during embryon-ic development (see Sect. 2), and the second derives from a microscopic view of the relationship between the menin-gioma, the meninges and nerve roots. The splitting of the dura near the meningioma involves delamination (Figs. 234-237; see Fig. 7) which has the advantage of interrupt-ing the arterial circulation within the layer. This procedure

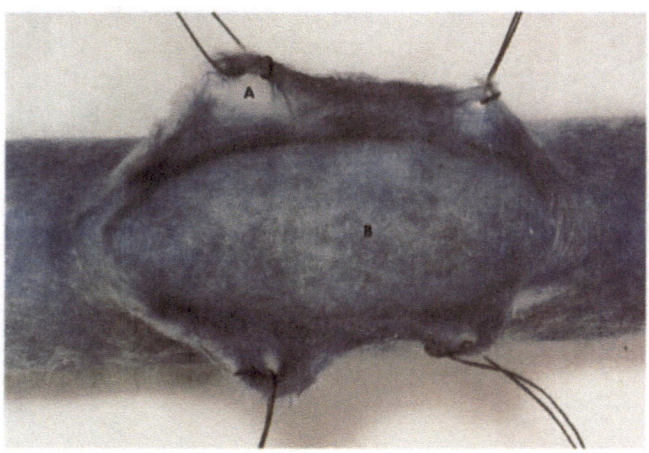

Fig. 234. Cotton model showing the splitting of the dura. *A*, The periosteal dural layer which is already freed and anchored above; *B*, surface layer of the deep dural leptomeningeal layer

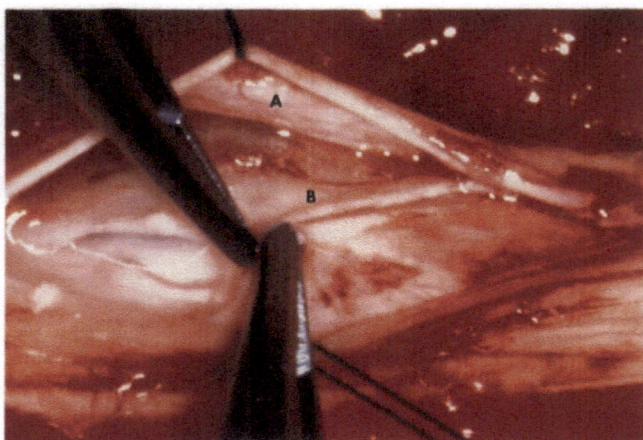

Fig. 236. Photograph from the operating microscope. The two for-ceps clinch the borders of the deep dural layer once the incision and anchorage to the upper periosteal layer on both sides has been performed

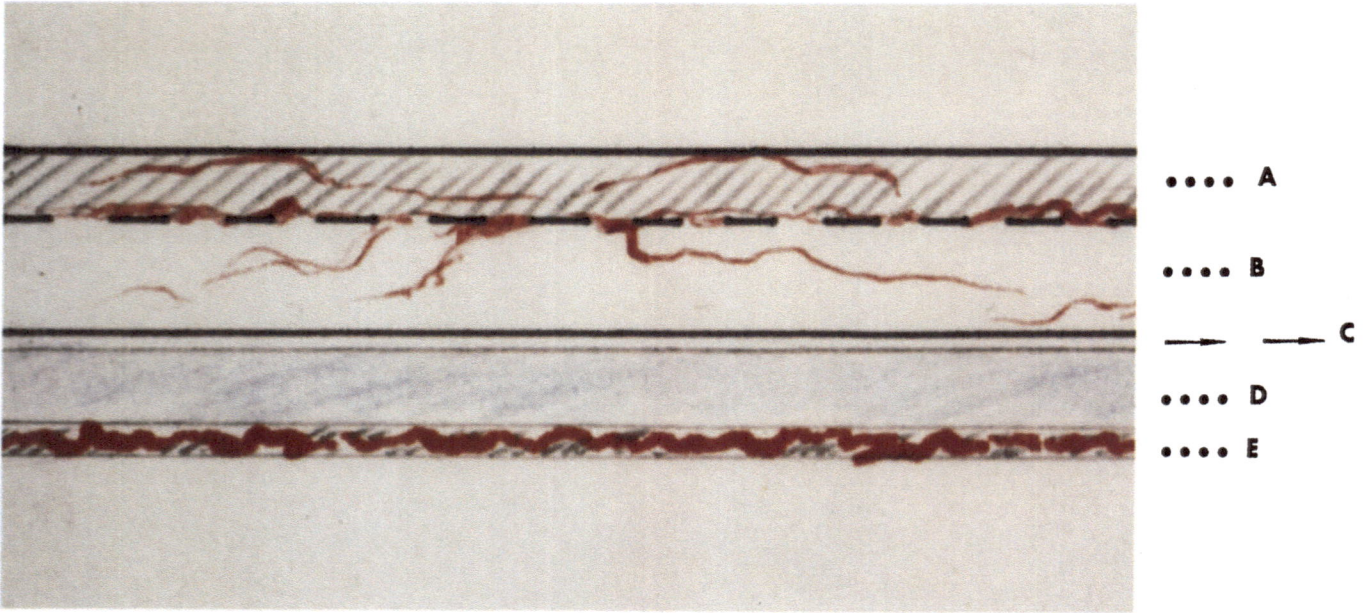

Fig. 235. Diagram of the meningeal layers. *A*, Dural periosteal layer; *B*, deep dural leptomeningeal layer; *C*, virtual subdural space; *D*, arach-noid and subarachnoidal space; *E*, pia mater

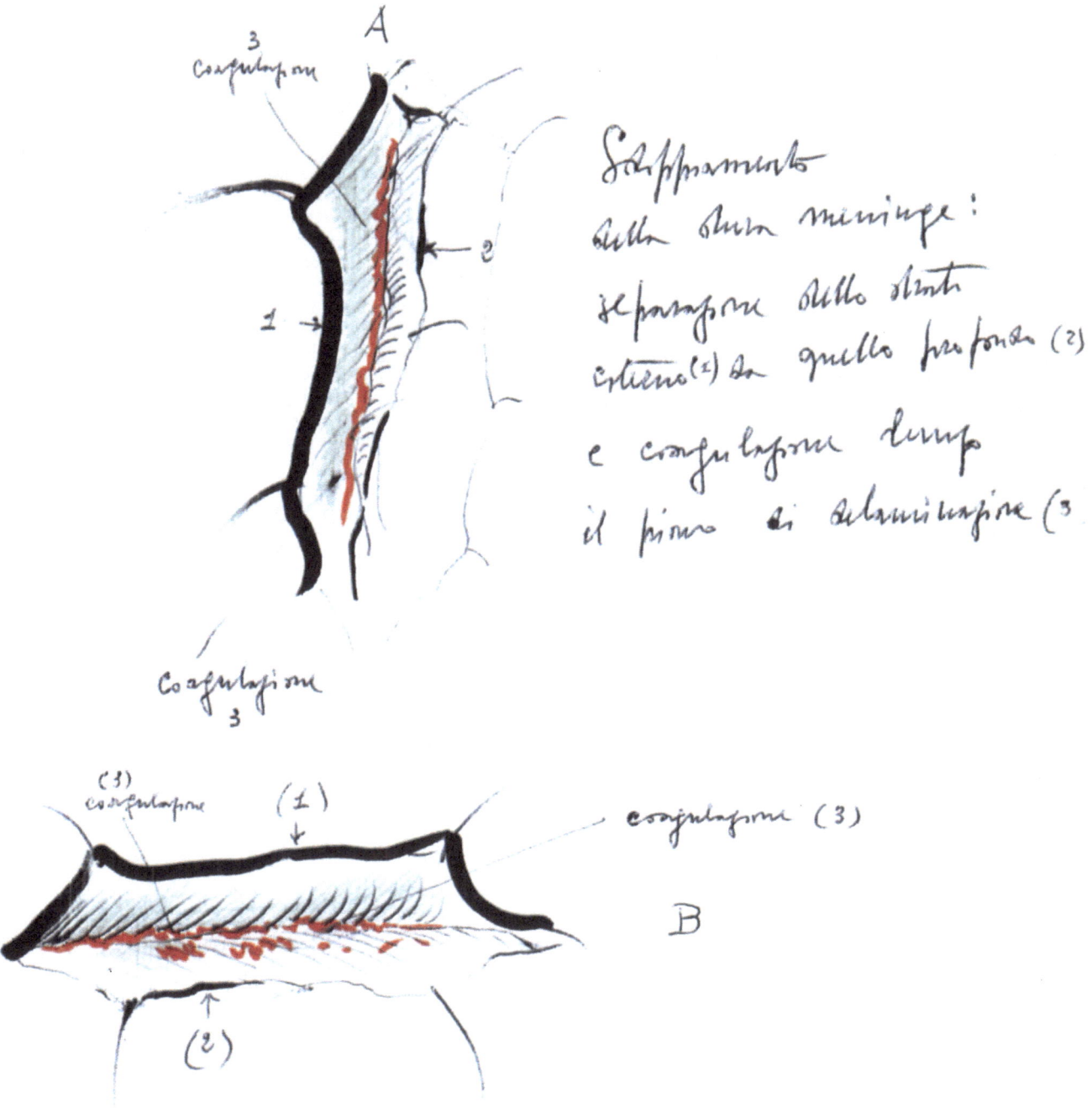

Fig. 237. The vertical (**a**) and horizontal (**b**) splitting of the dura. Separation of the external membrane (*1*) from the deep membrane of the dura (*2*) and coagulation along the delamination plane (*3*) (see Fig. 240)

reduces bleeding before isolating the tumour. The splitting of the dura is used in extramedullary meningiomas in posterior sites, in those with posterolateral development and partially in those with a lateroventral extension (Fig. 238).

Case No. 75: Transitional Meningioma
A 53-year-old woman (1994). Right posterolateral intradural extramedullary meningioma in D4.
Clinical Course. 10 years. Fastidious interscapular dorsal back pain and paraesthesias at the internal side of thigh and of the perineum. Three years before hospitalization she experienced lumbosciatica attacks on the left at S1 lasting 15 days. Six months before admission new lumbago attacks occurred with cruralgia and sciatica predominantly on the left. Paraesthesias of a cordal type at lower limbs, ascending to umbilical line. At the level of the pain syndrome hypostenia to left lower limb. Sphincter disturbances in the form of retention.
Neurological Examination. Slight hypotrophy of one-third of the lower left thigh. Reduced ankle jerk and left patella reflex. Walking with paraparetic gait and coordination disturbances. Slight hypovalidity on the toes. Superficial, tactile and painful hypoaesthenia in L2 area, reaching distal tract of left lower limb. Paraesthesias of a cordal type to lower limbs. Band of hyperaesthesia from D6-D7 at level of pain syndrome.
Rachicentesis. 0.37 g protein per thousand.
X-Ray of Dorsal Rachis. Slight convex scoliosis on the right (Fig. 239).
Dorsal MRI. In D4 expansive intradural-extramedullary lesion posterolaterally on the right. The cord was displaced forwards and to the left. The neoplasm was enhanced homogeneously (Fig. 240).
Myelo-CT. The expansive intradural-extramedullary lesion, non-homoeneously hyperdense, adhered to the right posterolateral dural wall. In D4 the cord pushed ventrally to the left (Figs. 241, 242).
Surgical Treatment. Hypervascularization of the muscular masses, paraspinous and of the laminae. Dural malformation as a plial-formed enlargement. No pulsations. Delamination of the dura which in some parts appeared thinned. Coagulation of the blood supply deep in the two dural layers at a distance from each other. Once opened in the leptomeningeal layer of the dura (Fig. 243), the meningomatous tissue seen, of a red-wine colour and of a soft consistency with a calcified attachment base in a right posterolateral position (Fig. 244). The arachnoid was opened and the tumour weighed down. The cord surface presented a clear mark laterally. Removal en bloc together with the calcified meningeal invasion (Fig. 245) and the deep dural layer. The ventral dural plane presented an irregular hypervascularization of the arterial network.
Results. After 2 weeks walking was possible but with ataxic gait. Hyperreflexia to lower limbs, distally to the knee, slightly and progressively improving. After 7 months no motor deficit with almost normal walking. Slight loss of strength in left lower limb. Complete regression of sphincter disturbances. After a recent check-up further improvement. (During the initial onset of the pain syndrome, apart from cord paraesthesia symptoms to lower limbs, the blocking painful attacks at L5 resembled a lumosciatica syndrome.)

Once the external layer of a posteriorly located meningiomas has been incised, the separation of the superficial layer (periostal spinal dura) from the deep layer (leptomingeal spinal dura) is performed easily by a gradual decollement using thin spatulas (Figs. 237, 238; see cases 8, 9). The external flap resembles the page of a book and is even now distant to the deep dural layer; however, it is still attached to the paravertebral muscles by a thread-like suspension. The gradual coagulation of the blood

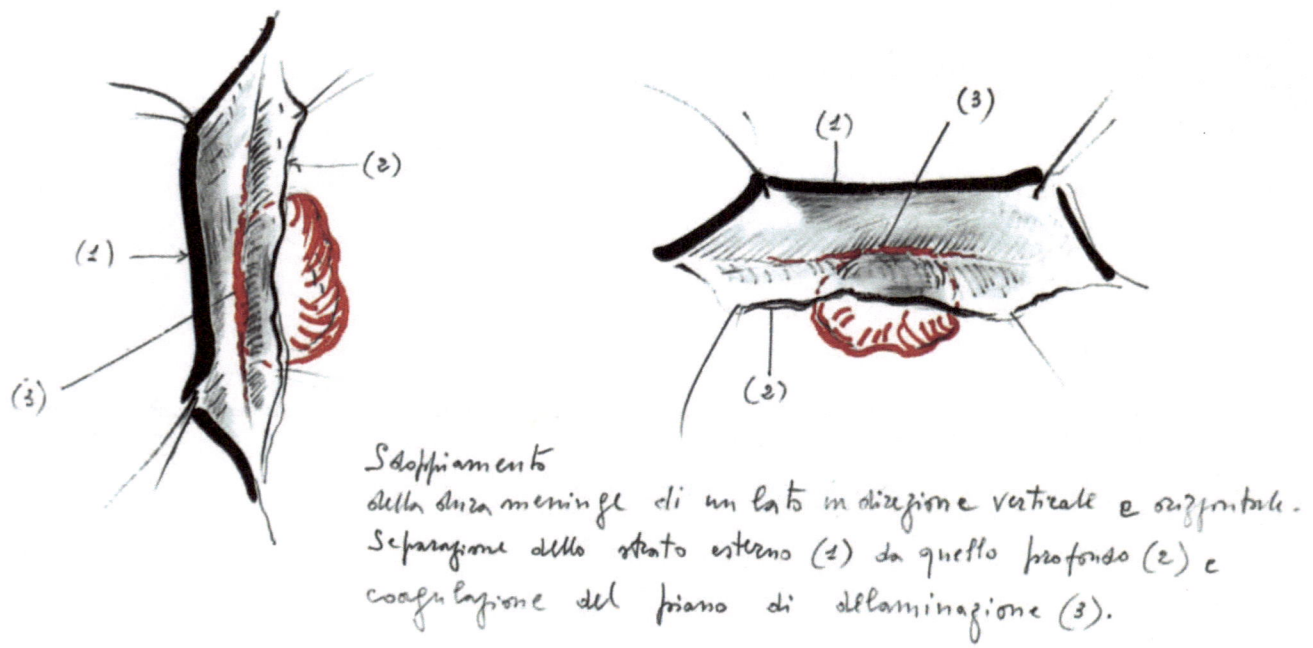

Sdoppiamento della dura meninge di un lato in direzione ventrale e sopportale. Separazione dello strato esterno (1) da quello profondo (2) e coagulazione del piano di delaminazione (3).

Fig. 238. Diagram of dural delamination, with the meningioma attachment below the dural leptomeningeal plane

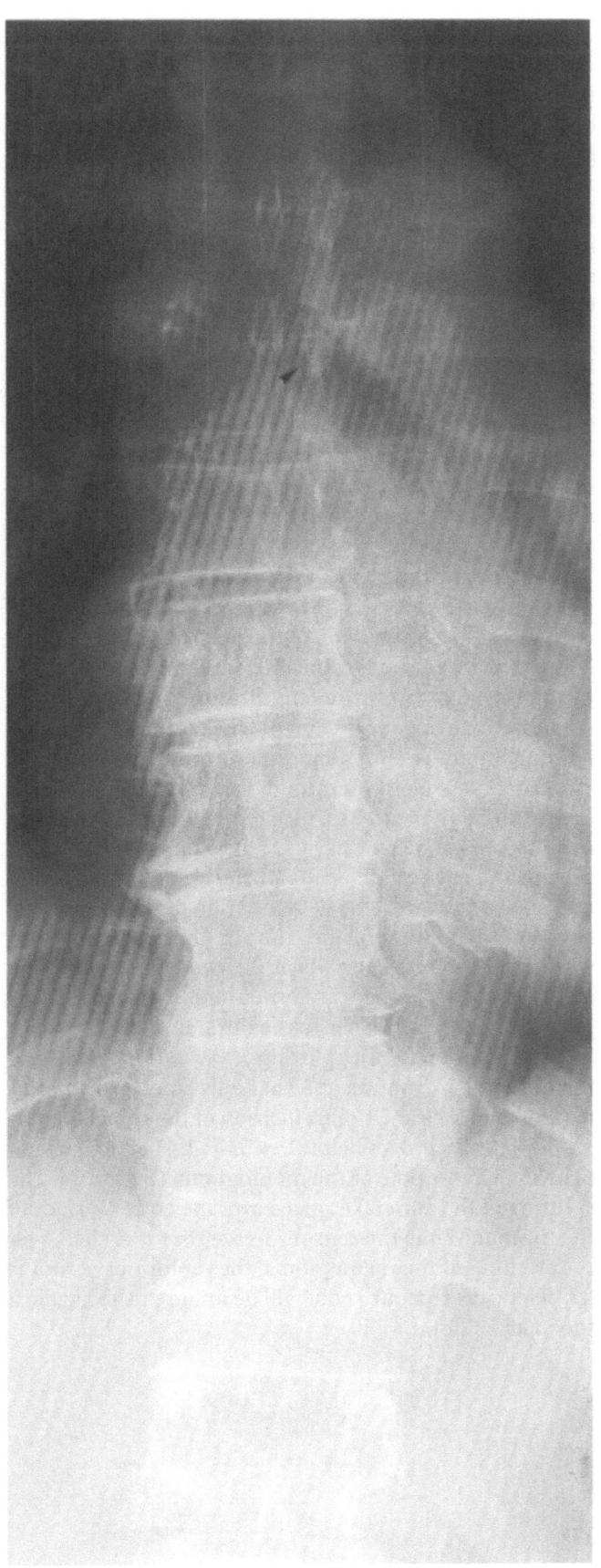

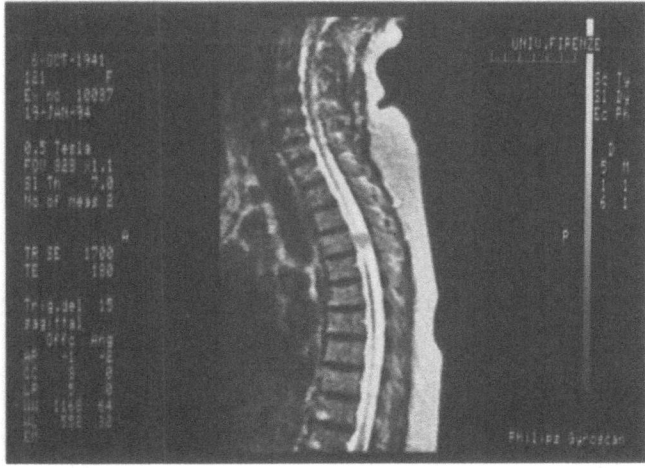

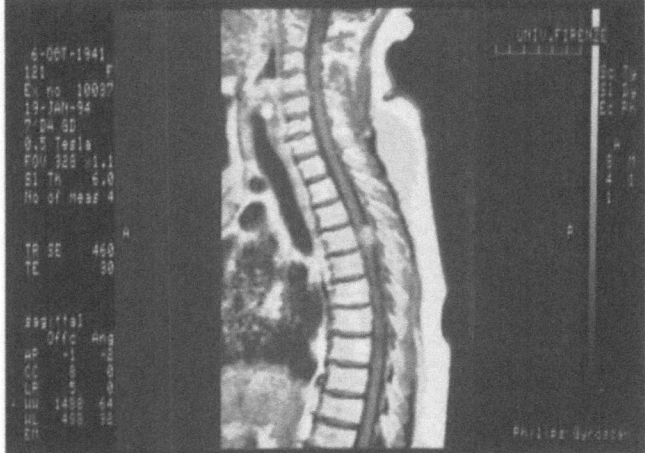

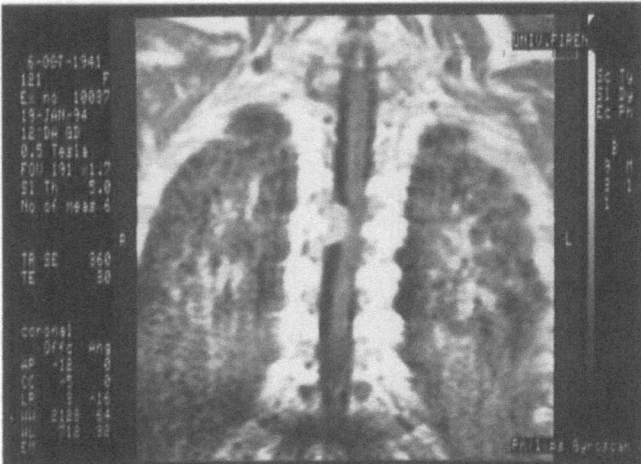

Fig. 240. MRI. Sagittal projection T2 (TR 1700 and TE 180). Sagittal and coronal T1 with contrast medium. Expansive process inside the canal in D4, which assumes the contrast medium homogeneously and leans onto the right-side articular pedicle

Fig. 239. X-ray dorsal rachis. Slight scoliosis at the medial upper dorsal tract with thinning of the articular pedicle of D5 on the left (*arrow*)

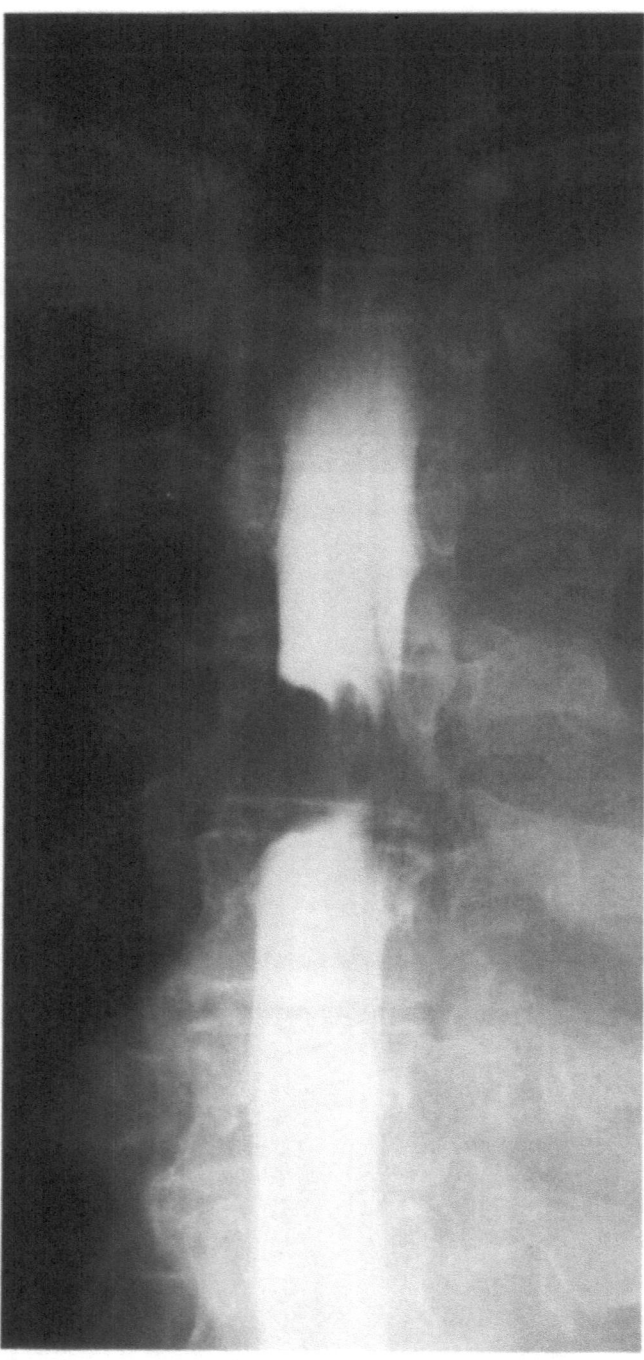

Fig. 241. Myelography via lumbar puncture. Transitory block in D4-D5 producing a filling defect on the right where the subarachnoidal space is enlarged, and the cord is displaced towards the right. The definition of the compression's upper pole appears irregular

vessels within the dural layer which is in continuity with the tumour attachment reduces bleeding at the operating field (see Fig. 6). In meningiomas with premedullary development the dura is split by partially reaching the lateral sheath near the nerve roots. The preparation of the two layers is preceded by a very lateral paramedial incision of the dura, thereby protecting the posterior myelitic area (Fig. 246). Anchorage towards the external periosteal dural layer finds more space at the level of arthrectomy and foraminotomy once these have been performed. The incision of the deep dural membrane falls exactly on the oblique course of the nerve bundles of the posterior nerve roots at their entry into the dural plane of the intravertebral foramen, revealing the medullary lateroventral region. Rotating the horizontal operating table slightly backwards makes it easier to reach the premedullary arachnoid and to uncover the capsulated part of the tumour.

After performing haemostasis between the two dural sides at the attachment base of the meningioma near the nerve roots comes invasion of the deep dural layer, which is intact until this stage, but the arachnoid membrane, through which the entire length of the meningioma is seen (see case no. 62; Fig. 91, 92), is left intact. Once the relationship of the meningioma to the myeloradicular structures has been identified, the arachnoid appears clearly along the entire surface of the tumour. When the meningioma shows transversal development and compresses the entire side of the posterior columns, which are pushed forwards, the delamination of the dura is followed by debulking of the tumour and fragmentation with small spoons especially at the two lateral sides. The invasion of laterally located meningiomas usually lies near the nerve roots close to the dural funnels.

Preparation for the splitting of the periosteal layer of the dura mater from the internal one is performed after paramedian incision. Contraincision of the spinal meninges sometimes proves helpful, with an L-shaped incision below the lower pole of the meningioma (Fig. 247). The splitting of the dura takes place over the entire surface of the tumour. While the sensory nerve root is arched over the swelling of the meningioma, the motor nerve root is hidden by the tumour and it will be found pushed against the internal dural wall.

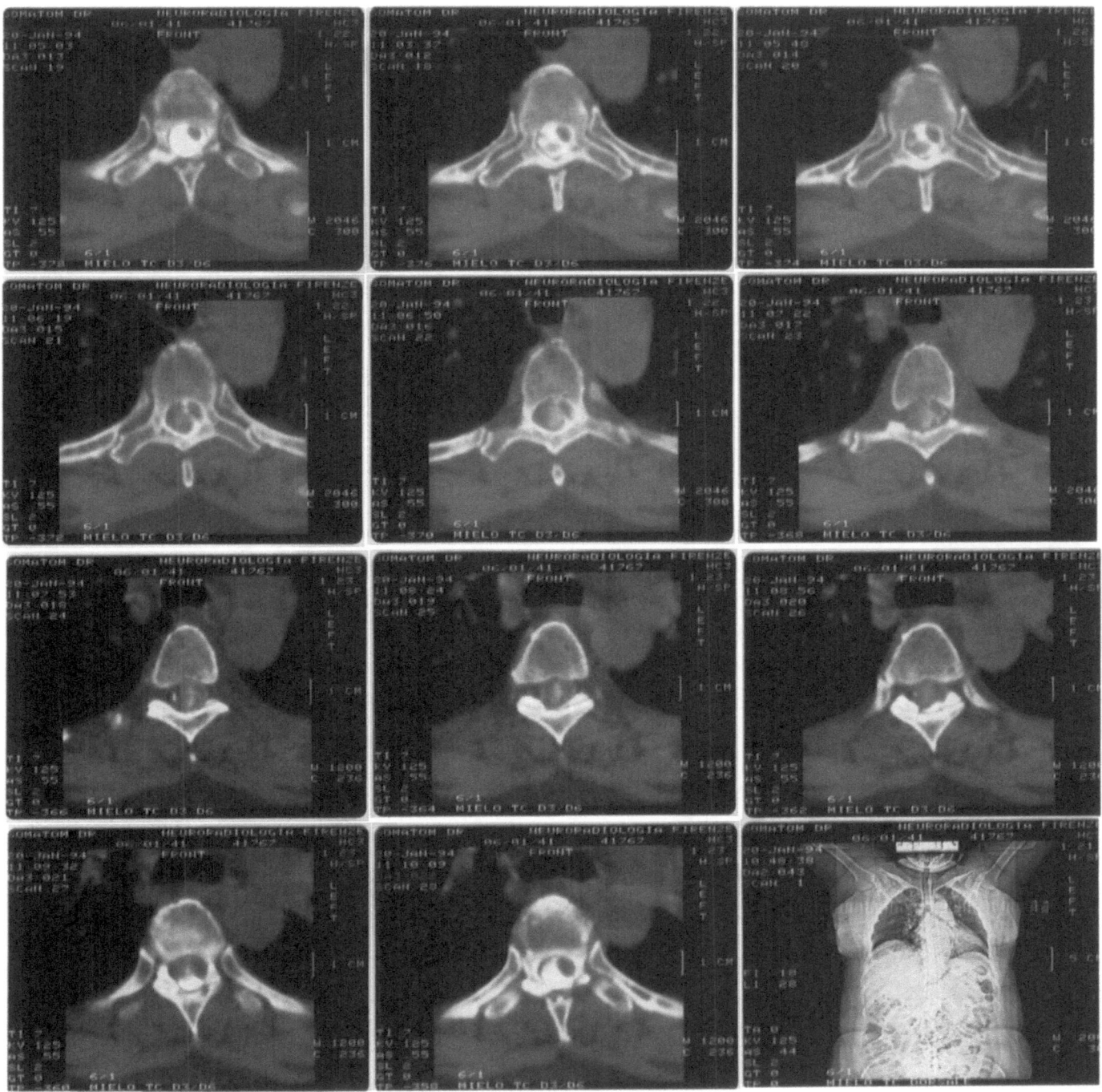

Fig. 242. Myelo-CT. A double roundish-shaped isodense image in D4-D5 is evident posteriorly to the right of the subarachnoidal space at the upper bilobed pole of the expansive lesion, which displaces the cord forwards and to the left. In lower sections the lesion occupies the canal almost entirely

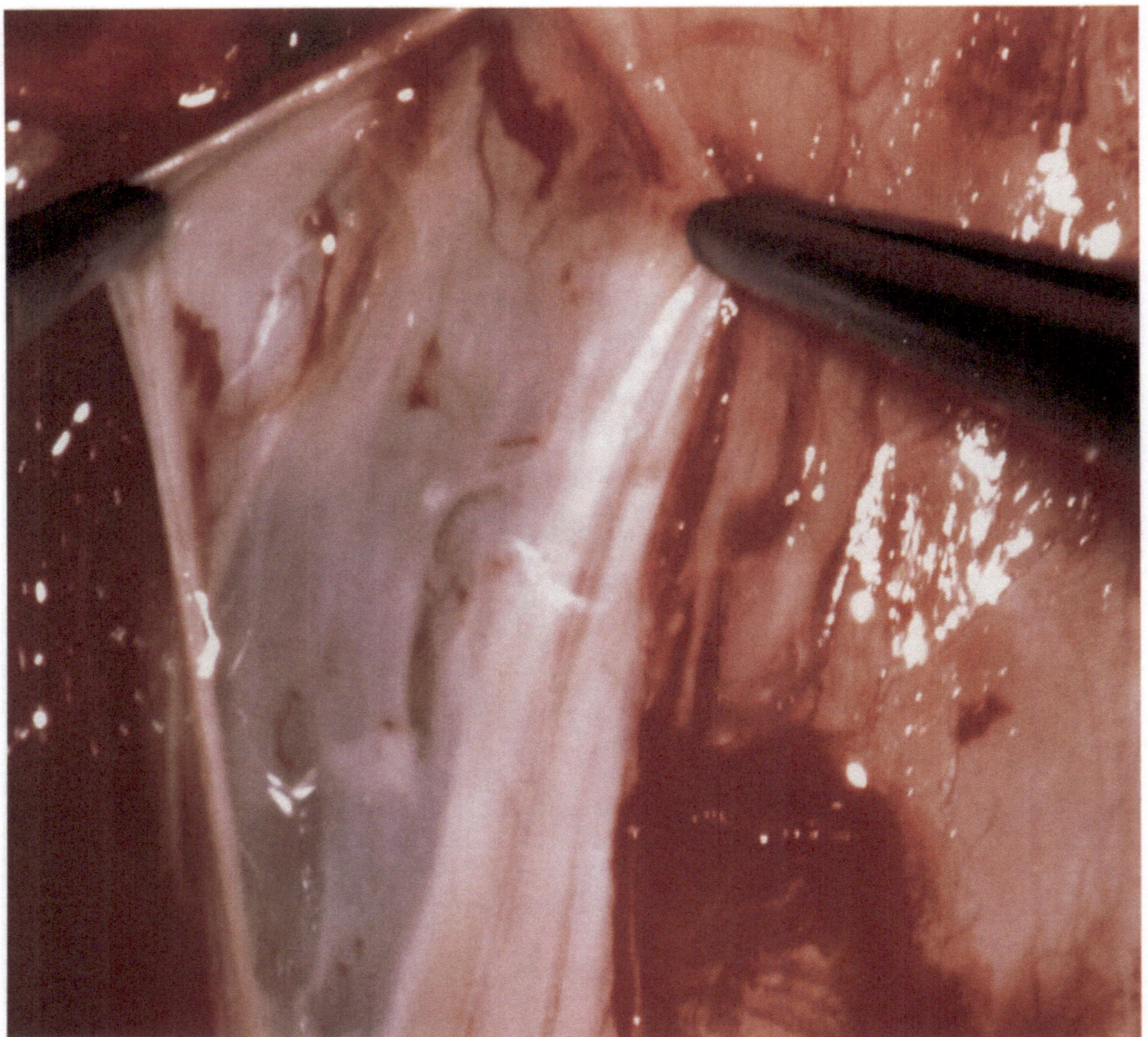

Fig. 243. The first stage of the dural splitting is performed with a left paramedian incision. In the centre an already evident longitudinal opening of the dura, leptomeningeal layer. Small arterial branches are seen towards the upper end deep in the two separated layers

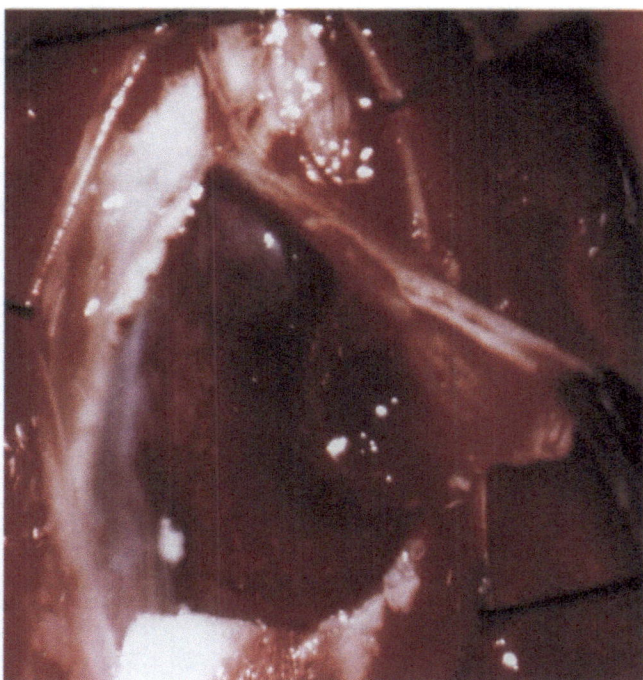

Fig. 244. The horizontal contraincision of the deep layer produces a flap stretched towards the right. This preparation allows a full view of the meningioma with its attachment, revealing the archnoidal relationship and that between surface layer and cord

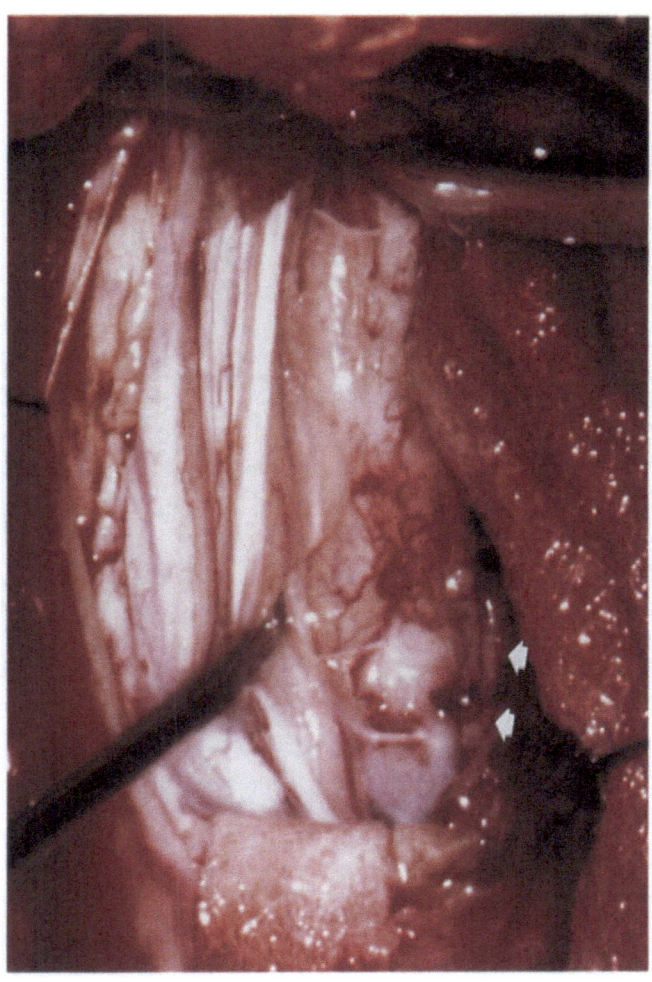

Fig. 245. The cord is displaced forwards. Excision has been possible, sparing the surface layer circulation in toto

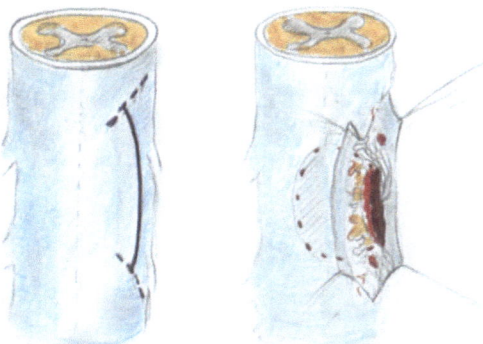

Fig. 246. A lateral, linear or arch-shaped incision with oblique contraincisions towards the upper or lower end until reaching the radicular funnels for premedullary meningiomas. This type of incision helps to protect the posterior medullary surface layer

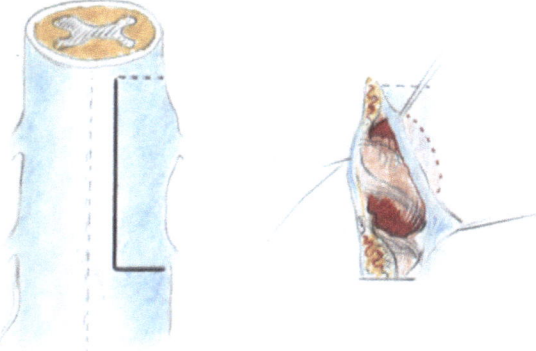

Fig. 247. A paramedian right or left L-shaped incision with the possibility of a contraincision at the upper end for posterolateral or lateroventral meningiomas invading a lateral dural surface near a radicular funnel

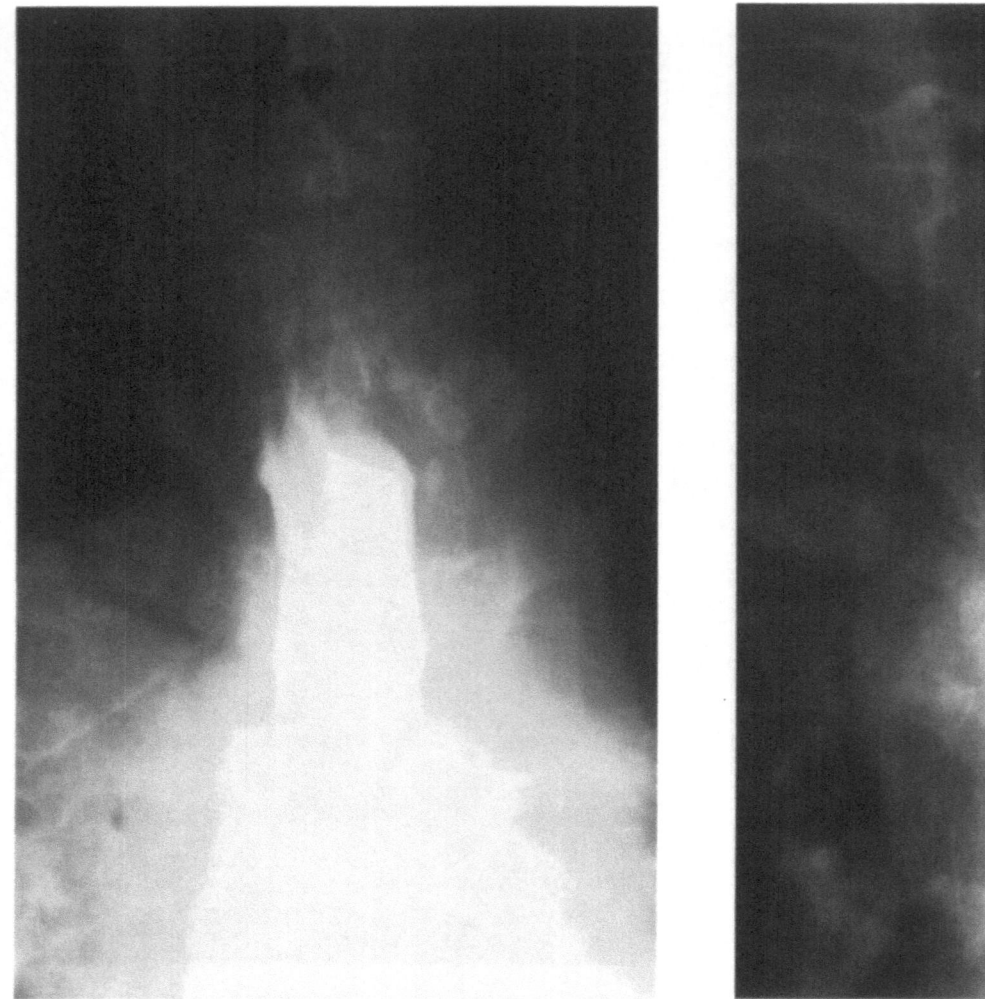
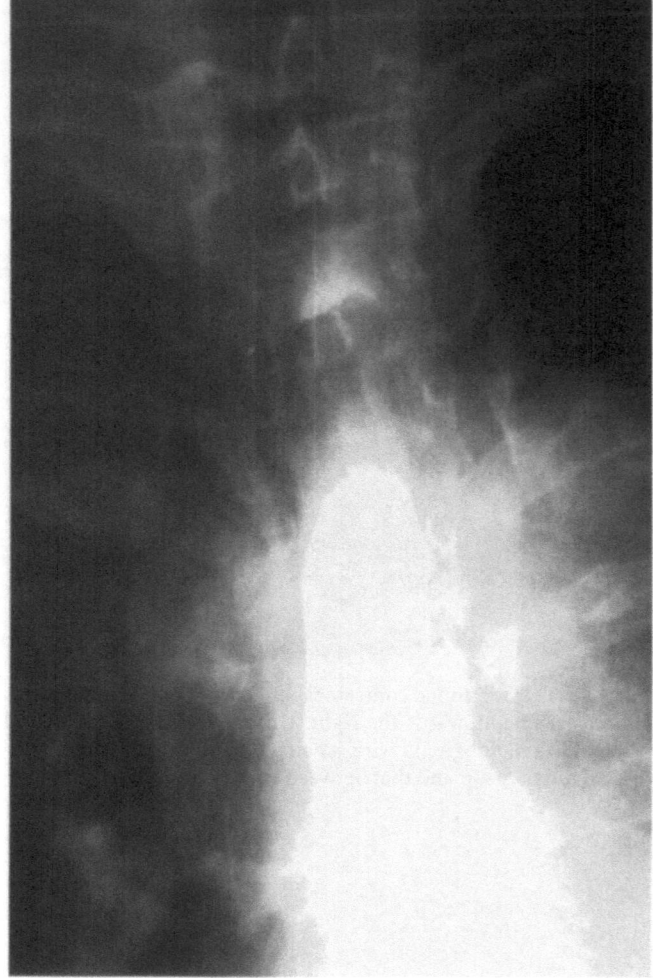

Fig. 248. Myelography via lumbar puncture. Block at D4 level with upper concave aspect which diminishes at the right. The subarachnoidal space appears enlarged at the left and the cord displaced to the right. A small amount of the contrast medium passes the block and defines the upper pole of the lesion with its extension

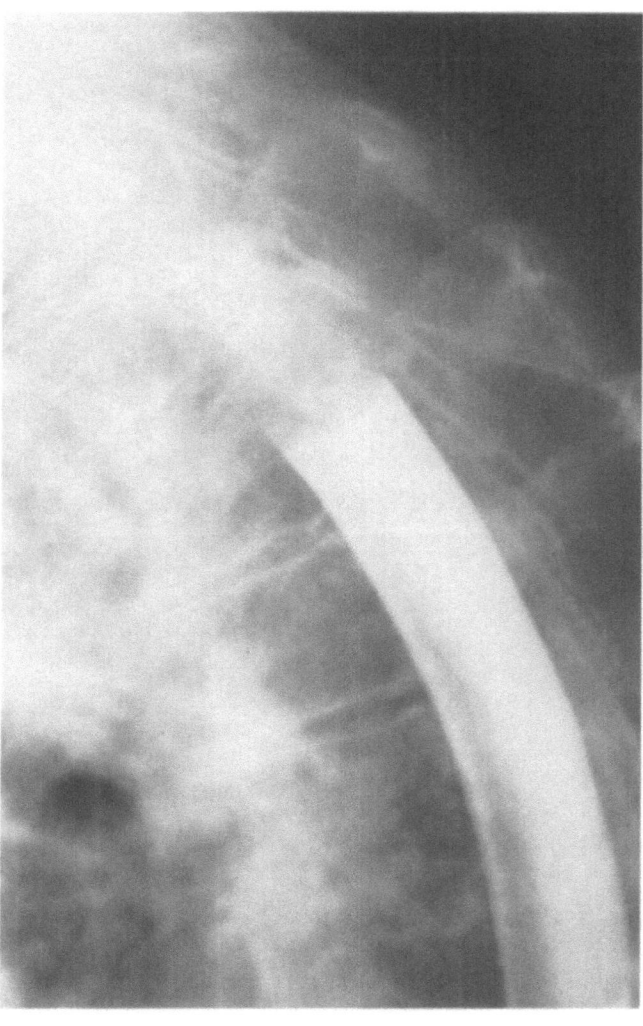

Fig. 249. Laterally the subarachnoidal space is wide posteriorly below the block

Case No. 85: Transitional Meningioma with Widespread Osseus Metaplasms

A 72-year-old woman (1993). Left posterolateral intradural-extramedullary meningioma in D3-D4.

Medical History. Surgery for the removal of mammary cysts at age 42 years.

Clinical Course. 30 years. Pain at dorsal tract becoming more intense in the previous 5 years. For 6 months there had been numbness of the skin rising towards the mammillary line. Progressive difficulty in walking.

Neurological Examination. Severe spastic paraparesis with hyperreflexia. Hypertrophy of lower third of the femoral quadricep and the gastrocnemius on the right. Anaesthesia of mammary line, superficial tactile and pain hypopallaesthesia at sternal region.

Rachicentesis. 1.40 g protein per thousand.

X-Ray of Dorsal Rachis. Scoliosis with dorsal kyphosis. The articular pedicle on the left of D4 appeared blurred at medial tract.

Myelography (via lumbar puncture). Wide subarachnoidal space in upper posterior dorsal area. Anteroposteriorly the iodine column passed the block at D4 and produced a filling defect on the right (Figs. 248, 249).

Myelo-CT. In D3-D4 expansive intradural-extramedullary structure with left posterolateral invasion. The cord was displaced forwards on the right (Fig. 250).

MRI. In D3-D4 expansive oval-shaped structure measuring at the most 2 cm in diameter and occuping left posterolateral part. The neoplasm had an isodense signal in T2 (Fig. 251).

Surgical Treatment. No pulsation emitted at the dural plane. Splitting of the dura with left paramedian incision of the only external dural layer and total coagulation of the circulation. Low horizontal contraincision conserving the dural plane along the entire calcified surface of the tumour. Once the deep layer of the dura was incised and anchored down on the left, the opening of the arachnoid was performed at the upper pole level and the medullary pulsatons reappeared. The cord was completely pushed forwards on the right. Total removal of adherent structures along the posterior surface of the meningioma. Lifting lower pole of neoplasm and freeing adherent structures to pia mater. On this side the root of D5 was elongated. A cleavage point was found on the calcified medial part of the tumour and was removed en bloc, clenching it from left to right. Haemostasis of invasion surface layer with removal of the internal dural membrane (Figs. 252, 253).

Results. Motor inhibition in the first 24 h. Gradual recovery leading to normal walking within 1 year.

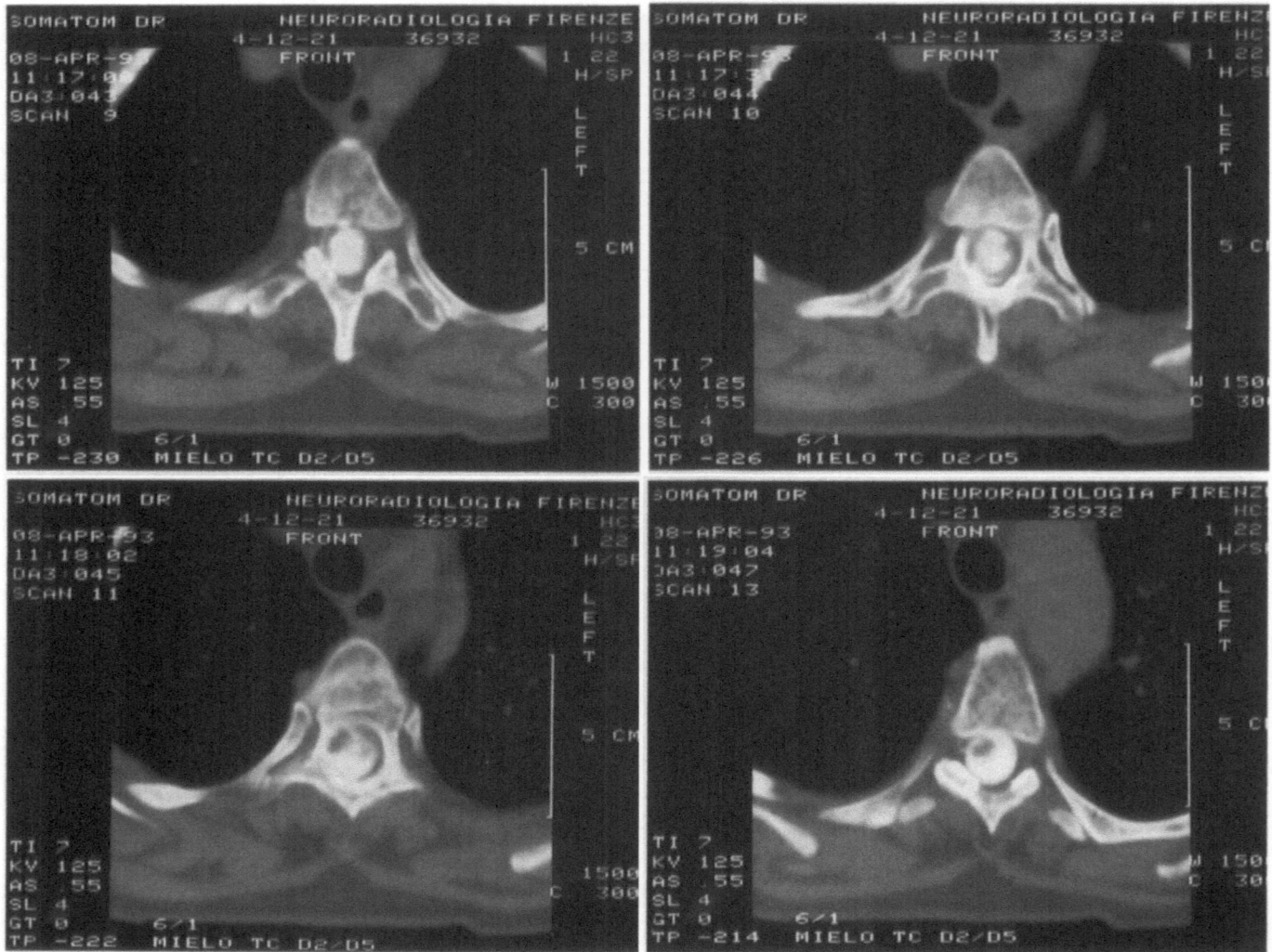

Fig. 250. Myelo-CT. A densely calcified lesion occupying the rachidian lumen, almost entirely displacing the cord forwards and to the right. The cord is seen surrounded by a large subarachnoidal space below the neoplasm

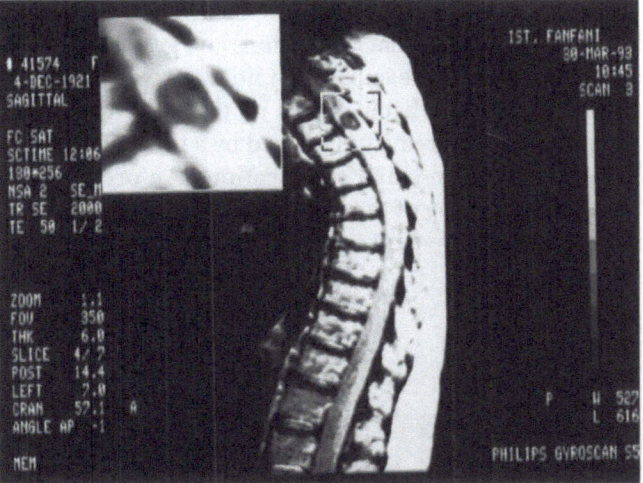

Fig. 251. MRI. Sagittal projection shows protonic density (TR 2000 and TE 50). The oval-shaped lesion at D3-D4 level appears non-homogeneous (hypointense externally with small hyperdense areas inside, in contrast to the spinal cord) which indicates a predominant calcium component

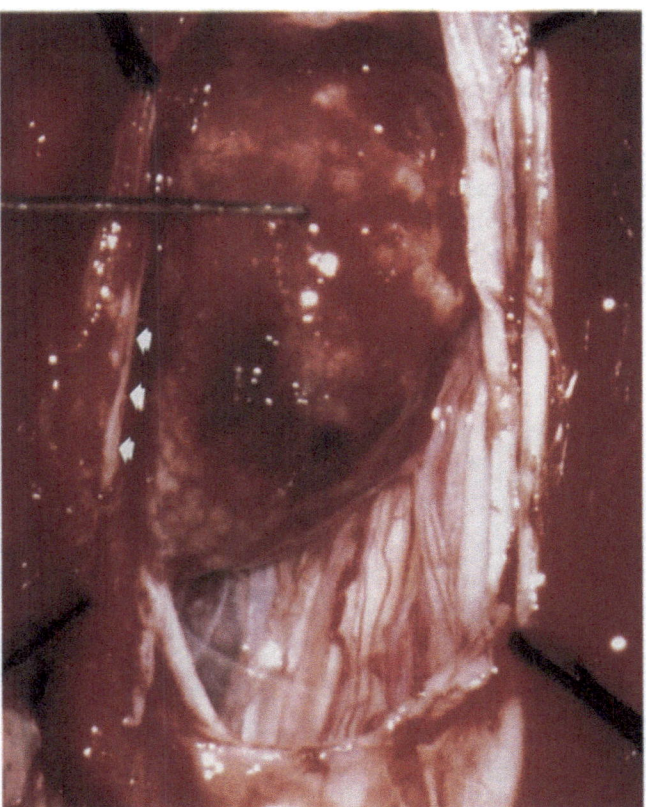

Fig. 252. The dural splitting is seen clearly on the right. The tumour is almost completely calcified and anchored with a hook when tilting to remove the arachnoid below. On the left the deep dural layer adheres to the whole length of the meningioma attachment (*arrow*)

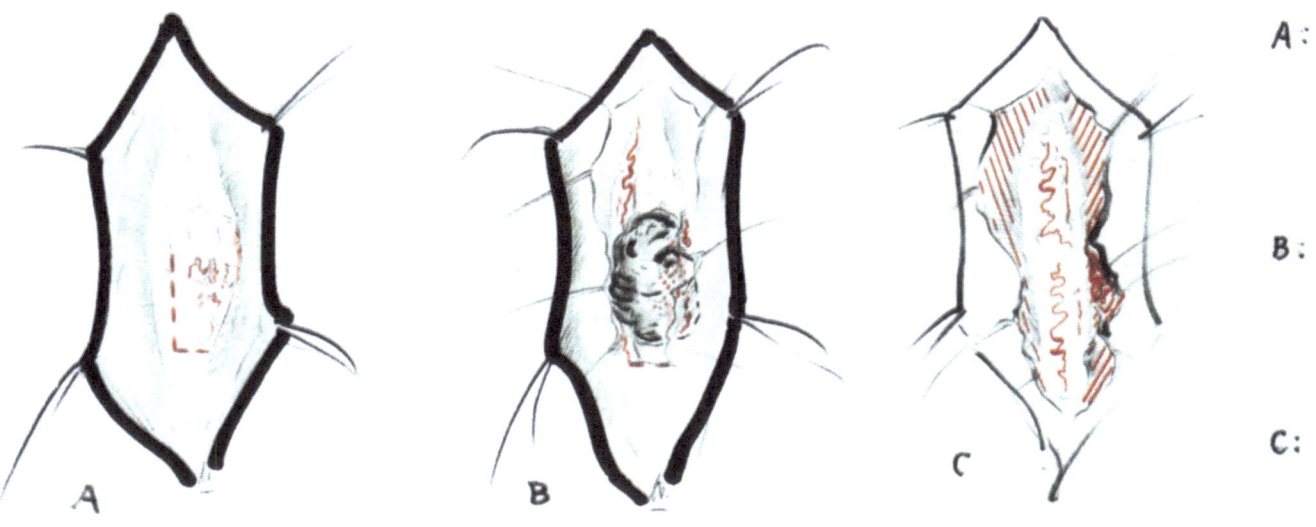

Fig. 253. Sequence of the surgical phases. *A*, Large bilateral opening of the external dural layer. The initial opening of the deep leptomeningeal layer is indicated. *B*, The splitting of the dura on both sides has been performed by passing the upper pole of the meningioma. On the right note the hypervascularization of the tumoral insertion. *C*, After total removal the cord has been reconducted to its axial position and the contralateral arachnoidal adherent structures removed. The area indicated is at the deep dural plane, with the tumoural insertion which will be removed on the right

167

9.7 Opening the Arachnoid

Before completely opening the arachnoidal membrane we usually pierce it in the most dilatated tract near the upper pole of the tumour. This is due first of all to the increase in pressure of the fluid above the compression and secondly, keeping the subarachnoidal space closed below the tumour lowers the probability of fluid pressure variations in the area where the cord is compressed and reduced in volume. Piercing the arachnoid stimulates recovery of the medullary pulsations and gradually reduces the tension in the subarachnoidal space. The arachnoidal process which forms in the vicinity of the meningioma's extremity is formed by a thickened tissue, particularly when small calcifications are present. The subsequent freeing of the arachnoidal membrane reveals the cord's displacement (see Fig. 257).

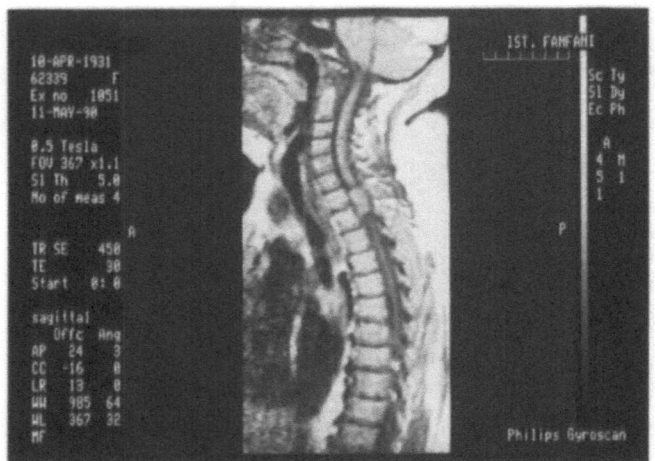

Fig. 254. MRI. Sagittal and coronal projections (see Fig. 255) T1 (TR 450 and TE ms) and axial projection with protonic density (TR 1700 and TE ms; see Fig. 256). At cervicodorsal passage level an expansive, roughly oval-shaped lesion occupies the right half of the vertebral canal and shows the same density as the cord, which is thinned by the compression and pushed to the left

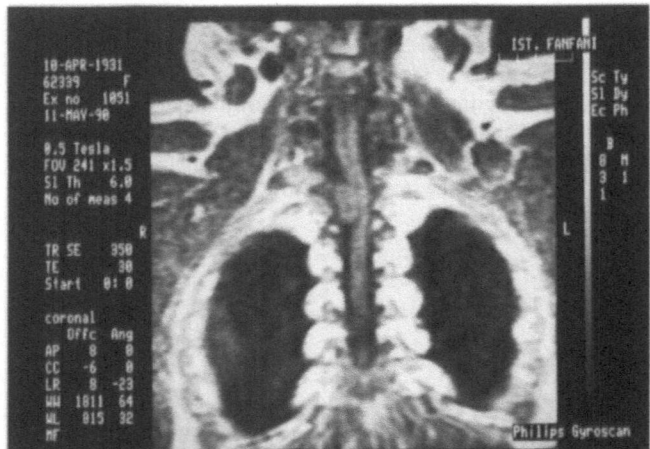

Fig. 255. MRI. Coronal projection

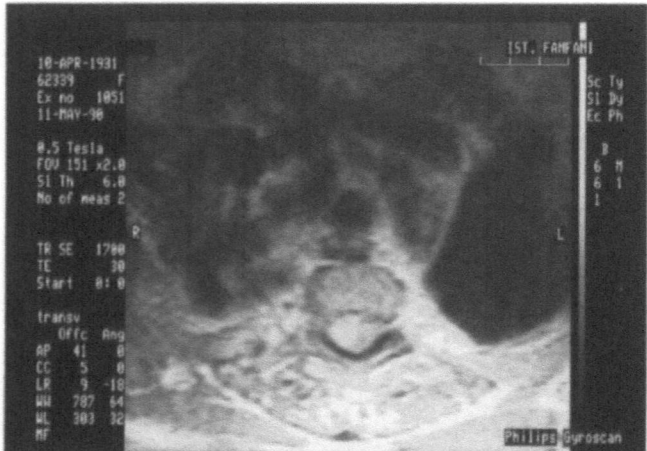

Fig. 256. MRI. Axial projection

Case No. 87: Transitional Meningioma

A 59-year-old woman (1990). Right ventrolateral intradural-extramedullary meningioma in D1.

Clinical Course. 15 years. Burning type of paraesthesias at upper dorsal level, pronounced when straining. The patient (weight 140 kg) had been walking with difficulty for the past 20 years. Three months prior to hospitalization she was affected by paraesthesias in both lower limbs to the right. In walking there was a tendency to lean to the right.

Neurological Examination. Severe spastic paraparesis with hyperreflexia of patellas and of Achilles tendons. Tactile and pain hypoaesthesia from D4 and pallaesthesia in sternal region.

Rachicentesis. 1.15 g protein per thousand.

Myelography (via lumbar puncture). Total block behind body in D4, with slight flow on the left. The image was atypical for a meningioma.

Myelo-CT. Displacement of cord posteriorly and towards the left. In D1 intradural-extramedullary tumour.

MRI. Ovaloid formation with a diameter of 2 cm situated laterally on the right of the rachidian canal in C7-D1. The cord was displaced towards the left. In coronal scans the neoplasm appeared laterally on the right. The cord was curved contralaterally (Figs. 254-256).

Surgical Treatment. On opening the dura, the encapsulated tumour was seen below the roots of C8 on the right and pushed the motor root forwards (Figs. 257, 259). The meningioma was also premedullary. Gradual removal of adherent arachnoidal structures. Coagulation of capsule and debulking of central part. Provisional tamponing of the central excavation with gelatine and haemostasis along the attachment on the internal surface of the dura near the upper poles. Coagulation of the base of attachment and total removal of the tumour.

Results. Slight motor inhibition during postoperative phase with a reduction in the hypoaesthesia level. After 10 days the patient had recovered good motility. Three months later walking proved possible but persisting anaesthesia to underarm region and internal side of right arm on C8 and D1.

In this surgical phase the adherent structures between meningioma and leptomeninges must be sectioned. Medullary malformations in relationship to compression correspond exactly to the MRI and CT images. Myelo-CT, however, offers a more precise topographical view of the tumour and the leptomeninges. These relationships are studied in the set of scans along the entire extention of the tumour.

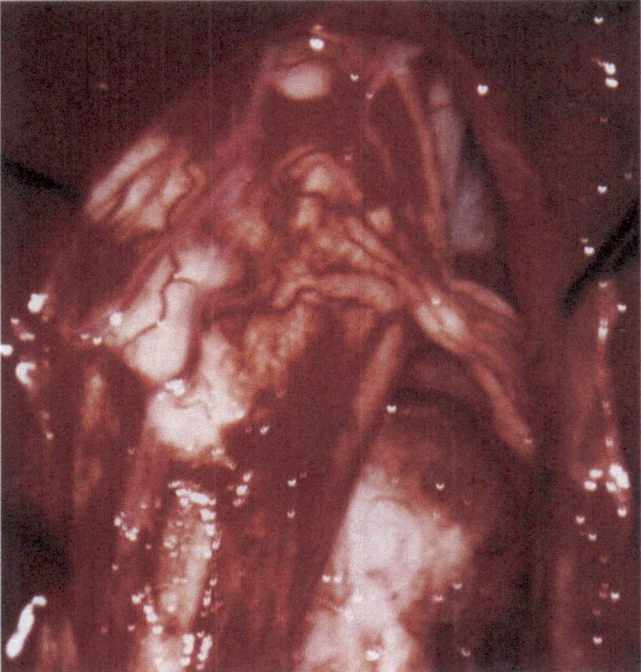

Fig. 257. The tumour is below the spinal root

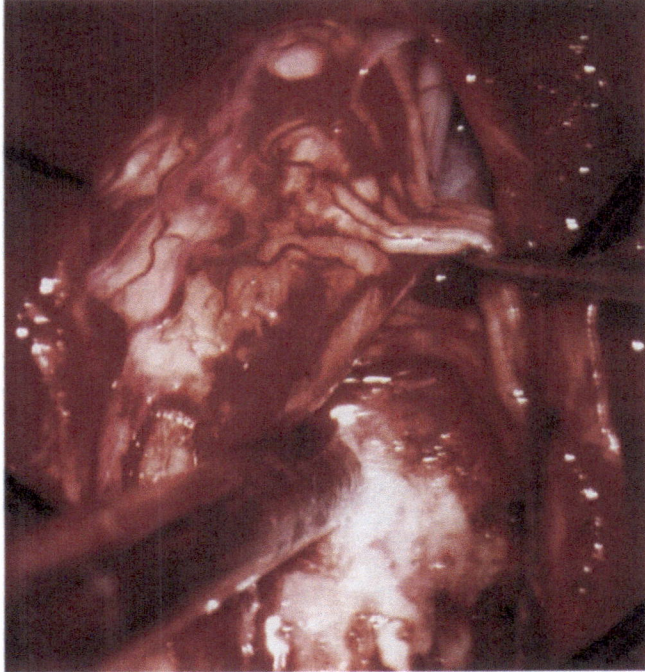

Fig. 258. The tumour pushes the motor root forward

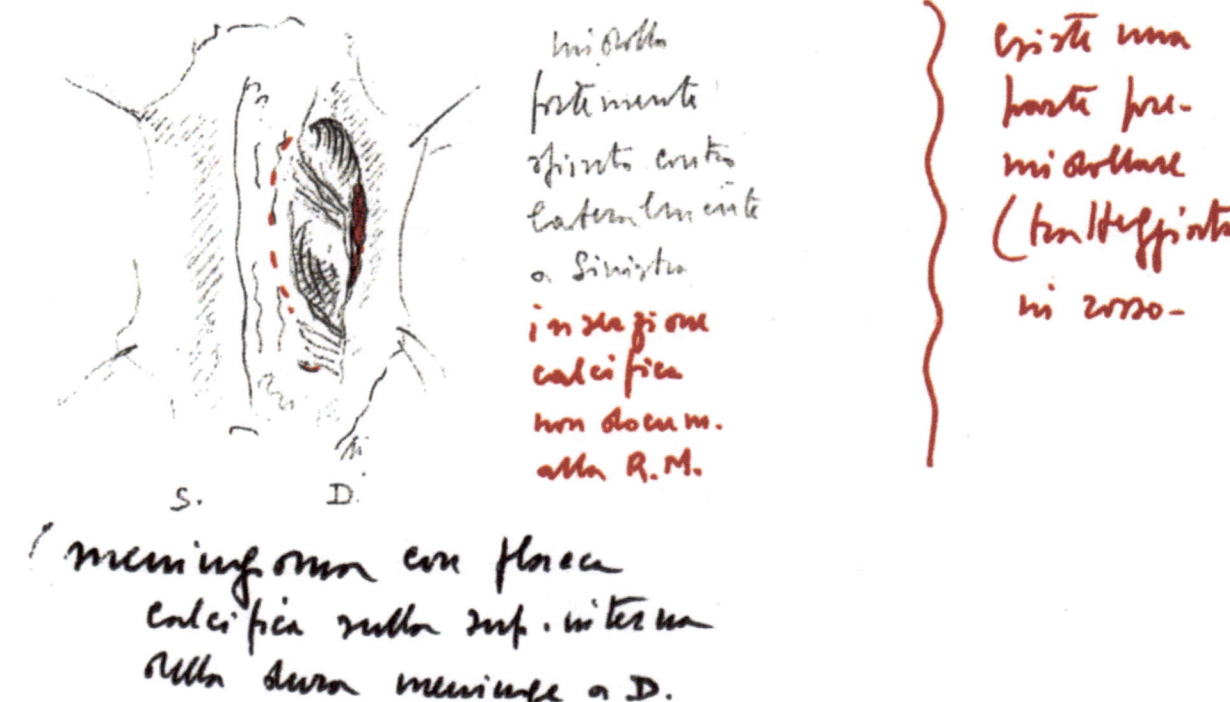

Fig. 259. Postoperative plan. The calcified attachment near the dural funnel of the C8 root is marked (*red*)

9.8 Radicotomy

When the meningioma shows a neighbouring relationship with more than one nerve root, it is easier to spare the one that covers the major part of the tumour, keeping it distant from the capsule. In cases in which the nerve root is enveloped by a tumour the decision to perform radicotomy depends only on the morphological features of vascular damage produced by this compression. If signs of degeneration are observed at the nerve root by the alteration of its characteristic pearly colouring to a greyish colour, radicotomy is justified and facilitates mobilization of the meningioma. In our series sensory nerve roots were sectioned 16 times; in five cases this made excision of the tumour easier (Table 16). In the other 11 cases the nerve root was enveloped by the tumour capsule. In the latter series only one nerve root showed signs of serious atrophy.

Case No. 88: Nonclassified Meningioma
A 43-year-old man (1975). Left posterolateral intradural-extramedullary meningioma in D7-D8.
Clinical Course. Dorsal, band-like pain on the left above the umbilical transverse line. Nocturnal exacerbation and when straining. One month before hospitalization there was irradiation to right. For 10 days stiffness to lower limbs with difficulty in walking.
Neurological Examination. Presence of pigmented cutaneous birthmark. Spastic-ataxic paraparesis to the left. Vivacious patellas polyphasic ankle jerk. Hypoaesthesia from D7-D8 with band-like anaesthesia in D8-D9. Sphincter disturbances in the form of retention.
Rachicentesis. 1.59 protein per thousand.
X-Ray of Dorsal Tract. Scoliosis and anomalies of the spinous processes of D7 which appeared tilted towards the left anteroposteriorly and with a wider base than normal.
Myelography (via lumbar puncture). Dome-shaped block in D7-D8. Above the compression the ondulated diagram revealed the dilatated arterial vascularization.

Surgical Treatment. On opening the dura, the cord was pushed forwards by a reddish-wine coloured subarachnoidal neoplasm. Opening of the arachnoid and radicotomy of the eighth dorsal root on the left which was atrophic. Removal en bloc of neoplasm.
Results. Immediate disappearance of pain symptoms. After 1 month walking was possible with support but an ataxic component persisted. Total recovery after 3 months.

When the nerve root is compressed but retains a good vascularization morphology, the radicular section can be carried out so as to spare the principal artery and to remove it from the nerve bundle. After isolating the tumour from the medullary surface it is possible to see the adherent structures with the motor roots by simply lifting the meningioma, and they are spared once they are at a distance from the arachnoid.

9.9 Modes of Excision

Cushing's techniques for removal of anterolateral meningiomas consisted in debulking the central part of the tumour after the incision of the capsule, which leads to a gradual reduction in the compression (Figs. 260-262). At this point the meningioma is reclined against the ventral

Table 16. Radicotomy performed on 125 meningiomas

Case no.	Level	Topography	Radicotomy
28	C1-C2	Right ventrolateral	C1
114	C1-C2	Right ventrolateral	C2
64	C4	Right ventrolateral	C5
54	C4-C6	Right ventrolateral	C6
65	C7-D1	Right ventrolateral	C8
92	C7-D9	Right ventrolateral	D2
91	D1-D2	Left ventrolateral	D2
112	D2	Left posterolateral	D6
60	D5-D6	Right ventrolateral	D6
115	D6-D7	Ventral	D8
44	D6-D7	Right posterolateral	D7
3	D7	Left ventrolateral	D7
88	D7-D8	Left posterolateral	D8
45	D7-D8	Right posterolateral	D7
111	D9-D10	Left posterolateral	D10
62	D12-L1	Ventral	L1

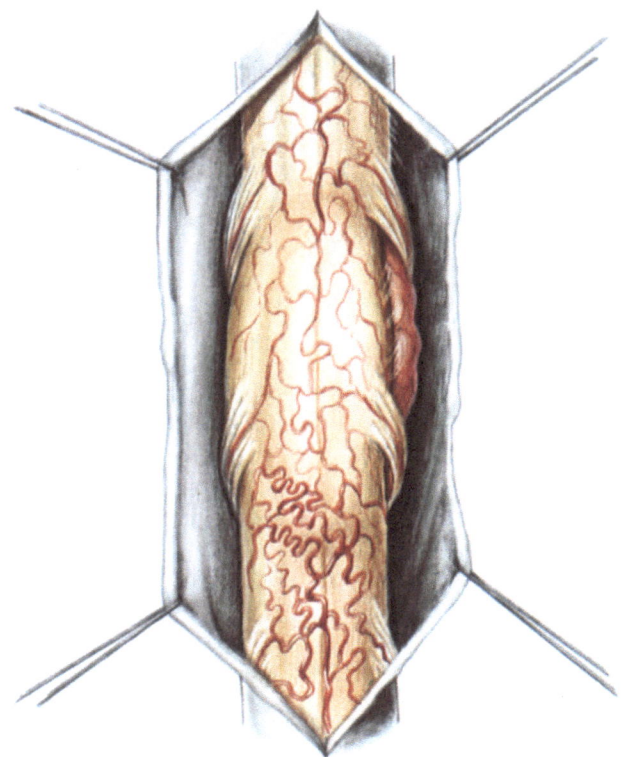

Fig. 260. Scheme from Cushing's technique

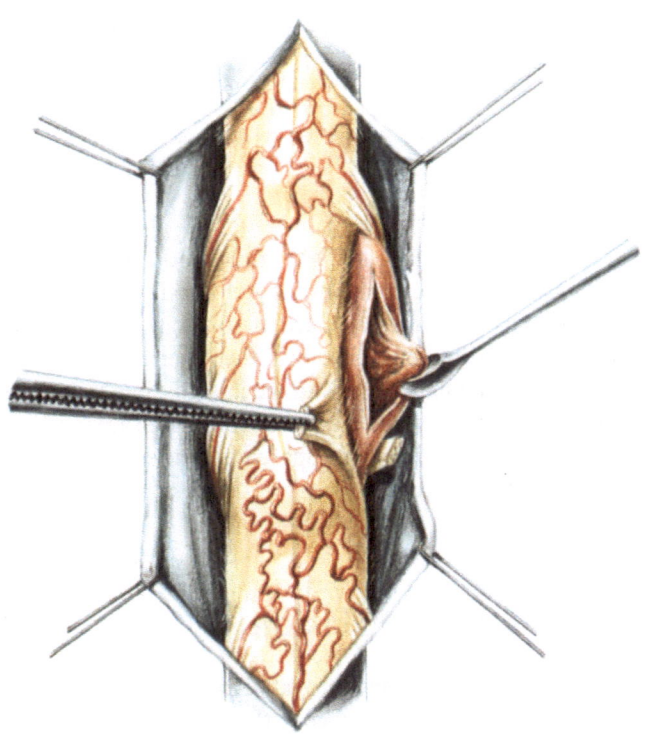

Fig. 261. The intracapsula debulking of the meningioma can be accompanied by a posterior radicotomy, which produces more space for the removal of a ventrally located tumour

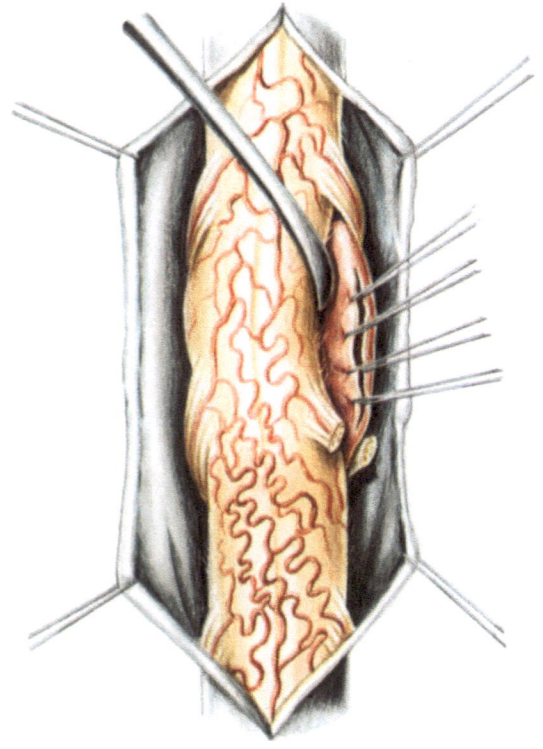

Fig. 262. Traction of the tumour's capsulae after debulking

plane of the spinal dura, leaving more space to view the arachnoidal septa, which is sectioned prior to removal. In some cases the defined invasion of the meningioma favours mobilization of the remaining part of the tumour on the opposite side for removal by fragmentation. In a paramedian site the incision of the dura may be by means of a linear, an arch-shaped or an L-shaped cut even in reoperated cases of premedullary relapses of other natures. This technique has proven valuable in intradural-premedullary lesions of a malignant nature. The patient in case no. 38 was operated on for neurosarcoma. In the first operation the patient was placed in a sitting position, and the dural incision was performed vertically. The operation was successful without deficit. Relapse resulted in a second operation, but here the patient was placed in a lateral decupitus position and the following procedure was performed. After preparation of the dura a lateral incision was made which helped protect the entire posterior side of the medullary surface without involving the adherent structures of the first operation. The total excision of the

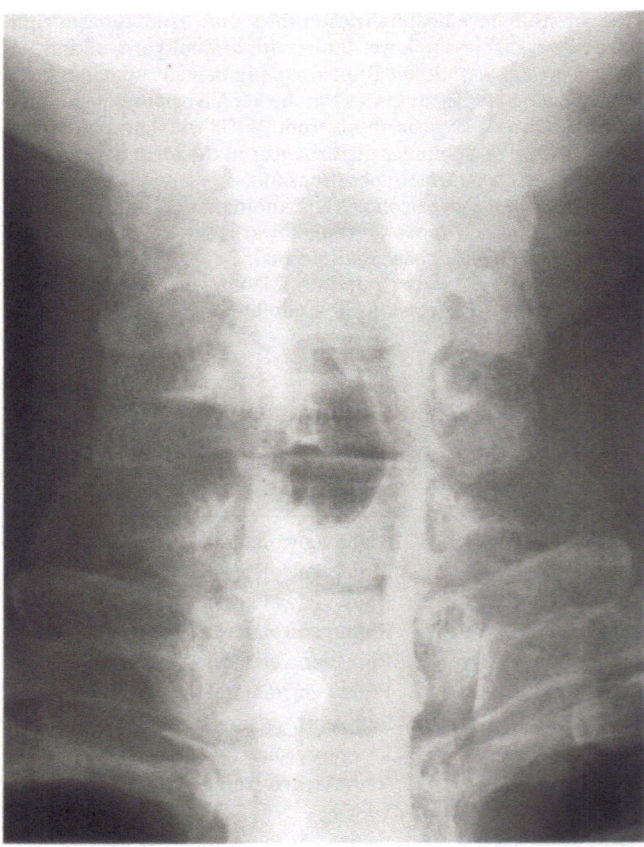

Fig. 263. Partial block on the right side. A clear linear reduction in the contralateral subarachnoidal space

172

relapse tumour resulted in partial regression of the severe tetraparesis and after 6 months the patient was able to walk without support. The hypoaesthesia of a Brown-Sequard nature remained unaltered (Figs. 263-267).

All methods for opening the meningeal sac follow the fundamental principles described by Guillaime et al. (1957): no manipulations of the cord, fragmented removal when total removal en bloc is not possible, stopping of all bleeding in the subarachnoidal space and, once the tumour has been freed from the leptomeninges, performing the various phases of the operation by preparing sufficient space to separate the meningioma from the myeloradicular structures, always noting arterial surface-layer blood supply. Cases of subarachnoidal meningioma in which it is essential to open the arachnoid before separating the tumour from the cord differ from other cases where observation under preoperative microscope reveals total extrarachidian development. This feature has been observed in some cases of globally calcified meningiomas and, according to Levy (1982), are extremely difficult to dissect (Figs. 145, 146).

Case No. 38: Psammomatous Meningioma

A 55-year-old man (1994). Posterolateral intradural-extramedullary, extraarachnoideal meningioma in D11 (almost totally calcified).

Clinical Course. 10 years. Lumbago attacks with irradiation of tingling sensation spreading in a band-like manner to the right up to the inguinal region at intervals. Three years before hospitalization accentuation of symptoms with sensations in a paravertebral, dorsolumbar site on the right; pain irradiating and paraesthesia to gluteal area, anterior and posterior thigh and posteriorly at leg to right foot. Fastidious dysaesthesia at inguinal area, right testicle

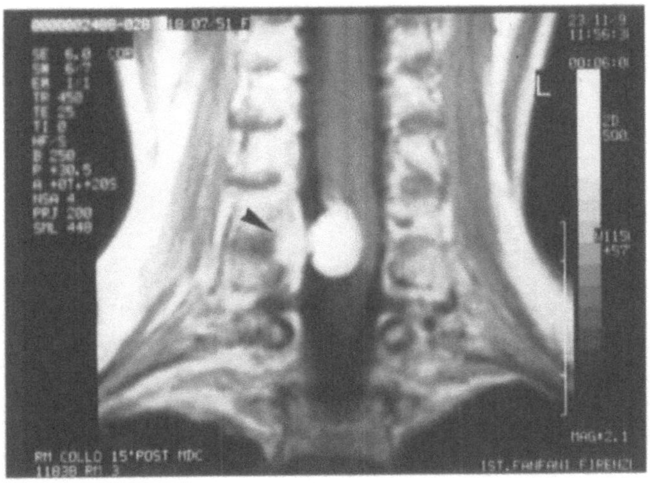

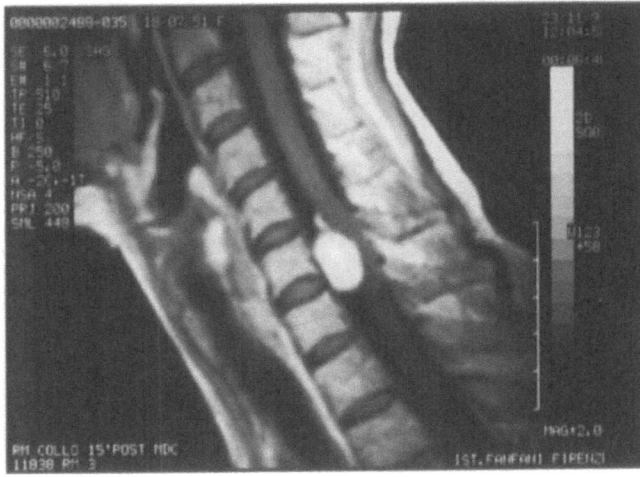

Fig. 264. Displacement of the medullary corridor towards the left is confirmed by MRI with gadolinium in a coronal projection. This scan shows a tumoral extention in the intravertebral foramen (*arrow*), clearly corresponding to the interruption on the external surface above and below the tumour, as already described by myelographic oblique image

Fig. 265. The scan clearly shows the anterior topography of the tumour

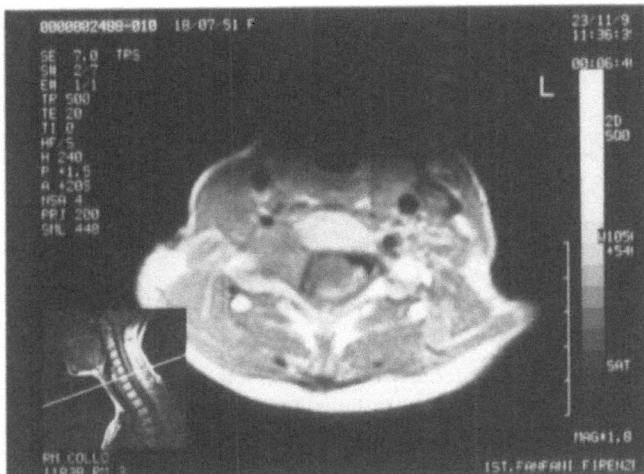

Fig. 266. Same case in axial projection

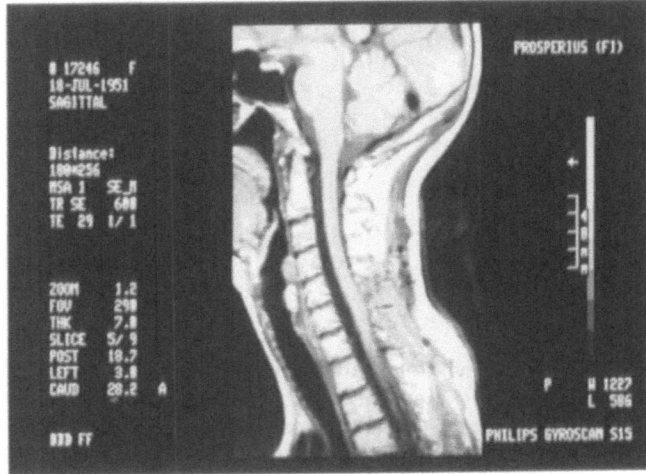

Fig. 267. A 6-month check

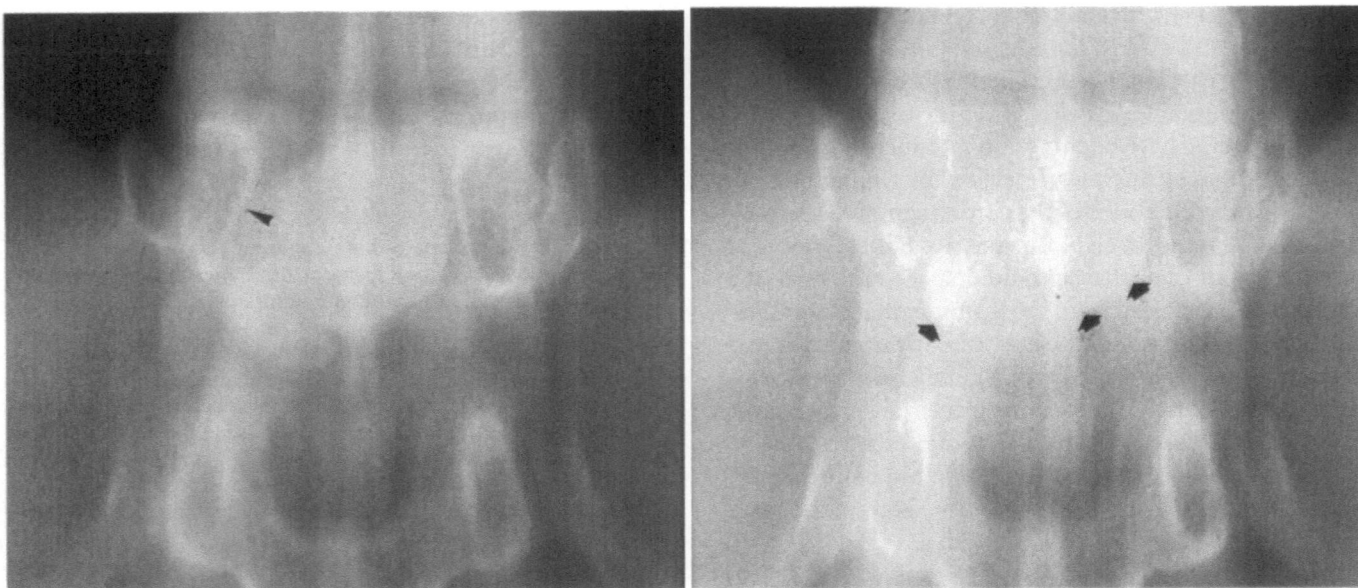

Fig. 268. The images, in stratigraphy, show the calcified tumour

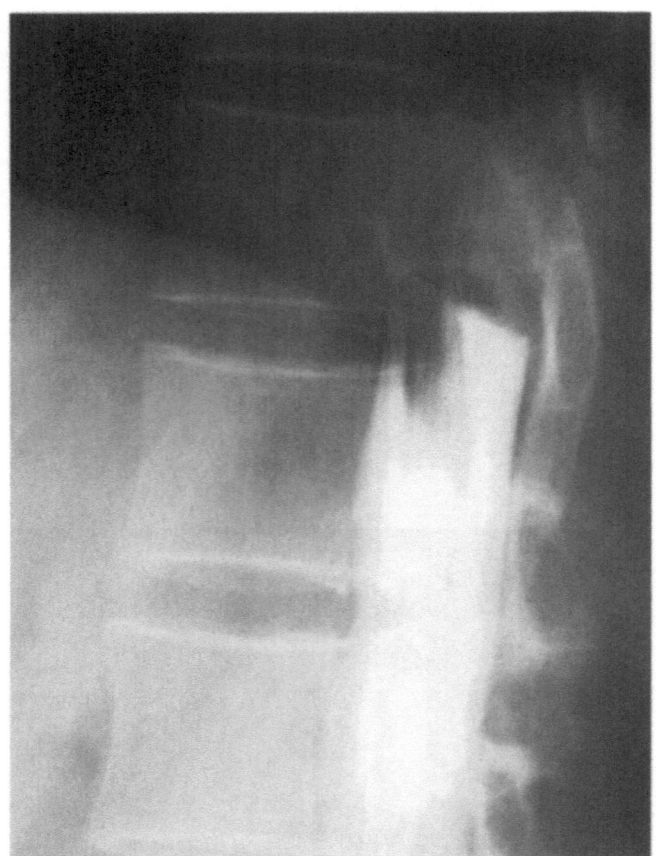

Fig. 269. Myelography. Total block in D11-D12; the medullary corridor is displaced forwards. The contrast medium enlarges the subarachnoidal space posteriorly and continues to define the whole ventral part of the calcified meningioma. This feature is important during surgery for locating the expansive and totally extra-arachnoidal process

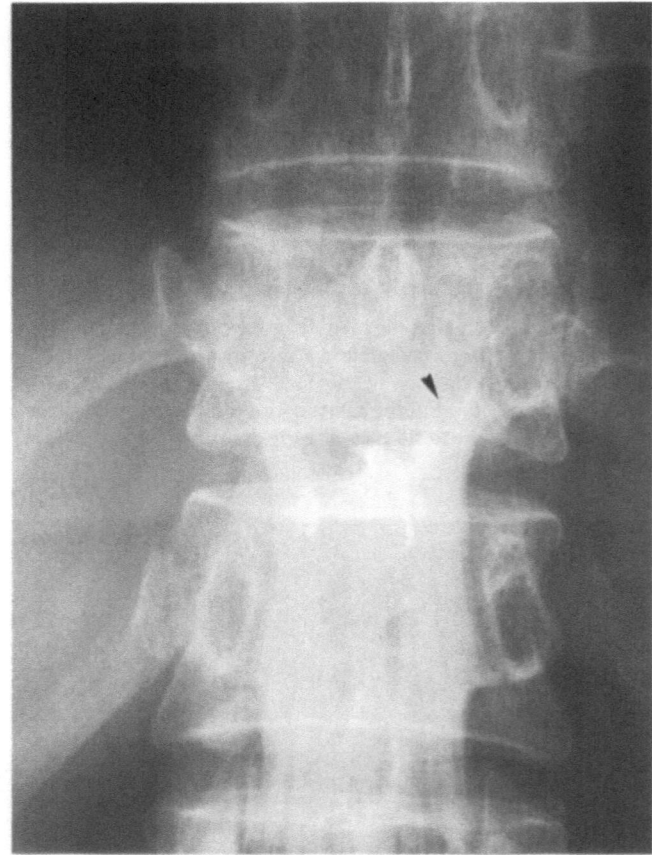

Fig. 270. Anteroposteriorly the irregular lower pole of the meningioma is defined. The contrast medium surrounds the lateral protrusions of the tumour particularly along its left surface (*arrow*)

and perineal region. For approx. 6 months further deterioration with paraesthesias to medial and lower abdomen on the right; motor incoordination to lower limbs. Sphincter and sexual disturbances in the form of urinary incontinence and frequent spontaneous nocturnal ejaculations.

Neurological Examination. Rigid lumbar rachis due to contracture of paravertebral muscles. Loss of strength in the right lower limb. Lively patella reflexes. Bilateral foot clonus. Ataxic gait. Superficial tactile and painful hypoaesthesia from D9-D12 on the right side. Sphincter disturbances in the form of incontinence.

Rachicentesis. 0.33 g protein per thousand.

X-Ray of Dorsal Tract. Image showed calcified tumour to the right in stratigraphy (Fig. 268) Segmental scoliosis. Alterations due to erosion of articular pedicles and of intravertebral foramens in D11-D12 on the right. Congenital dysmorphia of posterior arch of L5.

Myelography (via lumbar puncture). Contrast medium defined the entire lower surface and part of borders of tumour, identifying the true volume and the major calcified component on the right (Figs. 269, 270).

Myelo-CT. The tumour seemed to occupy the rachidian canal entirely. The iodine medium defined the lower right lateral border of the meningioma with foramenal layer (Figs. 271, 272).

MRI. In D11 within the vertebral canal roughly rounded lesion with nonhomogeneous structure and a relatively reduced signal. The tumour compressed and displaced the preterminal tract of the cord from the back to the front (Figs. 273, 274).

MRI with Gd-DTPA. The lesion was slightly enhanced in the most anterior peripheral area.

Surgical Treatment. Hypervascularization of the laminae with accentuation of the distance between spinous processes. The posterior arches were curved outwards with mega-apophysis. Accentuation of dural surface vascularization. The dura emitted no pulsations and felt taut on a mass below which there was a hard, stone-like consistency. The external side of the dura on the anterolateral right had already been invaded by tumourous tissue which reached the epidural venous plexes. Delamination of the dura at lower tract level of the neoplasm. Splitting of the meninges allowed coagulation deep in the dura, gradually checking haemorrhages between the external membrane and internal dural layer. On reaching the surface of the tumour gradual fragmentation deep in the calcified tissue. The vascular participation of the external layers differed from that of the deep layers: the most conspicuous blood supply still appeared to be in continuity with the meningiomas attachment which extended towards the intravertebral foramen on the right. In this case an ultrasound osteotome was used to facilitate the almost complete debulking of the tumour and reaching the capsule at the level of the intravertebral foramen which was wider than normal. This excavation to reduce compression against the cord revealed the

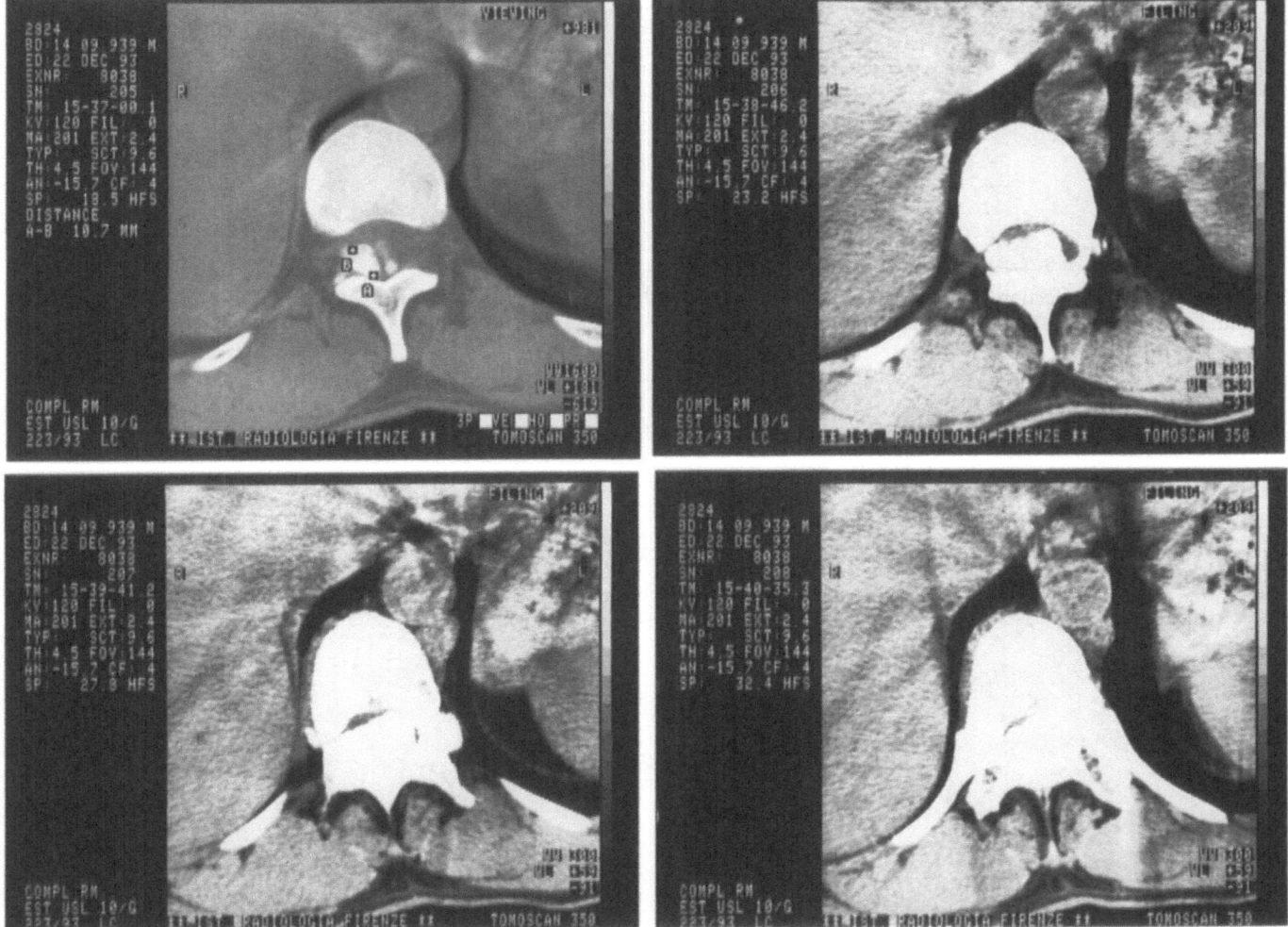

Fig. 271. CT. Calcified lesion which occupies the vertebral canal in D11-D12. Ventrally the residual space of the rachidian lumen is gradually reduced due to the large compact area of the tumour

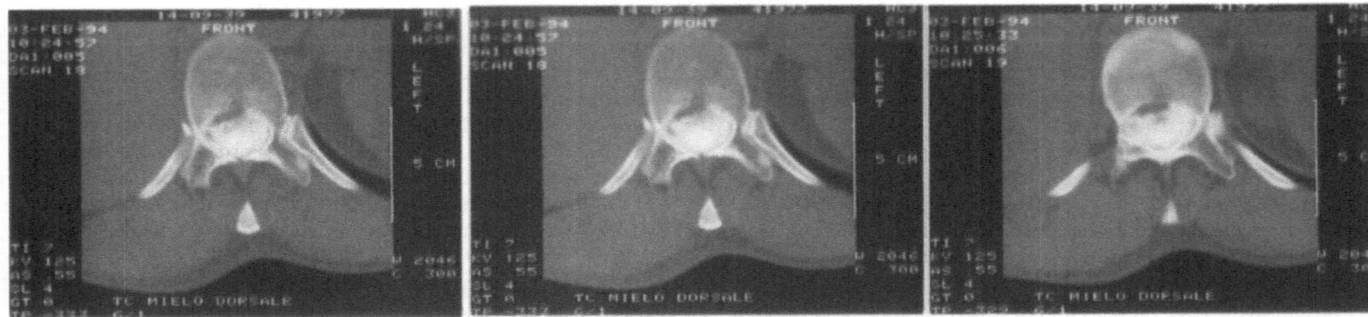

Fig. 272. Myelo-CT. The meningioma appears irregular and more calcified in the left posterior and lateral parts. The borders are more clearly defined, and its relationship with the displaced cord appears reduced to a lamella

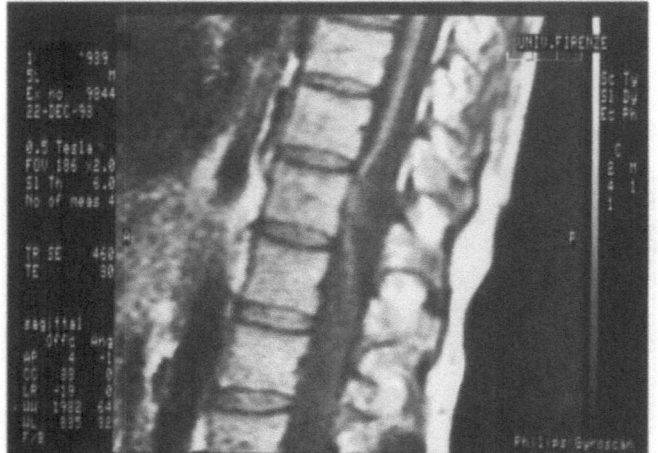
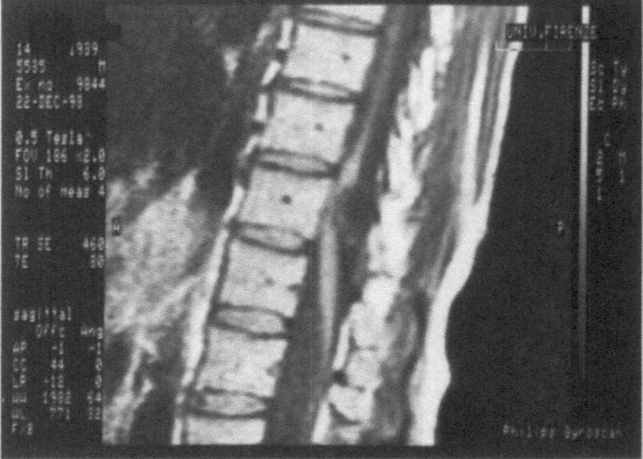

Fig. 273. MRI. Sagittal projection T1, sagittal and coronal T1 (TR 450 and TE 30 ms; see Fig. 274). The expansive roundish-shaped lesion is located behind the cord in D11-D12 and produces a nonhomogeneous hypointense signal indicating its calcified nature

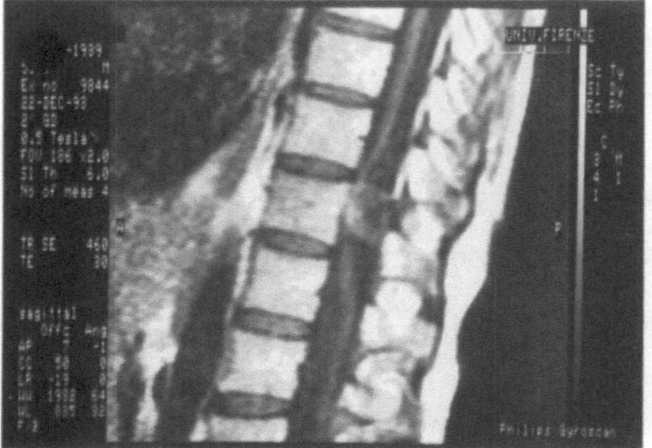
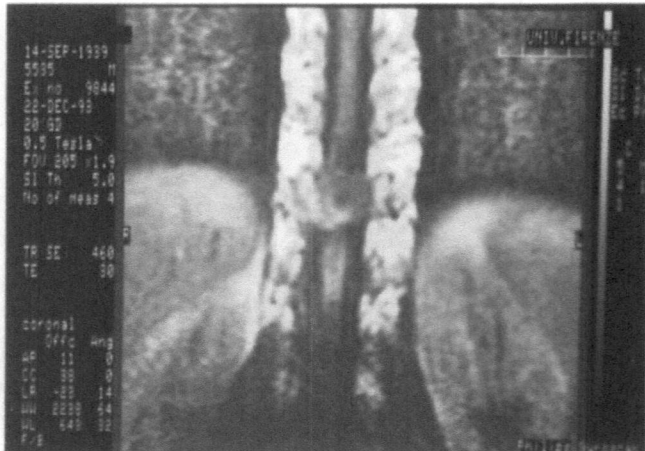

Fig. 274. The neoplasm assumes the paramagnetic contrast medium only in its anterior part

arachnoidal plane which appeared to be without interruption below the deep surface layer of the tumour (Fig. 275). Gradual tilting of the residual calcified part of the meningioma through the arachnoid revealed the cord to be reduced to a thin shred. Total removal together with the internal dural membrane along the entire length of the meningioma's invasion. After replacing the cord in an axial position, reconstruction with suture only of the external dural membrane.

Results. After slight persistence of paraesthesia irradiating bilaterally to the anterior side of thigh, complete regression of pain syndrome. Complete surgical recovery after 1 year.

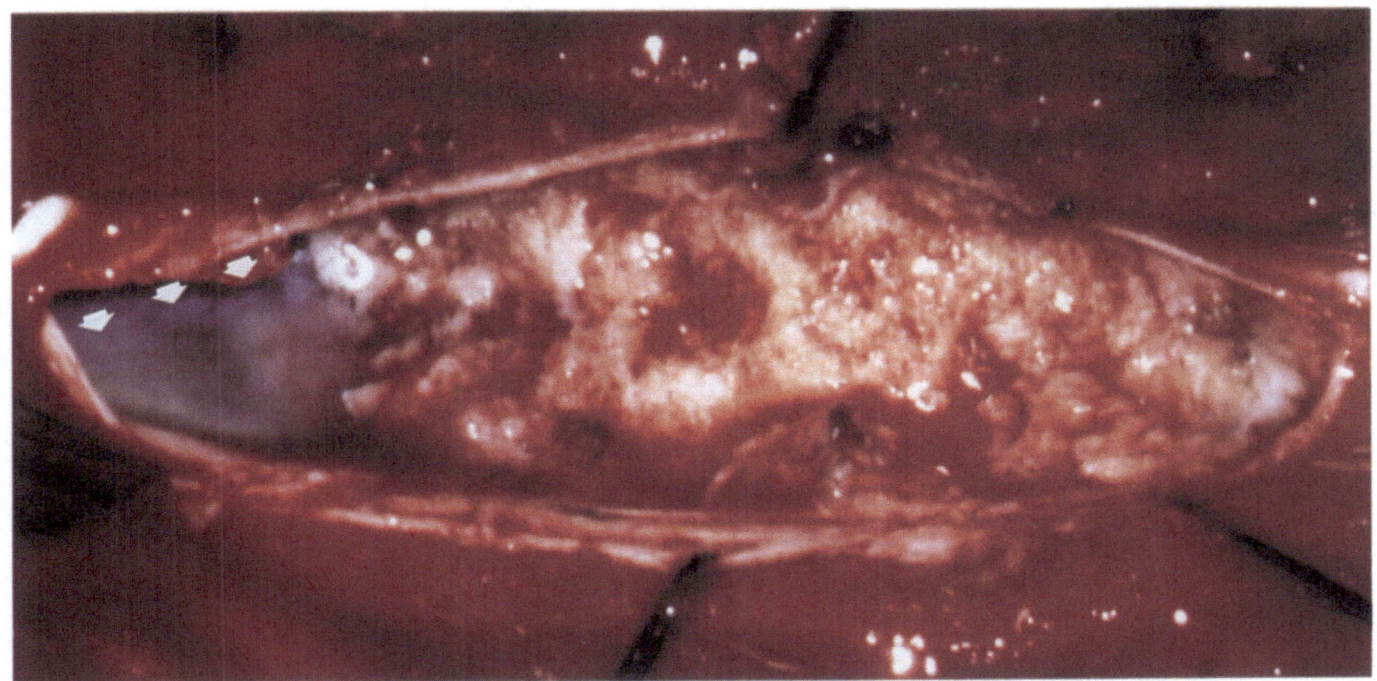

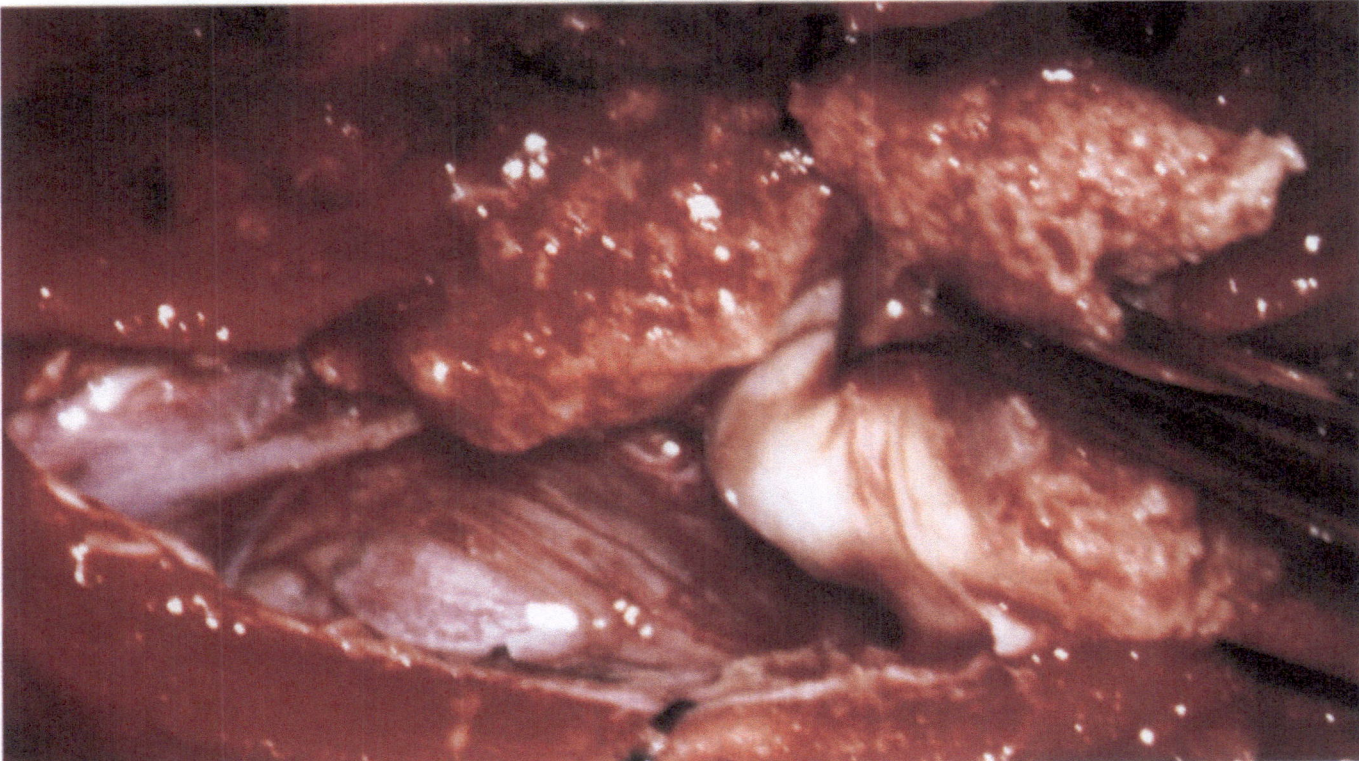

Fig. 275. *Arrows* (*left*), the arachnoidal plane which remains below the entire extension of the tumour. The central part of the enlarged meningioma reaches the intravertebral foramen and is clearly seen in the right paramedian MRI scan with gadolinium (see Fig. 274)

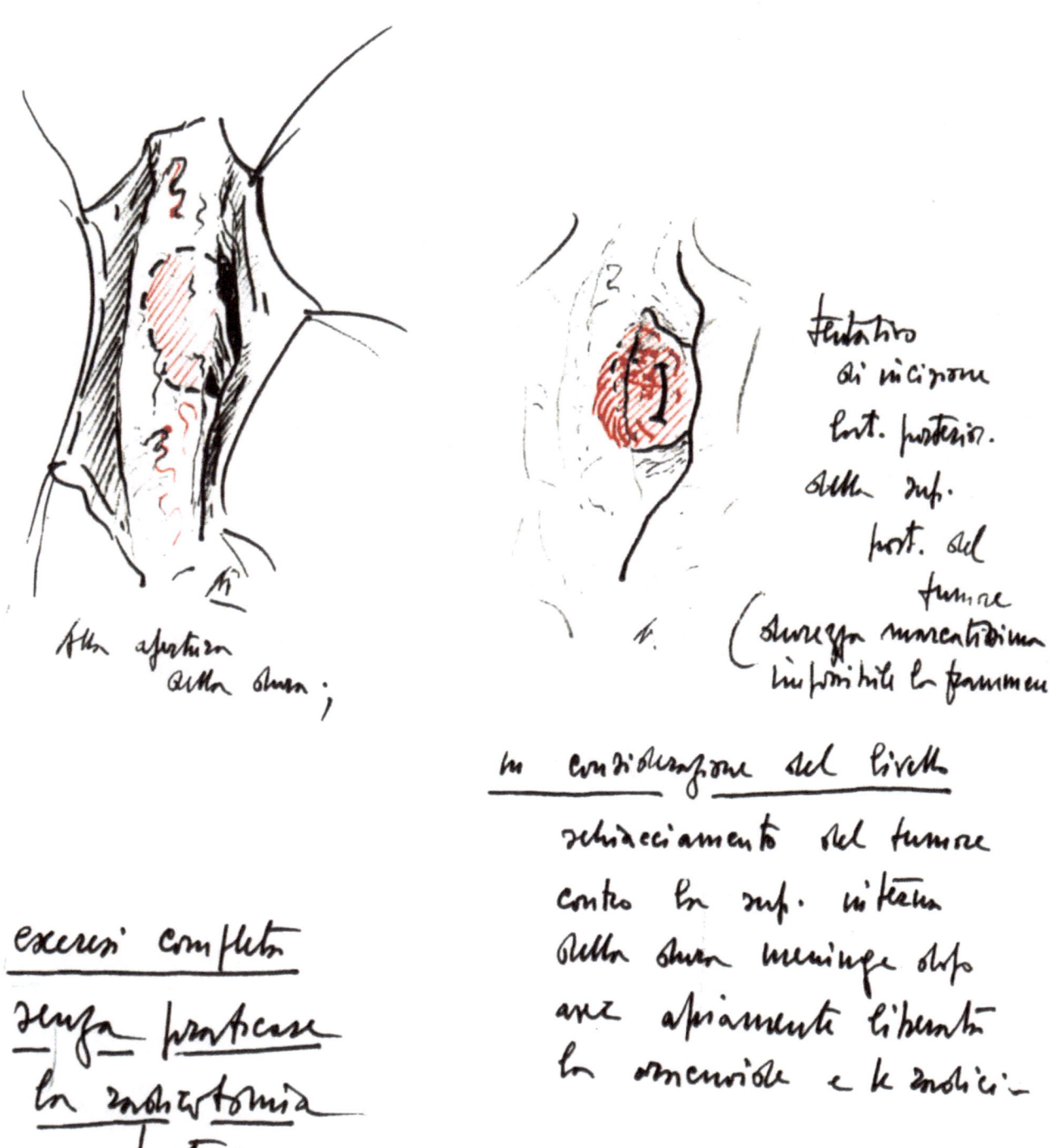

Fig. 276. The location of the almost totally premedullary lesion. The calcified capsule with a right attachment presented an obstacle in debulking the meningioma. In this case excision was performed by gradually pressing the tumour against the internal surface of the dura

Our experience shows that meningiomas with extra-arachnoidal development are easy to remove. The interposition of a small strip of cotton on the arachnoidal plane during the lifting of the meningioma leads to complete freeing of the meningioma without possibly traumatic manoevres for the cord. The arachnoidal membrane, while conserving the physiological relationship of the layers as a protective plane, prevents risk of arachnoidal haemorrhage. In the literature a number of haemorrhagic situations are noted that are defined as "haemorachis", but these complications no longer take place even if the meningioma is totally calcified. The manoevres during the gradual excision phase are facilitated by anchoring the most ventral calcified surface layer with the aid of a small hook. The most delicate point lies at the upper pole of the meningioma where it adheres to the oedematous tract of the cord. We can now obtain more detailed preoperative images from neuroradiological diagnostic data than was possible a few years ago, and this enables us to perform surgery by following a plan of anatomic relationships already prepared by CT and myelo-CT scans.

Cushing's technique of performing an incision on the capsule before removal is still a very valuable method but can be used only if the neoplasm tissue is friable and of a soft consistency (Fig. 276, case no. 38). Some authors, including Perria et al. (1983) and Jain (1983), recommend the use of laser surgery for excision of very calcified tumours. Both laser and ultrasound osteotomes facilitate the removal of a meningioma, but they must always be used with care to ensure that the medullary surface is protected. When the tumour attachment is formed by a calcified lamella, such as in en plaque meningiomas (Fig. 277, case no. 81) or by a bony spur within the dural layer, the excision must be made in the last phase of surgery because major bleeding usually occurs in the calcified areas of invasion. The calcified part of posteriorly located tumours can be excised by keeping the tumour raised above the medullary surface even during the first phase of surgery without running any risk for the cord. After removal of the meningioma the cord often does not seem to recover its pulsations in the tract where a myelitic mark is left by the compression. This is caused partly by the adherent structures which develop between the pia mater and arachnoid and weigh upon the contralateral internal dural side of the tumour site.

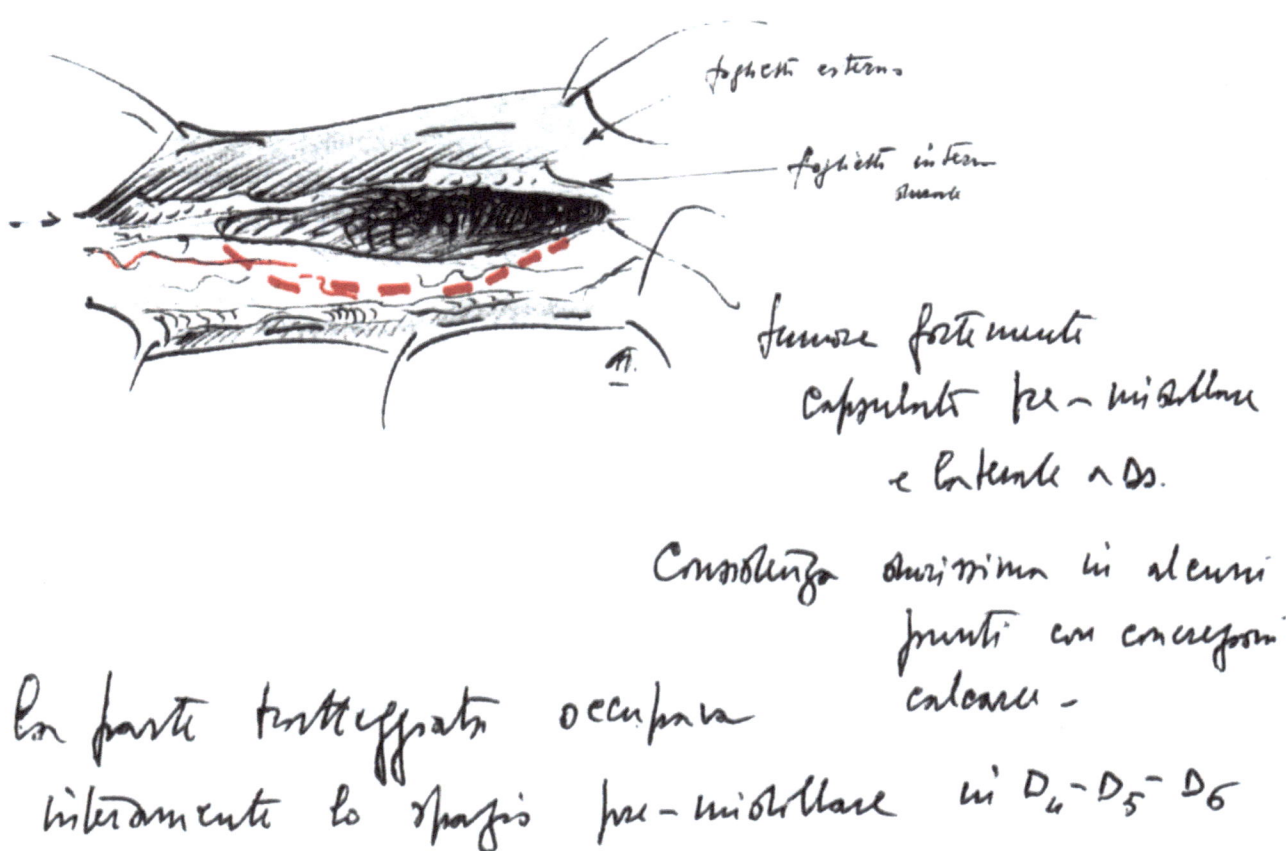

Fig. 277. Premedullary meningioma en plaque

Case No. 79: Transitional Meningioma
A 70-year-old female (1980). Left ventrolateral intradural-extramedullary meningioma in D8-D9.
Clinical Course. 15 years. Burning type of pain at left gluteal region. Five years before hospitalization the patient suffered sciatica for 15 days followed by paraesthesias to left lower limb. For 7-8 months pain on the right lateral side of thigh, leg and to the first two toes. In the latter period the patient reported cord pain to the legs.
Neurological Examination. Dorsal pain. Hypotrophy to quadriceps and gastrocnemius on the left. Lack of stength and paretic-spastic walking; pronounced ataxia on the left. Tactile and painful hypoaesthesia from D9 distally pronounced to the right. Sphincter disturbances in the form of the retention of urine.
X-Ray of Dorsal Rachis. Slight convex scoliosis and the narrowing of vertebral pedicle from D7-D8 (Fig. 278).
MRI. In D8-D9 in the central site and left paramedian compression, ovaloid in shape and measuring 2 cm; the meningioma was more developed in D9 and pushed the cord forwards to the right (Figs. 279, 280).
Surgical Treatment. The dural plane showed hypervascularization of the surface layer. Dural malformation on the left due to compression below. The enlargement of the meninges was close to the confluence point of the roots near the intravertebral foramen. Incision of dura with decollement only of external membrane and coagulation of pathological circulation along the invasion of the meningioma. After incision of the deep dural plane, opening of the arachnoid and raising of the tumour, keeping it at a distance from the cord. The meningioma, substantially posterior, also occupied the anterolateral region. The motor root adjacent to the ventral part of tumour was curved upwards and pushed forwards. Total excision together with dural leptomeningeal plane (Figs. 281-289).
Results. Great improvement in neurological picture after 4 months. Total recovery after 3 years.

After removal of the tumour it is advisable to reposition the spinal cord to an axial location and keep it at a distance from the tract which adheres to the spinal dura. Usually the ischaemic shell-shaped mark persists against the cord above and below the site of the compression.

Case No. 48: Transitional Meningioma
A 56-year-old female (1978). Left posterolateral intradural-extramedullary meningioma in D8.
Clinical Course. 3 months. Sudden sense of weakness at lower limbs with instability while walking followed by paraesthesias distally to lower limbs to the right.
Neurological Examination. Spastic-ataxic paraparesis with hyperreflexia. Radicular hypoaesthesia on D8-D9 and cord hypoaesthesia from L1.
X-Ray of Dorsal Rachis. Slight scoliosis.
Myelography (performed suboccipitally). Partial block in D8 producing a dome-shaped image.
Surgical Treatment. On opening the dura a left posterolateral subarachnoidal neoplasm was seen invading the internal surface of the dura near the intravertebral foramen of the ninth dorsal root. Excision en bloc (see Figs. 290-291).
Results. Rapid remission of clinical syndrome with complete recovery over the following 3 months.

If the manoevres to free the thickened leptomeninges prove difficult, it is advisable not to use excessive force but to refer to postoperative and MRI checks, so that per-

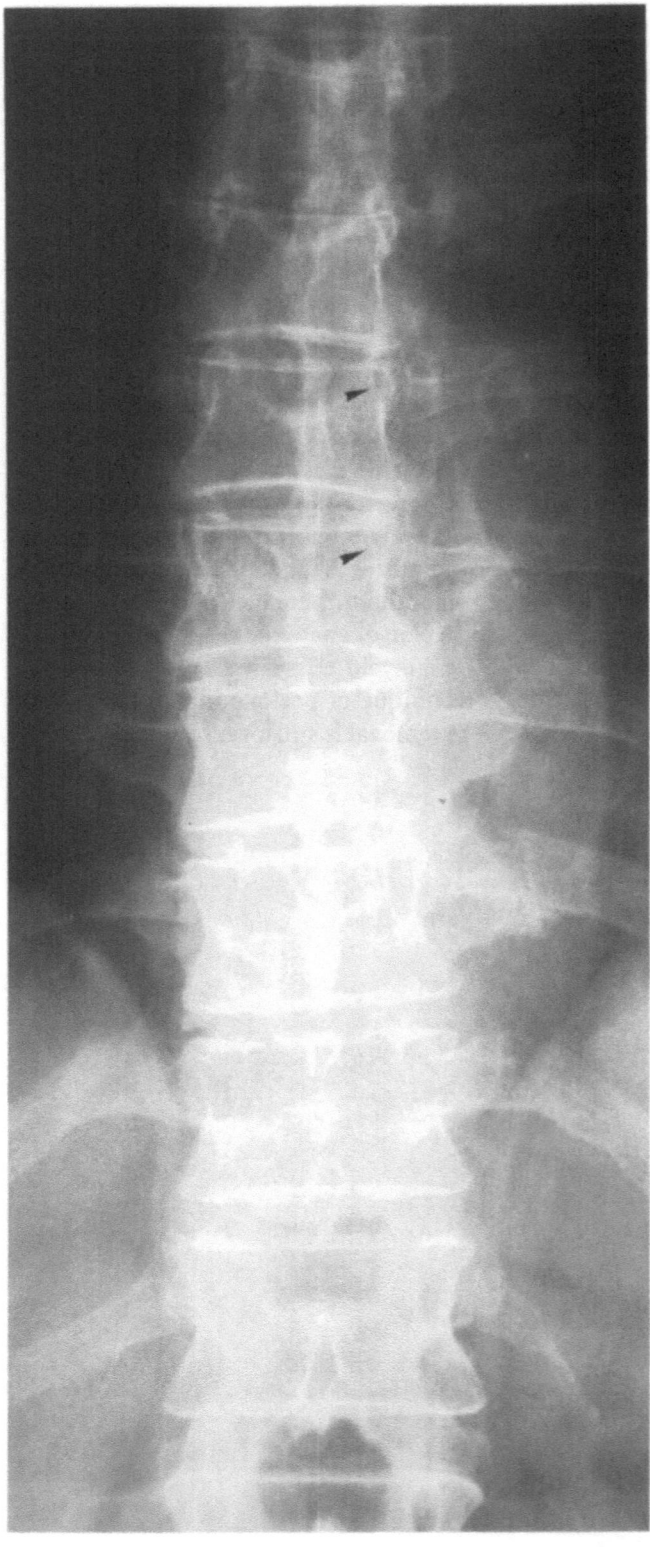

Fig. 278. X-ray. Anteroposteriorly, slight scoliosis and the thinning of the left articular facets in D7-D8 (*arrows*)

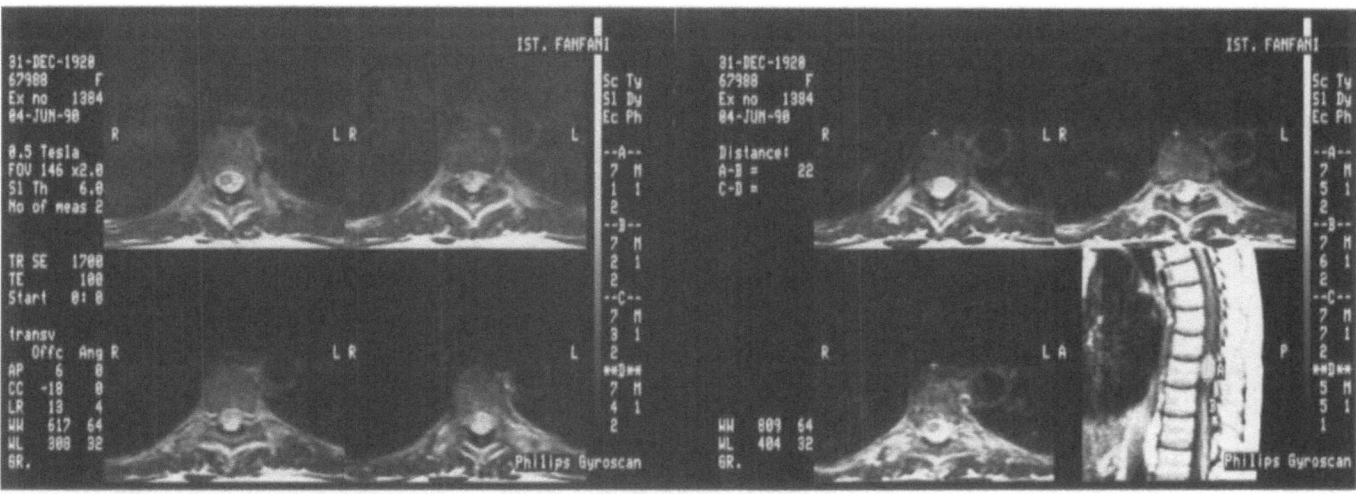

Fig. 279. MRI. Sagittal projection T1 with contrast medium and axial projection T2 (TR 1700 and TE 100 ms). Expansive oval-shaped process in D8-D9 shows sensitivity to the cord and hyperintensity with contrast medium. The tumour occupies a large part of the canal from the left posterior tract and is located in front and to the right of the cord

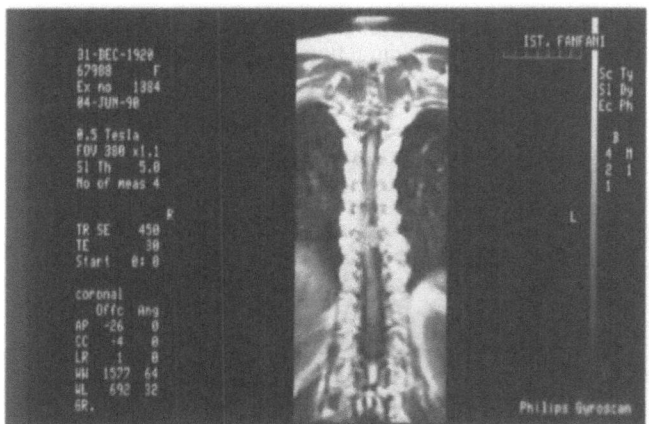

Fig. 280. MRI. Coronal projection T1 (TR 450 and TE 30 ms)

sistent malformations to the cord do not obstacle the patient's recovery. Some authors recommend excising the base attachment together with removal of the meningioma, sacrificing a part of the dura which is replaced by a dural plastic. This technique is not used frequently today: only once by Levy et al. (1982) in 97 meningioma cases and only twice by Solero et al. (1989) in 156 meningioma cases. Our technical variant splits the dura, without reducing the consistency of the external membrane, which is joined and sutured at different points.

Before the suture of the dura, the previously prepared deep dural layer is sectioned together with the tumoral attachment. Formerly we performed the excision of the dura after or together with the excision of the base attachment. Dural plastic was used with a lamina of amni-

on in seven cases (chapter 10, cases 6, 12, 13, 17, 22, 29, 93; see Fig. 292). However, we have not used this technique since 1971 in order to avoid postoperative complications recorded in the literature such as fluid, extrameningeal alterations and postoperative fluid fistulae (see Fig. 293).

Case No. 116: Psammomatous Meningioma
A 72-year-old woman (1980). Posterior intradural-extramedullary meningioma in D10-D11.
Clinical Course. 1 year. Weakness in both lower limbs with claudication to the right. Lumbago with irradiation to right gluteal region.
Neurological Examination. Spastic paraparesis with hyperreflexia. Instability while walking, of a spastic-paretic nature. Hypoaesthesia from D12.
Rachicentesis. 0.66 g per thousand.
X-Ray of Dorsal Rachis. Scoliosis.
Myelography (performed suboccipitally). Block in D10-D11 with dome-shaped filling defect and slight flow sideways on the left after 40 mins.
Surgical Treatment. Dural surface had a calcified area. Opening of the arachnoid below neoplasm and removal of small mass resembling an almond of a red-wine colour together with calcified base and a part of posterior dura.
Results. Walking with slight spasticity in the following 10 days. Clinical recovery after 3 years.

Long-standing spinal compression leads to the thinning of the spinal dura in the tract where the tumour has developed. One should remember that splitting of the dura is possible, along the entire invasion of the meningioma. This is indicated especially in cases with a dura greatly reduced in thickness and denser than the underlying pathological tissue. This condition can be seen under a preoperative microscope and is more evident in small lentil-like meningiomas than in larger tumours or in tumours with multiple locations such as in von Recklinghausen's

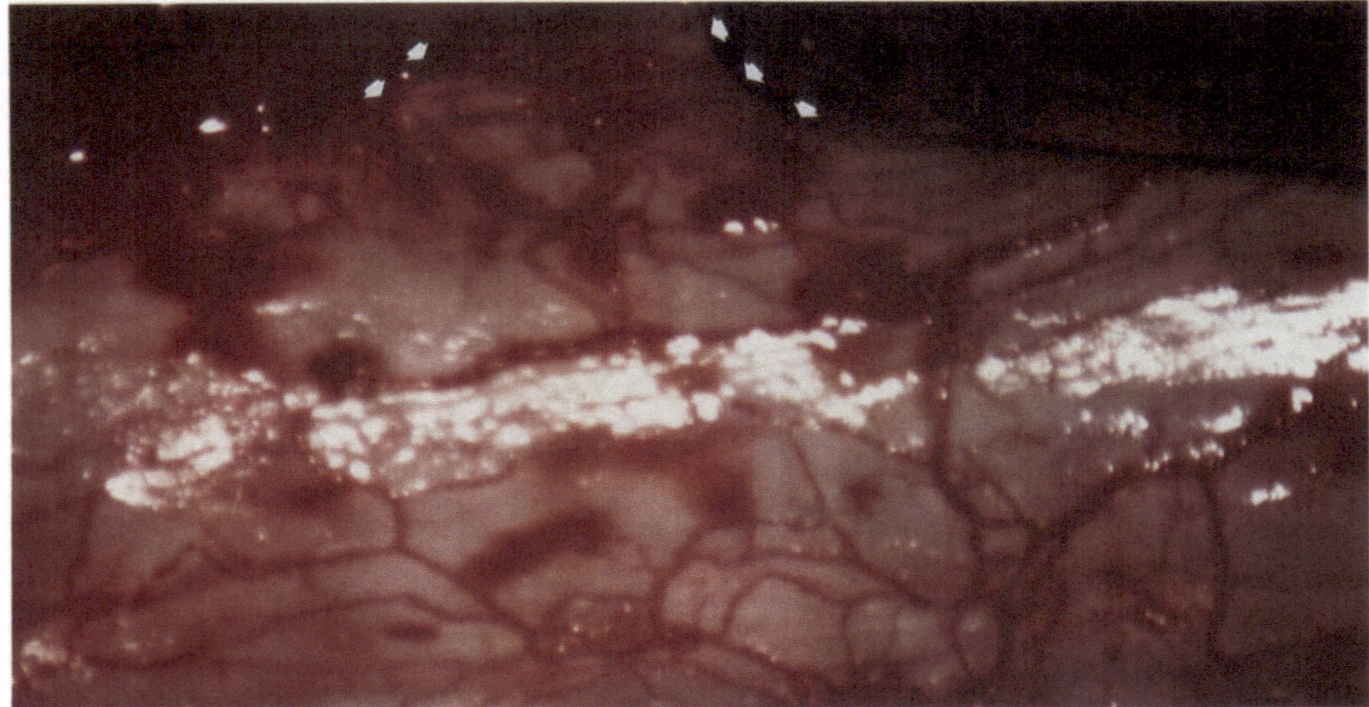

Fig. 281. Hypervascularization along the external layer of the dura at the malformed tract near the dural funnel on the left (*arrows*)

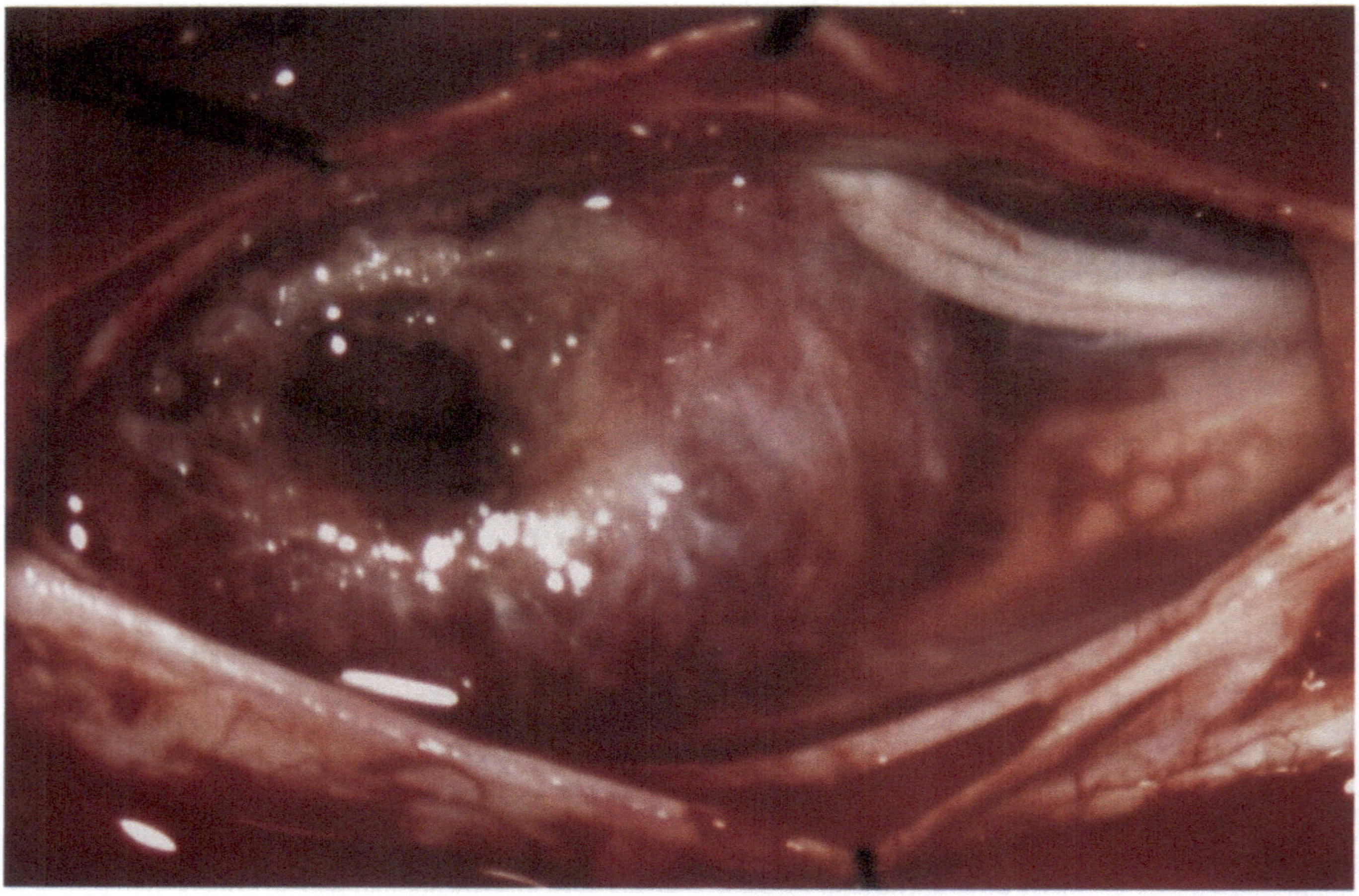

Fig. 282. The meningioma has already been partly debulked but is still surrounded by the arachnoid. The external dural layer has been anchored at the upper end allowing coagulation of the two dural membranes

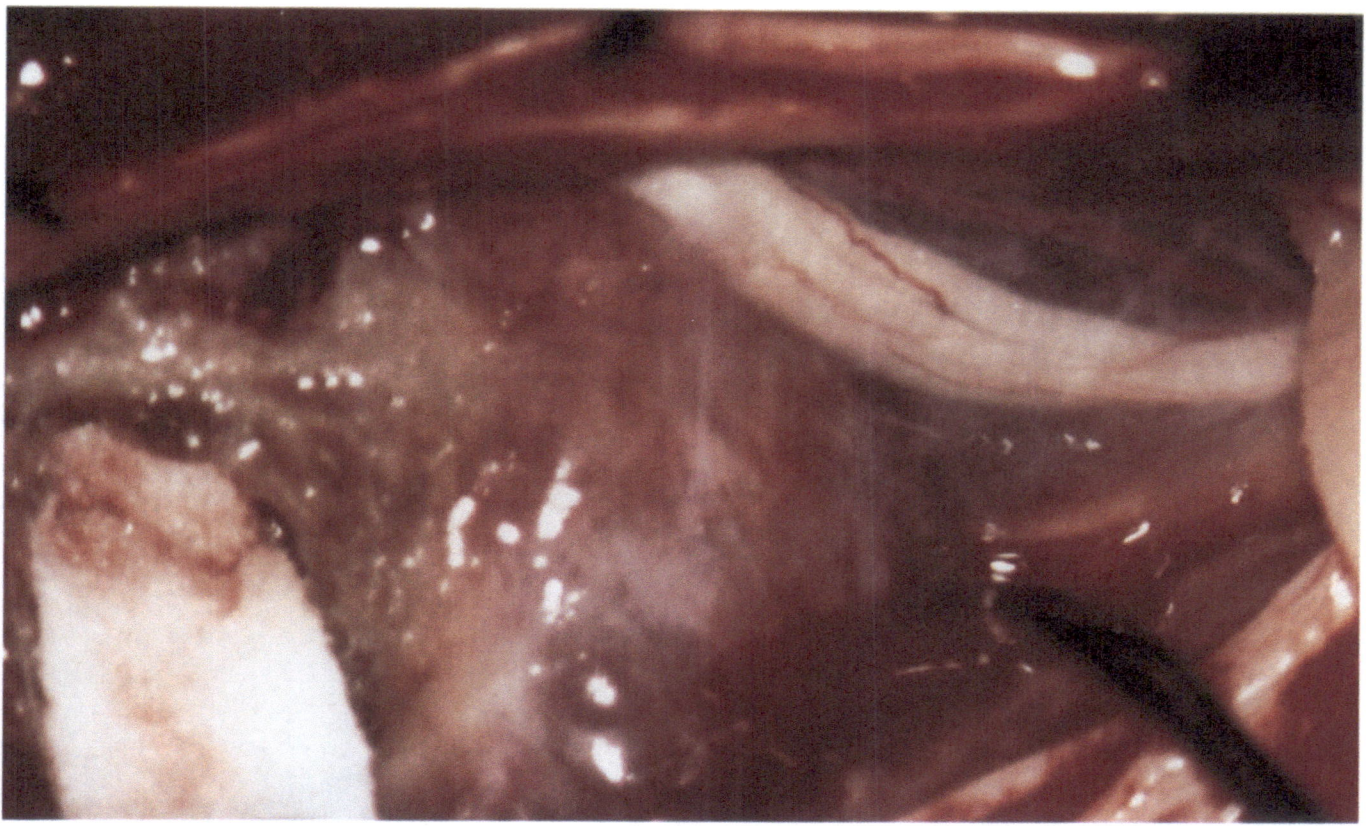

Fig. 283. The relationship between tumour, arachnoid and root is clearly seen. The root is at a distance from the surface layer of the cord which is displaced to the right

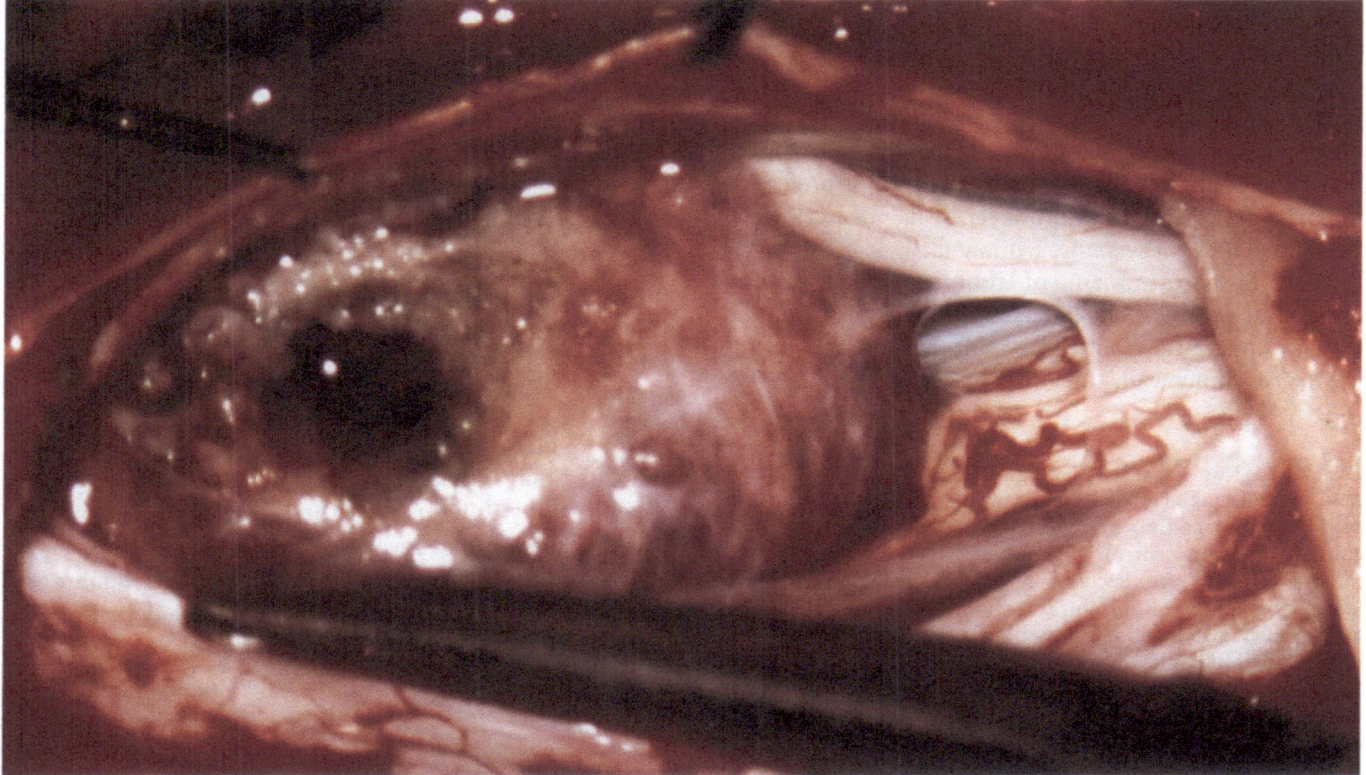

Fig. 284. The surgical phase of opening the arachnoid and removing it from the posterior surface of the tumour and from the left root of D9. The previous coagulation between the two dural layers has greatly reduced the haemorrhagic element during the operation

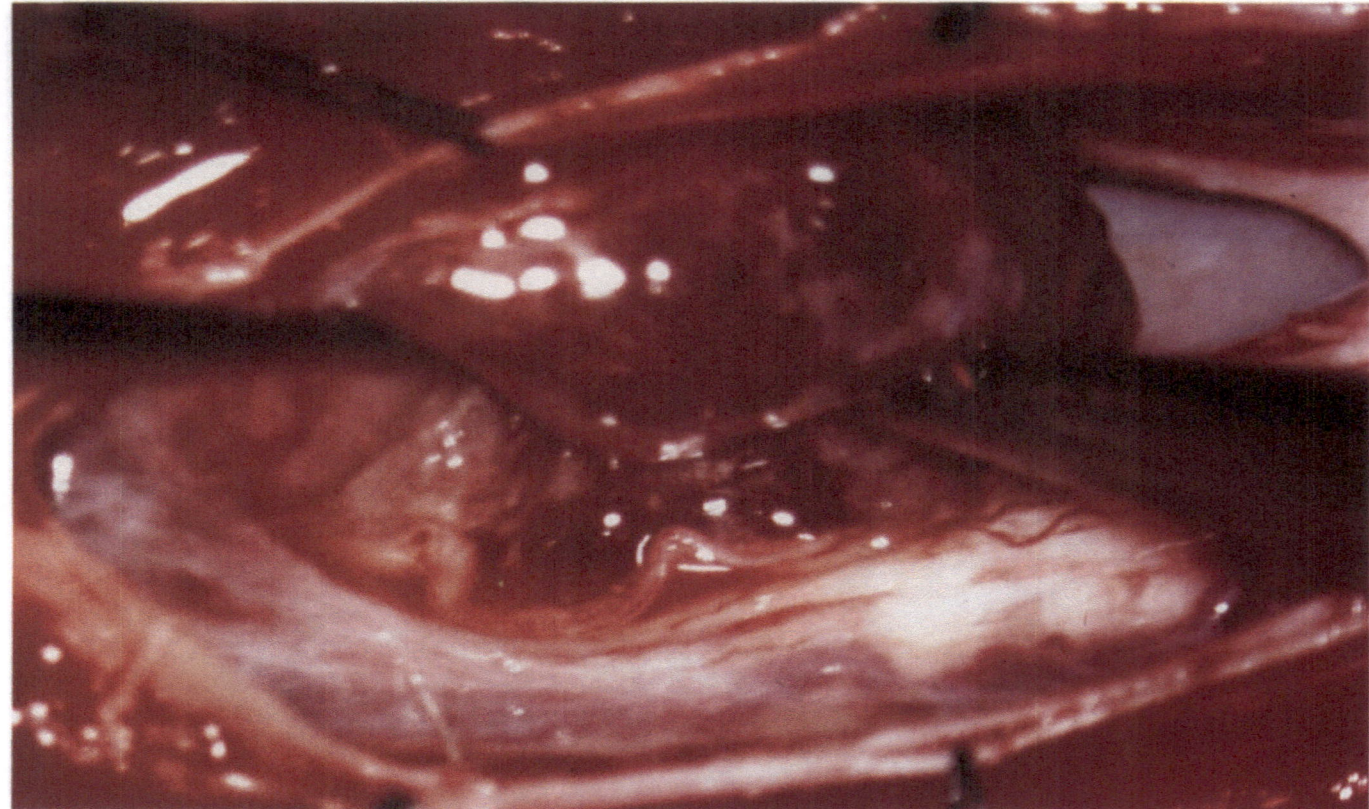

Fig. 285. Gradual lifting of the tumour against the internal left lateroventral dural plane

disease. Small meningiomas appear as simple swellings of the internal surface layer of the dura.

After removal of premedullary meningiomas it would be an error to suture the dura very tightly thereby forcing the medullary surface to tolerate a persistent state of compression. When medullary oedema occurs, it is preferable to cover the cord with a thin layer of haemostatic gelatine and make a loose suture without facing the meningeal borders. Some rare forms of tumours with intra- and extradural development can occur in these positions and they occupy a large tract of the epidural space and invade the nearest bony wall.

Case No. 66: Non-classified Meningioma

A 68-year-old man (1974). Right posterolateral intradural-extramedullary meningioma in L3-L4 (calcified at both ends with soft consistency in the centre).

Clinical Course. 30 years. Recurrent lumbosciatica attacks on the right leading to paralysis of the foot. Five months before hospitalization motor deficit also to left lower limb with deficitory deambulation to the right. Motor claudication on right.

Neurological Examination. (Previous diagnosis of neurofibromatosis together with scattered cutaneous stigmate such as pigmented stains of various sizes and birthmarks). Evident hypotrophy of anterior tibial, peroneal and lower third of the right thigh: areflexia of patella and ankle jerk. Hypoaesthesia in L2 that increased in dermatomes below. Anaesthesia on L5, S1. Urinary incontinence.

Rachicentesis. 2.18 g protein per thousand.

X-Ray of Lumbar Rachis. Erosion of posterior wall of vertebral bodies of L3 and L4 with erosion of the laminae, pedicles and articular facets. Densifying of the cortex (Fig. 294).

Myelography (performed suboccipitally). Block producing an irregular image in L2-L3.

Surgical Treatment. The laminae were of a compact consistency, appeared curved posteriorly and were hypervascularized. The dura had been invaded and on opening the dura the upper pole of the completely calcified tumour was observed. It adhered to the internal surface of the dura and enveloped more than one root, some of which were very thin, with others were displaced towards the left. Total excision and fragmentation of the calcified component.

Results. Walking was possible with support after 45 days but bilateral steppage persisted. Sphincter disturbances improved.

In these rare forms a laminectomy associated with an arthrectomy is performed along the eroded area to remove the bony remains near the intraforaminal canals. In meningiomas that invade almost exclusively the leptomeninges or those with intramedullary development the techniques are modified to suit each case depending on the extent of the myelotomy: separating the neoplastic tissue from the pia mater and the medullary columns and at the same time saving the surface-layer blood vessels as much as possible to avoid haemorrhaging. When the meningioma is intramedullary the myeloctomy is carried out in the area where the myelitic layer is less vascularized.

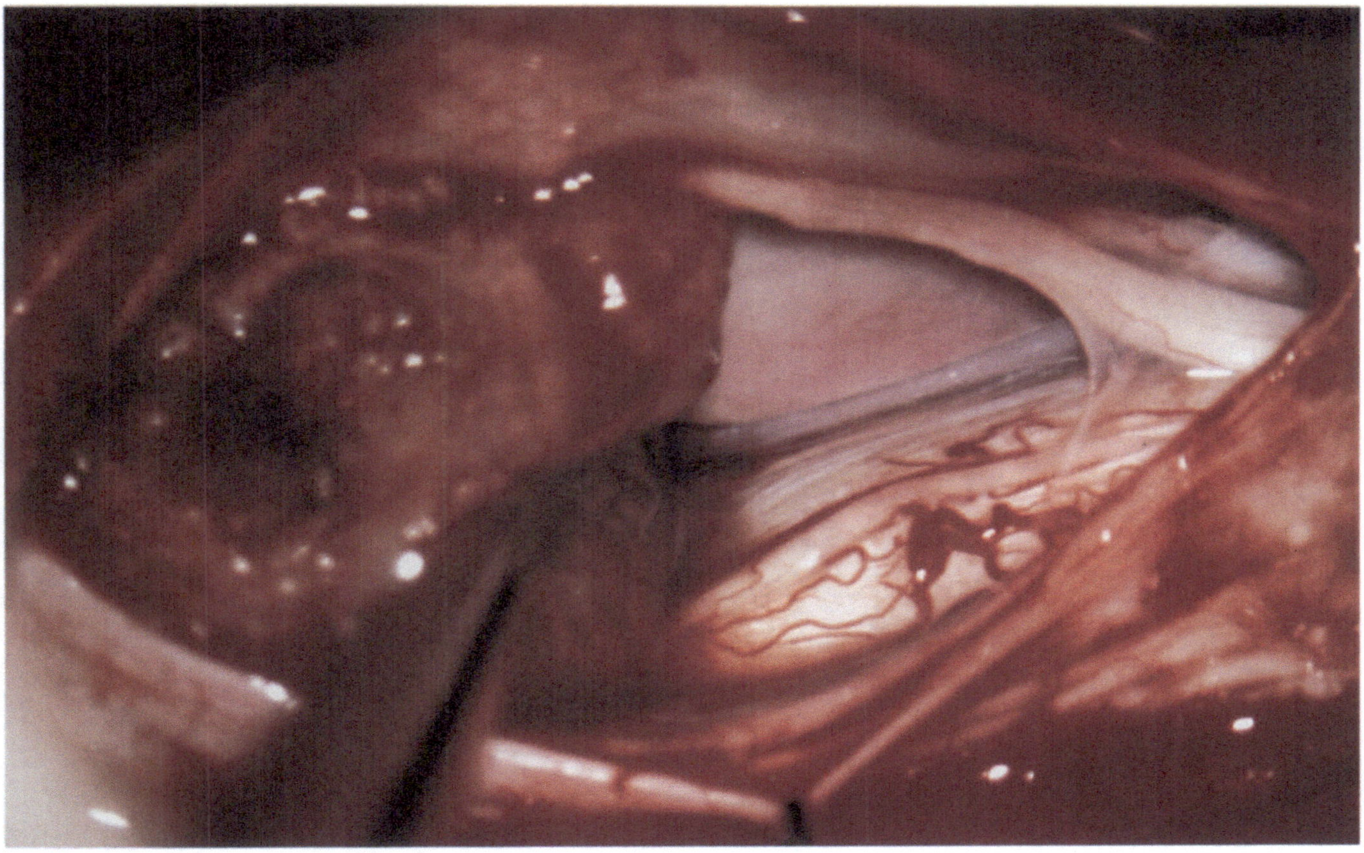

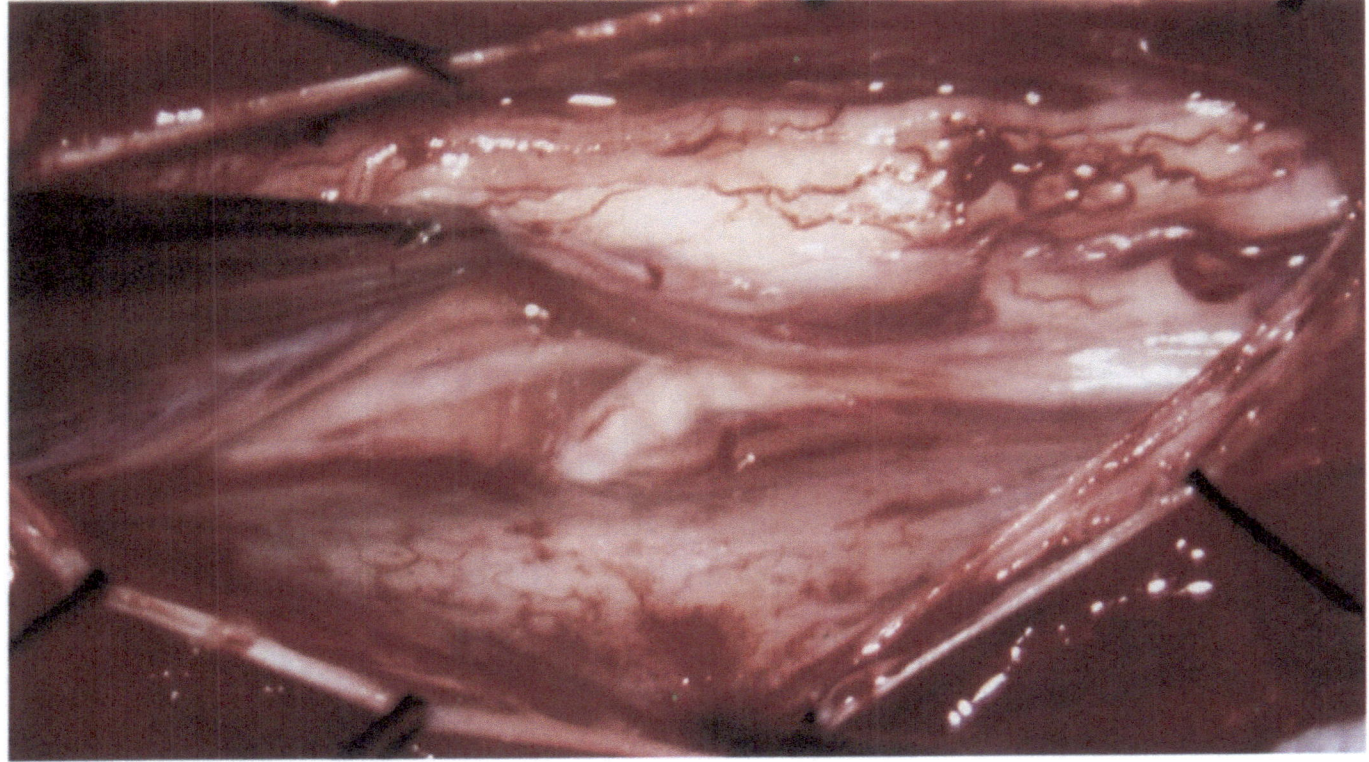

Fig. 286. The entire surface layer circulation has been spared. Immediately after excision the replenishment of the thin vessels near the myelitic ischaemic area can be seen in the operating microscope (see Fig. 287)

Fig. 287. Removal of the contralateral leptomeningeal adherent structures phase. The shadow left by the meningioma appears whitish in colour and ischaemic

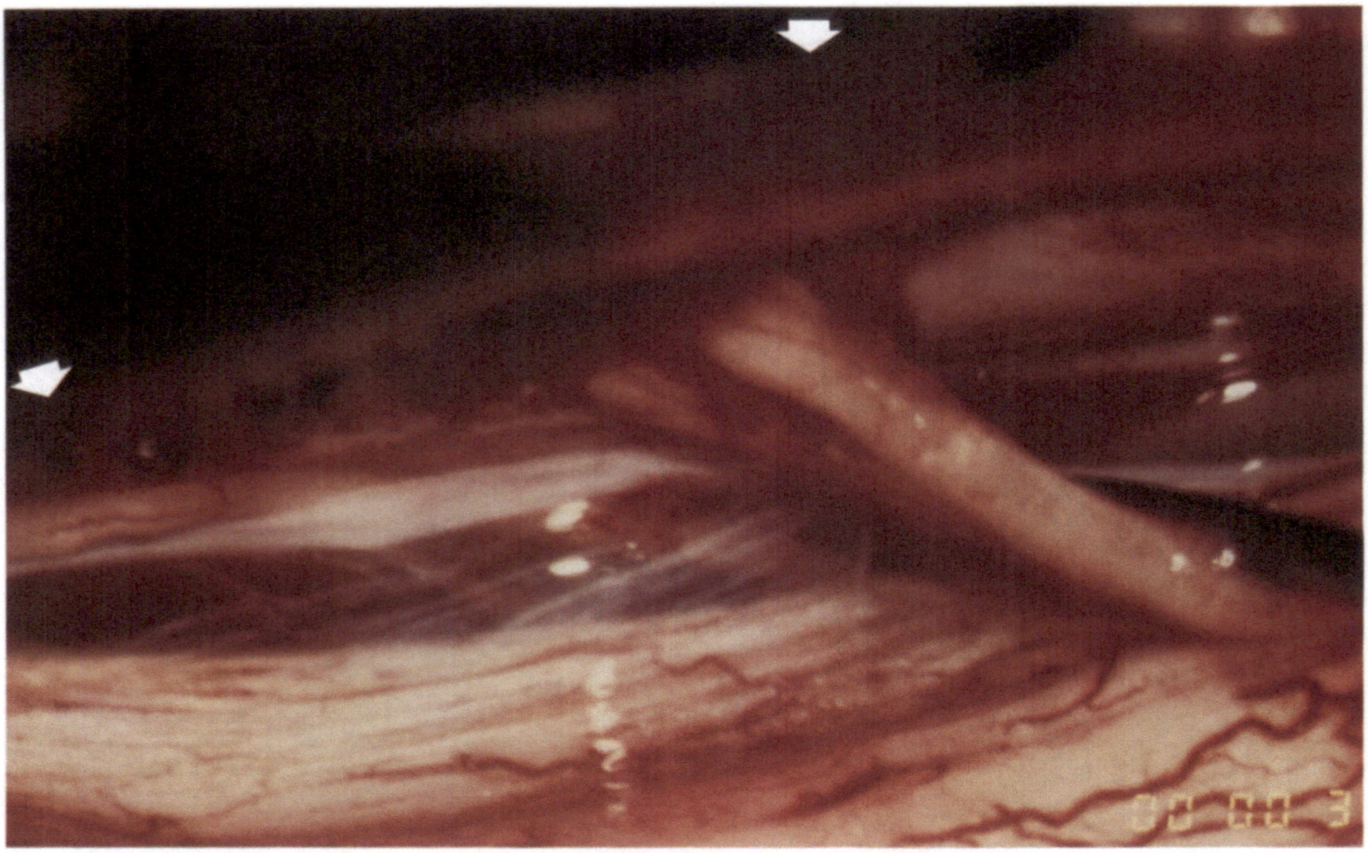

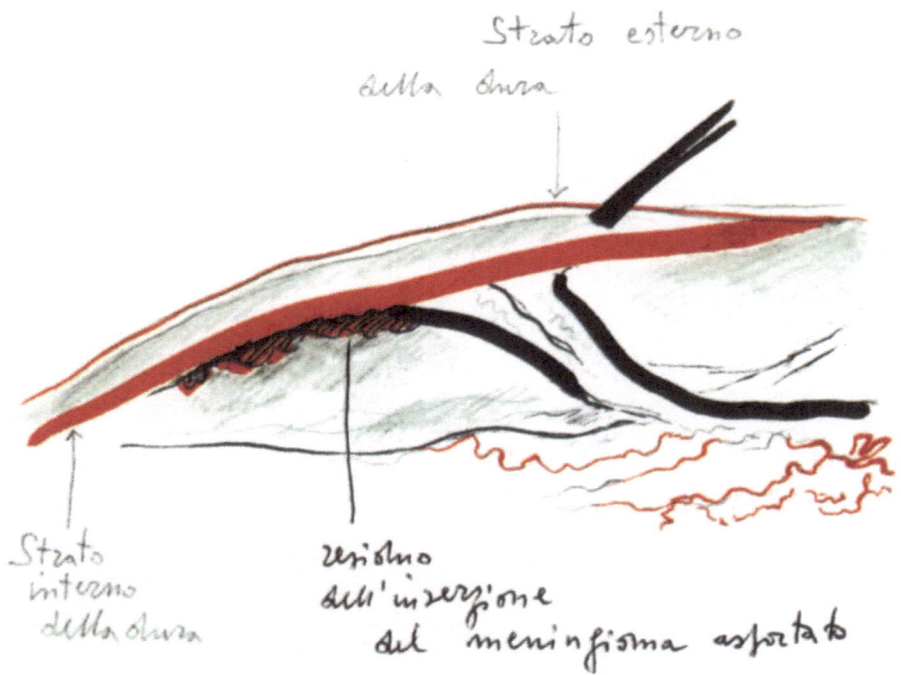

Fig. 288. *Above* (*arrow*), the external layer of the dura and the performed laminectomy. *Left* (*arrow*), the leptomeningeal plane of the dura. Ischaemic shadow on the left posterolateral surface of the cord. *Below*, the deep leptomeningeal plane of the dura; the residual attachment of the removed meningioma near the root's entry zone into the dural funnel (see Fig. 289)

Strato esterno
della dura

Strato
interno
della dura

residuo
dell'inserzione
del meningioma asportato

Fig. 289. Diagram of the splitting of the dura

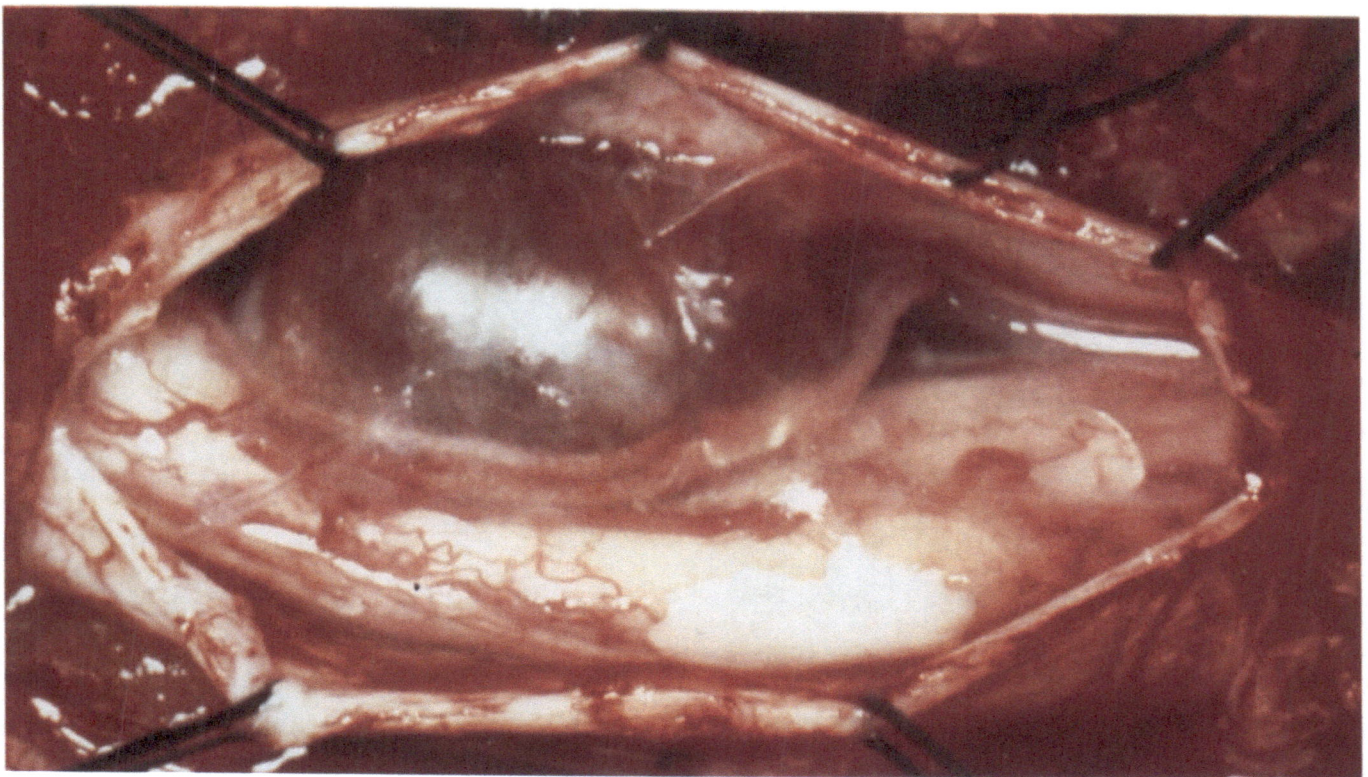

Fig. 290. The meningioma appeared to be enveloped by the arachnoid

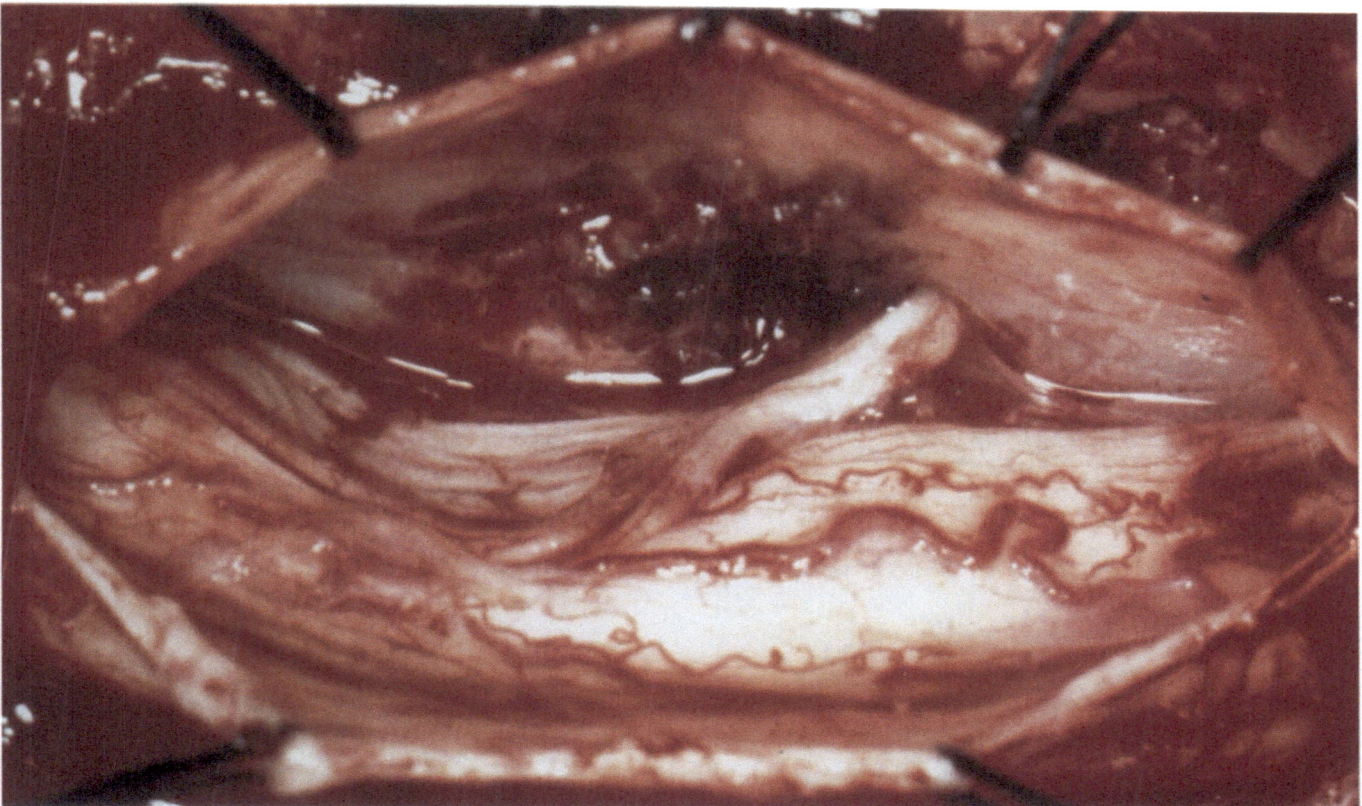

Fig. 291. The tumour is excised. The spinal cord is displaced controlaterally. It is possible to see the tumour inserction on internal surface of the dura

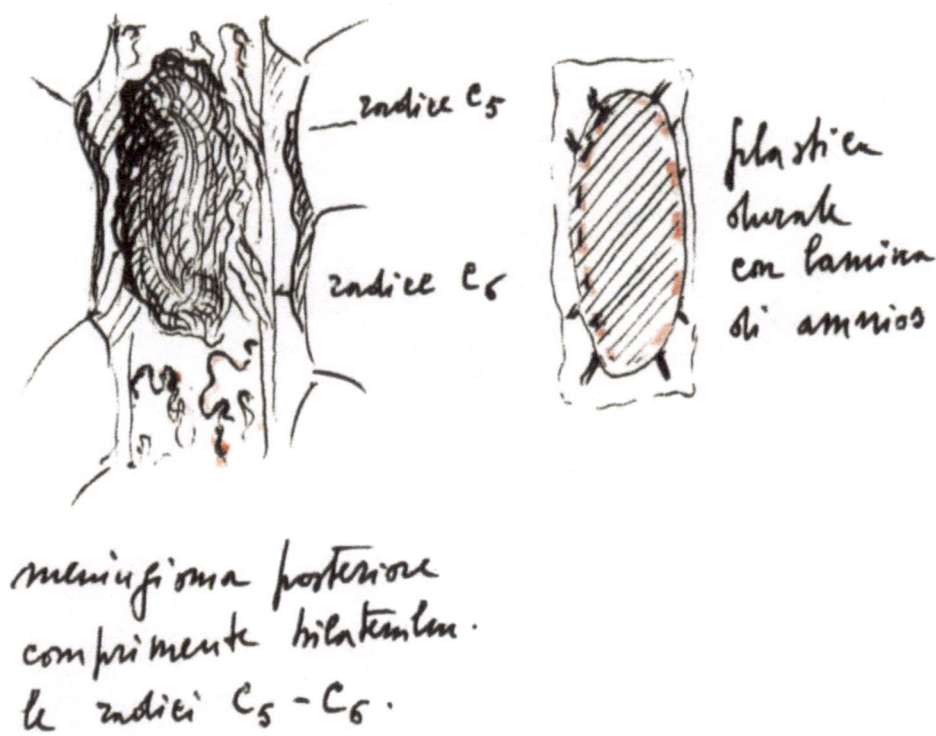

radice C_5

radice C_6

plastica
durale
con lamina
di amnios

meningioma posteriore
comprimente bilateralmente
le radici C_5 - C_6.

Fig. 292. Dural reconstruction with a lamina of amnios

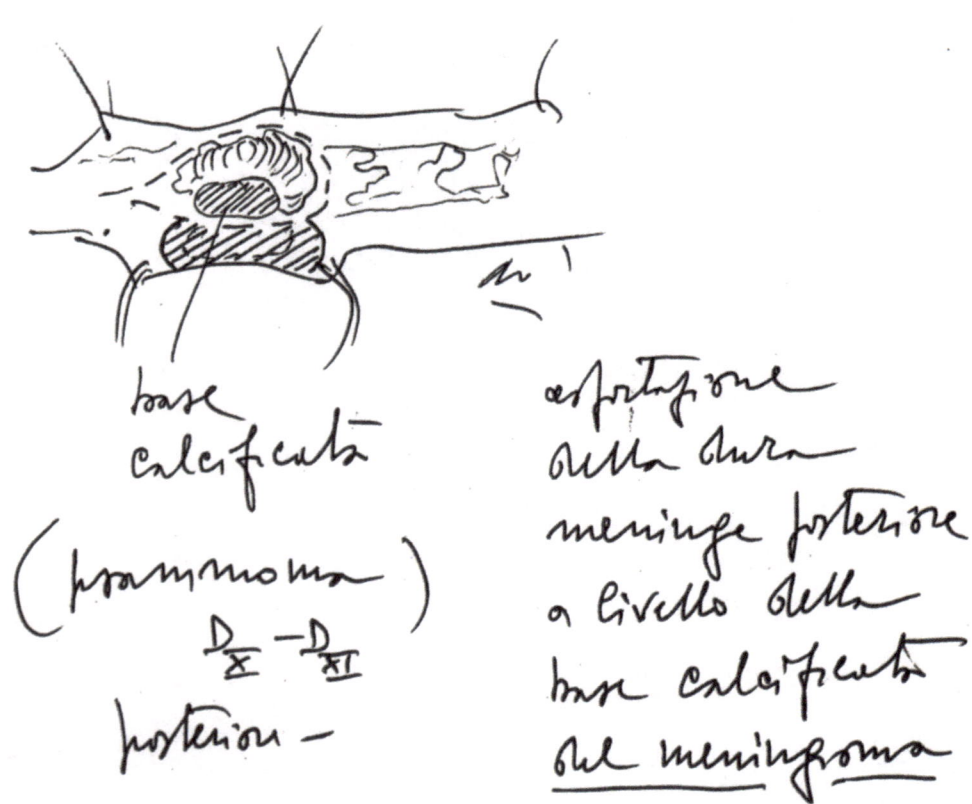

base
calcificata

(psammoma)

$\frac{D}{X}$ - $\frac{D}{XI}$

posterior -

asportazione
della dura
meninge posteriore
a livello della
base calcificata
del meningioma

Fig. 293. The calcified dura is excised at the level of inserction of the tumour

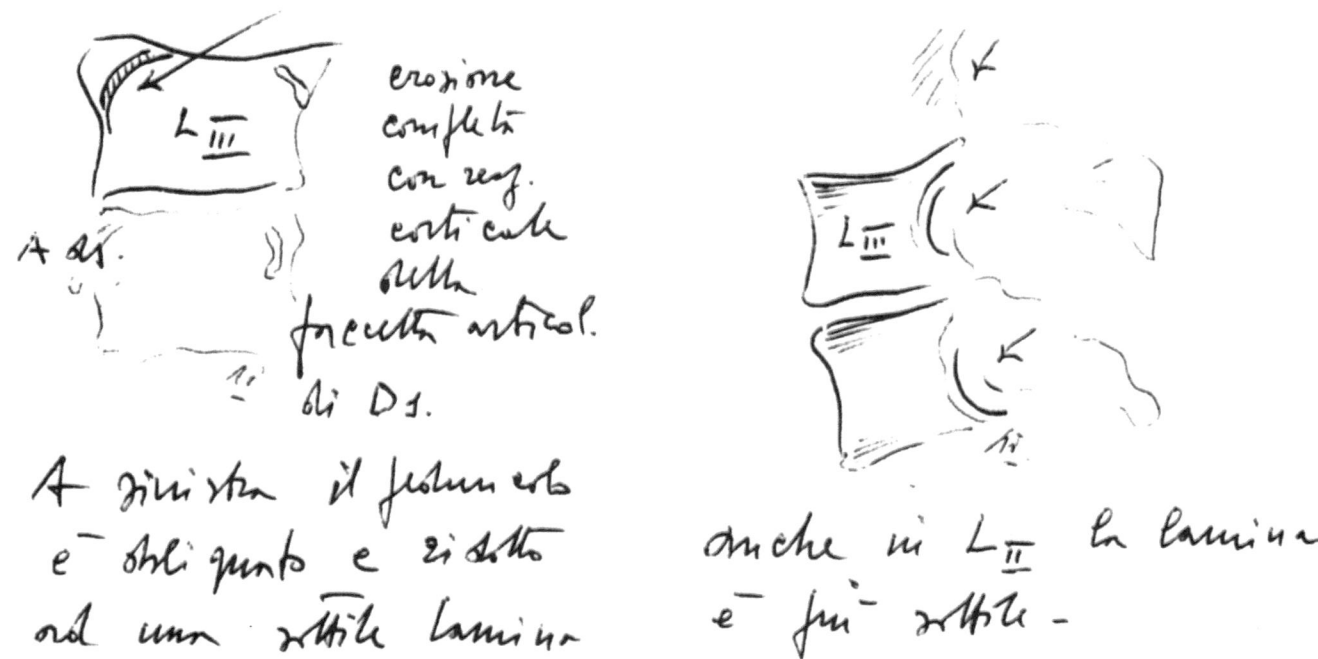

Fig. 294. Erosion of posterior wall of vertebral bodies of L3 and L4 with erosion of the laminae, pedicles and articular facets

9.10 Complications and Follow-Up

Nowadays surgical complications seldom arise in cases of spinal meningioma. Mortality is estimated at 1.30% (Pagni 1989; Malik 1991). While Learmonth (1927) and Cushing (1959) earlier found some 10%-12%, the mortality rate has recently been reported as 3 cases in 97 (3%) by Levy et al. (1982), 1 in 29 by Namer et al.(1987), 1 in 52 by Pagni (1989) and 2 in 174 (1.4%) by Solero et al. (1989). The causes of death are frequently reported in the literature as resulting from polmomary thromboembolus, cardiovascular respiratory insufficiency and bronchopneumonia. Less frequent causes include sceptic states, urinary infection and medullary vascular damage. Excep-

tionally rare cases of meningitis may also cause death. Guillame et al. (1957) reported a case where death on the operating table was due to vertebral breakage in a patient operated on for a relapse of an upper cervical meningioma. One of our patients died from a calcified intramedullary meningioma at the level of the bulbar-medullary junction after a clinical course lasting over 30 years and interpreted as disseminated sclerosis. Horwitz (1957) emphasised major surgical risks in meningioma cases located in the cervicobulbar passage.

We examined the postoperative course and types of complications responsible for the death of six patients in our series (two men and four women aged 63-76 years, mean 70.1). Five of these patients suffered from cardiac,

Table 17. Results of follow-up

	1 month		3 months		6 months		1 year		3 years		Longer	
	n	%	n	%	n	%	n	%	n	%	n	%
Recovered	25	21.6	12	10.3	8	6.9	2	1.7	2	1.7	1	0.9
Motory deficit improved	37	31.9	12	10.3	1	0.9	-	-	-	-	3	2.6
Sensory deficit improved	33	28.4	3	2.6	1	0.9	1	0.9	-	-	1	0.9
Unchanged	26	22.4	7	6.0	4	3.4	4	3.4	3	2.6	1	0.9
Deteriorated	18	15.5	2	1.7	1	0.9	-	-	-	-	2	1.7

Reccurence 2 (1.7%), deaths 7 (5.6%).

cerebrovascular and dysmetabolic pathologies, had been diabetic for a long period and were acutely decompensated during the postoperative phase.

The severity of the neurological picture, i.e. motor deficit, constitutes another risk factor (Pertuiset et al. 1960). In the preoperative phase four of our patients were paraplegic and incapable of standing upright or walking. Elderly patients with significant neurological disturbances show much slower recovery; the risk of bronchopulmonary complications is much higher than in those suffering from dorsal myelitic compression, which reduces thoracic mobility. However, three patients aged 81, 92 and 89 (meningiomas in D10, D11 and D12) had no postoperative bronchopulmonary complications, and therefore a rapid total recovery. This was also the case in an 80-year-old with a meningioma in the cervicodorsal passage. The oldest patient in our series, and in all the literature, suffered postoperative complications in the form of chronic subdural haematoma 1 month after surgery. She was operated on urgently and enjoyed total recovery of motility, which she still has today at the age of 95 years.

We analysed our results at follow-up periods of 1, 3 and 6 months and 1 and 3 years. To these we added a further group with a longer follow-up (3-13 years). The clinical course was considered in 116 of 125 patients (92.8%); in five (4%) there was insufficient information available for the 1-month follow-up and four (3.2%) were excluded because histological examinations showed malignant meningiomas. Of these, 109 remained under supervision at 1 month (94%), 50 at 3 months (43.1%), 30 at 6 months (29.9%), 10 at 1 year (8.6%) and 9 at 3 years (7.8%). Beyond this period there were 21 patients (18.1%): 3 at 4 years (2.6%), 6 at 5 years (5.2%), 2 at 6 years (1.7%), 1 at 7 years (0.9%), 3 at 8 years (2.6%), 3 at 9 years (2.6%) and one each at 10, 12 and 13 years (0.9%). The mean follow-up was 10.6 months. Seven patients died (5.6%): four due to cardiorespiratory insufficiency, one due to pulmonary embulus within 20 days of the operation, one due to diabetic hydroelectric decompensation and one due to bronchopneumonia. Of the 116 patients in the follow-up 50 were considered clinically cured (43.1%). Table 17 summarizes our results.

9.11 Conclusions

Increased vascularization in meningiomas is not restricted to tumoural tissues but affects the entire region where the tumour develops. The relationship between this hypervascularization and the arterial blood supply differs from that at the tumour site. This is also the case with the nerve structures as the cord is displaced contralaterally at the site of the meningioma and the motor nerve remains between the dural plane and the ventral part of the tumour. The posterior root often appears curved and stretched over the densest peripheral part of the meningioma in laterally located cases. In cervical positions where the roots are close together this radicular stetching can take place over several metameres. When the development of a meningioma corresponds to a great vertical or transversal extension some roots undergo some form of atrophy. Sometimes a root can be enveloped in the meningioma's major swelling. Although the pathological vertebromedullary vascularization in some meningiomas is not substantially changed, some haemorrhagic forms occur due to alterations in the dura and cord vascularization. As Al Mefty (1991) noted, "spinal meningiomas are noted for their vascularity".

Direct compression of the meningioma on the cord also produces ischaemia-related phenomena. This occurs slowly and gradually during the often chronic development of the tumour and alters the epidural venous vascularization at this level. In premedullary locations the compression affects the anterior spinal artery blood supply and on opening the dura one sees the narrowing of the arterial network of the posterior columns. Defined ischaemias, either more or less pronounced, depend on the level of the lesion and on the length and nature of minor or major consistency of the tumour. When the cord is displaced behind the medullary columns the posterolateral surface of the cord tolerates the resistance of the vertebral arches. Among the factors which intervene in the pathogenesis of myeloradicular, vascular modifications are the reactive, leptomeningeal adherent processes. These stabilize particularly at the upper and lower pole of the meningioma and contribute to the cause of compression on the subarachnoidal vessels on the side opposite to the compression. In meningiomas with extra-arachnoidal development the medullary vascularization is protected by the leptomeninges and during the gradual removal of the meningioma there may be a partial repletion by the small arteries which have not been completely compressed by the neoplastic tissue and continue up to the cord leaving an ischaemic shell-shaped shadow.

In evaluating myelitic damage we have considered the possibility of a demyelinization process. It is difficult to explain the rapid recovery of the neural structures once the mechanical cause has been eliminated. According to Al-Mefty (1991) it is difficult to attribute functional recovery to remyelinization. We are convinced, however, of the vascular origin of myelitic damage and find that after excision it is necessary to eliminate every single leptomeningeal adherent structure, not only on the side of the meningioma, but also on the opposite, perimedullary side where the myelitic surface lies close to the internal dural layer, and where the plial vessels have undergone vascular disturbance.

Every regional ischaemic form, to a greater or lesser degree, can be associated with an arterial vasodilatation picture above the compression. These conditions, already reported in other compressions at the same level, are confirmed by MRI. They present an irregular vascularization formed by dilatated ansas along the medullary tract above the meningioma site. The dilatation of this arterial vascularization increases the volume of the cord due to a concomitant pathological situation of diffused oedema to various myelomeres. The variations in myelitic vascularization as a consequence of the compression correspond to the tract where the cord has greater vascularization and in upper cervical sites and in the dorsolumbar passage. In the medial dorsal tract (D4-D8) the vasodilatation alterations above and below the meningioma are less than those identified by Lazorthes (1958) and Zulch (1962) in their research on medullary vascularization. In the lumbar tract major vascularization derives from Adamkievich's and Desproge-Gotteron arteries and do not produce important vascular alterations in the meningioma. These maintain an exclusively arachnoidal origin and diffuse with the following histopathological characteristics: (a) exclusively subdural, extramedullary, intra- and extra-arachnoidal meningioma, (b) intradural meningioma but with an extradural and sometimes intraosseus component, (c) meningioma without invasion of the dura, purely leptomeningeal, subarachnoidal with exclusively pia mater coinvolvement, and (d) intramedullary meningiomas.

Neuroradiological diagnosis by CT, myelo-CT and MRI allow us to plan surgical procedures before surgery with the help of the images produced by the scanners. Since the advent of CT and MRI the use of myelography and myelo-CT with hydrosoluble contrast medium remains extremely important because these techniques show the very variable features of the subarachnoidal space which during excision of the meningioma represents the most delicate structure in performing the global removal of the tumour.

Every operation can be helped by minimizing the traumatic manoeuvres of reclining the cord during excision to avoid blood flowing into the subarachnoidal space. The various techniques which we have introduced have greatly reduced bleeding; these include coagulation of the arterial blood flow deep along the entire area of the invasion of the meningioma. These techniques for removing premedullary meningiomas are partial and are performed along the lateral side only of the meningeal sac using a variety of incisions.

Diagnostic examinations used in previous surgical procedures allow us to approach and resolve the haemodynamic variations of the surface layer which have repercussions on the white and grey matter of the cord.

We cannot explain the regression of motor and sensory deficiency signs without referene to vascular variations, even in the meningioma cases with global calcification and which occupy the rachidian canal almost entirely.

Although posterior and lateral approaches are always used in surgery, on the basis of the technical principles described above we could not exclude the practice of locating medullary sites by using an anterior somatological approach.

10 Other Anatomical-Clinical Observations

Case No. 7: Psammomatous Meningioma
A 67-year-old woman (1962). Posterior intradural-extramedullary meningioma in D2-D3.
Medical History. Diabetes.
Clinical Course. 2 years. Paraesthesias to lower limbs, spreading upwards to the left. After 1 year motor deficit to lower limbs to the left. Two months prior to hospitalization the patient developed monoplegia on the left and severe motor deficit to right lower limb.
Neurological Examination. Spastic paraplegia. Hypoaesthesia from D3-D4 which increased distally. Sphincter disturbances in the form of incontinence.
Rachicentesis. 0.70 g per thousand.
X-Ray of Dorsal Tract. Severe kyphoscoliosis.
Myelography (performed suboccipitally). Total block in D2-D3 producing an irregular-shaped filling defect anteroposteriorly.
Surgical Treatment. Posterior neoplasm the size of a large almond covered by a calcified lamina and adhering to the internal surface layer of the dura. Arachnoidal adherent structures in the vicinity of the upper pole of the neoplasm.
Results. Postoperative motor inhibition to upper limbs followed by a gradual improvement which led to a complete recovery within 6 months.

Case No. 10: Transitional Meningioma
A 58-year-old man (1963). Posterior intradural-extramedullary meningioma in D6-D7.
Clinical Course. 6 months. Motor deficit to lower limbs to the right.
Neurological Examination. Spastic paraparesis to the right. Bilateral Babinski sign. Hypoaesthesia from D7-D8.
Rachicentesis. 2.20 g protein per thousand.
Surgical Treatment (under a local anaesthetic). The dural surface appeared very taut, haemorrhagic and hard to the touch. On opening the dura a calcified neoplasm was seen adhering very close to the posterior columns of the spine. The arterial blood supply above and below the tumour appeared dilatated. Excision en bloc after removing the adherent structures between the tumour and the posterior surface layer of the cord. The tumour was removed together with its dural insertion. Dural plastic.
Results. Initial motor inhibition to lower limbs with gradual recovery over 1 year. Total recovery verified after 6 years.

Case No. 4: Psammomatous Meningioma
A 51-year-old woman (1963). Intradural-extramedullary, premedullary meningioma in C7.
Clinical Course. 12 years. Surgery performed 12 years previously for removal of a meningioma in the same site, with regression of the clinical syndrome. For 6 years the patient complained of sensory impairment of the hemithorax and right lower limb. Two years prior to hospitalization this disturbance affected the left with a loss of strength in the legs.
Neurological Examination. Spastic paraparesis. Bilateral Babinski sign. Touch and painful hypoaesthesia at D6 level to the right hemithorax.
Rachicentesis. 0.35 g protein per thousand.
Myelography (performed suboccipitally). Transitional block in C6-C7, corresponding to upper border of previous laminectomy (C7-D1-D2). Contrast medium produced an irregular image.
Surgical Treatment. On opening the dura the adherent arachnoidal structures were seen. The seventh left cervical root was curved backwards. The flattened cord was pushed forwards and towards the right. After removing the arachnoidal adherent structure a tumour was seen the size of a large walnut and of hard consistency. Reclining the sensory root of C7 provided access to the capsule of the tumour and the tumour was debulked. The attachment of the tumour was at the radicular funnel in C7. Total excision.
Results. Initial motor inhibition followed by a gradual improvement leading to complete recovery in 6 months. Slight hypoaesthesia to right hemitrunk persisting even after 7 years.

Case No. 14: Fibroblastic Meningioma
A 64-year-old woman (1963). Intradural-extramedullary, premedullary meningioma in D9.
Clinical Course. 7 years. Motor deficit at lower limbs leading to paraplegia in the course of 1 year.
Neurological Examination. Spastic paraplegia. Foot and patella clonus. Bilateral Babinski sign. Hypoaesthesia affecting various forms of sensitivity from D9, increased distally. Sphincter disturbances in the form of incontinence.
Rachicentesis. 0.40 g protein per thousand.
Myelography via Lumbar Puncture (Lipiodol). Total block producing a dome-shaped feature in D9.
Surgical Treatment. The dura appeared taut and hard to the touch. On opening the dura the cord appeared whitish in colour, ischaemic and curved backwards. By slightly reclining the cord to the left a premedullary neoplasm could be seen the size of a small walnut, which invaded the anterior surface of the dura. Removal of the arachnoidal adherent structures above and below the tumour and excision en bloc. Coagulation of the base of attachment.
Results. Paraplegia persisting even after 2 years.

193

Case No. 1: Transitional Meningioma

A 62-year-old woman (1964). Right anterolateral intradural-extramedullary meningioma in C3-C4.

Clinical Course. 1 year. Tingling type of paraesthesias and slight loss of strength to the right hand and lower limb.

Neurological Examination. Right hemiparesis with Brown-Sequard syndrome at lower cervical level. Right Bernard-Horner syndrome.

Rachicentesis. 0.37 g protein per thousand.

X-Ray of Cervical Rachis. Anteroposterior image showed thinned articular features on the right of C6.

Myelography (performed suboccipitally). A lateral block in C3-C4 producing a cuneiform filling defect. Anteroposterior image showed slight flow on the right which formed a small roundish filling defect.

Surgical Treatment. By slightly reclining the sensory root of D3 a neoplasm of premedullary development was seen laterally and on the right, invading the anterior surface of the dura. Incision of the capsule and fragmented excision performed.

Results. Rapid regression of the neurological syndrome. Total recovery (at 5-year check).

Case No. 8: Transitional Meningioma

A 57-year-old woman (1964). Posterior intradural-extramedullary meningioma in D5-D6 (see. Chap. 9).

Case No. 2: Transitional Meningioma

A 48-year-old woman (1965). Posterior intradural-extramedullary meningioma in C4- C5 (see Chap. 9).

Case No. 16: Nonclassified Meningioma

A 60-year-old woman (1966). Lateroventral intradural-extramedullary meningioma in D12-L1 (see Chap. 9).

Case No. 15: Transitional Meningioma

A 60-year-old woman (1966). Left intradural-extramedullary meningioma in D11-D12.

Clinical Course. 5 years. Back pain with painful paraesthesias to lower limbs. Left painful paroxysms on L1 exacerbated by coughing and straining. Motor deficit to lower limbs for 2 years.

Neurological Examination. Spastic paraparesis with bilateral Babinski sign. Left hyperaesthesias on L1.

Rachicentesis. 0.53 g protein per thousand.

X-Ray of Dorsolumbar Tract. Laterally pronounced physiological lordosis. Anteroposteriorly right convex scoliosis at dorsolumbar passage.

Myelography (performed suboccipitally). Anteroposteriorly linear block, denser on the right in D11-D12. Laterally a dome-shaped filling defect.

Surgical Treatment. Subarachnoidal meningioma invading on left near the radicular funnel of D12. Excision by radicotomy of sensory component.

Results. Total recovery.

Case No. 22: Sarcomatous Meningioma

A 47-year-old man (1966). Left lateral intra- and extramedullary meningioma surrounding the root of L2 at the intravertebral foramen level.

Clinical Course. 6 months. Left lumbocruralgia and numbness of the skin type of paraesthesias on the same territory.

Neurological Examination. Evident signs of rigidity of the spine with antalgic attitude. Hypotrophy of left femoral quadricep. Loss of left patella reflex. Left hypoaesthesia on L1 and L2.

Rachicentesis. 4.90 g protein per thousand.

Myelography (performed suboccipitally). Total block in L1. The image produced was typical of an epidural lesion.

Surgical Treatment. Left epidural neoplasm at the intravertebral foramen of L1-L2. The tumour was of a lardaceous consistency and closely adherent to the dura, pushing the dural sac from left to right. Tumoural structure in the intravertebral foramen. On opening the dura the tumoral proliferation was seen to involve the internal surface of the dura. Excision together with the tumourous attachment. Dural plastic with amnion lamina.

Results. Regression of symptoms. After 1 month motor impairment syndrome to left lower limb leading to monoplegia with sphincter disturbances in the form of retention. The patient was reoperated on for a relapse on D12. The tumour had invaded the roots of the cauda.

Case No. 23: Sarcomatous Meningioma

A 45-year-old man (1966). Left lateral extradural meningioma in L5-S1-S2.

Clinical Course. 5 months. Relapsing lumbago irradiating with pain to posterior side of the legs to the left. Motor deficit to lower limbs for 1 week.

Neurological Examination. Evident rigidity of lumbar tract. Diminished ankle jerk. Sphincter disturbances in the form of incontinence.

Rachicentesis. 1.60 g protein per thousand.

Myelography (performed suboccipitally). Total block in L5-S1.

Surgical Treatment. Excision of a tumour of lardaceous consistency resembling a flow and adhering to the external surface of the dura surrounding the left roots of L5-S1-S2.

Results. During 1 month recovery of motor deficit to lower limbs. Three months later acute paraplegia. Second operation to locate malignant meningioma in D7-D8. After an initial recovery of the neurological picture and an improvement in walking the patient was again affected by paraplegia which lead to a third operation locating a malignant meningioma in D5-D6. Death occurred 3 months later.

Case No. 9: Psammomatous Meningioma

A 29-year-old woman (1968). Right posterolateral intradural-extramedullary meningioma in D5-D6.

Medical History. Luetic infection.

Clinical Course. 5 months. Loss of stength in lower limbs initially on the left then spreading to both sides, with paraesthesias for the previous month.

Neurological Examination. Spastic paraplegia. Patella and foot clonus. Bilateral Babinski sign. Hypoaesthesia in D6 with anaesthesia below.

Rachicentesis. 1.50 g protein per thousand.

Myelography (performed suboccipitally). Total block in D5-D6 producing an irregular half-moon shaped filling defect on the right.

Surgical Treatment. Subarachnoidal neoplasm the size of an almond posterolaterally on the right which displaced the spine contralaterally. Opening the arachnoidal layer and excision of tumour invading the internal surface of the dura near the intravertebral foramen. Once the neoplasm was removed a shell-shaped shadow created by the meningioma was visible posterolaterally to the cord on the right.

Results. Over 1 month the patient gradually recovered voluntary movements and 6 months later started walking. Total recovery after 1 year.

Case No. 6: Nonclassified Meningioma

A 51-year-old woman (1968). Posterior, intradural-extramedullary meningioma in D1-D2.

Clinical Course. 3 months. Cervical pain irradiating to right shoul-

der with paraesthesias to lower right limb and motor claudication.
Neurological Examination. Spastic paraparesis to the left. Bilateral Babinski sign. Brown-Sequard syndrome with partial loss of sensitivity from D1-D5.
Myelography (performed suboccipitally). Transitional block producing a dome-shaped filling defect in D1. Slight bilateral flow.
Surgical Treatment. Neoplasm invaded internal posterior surface of the dura. Total excision together with removal of dural attachment. Dural plastic with amnion lamina.
Results. Regression of paresis in 10 days. Clinical recovery after 1 year.

Case No. 11: Transitional Meningioma

A 60-year-old woman (1968). Right posterolateral intradural-extramedullary meningioma in D6-D7.
Medical History. Diabetes mellitus. Intoxication from mercury.
Clinical Course. 10 years. Pain at dorsolumbar tract, fatigue with walking. For 2 years she complained of painful paraesthesias to lower limbs and gradual motor impairment.
Neurological Examination. Spastic paraplegia. Patella and foot clonus. Bilateral Babinski sign. Anaesthesia from D7. Sphincter disturbances in the form of incontinence.
Rachicentesis. 3.05 g protein per thousand.
X-Ray of Dorsal Rachis. Widespread osteoporosis and signs of spondyloarthrosis.
Myelography (performed suboccipitally). Irregular block in D6-D7 with lateral flow on the left which produced a roundish-shaped filling defect.
Surgical Treatment. On opening the dura a neoplasm was seen invading the internal surface of the dura posteriorly on the right. Excision en bloc.
Results. Recovery of motility after 1 month. The patient was capable of walking after 6 months. Clinical recovery 1 year later.

Case No. 12 Fibroblastic Meningioma

A 69-year-old man (1968). Right posterolateral intradural meningioma in D6-D7.
Clinical Course. 1 year. Tingling sensation to right foot. One month later progressive loss of strength in right lower limb followed by paraesthesia to left foot.
Neurological Examination. Spastic paraparesis to the right. Bilateral Babinski sign. Tactile hypoaesthesia from D11, increased distally. Sphincter disturbances in the form of retention.
Rachicentesis. 1.20 g protein per thousand.
Myelography (performed suboccipitally). Total block in D6 with slight flow on both sides.
Surgical Treatment. Posterior neoplasm adhering to medullary surface. Excision together with the dural attachment. The arterial blood supply above and below the compression in stasis. Dural plastic with amnion lamina.
Results. Recovery of movements from the first day. Death occurred on the fourth day from a pulmonary embolus.

Case No. 13 Fibroblastic Meningioma

A 72-year-old woman (1968). Left posterolateral intradural-extramedullary meningioma in D7 adhering to the seventh dorsal root.
Clinical Course. 10 years. Painful paraesthesias to right lower limb. 1 year later, back pain with paraesthesias to the inguinal area. Motor impairment of lower limbs with difficulty in walking. In the previous 9 months this had grown progressively worse leading to paraplegia.
Neurological Examination. Spastic paraplegia with spinal automism. Bilateral Babinski sign. Anaesthesia level from D9. Sphincter disturbances in the form of incontinence.
Rachicentesis. 2.59 g protein per thousand.
Myelography (performed suboccipitally). Total block producing clear borders in D6-D9.

Surgical Treatment. Incision of dura at the sides of the dural attachment of the meningioma. Removal en bloc after removing the arachnoidal adherent structures between the meningioma and the medullary surface. Dural plastic with amnion lamina.
Results. Initial recovery including voluntary movements after 2 months but with persistence of hypotonia to both lower limbs.

Case No. 17: Transitional Meningioma

A 65-year-old woman (1969). Posterior, intradural-extramedullary meningioma in D6-D7.
Clinical Course. 5 years. Persisting back pain followed by gradual motor impairment to lower limbs.
Neurological Examination. Severe paraparesis to the left. Tactile hypoaethesia both superficial and painful in D7-D8 on the right, slightly lower on the left. Sphincter disturbances in the form of retention.
Rachicentesis. 0.98 g protein per thousand.
X-Ray of Dorsolumbar Tract. Severe kyphosis resulting from a previous fracture causing the compression of D12-L1. Spondylolisthesis L5-S1.
Myelography (performed suboccipitally). Total block in D6-D7 producing a slightly dome-shaped aspect.
Surgical Treatment. On opening the dura a posterior neoplasm was seen invading the internal surface of the dura. Excision together with the dural attachment. The spine appeared severely affected by atrophy. Dural plastic with amnion lamina.
Results. Signs of recovery of voluntary movements to lower limbs after only 2 days. One month later walking was possible with some difficulty. Recovery 3 months later.

Case No. 5: Meningothelial Meningioma

A 59-year-old woman (1969). Right ventrolateral intradural-extramedullary meningioma in C7-D1.
Clinical Course. 1 year. Motor impairment to lower limbs with distal paraesthesias to lower limbs to the right. Twenty days prior to hospitalization there was a rapid deterioration leading to paraplegia.
Neurological Examination. Spastic paraplegia. Hypoaesthesia in D1-D2 with anaesthesia from D6-D7. Sphincter disturbances in the form of incontinence.
Rachicentesis. 0.43 g protein per thousand.
Myelography (performed suboccipitally). Total block in C7-D1. The contrast medium flowed in a curve on the left side producing a blackberry-shaped image.
Surgical Treatment. The cord appeared reduced in volume and was severely flattened towards the left. Below the compression the cord's superficial blood flow appeared dilatated. Removal of one arachnoidal adherent structure from the tumour and total excision of the meningioma, which invaded the anterolateral surface of the dura.
Results. Slow recovery of voluntary movements to the left. Two months later walking was attempted. Total recovery (checked after 1 year).

Case No. 18: Transitional Meningioma

A 57-year-old woman (1969; Fig. 295). Right posterolateral intradural-extramedullary meningioma in D9-D10.
Clinical Course. 3 years. Back pain with sciatica irradiating towards the right. Three months prior to hospitalization the same symptoms appeared on the left leading to difficulty in walking.
Neurological Examination. Spastic paraparesis to the left. Hypoaesthesia from L1 affecting the various forms of sensitivity becoming gradually anaesthesia distally. Sphincter disturbances in the form of incontinence.
Myelography (performed suboccipitally). Block in D9-D10 produc-

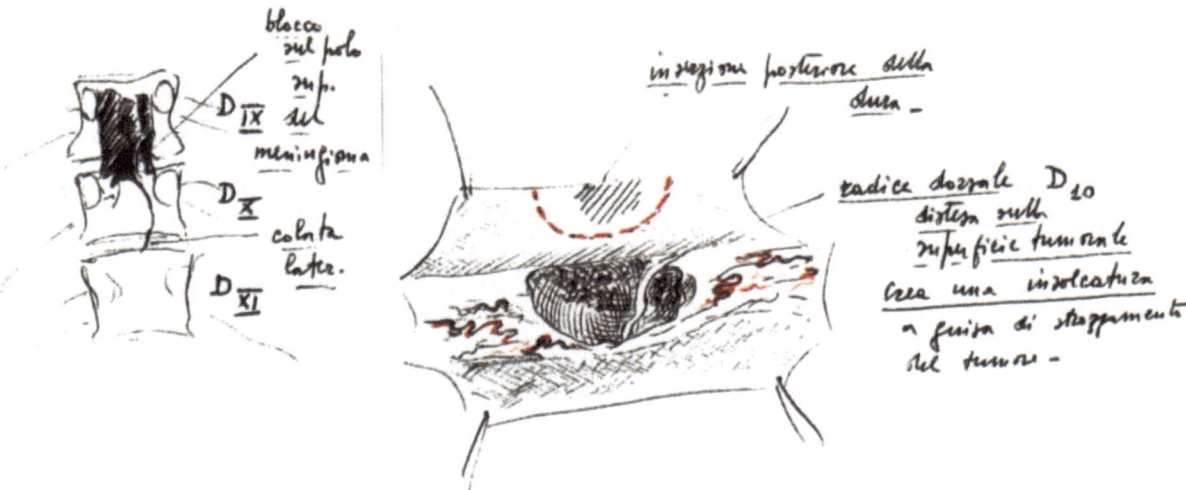

Fig. 295. Right posterolateral intradural-extramedullary meningioma in D9-D10

cing dome-shaped filling defect and slight convexity on the left.

Surgical Treatment. The meningioma invaded the internal posterior side of the dura towards the right. The cord was displaced towards the left. The tenth dorsal root on the right was stretched across a sulcus on the encapsulated part of the tumour. Removal of the arachnoidal adherent structures and excision en block. The dural invasion was thoroughly coagulated.

Results. Disappearance of the pain syndrome after 24 h. Three months later there was gradual recovery of active motility leading to almost normal walking after 1 month.

Case No. 20: Meningothelial Meningioma

A 70-year-old man (1969). Left anterolateral intradural-extramedullary meningioma in D6.

Clinical Course. 7 months. Back pain with sciatica irradiating to the left and later to the right. Two months later the patient was affected by motor impairment to the lower limbs.

Neurological Examination. Spastic paraparesis. Bilateral Babinski sign. Hypoaesthesia in the various forms of sensitivity from D5. Sphincter disturbances in the form of incontinence.

Rachicentesis. 1.19 g protein per thousand.

Myelography (performed suboccipitally). Total block in D7 with oblique cuneiform filling defect towards the right.

Surgical Treatment. Arched-shaped dural incision. The cord appeared atrophic and curved backwards, with an ischaemic area measuring 1 cm in length. The surface of the tumour presented a sulcus created by the dentate ligament, which was resectioned. Excision of the neoplasm and gently taking it towards the lateral wall of the dura. The part of the dura with the tumour attachment could not be spared. Plastic with amnion lamina.

Results. One week later there was a slight recovery of motility. One month later the patient began to walk. Clinical recovery after 3 months. Slight hyperreflexia persisted.

Case No. 19: Meningothelial Meningioma

An 80-year-old woman (1969; Fig. 296). Left anterolateral intradural-extramedullary meningioma in C7-D1.

Clinical Course. 1 year. Burning type of paraesthesias to right lower limb lasting all day and night. Ingravescent motor impairment to left lower limb.

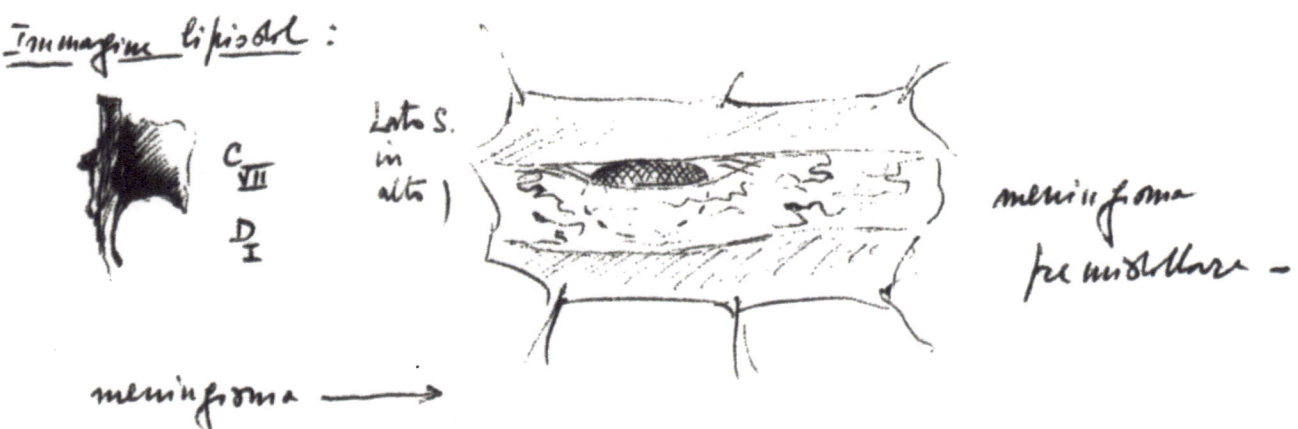

Fig. 296. Left anterolateral intradural-extramedullary meningioma in C7-D1

Neurological Examination. Spastic paraparesis to the left. Left Babinski sign. Band of hyperaesthesia on D8-D9 on the right.
Rachicentesis. 0.26 g protein per thousand.
Myelography (performed suboccipitally). Dome-shaped filling defect with slight flow on the right, convex externally and filling of radicular pocket in C7-D1.
Surgical Treatment. The cord was curved backwards and adhered to the internal side of the dura. The surface of the cord appeared of a whitish colour and ischaemic. The meningioma was of a premedullary development. Incision of the capsule and fragmented excision of the neoplasm. The dural invasion was coagulated.
Results. Immediate disappearance of cord paraesthesias. Clinical recovery 6 months later.

Case No. 21: Sarcomatous Meningioma

A 57-year-old woman (1969; Fig. 297). Left anterolateral intradural-extramedullary meningioma in C5-C6 enveloping the sixth cervical root.
Medical History. Operated on for removal of a fibroid.
Clinical Course. 8 months. Left cervicobrachial pain. For 2 months motor deficit to left hand and monoplegia at left lower limb.
Neurological Examination. Spastic tetraparesis to the left. Left Bernard-Horner syndrome. Severe motor deficit to left hand with atrophy of the first interosseous muscle. Bilateral Babinski sign. Hypoaesthesia in D1, hyperaesthesia in D2 and hypoaesthesia from D3-D4 which became anaesthesia distally. Sphincter disturbances in the form of retention.
Rachicentesis. 2.65 g protein per thousand.
X-Ray of Cervical Rachis. The spinal canal in C5-C6 showed widening, with thinning of pedicles on both sides.
Myelography (performed suboccipitally). Total block in C5-C6 and, by tilting, the contrast medium was encouraged to flow on the left.
Surgical Treatment. On opening the dura the neoplasm was seen occupying the left lateral region, curving the cord contralaterally. Tumour attachment invaded the internal surface of the dura. The neoplasm reached the premedullary region and enveloped the sixth cervical motor and sensory root on the left. Fragmented removal and radicotomy.
Results. Over 1 month there was a total recovery of the motility in the left lower limb with good recovery of the upper limb. Three months later the patient was affected by tetraplegia and died of widespread metastases affecting vertebrae and left lung.

Case No. 91: Transitional Meningioma

A 67-year-old woman (1970; Figs. 298, 299). Left anterolateral intradural-extramedullary meningioma in D1-D2.

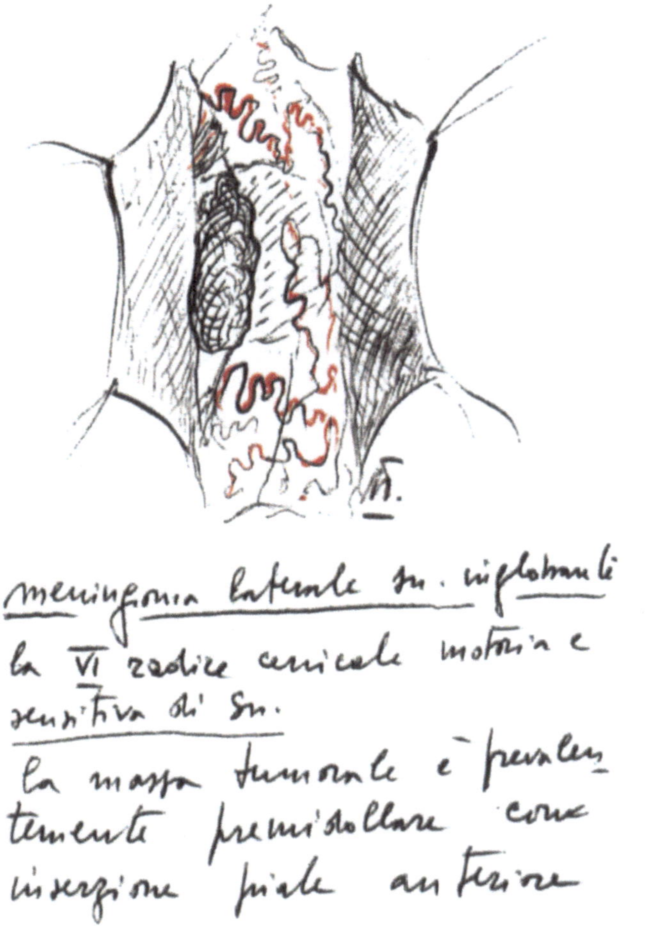

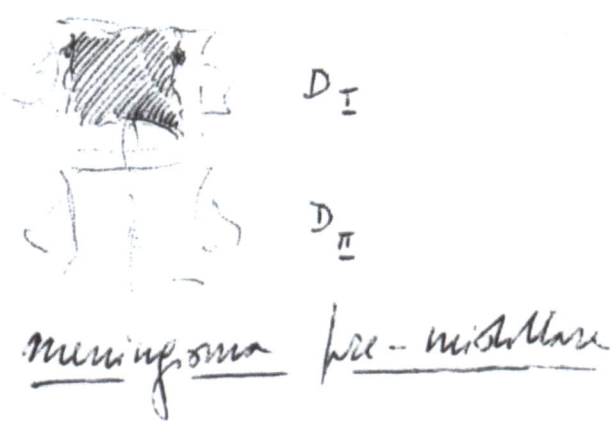

Fig. 298. Myelography. Total block in D1-D2

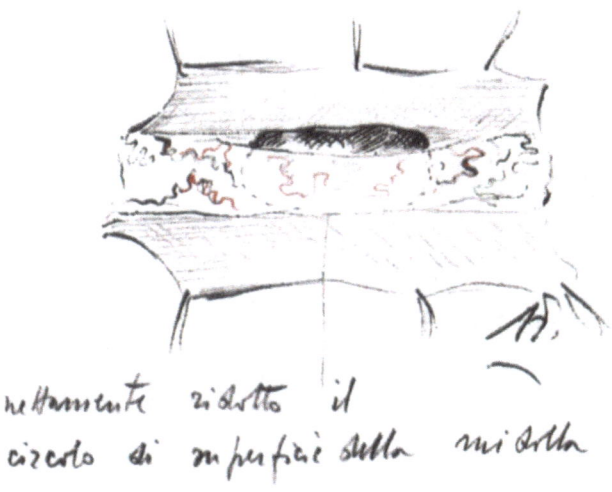

Fig. 299. Left anterolateral intradural-extramedullary meningioma in D1-D2

Fig. 297. Left anterolateral intradural-extramedullary meningioma in C5-C6

Clinical Course. 2.5 years. Pain at cervicodorsal passage irradiating to underarm and upper thorax, initially on the left then gradually affecting also the right. For 1 year weakness felt at lower limbs with motor claudication.

Neurological Examination. Spastic paraparesis to the left. Bilateral Babinski sign. Hypoaesthesia from D5 affecting the various forms of sensitivity to the right. Sphincter disturbances in the form of retention.

Rachicentesis. 1.63 g protein per thousand.

Myelography (performed suboccipitally). Total block producing a dome-shaped filling defect in D1-D2 with slight filling of the radicular funnels.

Surgical Treatment. The cord appeared ischaemic and curved posteriorly. The examination on the left lateral side revealed a premedullary neoplasm enveloping the second dorsal root. Fragmented gradual removal of the capsule from the ventral surface of the cord.

Results. Slight recovery of motility of the legs, with disappearance of sphincter disturbances in 2 days. After 10 days the patient was capable of fast walking.

Case No. 78: Angioblastic Meningioma

A 40-year-old man (1971; Fig. 300). Intramedullary meningioma in C2-C3.

Clinical Course. 10 years. Loss of strength with pain to right hemiside in the form of a burning sensation. Two years before hospitalization a laminectomy at C3-C7 was performed in another hospital, with diagnosis of an expansive intramedullary structure.

Neurological Examination. Right spastic hemiplegia. The right upper limb showed signs of atrophy at scapula-humerus level. Spontaneous semiflexion and abduction attitude of right arm. The digits were extended and clenching the fist was difficult due to contracture and spontaneous clonus tendency. Hypertonia of right leg with interotation in equinism of the foot. Right clonus and Babinski sign. Total anaesthesia of right upper limb involving C4-C7. Hyperaesthesia to right hemitrunk and lower limb affecting tactile sensitivity and to a lesser degree affecting hot, cold and pain. Abdominal disturbances in the form of retention of urine.

X-Ray of Cervical Tract. Evident kyphosis in C4-C5. The stratigraphic examination revealed a widening in the spinal canal at C4-C5 level. Thinning of pedicles in C4-C6.

Myelography (performed suboccipitally). Block producing cuneiform filling defect in C3 with slight sideways flow.

Surgical Treatment. The cord appeared increased in volume in upper tract. The superficial blood supply was thinned and presented a large, malformed median artery one cm below this artery at the C3 level; the medullary surface had been invaded by a lesion that reached the posterior columns, which were a red-wine colour. A myelotomy in a less vascularized area led to the view of a reddish-coloured neoplasm which was gradually removed. A slight demarcation was seen only deep in the lower part of the incision performed by the myelotomy.

Results. Reduction in hypertonia to right hemiside and improvement in voluntary motility. Walking was possible without support. Disappearance of sphincter disturbances.

Case No. 64: Transitional Meningioma

A 71-year-old woman (1971; Fig. 301). Left anterolateral intradural-extramedullary meningioma in C4.

Clinical Course. 1 year. Paraesthesias affecting hot and cold sensations at right lower limb, ascending to umbilical region. Simultaneous loss of strength in left hand. In the previous months paraparesis to the right.

Neurological Examination. Spastic paraparesis to the left. Accentuation of upper limb reflexes to the left. Band-like hypoaesthesia at mammary region on the right. Hypoaesthesia distally to left digits.

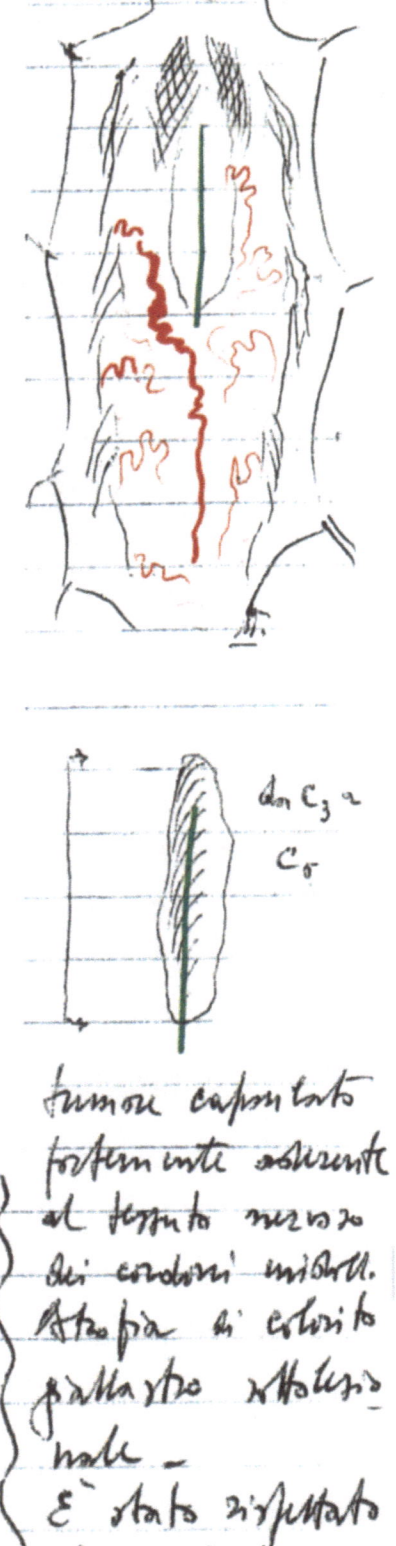

Fig. 300. Intramedullary meningioma in C2-C3

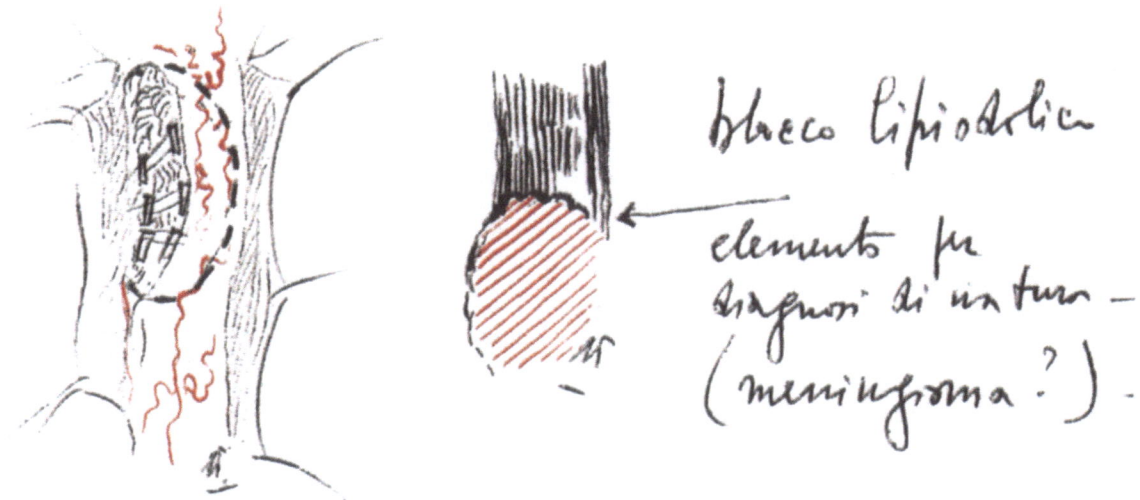

Fig. 301. Left anterolateral intradural-extramedullary meningioma in C4

Rachicentesis. 0.86 g protein per thousand.
X-Ray of Cervical Rachis. Thinning of articular facets of C5 on the left and slightly widened canal.
Myelography (performed suboccipitally). Total block in C4-C5 with slight flow on the right.
Surgical Treatment. The cord was flattened on the right, providing access to a neoplasm invading the left with sensory root wrapped around it. Opening of arachnoid and radicotomy of C5 sensory root. By reclining the tumour slightly to left, excision en bloc was performed with coagulation of the attachment contralaterally.
Results. Postoperative motor inhibition to the right lower limb. Gradual improvement leading to normal walking after 1 week.

Case No. 92: Meningothelial Meningioma
A 65-year-old woman (1971; Fig. 302). Right anterolateral intradural-extramedullary meningioma in C7-D1.
Clinical Course. 4 years. Cervical pain irradiating to interscapula area. Impediment in walking over the previous 6 months. Paraesthesias to lower limbs to the right for the last 4 months.
Neurological Examination. Spastic paraparesis to the right foot clonus. Bilateral Babinski sign. Painful hypoaesthesia from D5. Sphincter disturbances in the form of incontinence.
Rachicentesis. 0.25 protein per thousand.
Myelography (performed suboccipitally). Linear block in C7-D1.
Surgical Treatment. The cord appeared flattened towards the left, and the surface blood flow appeared in stasis. Opening of the arachnoid and radicotomy of sensory root of C4 enveloped by the neoplasm. Excision in toto of the meningioma which lay very close to the intravertebral foramen.
Results. The patient was capable of standing upright and walking within 1 week.

Case No. 110: Transitional Meningioma
A 62-year-old woman (1971). Right posterolateral intradural-extramedullary meningioma in C6.
Medical History. Luetic infection.
Clinical Course. 8 years. Back pain and loss of strength in lower limbs becoming gradually worse.
Neurological Examination. Spastic paraparesis with bilateral Babin-

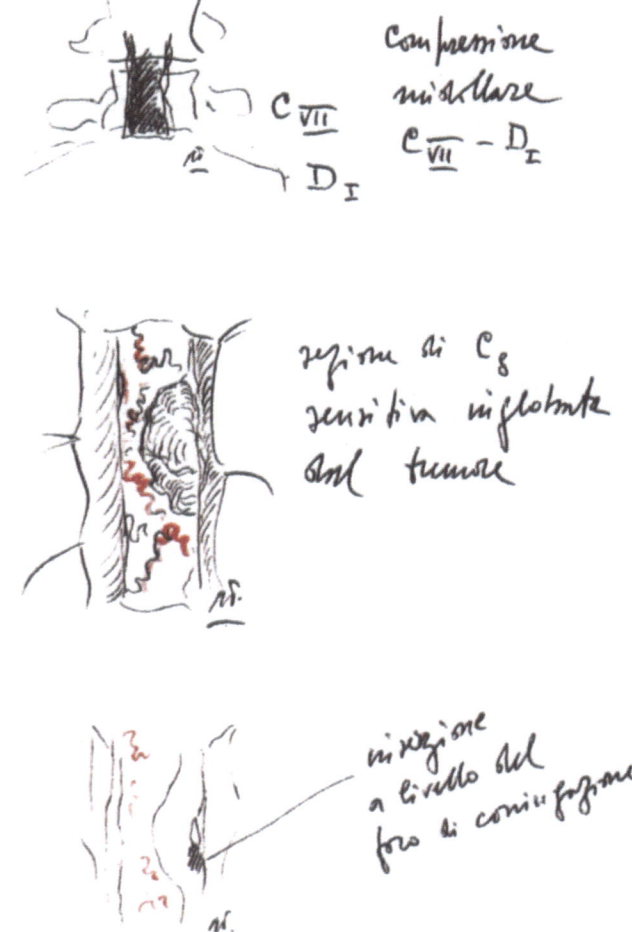

Fig. 302. Right anterolateral intradural-extramedullary meningioma in C7-D1

ski sign. Area affected by painful hypoaesthesia in D10. Sphincter disturbances in the form of incontinence.

Rachicentesis. 0.43 g protein per thousand.

X-Ray of Dorsal Tract. Scoliosis with spondyloarthrosis. Thinning of the articular pedicles in D6 on the left.

Myelography (performed suboccipitally). Total block on the right with dome-shaped filling defect.

Surgical Treatment. Neoplasm appeared adhering very closely to the internal dural surface in right posterolateral site. The cord appeared reduced in volume and flattened towards the left. Excision; the neoplasm left a shadow on the medullary surface.

Results. 10 days of walking practice. Complete recovery 1 month later.

Case No. 93: Nonclassified Meningioma

A 71-year-old woman (1971). Posterior intradural-extramedullary meningioma in C5-C6.

Family Medical History. The patient's son was affected by small subcutaneous lipomas and numerous skin fibromas.

Medical History. Operated on for left mammary fibroma.

Clinical Course. 40 years. Cervical pain with paraesthesias of a fastidious nature to upper limbs to the hands. Painful paraesthesias to left lower limb and slight motor claudication for 7 months.

Neurological Examination. Spastic paraplegia with bilateral Babinski sign. Hypoaesthesia from D5. Sphincter disturbances in the form of retention.

Rachicentesis. 2.70 g protein per thousand.

X-Ray of Cervical Tract. Thinning of pedicles in C5-C6 with osseous thickening in C6-C7.

Myelography (performed suboccipitally). Total block with dome-shaped filling defect in C5-C6 and slight bilateral flow.

Surgical Treatment. Posterior extra-arachnoidal neoplasm with invasion of internal dural layer. Excision together with dural invasion. Dural plastic with amnion lamina.

Results. Three days later, minor contracture of lower limbs. Persistence of paraesthesias to the hands. Regression of sensibility disturbances and disappearance of bladder retention. Neurological examination was negative after 3 years.

Case No. 65: Transitional Meningioma

A 66-year-old woman (1971; Fig. 303). Right anterolateral intradural-extramedullary meningioma in D1-D2.

Clinical Course. 3 months. Back pain irradiating slightly to interscapula area. Painful paraesthesias to right leg with gradual loss

of sensibility. Same symptoms but less severe to left lower limb and gradual loss of strength in lower limbs.

Neurological Examination. Spastic paraparesis to the right. Hypoaesthesia in D8-D9. Sphincter disturbances in the form of incontinence.

Rachicentesis. 0.70 g protein per thousand.

Myelography (performed suboccipitally). Total block with blackberry-shaped filling defect in D1-D2. Slight convex flow on the left.

X-Ray of Dorsal Rachis. Diffused spondyloarthrosis with ankylosed bone bridges.

Surgical Treatment. The posterior circulation of the cord appeared thinned for 2 cm. The tumour had a predominantly anterior attachment. Posterior radicotomy on D1 and D2 on the right. Fragmented excision. The base of the attachment on the internal ventral side of the dura presented small, calcified lamellae which were later removed and coagulated.

Results. Walking began after 15 days. Total recovery after 1 month.

Case No. 114: Meningothelial Meningioma

A 70-year-old woman (1971). Ventrolateral intradural-extramedullary meningioma predominantly on the right in C1-C2 (see Chap. 8).

Case No. 115: Psammomatous Meningioma

A 49-year-old woman (1972). Left intradural-extramedullary meningioma in D7 (see Chap. 6).

Case No. 96: Meningothelial Meningioma

An infant, 2 years 3 months old (1972). Posterior intradural-extramedullary meningioma invading medial raphe in D1-D2 (see Chap. 6).

Case No. 72: Meningothelial Meningioma with Lipomatous Component at Lower Pole Level

An infant, 2 years 3 months (1972). Intradural-extramedullary meningioma of filum terminale occupying the entire canal of L2 and S1 (see Chap. 6).

Case No. 119: Psammomatous Transitional Meningioma

A 72-year-old woman (1972). Intradural-extramedullary meningioma in D6-D7 (see Chap. 8).

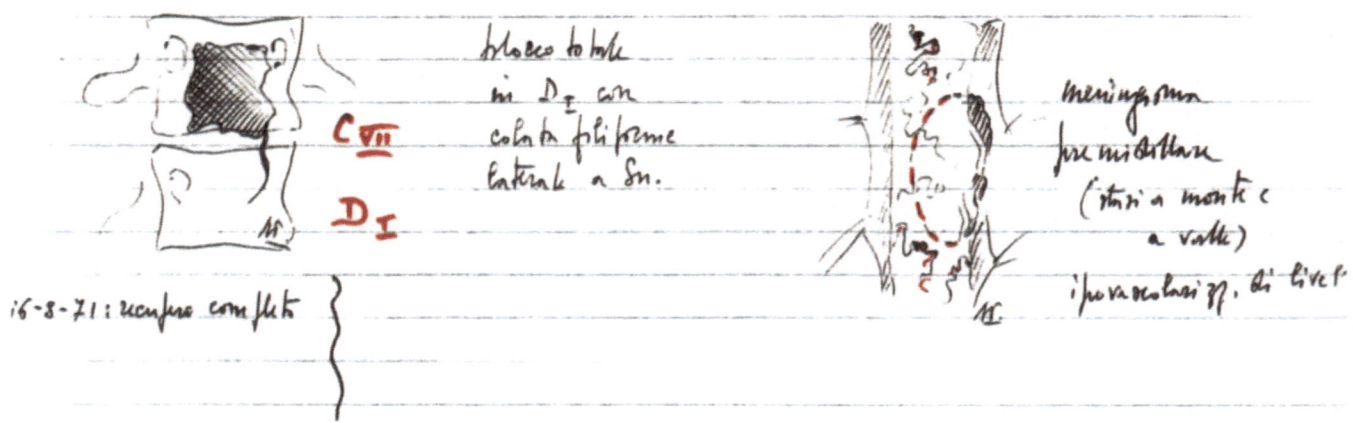

Fig. 303. Right anterolateral intradural-extramedullary meningioma in D1-D2

Case No. 44: Transitional Meningioma

A 69-year-old woman (1973). Intradural-extramedullary meningioma with right posterolateral development in D6-D7 (see Chap. 8).

Case No. 121: Transional Meningioma

An 69-year-old woman (1973; Fig. 304). Posterior intradural-extramedullary meningioma in D1-D2.
Medical History. Diabetes.
Clinical Course. 6 months. Burning type of paraesthesias to feet to the left. Constriction felt at abdomen. Weakness at lower limbs leading to severe paraparesis.
Neurological Examination. Severe spastic apaparesis. Hypoaesthesia from D3 becoming anaesthesia. Sphincter disturbances in the form of retention.
Rachicentesis. 1.20 g protein per thousand.
X-Ray Dorsal Tract. Scoliosis with osteoporosis and spondyloarthrosis signs. Thinning of articular facets in D2 on the left.
Myelography (performed suboccipitally). Total block in D1-D2. The contrast medium thickened in a uniform manner, flowing slightly sideways on the left and forming a concave filling defect towards the interior. Dome-shaped filling defect.
Surgical Treatment. Curved paramedian incision on the right along the margin of an area which was resistant to the touch. The neoplasm completely invaded the internal surface of the dura. Excision en bloc and coagulation of the attachment base.
Results. Ten days later the voluntary motility and sensibility disturbances showed great improvement. Total recovery 2 months later.

Case No. 82: Nonclassified Meningioma

A 23-year-old woman (1973). Right posterolateral intradural-extramedullary meningioma in D1-D2.
Clinical Course. 2 years. Hesitant walking with evident ataxia signs during the last months of pregnancy. One year prior to hospitalization, painful paraesthesias to lower limbs. In another hospital surgery was performed to remove a meningioma in the cervicodorsal passage. Regression of symptoms for 6 months. The return of motor disturbances led to paraplegia. Second operation performed in another hospital without any beneficial consequences.
Neurological Examination. Spastic paraplegia with foot clonus and bilaterally on patella. Bilateral Babinski sign. Hypoaesthesia from C3 becoming anaesthesia distally on both sides. Sphincter disturbances in the form of retention.
Rachicentesis. 2.30 g protein per thousand.
Myelography (performed suboccipitally). Irregular block with double flow in D2-D3.
Surgical Treatment. Leptomeningeal adherent structure which greatly reduced the cord's surface-layer circulation. The cord was displaced towards the left and strangulated, producing an hour-glass appearance. Excision of the thickened dura infiltrated by the neoplasm.
Results. Improvement in motility with incomplete regression of sensitivity disturbances.

Case No. 111: Transitional Meningioma

A 52-year-old woman (1973; Fig. 305). Left intradural-extramedullary meningioma in D10 enveloping the tenth dorsal root on the left.
Medical History. Diabetes.
Clinical Course. 10 months. Loss of strength of both lower limbs to the left, having an ingravescent nature with progressive impediment in walking and sense of instability.
Neurological Examination. Spastic-ataxic paraparesis (Levy grade 1). Foot clonus and bilateral Babinski sign. Hypoaesthesia from D7-D8 on the left from D12 on the right.
Rachicentesis. 2.33 g protein per thousand.
X-Ray of Dorsal Rachis. Right pedicle of D9 appeared thinned.
Myelography (performed suboccipitally). Block with dome-shaped filling defect in D10. A very slight flow defined the medial surface of the lesion. The location was posterolateral on the left.
Surgical Treatment. The tumour the size of an almond was of a red-wine colour and displaced the cord towards the right. The root of D10 on the left was enveloped by the tumour. Removal of leptomeningeal adherent structure. Radicotomy of D10 and excision in toto.
Results. Recovery of motor deficit but persistence of ataxic component.

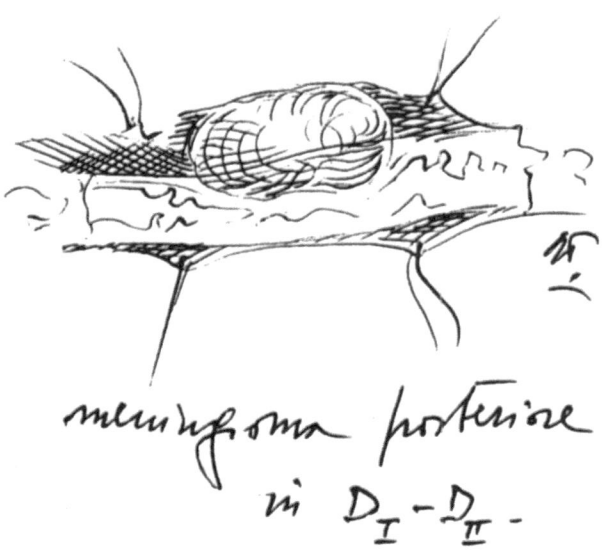

Fig. 304. Posterior intradural-extramedullary meningioma in D1-D2

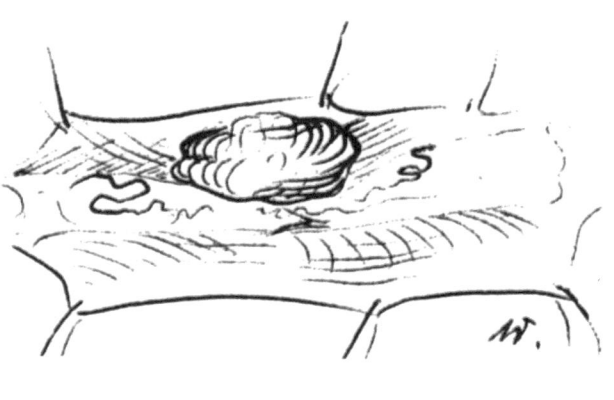

Fig. 305. Left intradural-extramedullary meningioma in D10 enveloping the tenth dorsal root on the left

Case No. 66: Nonclassified Meningioma

A 68-year-old man (1974). Right posterolateral intradural-extramedullary meningioma in L3-L4 (see Chap. 9).

Case No. 117: Psammomatous Meningioma

A 72-year-old woman (1974). Intradural-extramedullary, premedullary meningioma in D2.

Clinical Course. 1 year. Burning type of paraesthesias to right leg and after a few months monoparesis.

Neurological Examination. Spastic paraparesis to the left. Bilateral Babinski sign. Hypoaesthesias from D9.

Rachicentesis. 0.75 protein per thousand.

Myelography (performed suboccipitally). Slowing from C4 to C6; spondyloarthrosis with posterior marginal exostosis. Total block in D2 with dome-shaped filling defect and left lateral flow.

Surgical Treatment. On opening the dura the cord's surface-layer circulation was seen in stasis. In C7 the discal projection appeared calcified. After opening arachnoid the dentate ligament was cut and the cord gently reclined. The meningioma presented an irregular and partly calcified surface layer and was located in a premedullary site. Fragmented removal.

Results. Twenty days later voluntary motility was recovered only at right foot. Walking was unsteady even after 40 days; 9 months later walking was possible with one support. Persistence of cord paraesthesias.

Case No. 112: Fibroblastic Meningioma

A 51-year-old woman (1975; Fig. 306). Left posterolateral-extramedullary meningioma in D2.

Clinical Course. 3 years. Cervicodorsal pain irradiating to left in subscapula and mammary regions. One year later the same symptoms appeared on the right. For 3 months, motor impairment of lower limbs to the left.

Neurological Examination. Spastic paraplegia with foot clonus and Babinski sign. Hypoaesthesia from D3. Sphincter disturbances in the form of retention.

Rachicentesis. 2.18 g protein per thousand.

Myelography (performed suboccipitally). Total block in D1-D2 producing an irregular image.

Surgical Treatment. Posterior neoplasm located laterally to the left and having a reddish-wine colour. The tumour enveloped the second dorsal root. Fragmented removal with radicotomy of posterior sensory root of D2. Coagulation of attachment base.

Results. Over 1 week the patient gradually recovered motility until walking became normal. Complete recovery 2 months later.

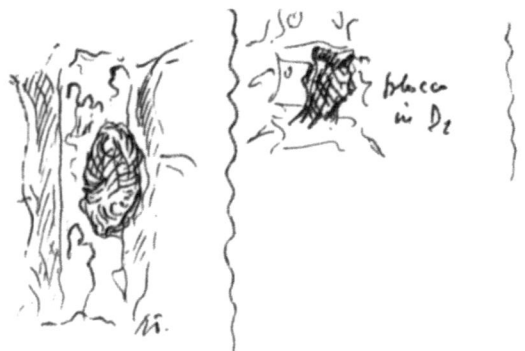

Fig. 306. Left posterolateral-extramedullary meningioma in D2

Case No. 55: Psammomatous Meningioma

A 61-year-old woman (1975). Posterior meningioma in D2.

Medical History. Operated on for the removal of uterine polyposis.

Clinical Course. 41 years. Persistent back pain forcing the patient to use a surgical corset. Three years prior to hospitalization the patient suffered from interscapula pain. Motor claudication at left foot, then to both.

Neurological Examination. Spastic paraparesis with foot clonus. Bilateral Babinski sign. Hypoaesthesia from D4. Shincter disturbances in the form of retention.

Diagnostic Rachicentesis. 2.68 g protein per thousand.

X-Ray Dorsal Tract. Accentuation of physiological kyphosis.

Myelography (performed suboccipitally). Block in D2 with thickening of contrast medium on the left.

Surgical Treatment. Tumoural component on meningeal surface with a hard consistency resembling a meningioma en plaque and with a partly intra- and extradural development. Total excision of neoplasm.

Results. Improvement in sensitivity from the very first postoperative days. Recovery of motility during the following 10 days. Normal walking 3 months later.

Case No. 3: Transitional Meningioma

A 61-year-old woman (1975; Fig. 307, 308). Left ventrolateral intradural-extramedullary meningioma in D7-D8.

Clinical Course. 1 year. Dorsal pain radiating to left hip. Tingling type of paraesthesias to left lower limbs with motor deficit also to the right shortly after.

Neurological Examination. Spastic-ataxic paraparesis to the left. Foot clonus and bilateral Babinski sign. Hypoaesthesia from D6-D7. Sphincter disturbances in the form of retention.

Rachicentesis. 0.60 g protein per thousand.

Myelography (performed suboccipitally). Block in D7-D8 with right lateral flow.

Surgical Treatment. The cord was reduced in volume and displaced towards the right. The circulation of the arterial surface layer appeared in stasis. After opening arachnoid a lateral premedullary neoplasm was seen on the left with the attachment base near the radicular funnel of the eighth root. Fragmented excision after radicotomy, then coagulation of the calcified attachment.

Results. Walking was attempted after 10 days. Motility returned to normal 2 months later but slight constriction still felt at the thorax.

Case No. 88: Nonclassified Meningioma

A 43-year-old man (1975). Left posterolateral intradural-extramedullary meningioma in D7-D8 (see Chap. 9).

Case No. 54: Psammomatous Meningioma

A 70-year-old woman (1976). Right anterolateral intradural-extramedullary meningioma in C4-C5-C6 (see Chap. 6).

Case No. 108: Psammomatous Meningioma

A 49-year-old woman (1976; Fig. 309). Left anterolateral intradural-extramedullary meningioma in D7-D8.

Clinical Course. 12 years. Dorsal pain with painful paraesthesias to right lower limb and later spreading to the left. Pain with girdle pattern at medial thoracic region bilaterally. Motor weakness at both lower limbs. Nine years previously the patient had successfully undergone surgery for the partial removal of a meningioma in D7 in another hospital. Three years later she began to suffer from back pain again, together with distal paraesthesias to lower limbs and ingravescent motor impairment.

Neurological Examination. Spastic paraparesis. Bilateral patella

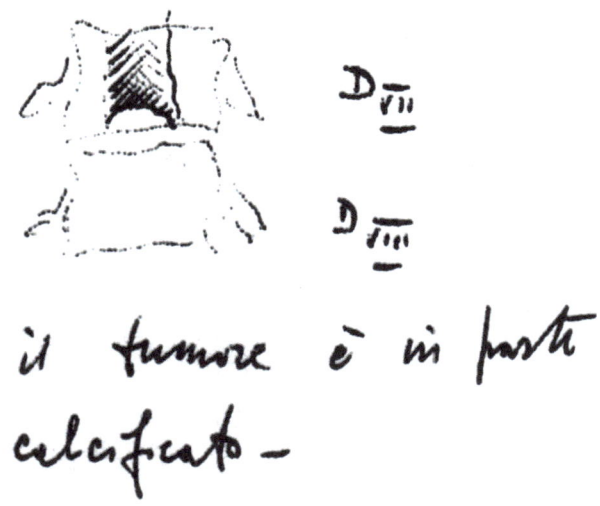

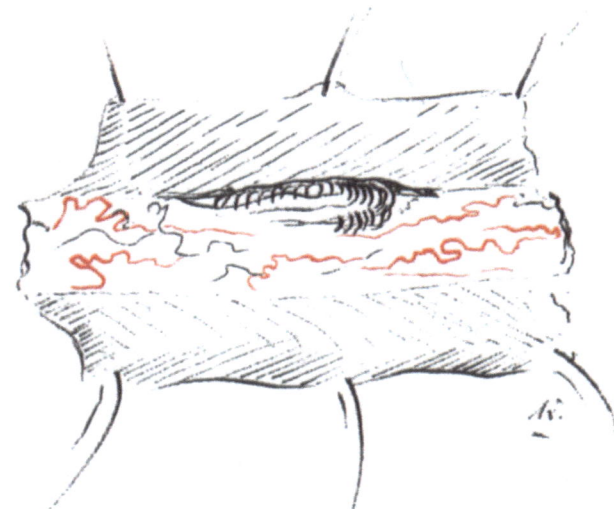

Fig. 307. Myelography: block in D7-D8

Fig. 308. Left ventrolateral intradural-extramedullary meningioma in D7-D8

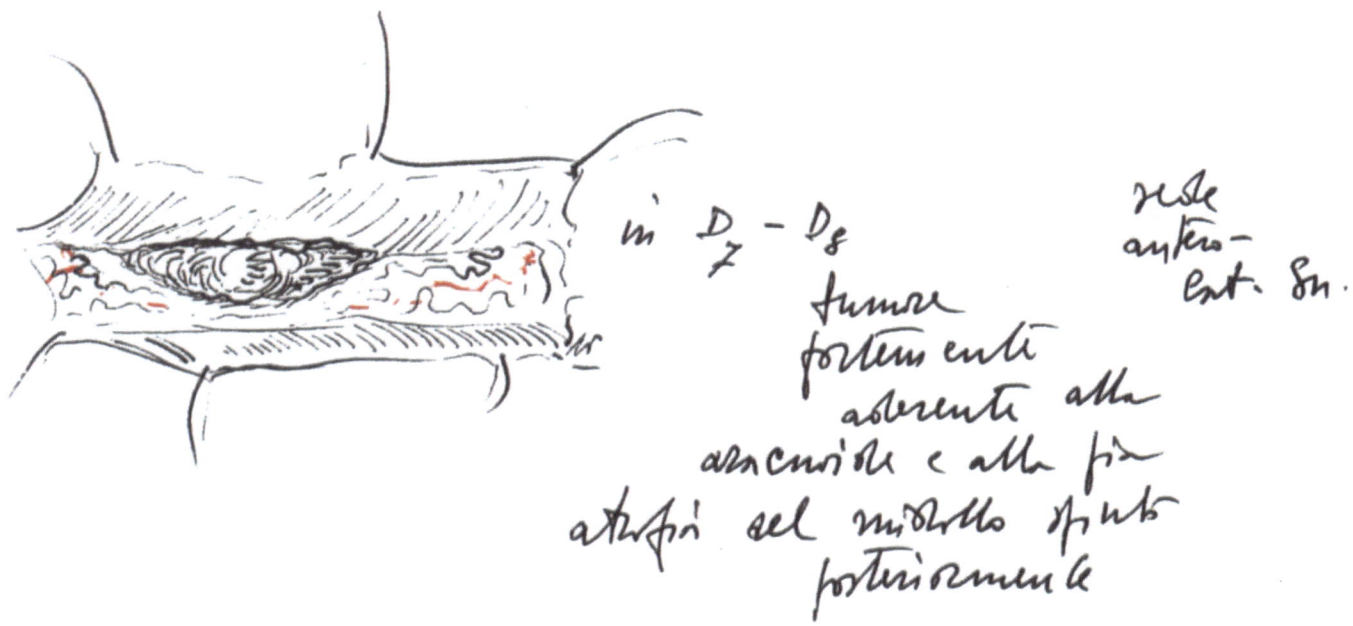

Fig. 309. Left anterolateral intradural-extramedullary meningioma in D7-D8

and foot clonus. Hypoaesthesia from D6-D7. Sphincter disturbances in the form of retention.
Rachicentesis. 1.15 g protein per thousand.
Myelography (via lumbar puncture). Block at D7-D8 level (previous laminectomy site) producing an oblique cuneiform image from left to right.
Surgical Treatment. Tumour measured 2 cm in length, adhering to internal anterolateral left surface of dura. The cord appeared atrophic and displaced to right. Total fragmented excision.
Results. Walking was attempted 15 days later. Slight ataxic component persisted.

Case No. 39: Transitional Meningioma
A 59-year-old woman (1976). Posterior intradural-extramedullary meningioma in D5-D6.
Clinical Course. 7 months. Dorsal pain radiating below, girdle-like to the inguinal region. Motor impairment to lower limbs to the left.
Neurological Examination. Spastic-ataxic paraparesis. Band of hypoaesthesia in D11 and anaesthesia affecting various forms of sensitivity at lower levels. Sphincter disturbances in the form of retention.
Rachicentesis. 1.50 g protein per thousand.
X-Ray Dorsal Tract. Kyphoscoliosis. Reduction in height of D11-D12.

Myelography (performed suboccipitally). Block almost producing dome-shaped filling defect in D11-D12 with slight sideways flow on the left.

Surgical Treatment. Posterior meningioma adhering to internal surface layer of dura. Excision and coagulation of the attachment base. The cord appeared flattened and pushed forwards with the surface-layer circulation in stasis above and below the tumour.

Results. Walking was possible after 2 months. Disappearance of sphincter disturbances. Clinically negative at 5-year examination.

Case No. 106: Syncytial Meningioma

A 61-year-old woman (1976; Fig. 310). Posterior intradural-extramedullary meningioma in D3-D4.

Clinical Course. 4 years. Shooting pain in left precordial region. Burning type of paraesthesias for 6 months to lower limbs ascending to mediothoracic region. Stiffness sensation to lower limbs to the left, with cramps at toes of right foot.

Neurological Examination. Spastic paraparesis with patella and foot clonus bilaterally. Hypoaesthesia on D5-D6 with anaesthesia below. Sphincter disturbances in the form of retention.

Rachicentesis. 0.33 g protein per thousand.

X-Ray of Dorsal Rachis. Right convex scoliosis.

Myelography (performed suboccipitally). Block in D3-D4 with slight flow on left.

Surgical Treatment. The dura appeared thickened along a 2 cm length. Opening of dura and decollement of neoplasm adhering to cord's surface. The cord was atrophic and flattened forwards with a reduction in the surface-layer circulation.

Results. Gradual improvement until normal walking was achieved in 15 days. The patient's condition remained stable after 1 month.

Case No. 30: Fibroblastic Meningioma

A 56-year-old woman (1976; Fig. 311). Premedullary, intradural-extramedullary meningioma in D2.

Clinical Course. 3 years. Burning type of paraesthesias to lower limbs at night and for 1 year the patient was affected by paraesthesias to the thighs and in the hypogastric region.

Neurological Examination. Hyperreflexia of patellas and ankle jerk. Hypoaesthesias from D7-D8.

Rachicentesis. 0.20 g protein per thousand.

X-Ray of Lumbosacral Rachis. Schistais in L5 and S1 with asymmetry of the laminae and spinous processes.

Myelography (performed suboccipitally). Block in D1-D2 producing a dome-shaped image.

Surgical Treatment. The cord appeared slightly curved backwards and covered the tumour in a premedullary site. The attachment extended to the ventral surface of the dura. Fragmented excision.

Results. One week later the patient was able to walk with some ataxic signs. Total recovery after 2 months.

Case No. 120: Calcified Meningioma

A 57-year-old woman (1976). Posterior extramedullary meningioma in D10-D11.

Clinical Course. 5 years. Pain distributed girdle-like at dorsolumbar passage to the right, increased with straining. Loss of strength in lower limbs for 7 months.

Neurological Examination. Dyschromic mark at upper right quadrant of abdomen. Harmonic hypotrophy at left lower limb with valgus of the foot, which had only three toes. Spastic paraparesis and equinism attitude of feet. Foot clonus with Babinski sign on the right. Hypoaesthesia from D10 distally.

Rachicentesis. 0.40 g protein per thousand.

Myelography (performed suboccipitally). Block in D10-D11. Central oval-shaped filling defect. Slight linear flow on the left.

Surgical Treatment. Completely calcified extradural neoplasm surrounding the dura. Excision en bloc.

Results. Very slight recovery of the voluntary movements with persistence of very marked hypertonia.

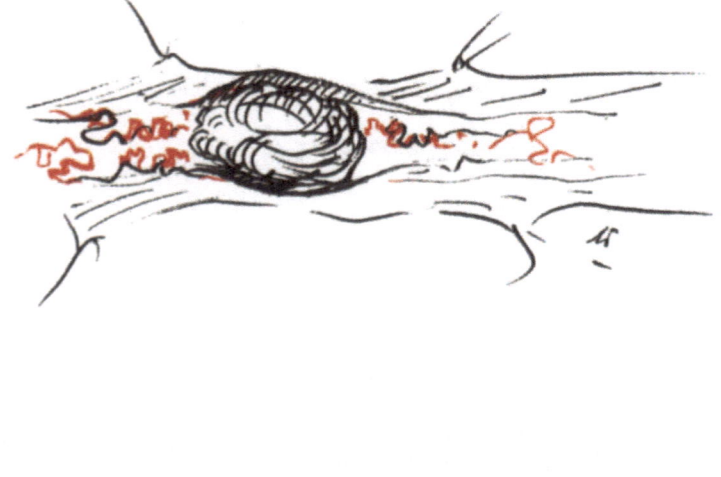

Fig. 310. Posterior intradural-extramedullary meningioma in D3-D4

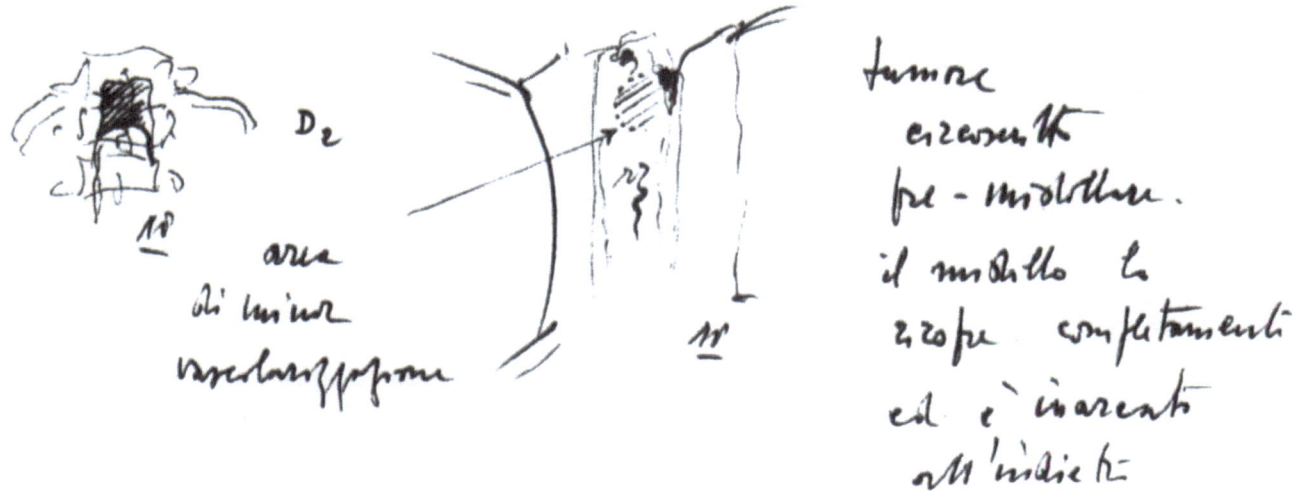

Fig. 311. Premedullary intradural-extramedullary meningioma in D2

Case No. 49: Meningothelial Meningioma
A 64-year-old woman (1977). Left posterolateral extramedullary meningioma in C4-C5 (see Chap. 8).

Case No. 53: Transitional Meningioma
A 52-year-old woman (1977; Fig. 312). An intradural premedullary meningioma in D11-D12.

Medical History. Hysterectomy due to fibroid.
Clinical Course. 3 years. Distal paraesthesias to lower limbs. Back pain and instability in walking.
Neurological Examination. Spastic paraparesis to the left, with ataxic signs. Foot clonus and bilateral Babinski sign. Hypoaesthesia in girdle-like pattern in D11-D12. Sphincter disturbances in the form of retention.
X-Ray of Spinal Column. Sinostosis of C2-C3 with fusion of the

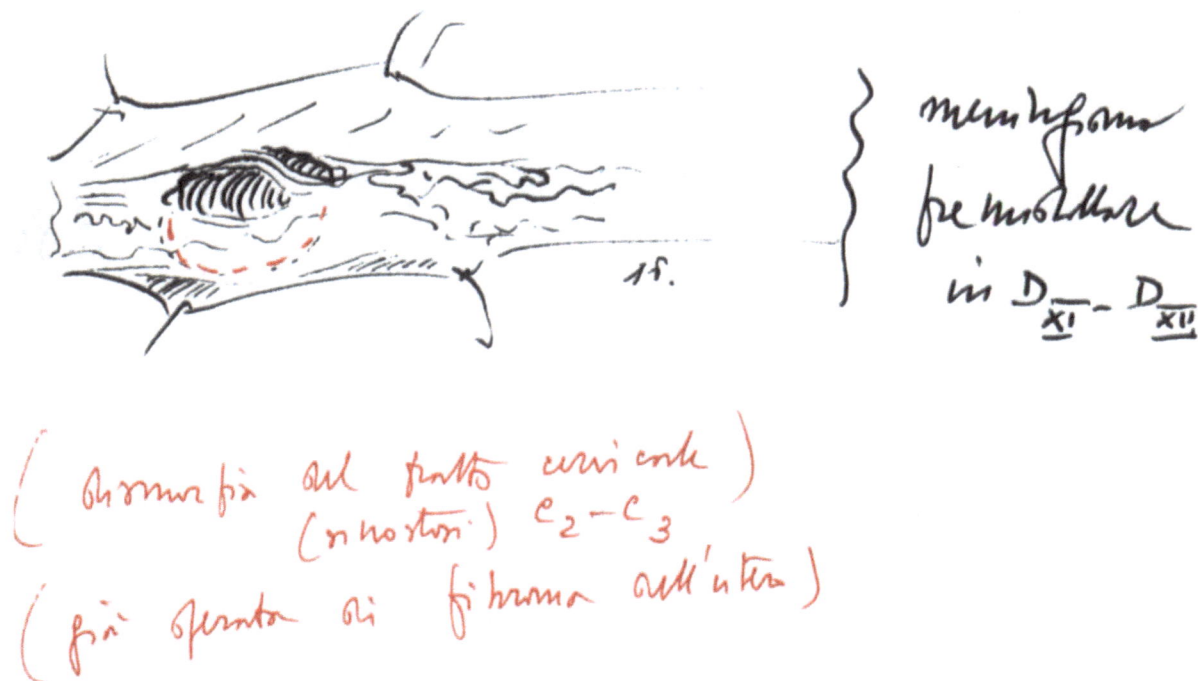

Fig. 312. Intradural premedullary meningioma in D11-D12

laminae into one spinous process.

Surgical Treatment. On opening the dura the cord appeared flatte-ned and displaced posteriorly by a reddish-wine coloured tumour the size of a small nut and adhering to the anterior internal surface of the dura. The left 12th dorsal root was raised by the tumour. Removal by fragmentation and coagulation of the attachment.

Postoperative Course. Motor inhibition for 10 days. After 1 month recovery of flex-extention movements of both lower limbs to the right. Exercising and walking 1.5 months later. An examination 7 months later showed patient to be walking normally.

Case No. 113: Transitional Meningioma

A 59-year-old woman (1977; Fig. 313). Left posterior intradural-extramedullary meningioma in D1.

Clinical Course. 30 years. Persistent attacks of back pain. One year prior to hospitalization burning paraesthesias to right foot and loss of sensibility at lower limb and to hypogastric region. One

month later sphincter disturbances in the form of retention. Two months prior to hospitalization motor impairment to the left. The back pain radiated to subscapula and underarm region on the left.

Neurological Examination. Spastic paraparesis to the left. Hypoae-sthesia from D8 to the right becoming anaesthesia distally.

Rachicentesis. 0.72 g protein per thousand.

Myelography (performed suboccipally). Total block in D1 with lateral flow on the right.

Surgical Treatment. Small neoplasm adhering to internal dural sur-face on the left posterolateral site. The lesion compressed the cord contralaterally, raising and bending the first dorsal root on the left. Excision en bloc after opening the arachnoid and freeing the root.

Results. Recovery after 1 month.

Case No. 26: Transitional Meningioma

A 37-year-old woman (1978; Fig. 314). Posterior intradural-extra-medullary meningioma in D2-D3.

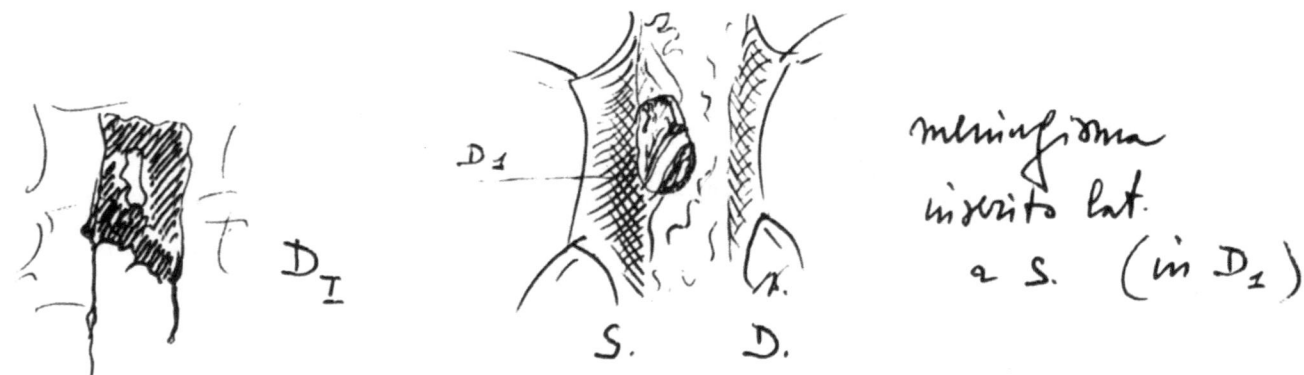

Fig. 313. Left posterior intradural-extramedullary meningioma in D1

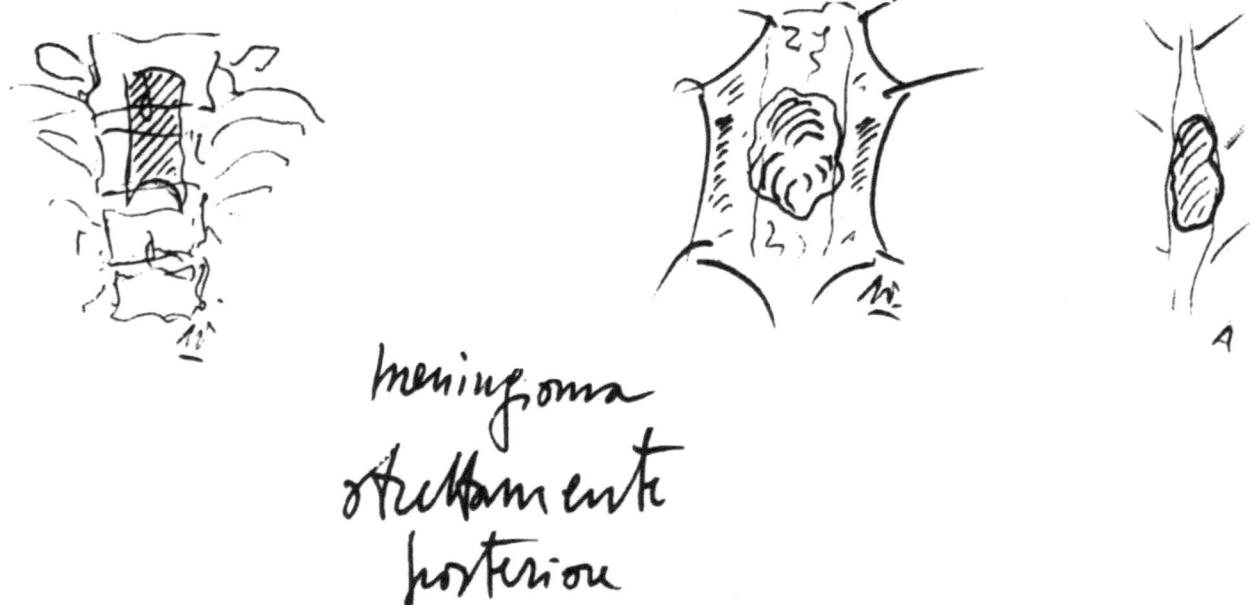

Fig. 314. Posterior intradural-extramedullary meningioma in D2-D3

Clinical Course. 5 months. Cervicodorsal pain radiating occasionally to subclavian area and to the last two digits on the left hand. Motor deficit appearing initially at left lower limb and then on right. Paraesthesias to feet of an ascending nature.
Neurological Examination. Pigmented birthmark on face. Spastic paraparesis to the left, with bilateral patellar and foot clonus. Bilateral Babinski sign. Hypoaesthesia from D3-D4 to the left. Sphincter disturbances in the form of retention.
Myelography (via lumbar puncture). In D2-D3 dome-shaped image at both upper and lower pole level.
Surgical Treatment. Small posterior neoplasm adhering to internal dural surface.
Results. Over the following 15 days the patient started walking. One month later, a neurological examination was negative. This condition persisted for 16 years.

Case No. 122: Psammomatous Meningioma

A 63-year-old woman (1978). Posterior intradural-extramedullary meningioma in D8-D9.
Clinical Course. 2 years. Burning type of paraesthesias to right leg, to sole of foot (operated on in another hospital for herniated disc 2 years previously). Subjective motor weakness to right lower limb then to left. Paraesthesias of an ascending nature.
Neurological Examination. Severe spastic paraparesis with foot clonus and bilateral Babinski sign. Hypoaesthesia from D10. Sphincter disturbances in the form of incontinence.
X-Ray of Dorsal Rachis. Slight scoliosis.
Myelography (via lumbar puncture). Total block in D9 without producing the characteristic image.
Surgical Treatment. Hypervascularization of the laminae. On opening the dura the subarachnoidal neoplasm adhered to the internal surface of the dura. Excision en bloc of the meningioma. The cord presented a shadow corresponding to the site of the tumour.
Results. Recovery of voluntary movements in only 10 days. Condition persisted after 8 months.

Case No. 48: Transitional Meningioma

A 56-year-old woman (1978). Left posterolateral intradural-extramedullary meningioma in D8 (see Chap. 9).

Case No. 43: Transitional Psammomatous Meningioma

A 75-year-old woman (1978). Premedullary intradural-extramedullary meningioma (see Chap. 6).

Case No. 69: Meningothelian Meningioma

A 56-year-old woman (1978). Left intra- and extradural meningioma with extrarachidian extension in a posterolateral site in L1-L3 (see Chap. 8).

Case No. 107: Meningothelial and Psammomatous Meningioma

A 57-year-old woman (1978). Left posterolateral intradural-extramedullary meningioma in D7 (see Chap. 8).

Case No. 102: Psammomatous Meningioma

A 49-year-old woman (1979). Left lateral intradural-extramedullary meningioma in D3-D4.
Medical History. Hypertension for 10 years.
Clinical Course. 1 year. Back pain with painful paraesthesias to lower limbs (plain laminectomy performed in another hospital with a diagnosis of discoarthrosis at D3-D4 level). Motor impairment at right lower limb spreading to left limb. Twenty days prior to hospitalization the patient complained of a feeling of constriction to the upper thoracic region irradiating to left scapula.
Neurological Examination. Paraplegia with bilateral foot clonus and Babinski sign. Hypoaesthesia from D4-D12 bilaterally.
X-Ray of Dorsal Rachis. Scoliosis of upper dorsal tract with thinning of articular facets of D3 on the right.
Myelography (performed suboccipally). Total block in D3 producing an irregular dome-shaped image.
Surgical Treatment. On opening the dura the neoplasm appeared to invade the internal surface of the dura on the left near the fourth dorsal root's entry zone. Removal in toto.
Results. For 1 month contracture was diminished and voluntary motility appeared. After 3 months walking began. Recovery 6 months later.

Case No. 41: Transitional Meningioma

A 63-year-old woman (1979; Fig. 315). Right anterolateral intradural-extramedullary meningioma in D11-D12.
Clinical Course. 5 months. Paraesthesias distally to feet of an ascending nature. Motor deficit to lower limbs and instability in walking.
Neurological Examination. Spastic-ataxic paraparesis. Hypoaesthesias bilaterally from D12.
Rachicentesis. 0.54 g protein per thousnd.
X-Ray of Dorsal Rachis. Anomaly in spinous processes of D8 and D9, obliquely towards the left, and of D10 on the right.
Myelography (performed suboccipally). Total block producing a

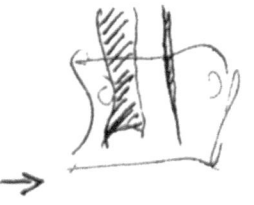
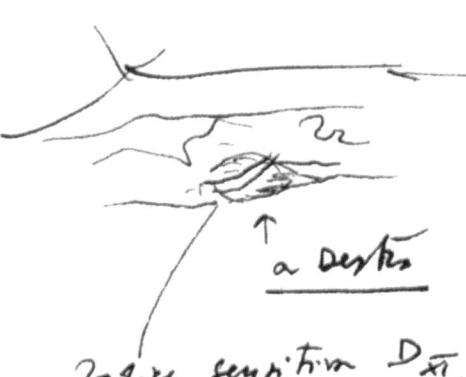

Fig. 315. Right anterolateral intradural-extramedullary meningioma in D11-D12

dome-shaped image and slight lateral flow on the left.

Surgical Treatment. On opening the dura the cord was displaced to the left by a laterally located neoplasm. The 11th dorsal root surrounded the tumour as a band. Total excision and coagulation of the base of attachment.

Results. Walking returned to normal in 10 days. Total recovery after 4 months.

Case No. 67: Meningothelial Meningioma

A 64-year-old man (1979; Fig. 316). Right posterolateral intradural-extramedullary meningioma in D1.

Medical History. Vascular-based encephalopathy.

Clinical Course. 1 year. Motor deficit to lower limbs and instability in walking.

Neurological Examination. Severe spastic paraparesis with bilat-

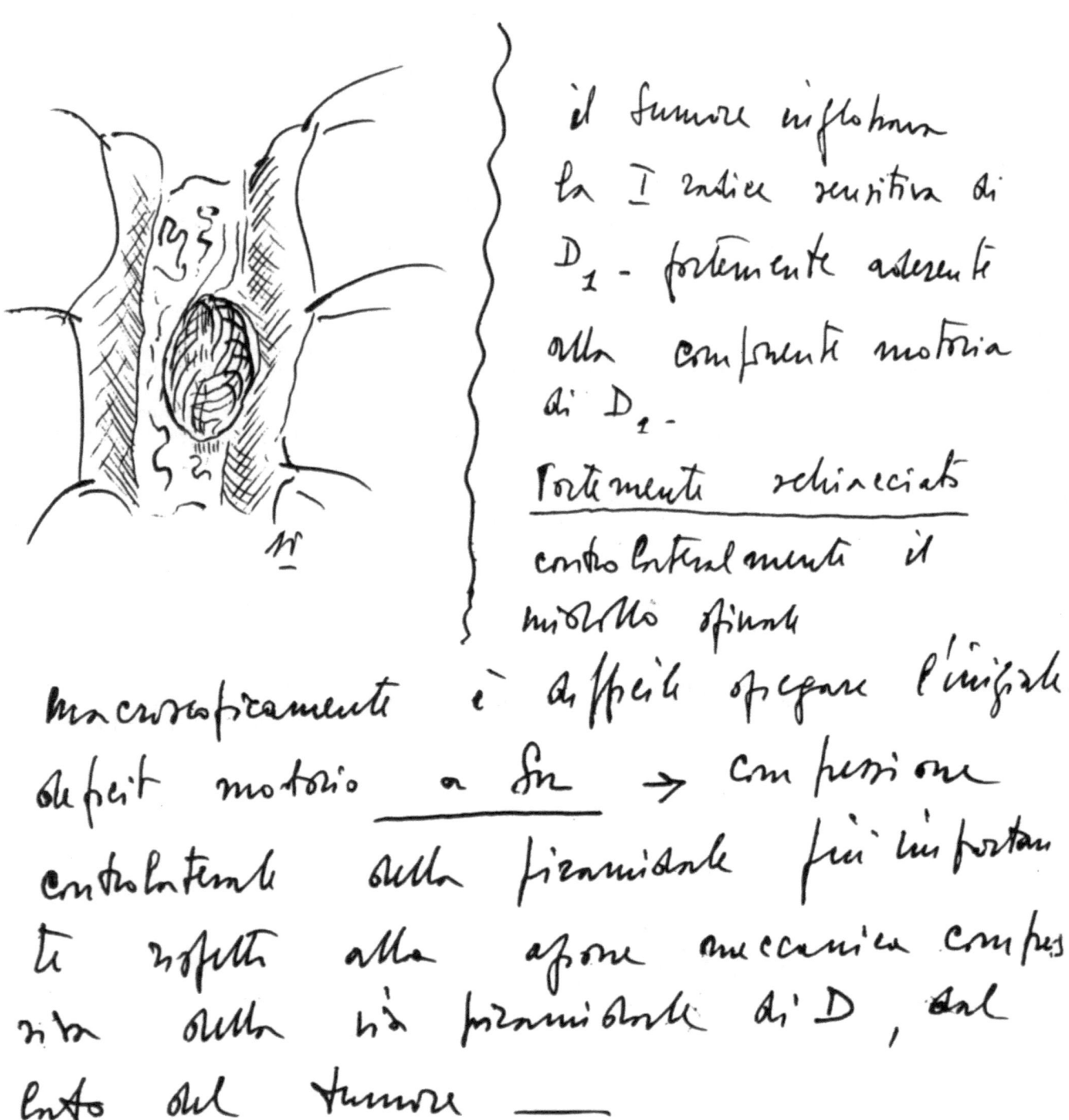

Fig. 316. Right posterolateral intradural-extramedullary meningioma in D1

eral foot clonus. Hypoaesthesia affecting superficial tactile and pain sensitivity from D5. Anaesthesia from D8. Sphincter disturbances in the form of incontinence.

Myelography (performed suboccipitally). Total block enlarged in D1 producing a dome-shaped image.

Surgical Treatment. On incising the dura a tumour was seen in a posterolateral site adhering to the medullary surface up to the radicular funnel. The cord appeared arched towards the left. The neoplasm was 2 cm long and pushed the motor root forwards. Excision of the meningioma in toto after a radicotomy of D1.

Results. After 20 h there was improvement, with less heaviness felt in the legs. After 2 days comatous state with hemiparesis on the left. CT on the cranium showed a greater ventricular dilatation on the right. Death occurred 25 days later due to bronchopneumonia, hyperthermia and high glycaemia level.

Case No. 116: Psammomatous Meningioma

A 72-year-old woman (1980). Posterior intradural-extramedullary meningioma in D10-D11 (see Chap. 9).

Case No. 73: Psammomatous Meningioma

A 60-year-old man (1980). Intramedullary meningioma in C1 (see Chap. 8).

Case No. 97: Transitional Meningioma

A 71-year-old woman (1980). Anterior intradural-extramedullary meningioma in D11 (see Chap. 8).

Case No. 27: Fibroblastic Meningioma

A 57-year-old woman (1980; Fig. 317). Premedullary intradural-extramedullary meningioma in D8-D9.

Medical History. Diabetes.

Clinical Course. 15 years. Occasional back pain. Two years prior to hospitalization burning type of paraesthesias and motor deficit to lower limbs to the right. Painful radicular syndrome to left hip.

Neurological Examination. Syndactylia of second and third toes of left foot. Severe spastic paraparesis with equinism attitude of feet. Left foot clonus. Bilateral Babinski sign. Band of hypoaesthesia in D11-L1. Sphincter disturbances in the form of incontinence.

Rachicentesis. 1 g protein per thousand.

X-Ray of Dorsal Rachis. Scoliosis. The left articular facet in D9 appeared thinned. A small roundish calcification was seen at the upper, somatic margin of D10.

Myelography (performed suboccipally). Dome-shaped block slightly irregular a little above the intersomatic space of D8-D9.

Surgical Treatment. On opening the dura the medullary circulation appeared in stasis. The cord was thinned and covered the tumour which was of a hard consistency and closely adhered to its surface. Removal by fragmentation.

Results. During the following 15 days the patient started walking. Recovery 1 month later.

Case No. 105: Psammomatous Meningioma

A 69-year-old woman (1981). Left posterolateral intradural-extramedullary meningioma in D1-D2 adhering to the left root of D2 (see Chap. 6).

Case No. 24: Meningothelial Meningioma

A 28-year-old woman (1981). Right anterolateral intradural-extramedullary meningioma in D2.

Medical History. Operated on for left mammary fibro-adenoma.

Clinical Course. 10 years. Fastidious paraesthesias at upper dorsal tract irradiating anteriorly, girdle-like to right mammary region. Seven months prior to hospitalization and in the sixth month of pregnancy a heaviness felt at the right lower limb. After the birth she

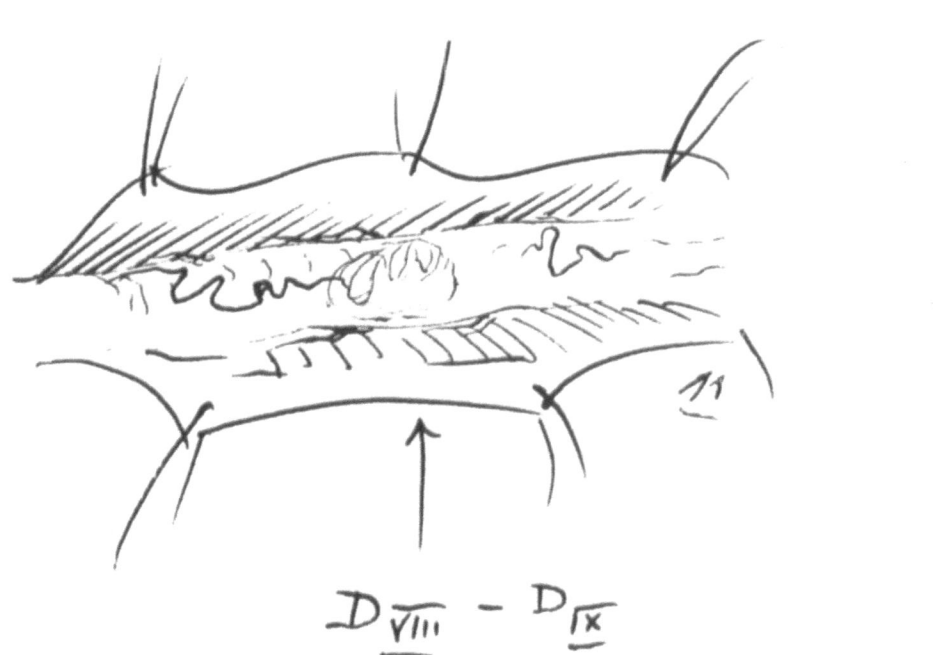

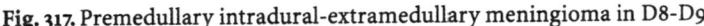

Fig. 317. Premedullary intradural-extramedullary meningioma in D8-D9

was affected by painful paraesthesias to the right lower limb and ingravescent motor weakness.

Neurological Examination. Flaccid paraplegia. Lack of patella reflex and ankle jerk. Hypoaesthesias from D4 becoming anaesthesia distally to lower limbs for the various forms of sensitivity. Sphincter disturbances in the form of retention.

X-Ray of Dorsal Rachis. Slight scoliosis of the upper dorsal tract.

Myelography (performed suboccipally). Block in D2 producing a dome-shaped image on the right, while the contrast medium tended to flow towards the external left side.

Surgical Treatment. The dural sac appeared swollen posteriorly. On incising the dura the medullary surface was whitish in colour and ischaemic. In front of the posterior root of D2 the meningioma invaded the internal anterolateral surface of the dural sac. Part of the tumour lay below. Removal by fragmentation and coagulation of the dural attachment.

Results. After 1.5 months reappearance of some voluntary flexion movements. Thirteen years later walking was possible with right hypertonia.

Case No. 25: Transitional Meningioma

A 63-year-old woman (1981; Fig. 318). Left ventrolateral intradural-extramedullary meningioma in D7-D8.

Clinical Course. 6 months. Painful paraesthesias to right lower limb followed by motor deficit to both lower limbs. One month prior to hospitalization the patient complained of precordial pain which seemed a myocardial disorder.

Neurological Examination. Severe spastic paraparesis. Hypoaesthesia from D7 bilaterally. Sphincter disturbances in the form of incontinence.

X-Ray of Dorsal Rachis. Right convex scoliosis with fulcrum in D7-D8.

Myelography (performed suboccipally). Block in D7-D8 with a thickened left side flow. Slight inclination towards the right. The subarachnoidal space above the block appeared dilatated.

Surgical Treatment. The left posterolateral tract of the dura appeared hypervascularized and yielded no pulsations. On incising the dura the neoplasm was gradually extricated. It appeared to be partly of a friable and partly of a hard consistency. Excision by fragmentation after freeing the arachnoidal layer which adhered to the ventral surface of the meningioma. Its attachment invaded the internal surface of the dura. After excision there was an evident shell-shaped shadow on the medullary surface left by the meningioma.

Results. Over the following 20 days the patient started walking. After 9 months he was considered clinically recovered. Residual slight spastic component to right lower limb (site corresponding to the onset of symptoms).

Case No. 74: Psammomatous Meningioma

A 60-year-old male (1981; Fig. 319). Right posterolateral intradural-extramedullary meningioma in D2-D3 (1981).

Relapse. Angioblastic meningioma (1989).

Clinical course. 1 year. Hot and cold paraesthesias at lower limbs to the left. Motor deficit to lower limbs to the right with impediment in walking (laminectomy at D5-D6 performed in another hospital).

Neurological Examination. Spastic paraparesis to the right. Lack of abdomenal reflexes bilaterally. Hypoaesthesia from D6 to the left. Sphincter disturbances in the form of imperious micturation.

Rachicentesis. 2.4 g protein per thousand.

X-Ray of Dorsal Rachis. Partial laminectomy of D4 and total of D5 and D6.

Myelography (performed suboccipally). Block producing an irregular image in D1.

Myelography (via lumbar puncture). Total block in D3.

Surgical Treatment. On opening the dura a neoplasm of a hard consistency was seen to invade the internal surface of the dura. The cord appeared atrophic, showed signs of ischaemia and was displaced to the right. Removal en bloc without a radicotomy.

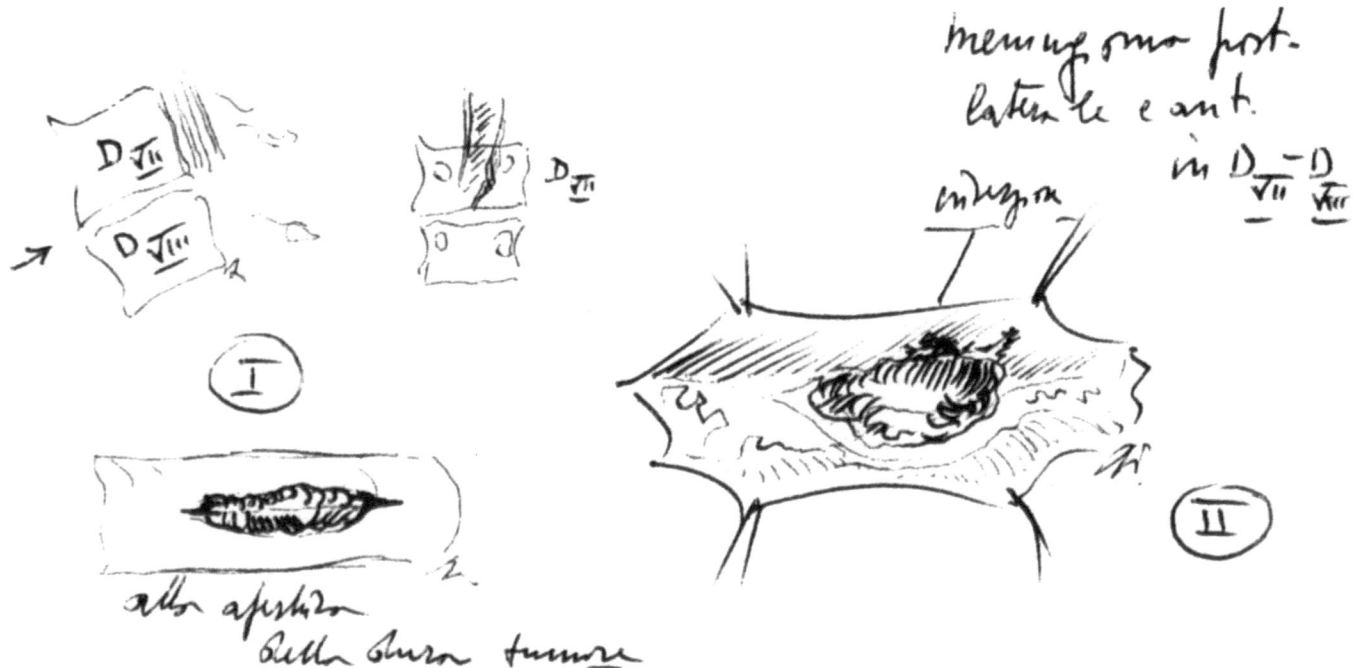

Fig. 318. Left ventrolateral intradural-extramedullary meningioma in D7-D8

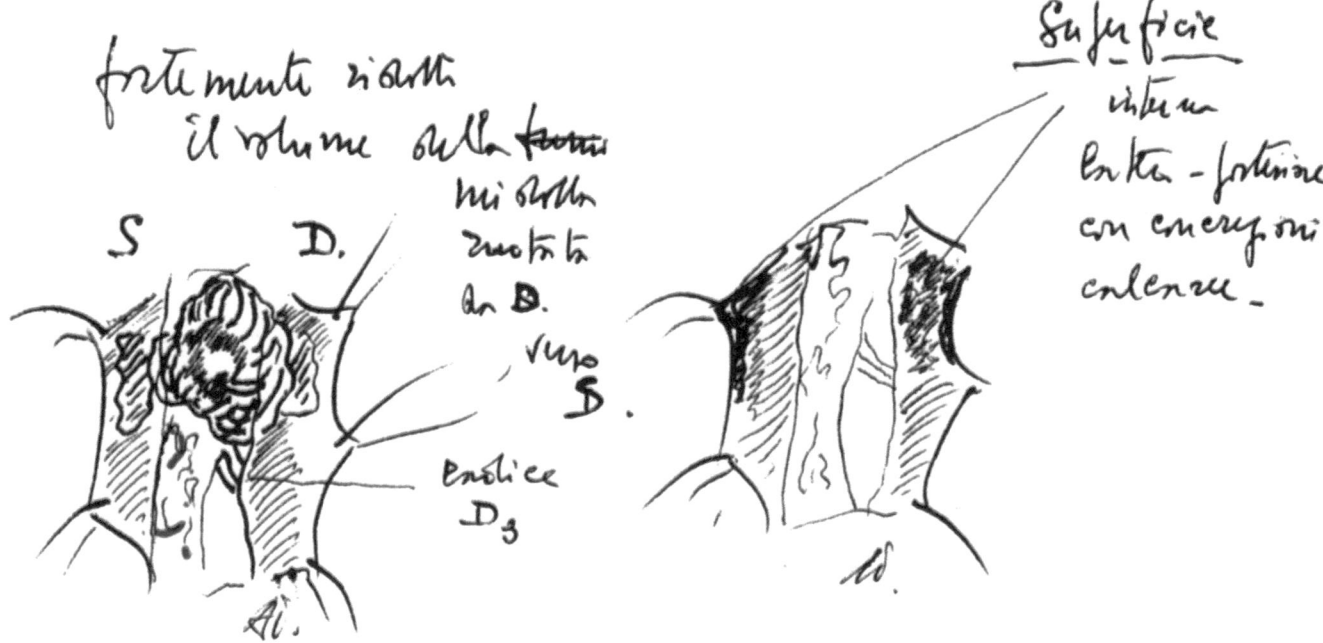

Fig. 319. Right posterolateral intradural-extramedullary meningioma in D2-D3

Results. Improvement in walking after 15 days. The patient was considered clinically recovered after 3 months.

The patient's condition remained stable for 8 years. Nine months before the second operation he was affected by motor weakness again to the right with paraesthesias to the left.

Neurological Examination. Spastic paraparesis with foot clonus. Bilateral Babinski sign. Hypoaesthesia left.

Rachicentesis. 0.80 g protein per thousand.

X-Ray of Dorsal Rachis. Left laterally located calcified area at the level of the laminectomy.

Myelography. Filling defect below the level of the laminectomy.

Myelo-CT. Partial block from D1-D3 showing an apparently intradural formation in a posterolateral site which displaced the cord towards the left.

Surgical Treatment. On opening the dura there was a tumour recurrence with an evident compression of the cord towards the left. Total removal together with a great part of the dura.

Results. Postoperative motor inhibition. After 2 months an initial recovery of voluntary movements of the lower limbs.

Case No. 86: Fibroblastic Meningioma

A 73-year-old woman (1981). Premedullary, intradural-extramedullary meningioma in D6-D7.

Clinical Course. 1 year. Constriction type of paraesthesias to the right leg followed by loss of strength to right lower limb with motor claudication. Back pain arose as the last symptom.

Neurological Examination. Spastic paraparesis to the right. Hypoaesthesia from D8 bilaterally.

Myelography. Total block producing a dome-shaped image showing the upper and lower poles of the tumour.

Surgical Treatment. The cord appeared atrophic and displaced posteriorly, reduced to a thin thread. Gradual splitting of tumour to reveal the capsule, which was incised. Fragmented excision, reclining the meningioma against the dural plane.

Results. In the first postoperative days the patient felt a slight heaviness to the right lower limb. Twenty days later walking proved satisfactory. Complete recovery after 1 month.

Case No. 32: Transitional Meningioma

A 74-year-old woman (1981). Ventral intradural-extramedullary meningioma in D9-D10.

Clinical Course. 6 years. Sudden loss of strength in the right lower limb. The same occurred in the left limb and resulted in a fall and a fracture of left malleolus. Four months prior to hospitalization the patient fell and fractured right foot.

Neurological Examination. Flaccid paraplegia. Hypoaesthesia from D10 becoming anaesthesia on the left on L1 and from L2 on the right.

X-Ray Dorsal Tract. Scoliosis.

Myelography (performed suboccipitally). Total dome-shaped block on the left in D9-D10.

Surgical Treatment. The cord had lost its surface-layer vascularization and resembled a thin lamina pushed and curved posteriorly. The meningioma adhered to the ventral surface of the dura. Freeing of the arachnoidal adherent structures and fragmented removal of the neoplasm.

Results. The neurological picture was unchanged. Some flexion movements appeared on the right leg after 1 month. Flex extention movements on the left were good 4 months later and 1 year later the patient was able to walk with support.

Case No. 101: Transitional Meningioma

A 78-year-old woman (1981; Fig. 320). Premedullary intradural-extramedullary meningioma in D10-D11.

Clinical Course. 3 years. Fastidious dorsolumbar sensations. Progressive motor weakness in lower limbs to the left leading to paraplegia.

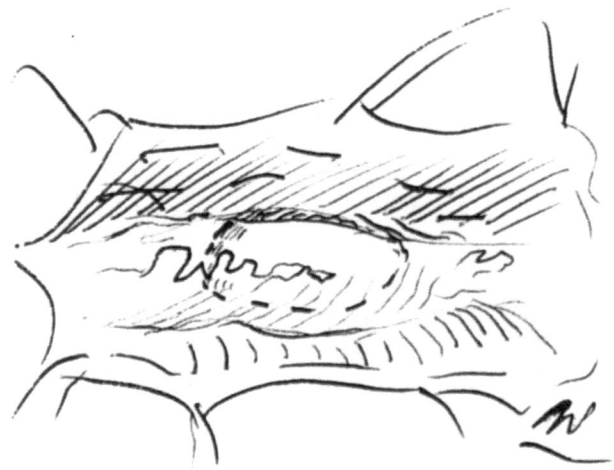
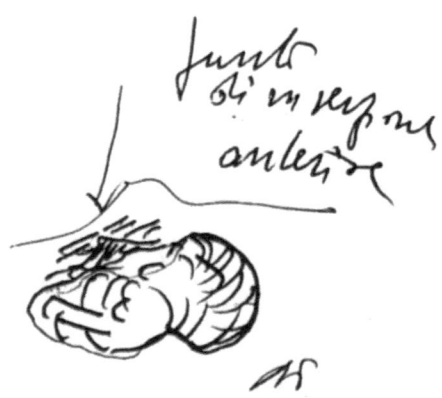

Fig. 320. Premedullary intradural-extramedullary meningioma in D10-D11

Neurological Examination. Severe spasticity with bilateral foot clonus. Hypoaesthesia from L1 to L4 with anaesthesia below. Sphincter disturbances in the form of retention.
Rachicentesis. 1.40 g protein per thousand.
X-Ray of Dorsolumbar Tract. Scoliosis with fulcrum in D9-D10.
Myelography. Total block in D11-D12. Dilatation of the arachnoidal space above the lesion. The corridor corresponding to the cord was dispalced to the right.
Surgical Treatment. Opening the arachnoid the posterior circulation of the cord appeared dilatated. Freeing the arachnoid revealed the site of the meningioma. Incision of the capsule and fragmented removal with coagulation of the anterior base of attachment.
Results. No changes in the neurological picture after 1 month.

Case No. 60: Psammomatous Meningioma
A 62-year-old woman (1982). Right anterolateral intradural-extramedullary meningioma in D5-D6 (see Chap. 6).

Case No. 34: Meningolethial Meningioma
A 66-year-old woman (1982). Right posterolateral intradural-extramedullary meningioma in D6-D7 (see Chap. 6).

Case No. 103: Fibroblastic Meningioma
A 58-year-old woman (1982). Left anterolateral intradural-extramedullary meningioma in D2-D3.
Clinical Course. 3 months. Pain at posterior side of left leg and weakness. Claudication with paraesthesias also on the right.
Neurological Examination. Severe spastic paraparesis to the left. On this side the lower limb was almost plegic. Bilateral foot clonus and Babinski sign. Hypoaesthesia on D5-D6 and total anaesthesia from D7. Retention of urine.
X-Ray of Dorsolumbar Tract. Scoliosis with thinning of right peduncle of D2.
Myelography (performed suboccipitally). Block in D2-D3. Slight flow on the right.
Surgical Treatment. Left ventrolateral tumour which displaced the cord towards the right. Fragmented removal.
Results. Improvement in motor deficit only at right. One month later reflexes on the left responded to stimulation. Improved sphincter disturbances. Satisfactory recovery of walking after 2 months.

Case No. 60: Transitional Meningioma
A 62-year-old woman (1982). Right anterolateral intradural-extramedullary meningioma in D5-D6.
Clinical Course. 1 year. Dorsal pain irradiating girdle-like to the right. For 6 months reduced sensitivity to thorax to the right and motor impediment at the legs.
Neurological examination. Spastic-ataxic paraparesis to the right. Bilateral foot clonus and Babinski sign. Hypoaesthesia from D7. Retention of urine.
X-Ray of Dorsal Rachis. Alterations in vertebral bodies of D5 in a slight calcified area of the right lower lateral portion.
Myelography (via lumbar puncture). Block on the right in D5-D6, producing a dome-shaped filling defect. A small amount of contrast medium passed the block defining an oval-shaped area.
Surgical Treatment. Opening the dura the cord was curved towards the left and the right presented the surface of the neoplasm with a sensory root wrapped round it. After opening the arachnoid the capsule was incised and the tumour debulked. The surface-layer circulation was thinned.
Results. During the following 15 days the patient was able to walk; walking became normal after 3 months. This condition remained stable after 1 year. Residual slight submammary pain on the right.

Case No. 61: Fibroblastic Meningioma
A 64-year-old woman (1982). Left posterolateral and anterior intradural-extramedullary meningioma in D12-L1.
Clinical Course. 7 years. Occasional back pain. One year before hospitalization, pain irradiating to left hip and inguinal area. Motor claudication and tingling paraesthesias distally in both lower limbs to the left.
Neurological Examination. Severe flaccid paraparesis. Left Babinski sign. Band of hyperaesthesia from D10 to L1. Hypoaesthesia from L1 becoming anaesthesia from L4 bilaterally. Sphincter disturbances in the form of retention.
Rachicentesis. 1.30 g protein per thousand.
X-Ray of Dorsolumbar Tract. The vertebral body of D12 appeared less clear and less calcified than the right lamina and the articular facets. In L1 the right articular facet was also thinned.
Myelography (via lumbar puncture). Total block in D12-L1.
Surgical Treatment. Opening the dura, a tumour of a reddish-wine colour and adhered to the internal surface of the dura. Large invasion along the internal anterior dural surface. The cord appeared

reduced in volume and compressed towards the right. Fragmented excision and total removal of arachnoidal adherent structures from the medullary surface contralaterally.

Results. Two weeks later the patient started walking. Clinical recovery after 6 months.

Case No. 63: Psammomatous Meningioma

A 77-year-old woman (1982). Left posterolateral intradural-extramedullary meningioma in D5-D6.

Clinical Course. 1 year. Tingling parasthesias at feet. Ingravescent motor deficit with motor claudication. Retarded constriction sensations as a band in the submammary region.

Neurological Examination. Severe spastic paraparesis to the left. Right Babinski sign. Hypoaesthesia from D4. Anaesthesia from D6-D7. Sphincter disturbances in the form of retention.

X-Ray of Dorsal Tract. Widespread spondyloarthrosis. The articular facets in D6 seemed diminished.

Myelography (performed suboccipitally). Block in D5-D6 producing a cuneiform image.

Surgical Treatment. Opening the dura the tumour appeared the size of an almond and did not adhere to the internal surface of the dura but showed left posterolateral invasion of the pia mater. Fragmented excision.

Results. Initial motor inhibition. After 15 days a few voluntary movements were made by the left lower limb. Two months later satisfactory improvement in movements. Walking was possible with support after 6 months.

Case No. 104: Transitional Meningioma

A 74-year-old woman (1982). Right anterolateral intradural-extramedullary meningioma in D4.

Clinical Course. 3 years. Band type of constriction at submammary area. Back pain and motor deficit at legs.

Neurological Examination. Spastic paraplegia. Hypoaesthesia from D2-D3 bilaterally with anaesthesia from D4. Retention of urine.

Rachicentesis. 3 g protein per thousand.

X-Ray of Dorsal Tract. Scoliosis with slight erosion of articular pedicle of D3 and D4.

Myelography (performed suboccipitally). Dome-shaped block in D3-D4. Slight flow on the left which defined the neoplasm.

Surgical Treatment. The cord was curved backwards and appeared flattened. Opening of the arachnoid and examining the right showed a premedullary neoplasm. Fragmented excision.

Results. Satisfactory recovery of the flex-extention voluntary movements on 20th day. Better on the left.

Case No. 62: Meningothelial Meningioma

A 62-year-old woman (1982; Fig. 321). Premedullary intradural-extramedullary meningioma in L1.

Clinical Course. 15 years. Lumbago without irradiation; more intense in the previous 2 years. For 6 months the patient had suffered from true bilateral pain to the hip and to the inguinal area. For 2 months, sciatica on both sides with motor deficit to lower limbs.

Neurological Examination. Slight spastic paraparesis with hyperreflexia without signs of sensory deficit.

X-Ray of Dorsolumbar Tract. Scoliosis of the dorsolumbar passage. Erosion of the posterior margin of the vertebral body of L1 with thinning of the lamina and increased interlamina space. Erosion of the peduncle of L1 on the right while L2 appeared thicker.

Rachicentesis. 0.39 g protein per thousand.

Myelography (performed suboccipitally). Dome-shaped block on the right in L1.

Surgical Treatment. Opening the dura the surface-layer circulation of the conus and entry zone of the roots appeared very thin. The medullary cone was reclined showing a ventral well-capsulated neoplasm. A root was enveloped by the tumour. Incision of the capsule and fragmented excision after performing a radicotomy.

Results. Regression of lower limb paralysis over 15 days and walking became possible. Clinical recovery in 3 months. The patient's condition remained stable after 2 years.

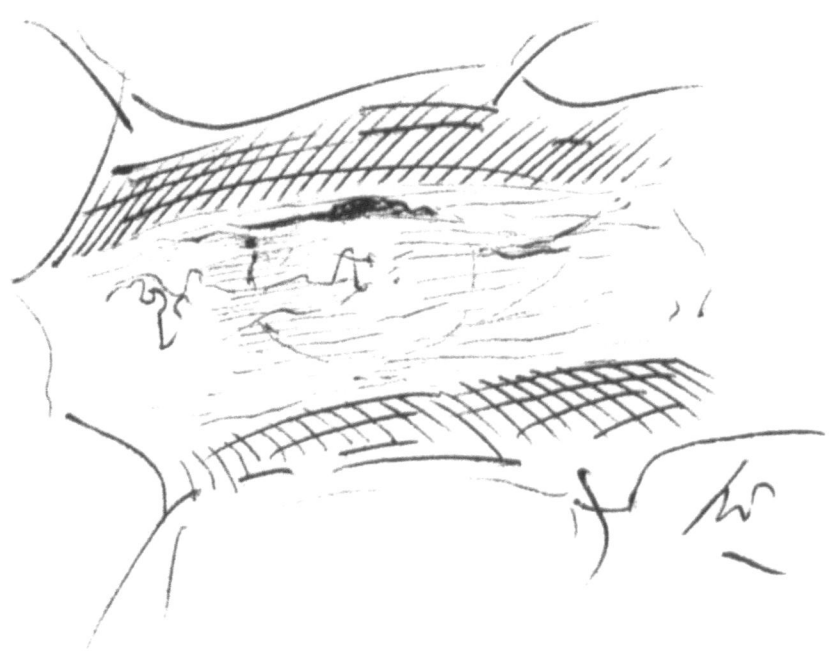

Fig. 321. Premedullary intradural-extramedullary meningioma in L1

Case No. 98: Nonclassified Meningioma

A 65-year-old woman (1982). Left anterolateral intradural-extramedullary meningioma in D2-D3.

Clinical Course. 2 years. Burning type of paraesthesias to lower limbs: gluteus, anterior side of left thigh and posteriorly down to the feet to the left. Motor claudication to right knee. Retarded constriction as a band to the submammary area.

Neurological Examination. Spastic paraparesis with right foot clonus. Hypoaesthesia from D2 bilaterally. Urine incontinent.

X-Ray of Dorsal Rachis. Thinning of articular facets in D1-D2.

Myelography (performed suboccipitally). Transitory block in D2-D3. Slight flow on the left was curved towards the exterior.

Surgical Treatment. Opening the dura the cord appeared atrophic. After freeing the arachnoid the cord was gently reclined towards the right. Incision of the capsule and fragmented excision. The left anterolateral invasion appeared calcified.

Results. Complete motor inhibition for 15 days. After 1.5 months good motility to left lower limb but persisting extention contracture on the right. Four months later walking was possible with bilateral support.

Case No. 36: Transitional Meningioma

An 82-year-old woman (1984). Posterior intradural-extramedullary meningioma in D5-D6 (see Chap. 8).

Case No. 109: Transitional Meningioma

A 75-year-old woman (1984). Posterior intradural-extramedullary meningioma in D8-D9.

Clinical Course. 2 years. Ascending paraesthesias to lower limbs to the right, with loss of strength to the left.

Neurological Examination. Spastic paraparesis with bilateral clonus of the patellar. Hypoaesthesia from D11 with band of hyperaesthesia from D8 and D10 on the right and on D11 on the left. Hypopall-

aesthesia from iliac crests.

Rachicentesis. 0.80 g protein per thousand.

X-Ray of Dorsolumbar. Scoliosis.

Myelography (via lumbar puncture). Block in D9. Dilatation above the subarachnoidal space on the left.

Surgical Treatment. The cord appeared atrophic and the surface-layer circulation extremely thinned. The tumour invaded the internal surface of the dura and the cord was displaced forwards. Excision en bloc.

Results. In 1 week the patient was able to stand upright. Clinical recovery in 2 months.

Case No. 50: Transitional Meningioma

A 63-year-old woman (1983; Fig. 322). Right posterolateral intradural-extramedullary meningioma in D3-D4.

Clinical Course. 6 months. Sensory cord disturbances with burning type of paraesthesia to anterior side of left thigh, of an ascending nature up to the left hemithorax. Later, stiffness to both lower limbs with progressive motor deficit to the left.

Neurological Examination. Severe spastic paraparesis with left foot clonus and bilateral Babinski sign. Painful hypoaesthesia from D6 bilaterally and thermal from D4 on the right. Pallaesthetic anaesthesia from D6. Sphincter disturbances in the form of retention.

Rachicentesis. 0.42 g protein per thousand.

X-Ray of Dorsal Rachis. Scoliosis and thinning of articular facets of D3-D4 bilaterally.

Myelography (via lumbar puncture). Transitional block producing a dome-shaped image in D3-D4 on the right.

Surgical Treatment. Opening the dura a neoplasm was seen lying in the subarachnoidal area which pushed the flattened cord towards the left. The subarachnoidal space was wide and the tumour passed the right dentate ligaments which tended to be particularly expanded. Total excision.

Results. The patient started walking during the first month but retained slight spasticity. Clinically recovered in 10 months.

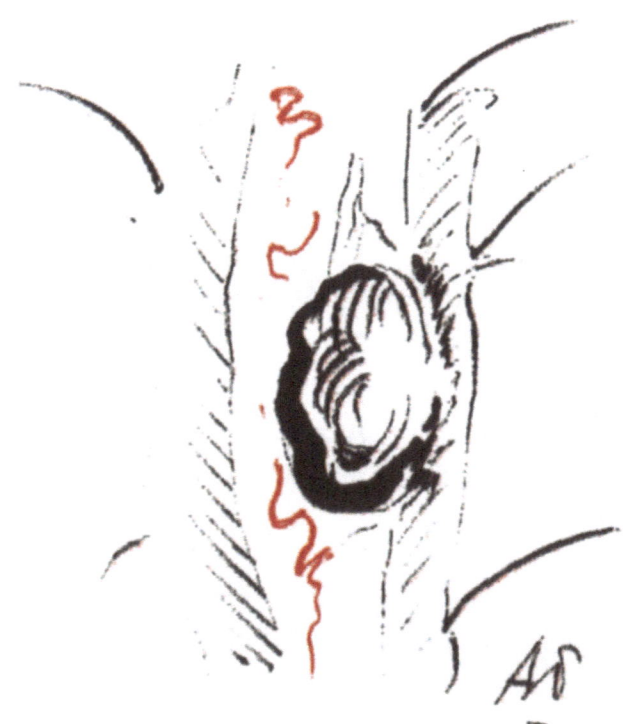

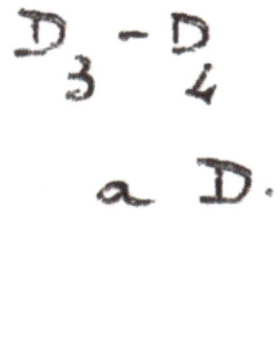

Fig. 322. Right posterolateral intradural-extramedullary meningioma in D3-D4

Case No. 126: Transitional Meningioma

A 27-year-old woman (1984; Fig. 323). Premedullary-intradural meningioma in D5-D6.

Medical History. Operated on for cutaneous angioma at the lower dorsal tract level in the first months of life.

Clinical Course. 10 years. Burning type of paraesthesias at lower limbs and loss of strength to the left.

Neurological Examination. Spastic paraparesis to the left. Foot clonus and bilateral Babinski. Hypoaesthesia from D6 and D8 on the left.

Myelography (via lumbar puncture). Dome-shaped block in D5 with slight lateral flow on the left.

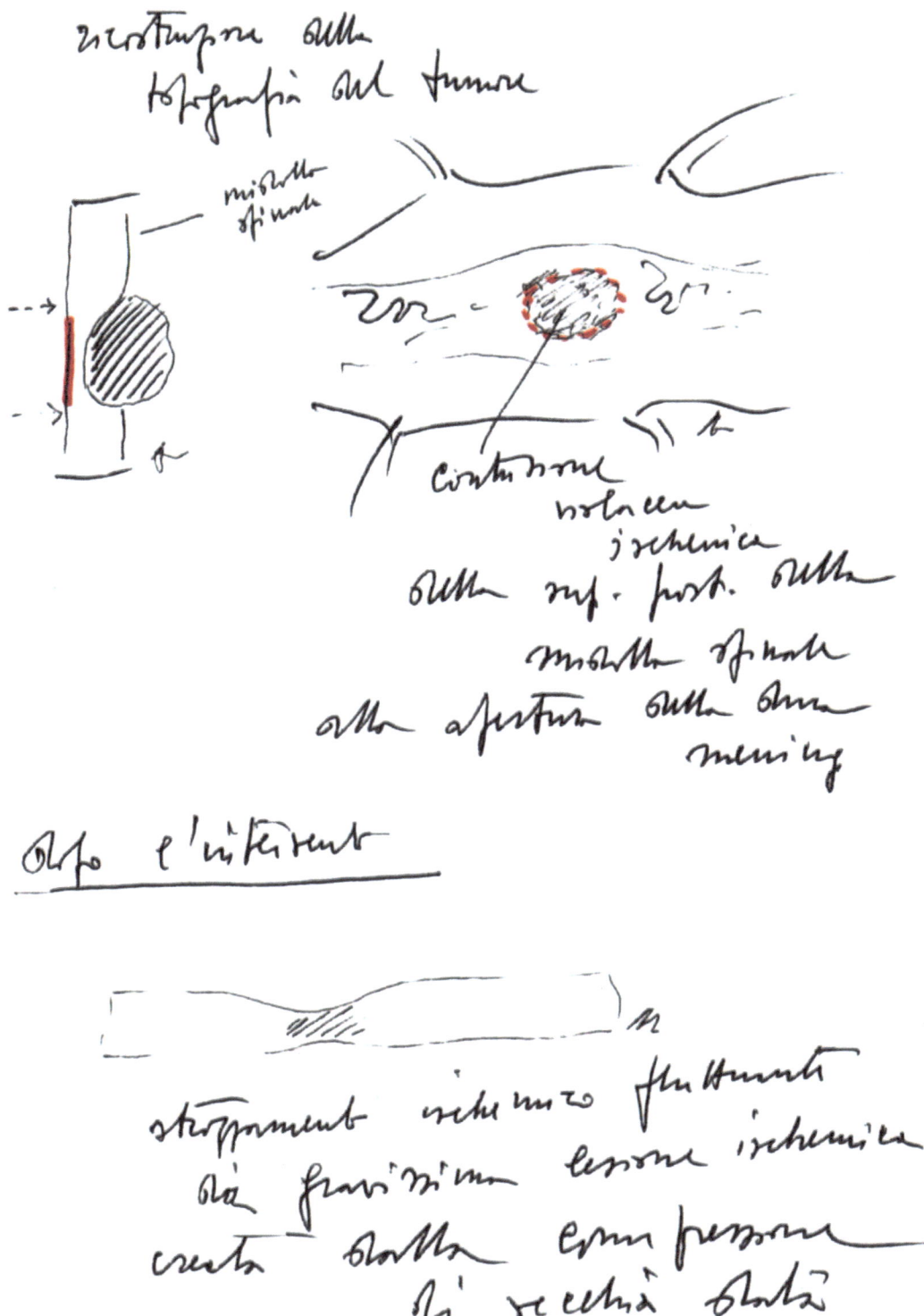

Fig. 323. Premedullary intradural meningioma in D5-D6

Surgical Treatment. The cord of a violet colour on the posterior side was curved towards the back and resembled a thin lamella. Incision of the capsule adhering to the right sixth motor dorsal root. Debulking of the tumour and total excision.

Results. The severe spastic paraparesis did not regress even after 1 year.

Case No. 125: Psammomatous Meningioma

A 61-year-old woman (1984; Fig. 324). Posterior and lateral intradural-extramedullary meningioma on both sides in D10-D11.

Clinical Course. 3 years. Motor weakness to the legs with initial distal slight motor claudication.

Neurological Examination. Spastic paraparesis. Hypotrophy of the inferior third of the right femoral quadricep. Slight bilateral patella and foot clonus. Bilateral Babinski sign. Hypoaesthesia from D11 distally. Hypopallaesthesia from the iliac crests.

Rachicentesis. 0.23 g prorein per thousand.

Myelography (performed suboccipitally). Block in D9-D10. Slight lateral flow on the left.

Surgical Treatment. Dural incision revealed a completely calcified neoplasm in a posterior site. Total fragmented removal. The cord was thinned.

Results. Rapid improvement and walking was possible after 2 months.

Case No. 59: Ossified Transitional Meningioma

A 63-year-old man (1985). Left posterolateral intradural-extramedullary meningioma in D11-D12 (see Chap. 8).

Clinical Course. 10 years. Constricted band-like back pain to left submammary. Tingling paraesthesias to lower limbs and motor weakness to the left. Two years prior to hospitalization the patient was affected by saddle-like paraesthesias.

Neurological Examination. Spastic paraparesis to the left with bilateral Babinski sign. Hypoaesthesia for the various forms of sensitivity from L1 on the left and L3 on the right. Urinary incontinence.

X-Ray of Dorsal Tract. Increase in interpeduncular distance in D12-L1.

Myelography Performed Laterocervically. Transitional block in D11-D12. The contrast medium defined the upper and lower poles of the neoplasm which was more developed on the left.

Surgical Treatment. The reddish-wine coloured tumour compressed the conus terminale forwards and invaded the internal surface of the dura in a left posterolateral site. Fragmented excision after removing the ventral surface of the tumour from the leptomeninges.

Results. The patient started walking in 10 days. Complete recovery in 1 year.

Case No. 71: Transitional Meningioma

A 64-year-old woman (1985; Fig. 325). Right posterolateral intradural-extramedullary meningioma in D1-D2.

Clinical Course. 10 years. Frequent back pain attacks. For 2 years, loss of strength to right lower limb and later to the left limb with motor claudication. Ascending tingling type of paraesthesias to feet spreading to the inguinal region.

Neurological Examination. Spastic paraparesis with foot clonus and bilateral Babinski sign. Hypoaesthesia from D7 bilaterally and

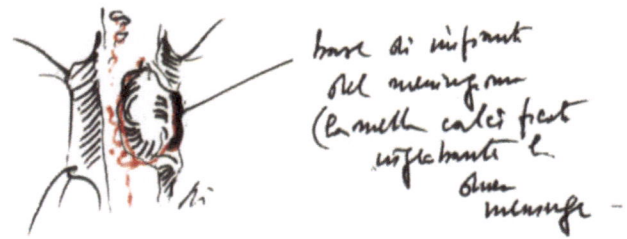

Fig. 325. Right posterolateral intradural-extramedullary meningioma in D1-D2

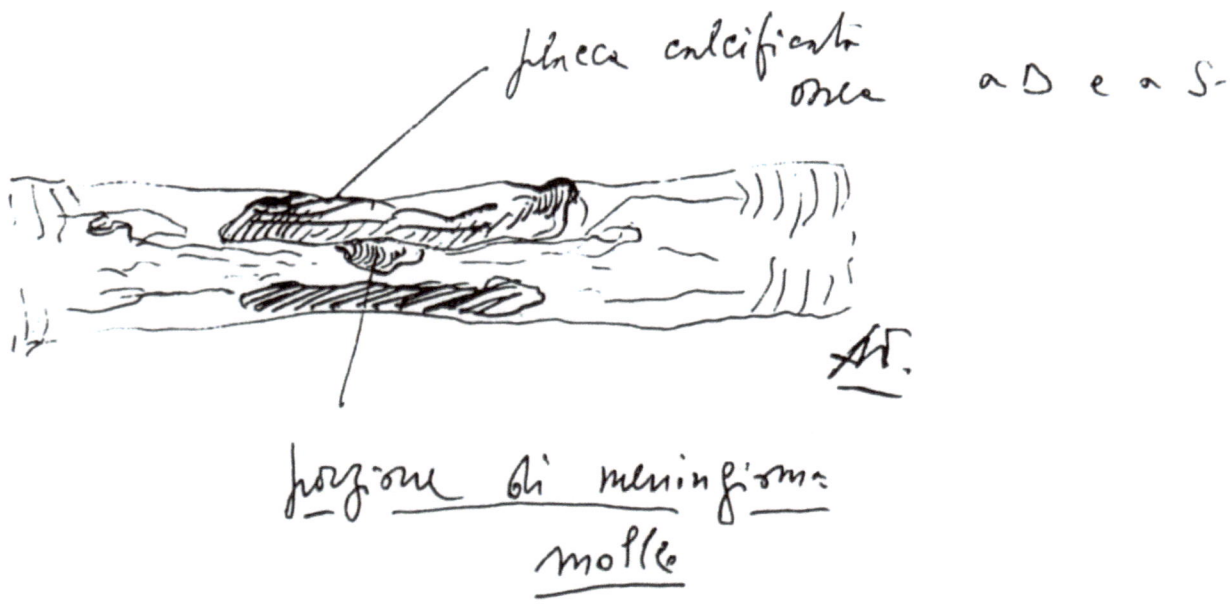

Fig. 324. Posterior and lateral intradural-extramedullary meningioma in D10-D11

hypopallaesthesia from iliac crests. Sphincter disturbances in the form of incontinence.

Rachicentesis. 0.65 g protein per thousand.

X-Ray of Dorsal Rachis. Slight scoliosis.

Myelography (via lumbar puncture). Transitory block in D1 defining the upper and lower poles of the neoplasm.

Surgical Treatment. Paramedian opening of the dura: the cord was displaced to the left by a lateral right neoplasm which adhered to the lateroventral surface of the cord. The right second dorsal root was pushed forwards. The base of attachment of the meningioma was formed by a calcified lamella on the internal surface layer of the dura.

Results. Walking was normal in a few days. The condition persisted after 2 years.

Case No. 51: Fibroblastic Meningioma

A 53-year-old woman (1985; Fig. 326). Left anterolateral intradural-extramedullary meningioma in D4.

Clinical Course. 5 years. Some attacks of back pain. Three years prior to hospitalization the patient suffered sphincter disturbances in the form of incontinence (surgery for plastic bladder without results). Tingling type of paraesthesias to anterior side of the thigh bilaterally, reaching the abdomen. One year prior to hospitalization motor deficit in both inferior limbs to the left and girdle-like constriction at left mammary region.

Neurological Examination. Spastic paraparesis to the right. Right foot clonus. Bilateral Babinski sign. Hypoaesthesia from D6 bilaterally, pronounced from D8. Persistence of incontinence.

Rachicentesis. 1.96 g protein per thousand.

Myelography (via lumbar puncture). Transitory block in D4 defining even the upper pole of the tumour.

Myelo-CT. Left paramedian intradural-extramedullary neoplasm pushing the cord against the bony wall of D4.

Surgical Treatment. Opening the dura the subarachnoidal neoplasm was seen. Coagulation of the anterior dural invasion and excision en bloc.

Results. The patient started walking normally after 29 days. Clinical recovery after 2 months.

Case No. 28: Transitional Meningioma

A 68-year-old woman (1985). Right anterolateral intradural-extramedullary meningioma in C1-C2.

Clinical Course. 10 years. (The patient underwent surgery in 1979 for a distinct cervical spondyloarthrosis via median longitudinal somatomy. Anterior arthrodesis performed from C4 to C6. There was a distinct improvement in the deficiency syndrome affecting all four limbs. Four years later the motor and sensory deficiency syndrome reappeared to the right together with a spastic tetraparetic picture. In 1984 the second operation consisted of a plain laminectomy from C2 to C4 in the presence of posterior spondyloarthrotic stenosis. The clinical picture deteriorated during the following 3 months).

Neurological Examination. Spastic tetraplegia to the right. Only some voluntary movements of the left shoulder and arm. Band of hypoaesthesia in C3 and total anaesthesia from C4. Retention of urine.

Rachicentesis. 0.38 g protein per thousand.

Myelography (via lumbar puncture). Block in C2 producing an upward concave image.

Surgical Treatment. Operated on for a right anterolateral meningioma in C1-C2. In C1 in the dural sac there was a transversal widening and a mass hard to the touch on the right. Opening the dura in a right lateral site a partly premedullary reddish tumour was seen as large as a big cherry. The meningioma adhered to the anterior surface of the dura and left a shadow on the cord, displacing it to the left. The surface-layer circulation of the lateroventral columns was extremely thin. A right posterior radicotomy was of C1 and C2 performed and mobilization of the anterior part of the tumour towards the exterior. Total excision and sparing of all the plial arteries was possible.

Results. Improvement in the movements of all four limbs as soon as the patient woke up. Subsequent motor and sensory improvement was more rapid in the upper limbs, especially on the left. One month later the patient was able to take a few steps and after 8 months could walk normally. The improvement was also in movements of the upper limbs. The patient's condition remained stable even at a 9-year check.

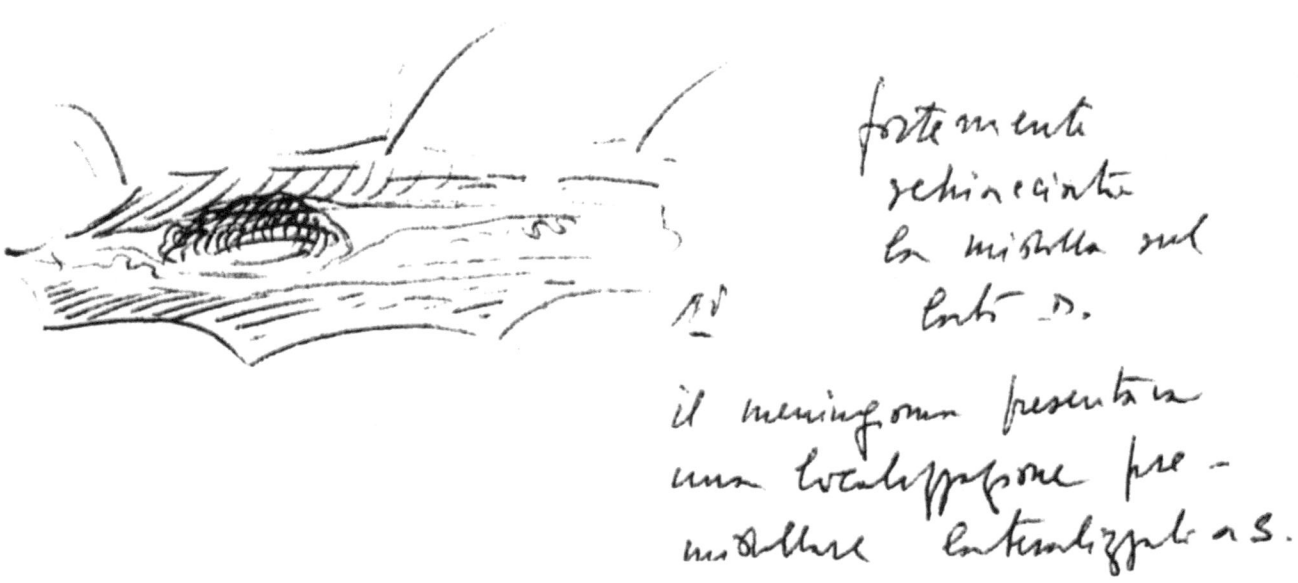

Fig. 326. Left anterolateral intradural-extramedullary meningioma in D4

Case No. 124: Sarcomatous Meningioma
A 45-year-old woman (1985). Right anterolateral extradural meningioma in S1.
Clinical Course. 4 years. Right lumbago and sciatica on S1 with tingling paraesthesias at the external margin of the foot. One month prior to hospitalization the patient felt fastidious saddle-like sensations.
Neurological Examination. Rigid lumbar rachis. Great pain felt on the right of the lumbosacral passage when touched. Loss of strength in plantar flexion of the right foot. Loss of ankle jerk on the right. Right hypoaesthesia on S1-S3
Rachicentesis. 0.64 g protein per thousand.
Lumbosacral Stratigraphy. Right oval-shaped osteolytic area in L5-S1 with thickened peripheral area.
Radicolography. A beak-shaped image which showed the right lateral portion of the terminal sac cut and the corridor of S1-S2 completely disappeared.
CT. Large intra- and extradural neoformation in S1 to the right. The lesion extended below for 6 cm involving the lateral wall of the sacrum.
MRI. A tumour from S1-S2 which extended across the depth of the sacrum and approached the wall of the rectum.
Surgical Treatment. The last tract of the meningeal sac was compressed from right to left. The tumoral mass which adhered to the first two sacral roots appeared in an osteolytic shell-shaped recess. The tumour was debulked and its presacral part removed.
Results. After an initial improvement in the pain and paraesthetic symptoms the patient was prepared for radiotherapy. She died 4 months later.

Case No. 57: Transitional Meningioma
A 56-year-old woman (1986). Right posterolateral intradural-extramedullary meningioma in D8-D9 (see Chap. 6).

Case No. 31: Psammomatous Meningioma with Numerous Calcifications
A 48-year-old woman (1986; Fig. 327). Left lateral intradural-extramedullary meningioma in D9-D10.
Medical History. Right mammary fibroadenoma.
Clinical Course. 6 months. Back pain with irradiation girdle-like to lower left dorsal tract. Motor claudication to the left with fastidious paraesthesias distally to lower limbs.
Neurological Examination. Severe spastic paraparesis to the left. Bilateral foot clonus and Babinski sign. Hypoaesthesia for the various forms of sensitivity from D11, pronounced distally. Hypopallaesthesia of the iliac crests which became anaesthesia distally.
Rachicentesis. 0.96 g protein per thousand.
X-Ray of Dorsal Rachis. Right convex scoliosis with thinning of peduncles of D9 on the left.
Myelography (via lumbar puncture). Dilatation of the subarachnoidal space in D11-D12 with upper concave block in D10. Slight flow producing a roundish-shaped filling defect on the right and defining a dome-shaped image corresponding to the upper pole of the neoplasm.
Myelo-CT. Confirmation of myelographic findings. Cortical reaction with a small area of erosion along the posterior wall of the vertebral body of D10. A scan showed the full view of the neoplasm presenting internal irregular calcified areas.
MRI. Expansive intradural-extramedullary structure in D9-D10 which displaced the cord towards the right. An axial scan showed the border of the irregular vertebral body.
Surgical Treatment. The dura was hypervascularized and swollen on the left, corresponding to the neoplasm below. The tumour adhered to the *left lateral internal surface near the dural funnel of the tenth dorsal root.* Confirmation of the calcified areas in richly vascolarized tissues. Removal by fragmentation. After excision a shell-

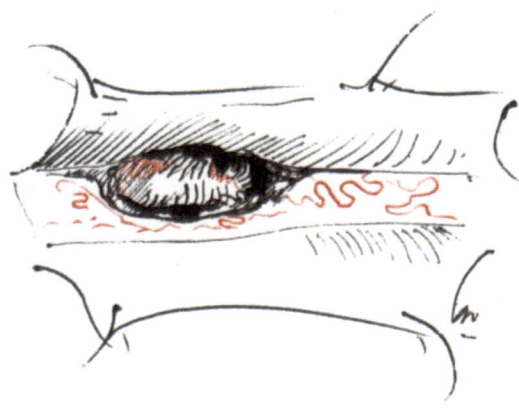

Fig. 327. Left lateral intradural-extramedullary meningioma in D9-D10

shaped shadow was seen deep in the cord.
Results. The patient gradually achieved normal walking over a 2-month period.

Case No. 56: Transitional Meningioma
A 75-year-old woman (1987). Right posterolateral intradural-extramedullary meningioma in D7-D8 (see Chap. 8).

Case No. 58: Transitional Meningioma
A 76-year-old woman (1987). Right posterolateral intradural-extramedullary meningioma in D2-D3 (see Chap. 8).

Case No. 29: Transitional Meningioma
A 63-year-old woman (1987). Left ventrolateral intradural-extramedullary meningioma in D5-D6 (see Chap. 8).

Case No. 45: Meningothelial Meningioma
A 59-year-old woman (1987). Right posterolateral intradural-extramedullary meningioma in D5-D7 (see Chap. 9).

Case No. 52: Fibroblastic Meningioma
A 73-year-old woman (1987). Right ventrolateral intradural-extramedullary meningioma in D1-D2 (see Chap. 8).

Case No. 123: Psammomatous Meningioma
A 76-year-old woman (1987). Right posterolateral intradural-extramedullary meningioma from C2-C6 (see Chap. 8).

Case No. 33: Transitional Meningioma
A 74-year-old man (1987; Fig. 328). Right posterolateral intradural-extramedullary meningioma in D9-D10.
Clinical Course. 10 years. Occasional back pain. Motor weakness with electric shock type of paraesthesias to right lower limb.
Neurological Examination. Monoplegia to right lower limb and severe paresis on the left. Tactile, thermal and painful hypoaesthesia from D8-D9; hypopallaesthesia from the iliac crests, increased distally to the right. Sphincter disturbances in the form of retention.

Rachicentesis. 0.69 g protein per thousand.
X-Ray of Dorsal Tract. Dorsolumbar scoliosis. Reduction in height of the vertebral body of D8 and spondyloarthrosis in D9.
Myelography (via lumbar puncture). Dome-shaped block near the space D9-D10.

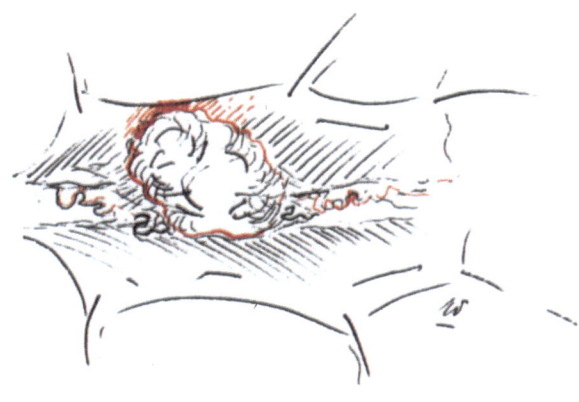

Fig. 328. Right posterolateral intradural-extramedullary meningioma in D9-D10

CT. The cord was compressed ventrally by a right posterolateral neoplasm of an irregular shape, nonhomogenous and thicker on the right.
Surgical Treatment. Opening the dura presented a reddish-wine coloured tumour surrounded by the arachnoid and invading the right internal posterolateral surface of the dura. The cord was flattened forwards. Opening the arachnoid and fragmented removal of the neoplasm. The cord was reduced in volume but with the surface-layer circulation in stasis.
Results. Over the next 20 days the patient started walking. Complete recovery at a 6-month check.

Case No. 68: Transitional Meningioma
An 82-year-old woman (1988). Right anterolateral intradural-extramedullary meningioma in C2 (see Chap. 6).

Case Nos. 76, 77: Fibroblastic and Transitional Meningiomas
A 28-year-old woman (1988). Multiple meningiomas in neurofibromatosis (see Chap. 6).

Case No. 100: Transitional Meningioma
A 73-year-old woman (1988). Right ventrolateral intradural-extramedullary meningioma in D2-D3 (see Chap. 8).

Case No. 40: Fibroblastic Meningioma
A 74-year-old man (1988). Premedullary-intradural-extramedullary meningioma in D2 (see Chap. 8).

Case No. 94: Transitional Meningioma
A 73-year-old woman (1988). Right ventrolateral intradural-extramedullary meningioma in C4-C5.

Medical History. Hypertension. Diabetes.
Clinical Course. 3 months. Loss of strength in upper limbs to the right with distal paraesthesias to the hand. Motor claudication to right lower limb.
Neurological Examination. Monoparesis in right upper limb and worse distally. Spastic paraparesis to the right. Severe hypoaesthesia from C5-C6 bilaterally for the various forms of sensitivity and anaesthesia in left lower limb. Sphincter disturbances in the form of retention.
X-Ray of Cervicodorsal Rachis. Scoliosis in upper dorsal tract. Alterations in pedicles in C4, C5 and C6 with an increase in the interpeduncular distance.
CT. The tumour occupied the entire canal in C5; no right radicular image.
MRI. The intradural-extramedullary neoplasm in C4-C5 appeared in arthrotic stenosis of the canal. In coronal scans the global image of the tumour was seen mainly on the right and reduced the volume of the cord which resembled a plain lamella curved towards the left.
Surgical Treatment. The lamina of C4 was eroded by the right compression. The dura felt taut and thin to the touch due to the mass below. Paramedian dural incision showed a neoplasm compact to the right which occupied the canal almost entirely. Incision of the capsule and removal of the posterior surface of the tumour. Fragmented excision of the neoplasm. Freeing and reclining the remaining capsule towards the exterior.
Results. The patient on awaking found an improvement in the movements of upper limbs to the left. During the following 2 months she was able to take short steps. Five months later, great improvement in all four limbs. Still slight difficulty in clenching a fist in the right hand. The condition lasted 4 years until gradual deterioration with hypostenia, associated was fastidious paraesthesias in all four limbs. Rapid deterioration over 1 month with impossibility of walking.
Neurological Examination. Severe spastic paraparesis to the right. Severe hypoaesthesia from C6 bilaterally.
MRI. Previous operation at C4-C5 level where the cord was pushed towards the right and was surrounded by scarred homogeneous tissue which underwent impregnation after the infusion of contrast medium. At the same level the cord showed a discreet and diffused modification of the signal on the basis of chronic ischaemia. Small focal ischaemic lesion in the bridge.
Surgical Treatment. Operation postponed due to the reappearance of cardiac rythm disturbance during the administration of the anaesthetic. A pace-maker was installed. At the operating field a scarred structure was found with ischaemic phenomena without tumour recurrence. Neurolysis at the operating microscope using microsurgery and the recovery of good medullary palpitations.
Results. Immediate regression of motor deficit and the patient started walking with a slight ataxic gait during the following 15 days. On the 18th days she was affected by arterial hypertension and diabetic decompensation. She died after an apoplectic ictus.

Case No. 90: Transitional Meningioma
A 57-year-old woman (1989). Left posterolateral intradural-extramedullary meningioma in C7-D1 (see Chap. 8).

Case No. 47: Ossified Transitional Meningioma
A 60-year-old woman (1989). Left anterolateral intradural-extramedullary meningioma in D4-D5 (see Chap. 8).

Case No. 42: Meningothelial Meningioma
A 60-year-old woman (1989). Right extramedullary meningioma occupying the intravertebral foramen in D9-D10 (see Chap. 8).

Case No. 99: Transitional Meningioma

A 79-year-old man (1989). Left ventrolateral intradural-extramedullary meningioma in D4 (see Chap. 8).

Case No. 95: Fibroblastic Meningioma

An 89-year-old woman (1989). Right posterolateral intradural-extramedullary meningioma in D12 (see Chap. 8).

Case No. 118: Transitional, Psammomatous Meningioma

A 63-year-old woman (1989). Right anterolateral intradural-extramedullary meningioma in D1-D2.
Medical History. Uterine polyposis.
Clinical Course. 2 years. Burning paraesthesias in right underarm region and upper thoracic quadrant. For 1 year a heaviness was felt in the lower limbs and for 3 months motor claudication to the right.
Neurological Examination. Severe spastic paraparesis to the right. Foot clonus and bilateral Babinski sign. Hypoaesthesia from D1-D2 on the right and from D3 increasing distally on the left. Sphincter disturbances in the form of incontinence.
X-ray of Lumbar Rachis. Spondyloarthrosis L5-S1.
MRI. Neoplasm in D1-D2 measuring 2.5 cm in length which left a shadow and displaced the cord posteriorly.
Surgical Treatment. After opening the dura the cord was seen to be curved towards the back and to the left by a reddish-wine coloured neoplasm which was covered by the right second dorsal root. On opening the arachnoid the root was reclined and the neoplasm removed by fragmentation. Coagulation of the base of attachment. The cord was atrophic and had an extremely thin surface-layer circulation.
Results. The patient gradually started walking within a few days. Complete recovery at a 5-year check.

Case No. 79 Transitional Meningioma

A 70-year-old woman (1990). Left ventrolateral intradural-extramedullary meningioma in D8-D9 (see Chap. 9).

Case No. 87: Transitional Meningioma

A 59-year-old woman (1990). Right ventrolateral intradural-extramedullary meningioma in D1 (see Chap. 9).

Case No. 46: Ossified Transitional Meningioma

A 36-year-old woman (1990). Posterior intradural-extramedullary and calcified meningioma in D2-D3 (see Chap. 8).

Case No. 81: Psammomatous Meningioma

A 51-year-old man (1991). Right anterolateral intradural-extramedullary meningioma in D4-D5-D6.
Medical History. Operated on in 1984 for dorsal stenosis in D7-D8 in severe kyphoscoliosis.
Clinical Course. 1 year. The patient, already affected by spastic paraparesis, had shown progressive deterioration over the previous 6 years. In the past 4 years he was unable to walk. For 2 years suffered a tingling type of paraesthesias irradiating girdle-like to the upper abdomen level.
Neurological Examination. Spastic paraplegia. Patella and foot clonus with bilateral Babinski sign. Painful hypoaesthesia from D8 and pallaesthesia from the iliac crests. Sphincter disturbances in the form of incontinence.
Rachicentesis. 1 g protein per thousand.
Plain MRI and with Gadolinium. Increase in the volume of the cord from D4 and D8-D9, with evident nonhomogeneous medullary structure. At this level analogous impregnation of contrast medium visible at the cord after an intravenous injection of gadolinium (incorrect diagnosis of intramedullary tumour). After neuroradiological examinations the patient was advised to undergo surgery, which was agreed to after 1 year.
Surgical Treatment. The cord appeared ischaemic and curved posteriorly towards the right by a left lateral premedullary tumour. Incision of the capsule and the haemorrhagic and hard-consistency tumour was debulked by fragmentation. A small encapsulated part of the tumour which adhered to the posterior columns was not removed.
Results. No changes in spastik paraplegia.

Case No. 37: Transitional Meningioma

A 64-year-old woman (1991). Left posterolateral intradural-extramedullary meningioma in D8.
Medical History. Arterial hypertension and angina pectoris.
Clinical Course. 10 years. Mediodorsal back pain irradiating girdle-like and bilaterally to the right. Hot paraesthesias on the left. Six months prior to hospitalization the paraesthesias spread to the right lower limb and to the anterior side of the left thigh. Motor weakness in both lower limbs to the right.
Neurological Examination. Spastic paraplegia with foot clonus and bilateral Babinski sign. Hypoaesthesia for the various forms of superficial, tactile, pain and pallaesthesia from D9 on the left and from D7 on the right. Sphincter disturbances in the form of retention.
X-Ray of Dorsal and Lumbar Rachis. Right convex scoliosis. Erosion of the articular facets in D8 on the right. Angiomatous aspect of the vertebral body of D11. Signs of stenosis of the rachidian canal in L1-L2. Sacralization of L5.
Plain MRI and with Gadolinium. Expansive intradural-extramedullary structure measuring 1 cm in diameter and situated on the posterior surface of the canal at D8 level which compressed and displaced the cord. Partial impregnation after intravenous administration of gadolinium. Angiomatous vertebra in D11.
Surgical Treatment. The dura appeared taut and nonpulsating. Dural delamination and coagulation of the deep dural circulation. The lower pole of the meningioma was seen and the internal dural layer was incised, sparing the arachnoid. The cord distinctly appeared moved forwards, very reduced in volume and marked by the neoplasm. The anterior part of the tumour was the only part that was not calcified and became soft. The same techniques were used for the upper pole of the meningioma and excision was performed by reclining the neoplasm towards the exterior.
Results. Initial motor inhibition at lower limbs. After 1 month the patient started walking. Two years later she walked normally. Slight hypertonia persisted to the right.

Case Nos. 83, 84: Psammomatous Meningioma in Two Sites

A 48-year-old woman (1992). Left posterolateral meningioma in D9-D10 and a right premedullary meningioma in D11 (see Chap 8).

Case No. 85: Transitional Meningioma with Widespread Osseus Metaplasms

A 72-year-old woman (1993). Left posterolateral intradural-extramedullary meningioma in D3-D4 (see Chap. 9).

Case No. 80: Transitional Meningioma

A 69-year-old woman (1993). Right posterolateral intradural-extramedullary meningioma in D10-D11 (see Chap. 6).

Case No. 70: Transitional Meningioma
An 81-year-old woman (1994). Right posterolateral intradural-extramedullary meningioma in D10 (see Chap. 8).

Case No. 38: Psammomatous Meningioma
A 55-year-old man (1994). Intradural-extramedullary meningioma and posterolateral extra-arachnoidal meningioma in D11 (almost entirely calcified) (see Chap. 9).

Case No. 75: Transitional Meningioma
A 53-year-old woman (1994). Right posterolateral intradural-extramedullary meningioma in D4 (see Chap. 9).

References

Abbe R (1890) Spinal surgery - a report of eight cases. Med Rec 38: 85-92

Abbott M, Killefer FA, Crandall PH (1968) Melanotic meningioma. Case report. J Neurosurg 29:283-286

Abbruzzese G, Dallagata D, Morena M et al (1988) Electrical stimulation of the motor tract in cervical spondylosis. J Neurol Neurosurg Psychiatry 51:796-802

Adamkiewicz A (1882-1885) Die Blutgefässe der menschlichen Rückenmarkesoberfläche. Sitzung Akade Wissensch. Wien Math Natural Klasse, p. 101

Adams EF, Schrell UMH, Fahlbusch R (1990) Hormonal dependence of human meningiomas. Part II: In vitro effect of steroids, bromocriptine, and epidermal growth factor on the growth of meningiomas. J Neurosurg 73:750-755

Adelman LS, Aronson SM (1972) Intramedullary nerve fiber and Schwann cell proliferation within the spinal cord (schwannosis). Neurology 22:726-731

Adson AW (1925) Diagnosis and treatment of tumors of the spinal cord. Northwest Med 24:309-317

Adson AW (1938) Intraspinal tumors. Surgical considerations: collective review. Int Abstr Chir 67:225-237

Adson AW (1939) Tumors of the spinal cord. Diagnosis and treatment. Can Med Assoc J 40:448-459

Adson AW (1950) Surgical consideration of intraspinal tumors. J Int Coll Surg 14:1-11

Adson AW, Ott WO (1925) Results of the removal of tumors of the spinal cord. Arch Neurol Psychol 8:520-538

Aghadiuno PU, Adeloye A, Olumide AA, Nottidge VA (1985) Intracranial neoplasms in children in Ibadan, Nigeria. Childs Nerv Syst 1:39-44

Agnoli A, Bonamini F, Frasconi F, Farina P, Tartarini E (1963) Tumori spinali (Parte I: studio clinico, anatomopatologico e radiologico di 75 casi). Riv Neurobiol 9:685-746

Agrifoglio E (1951) Meningioma fibroblastico del filum terminale. Minerva Chir 6:10

Aki T, Toya S (1994) Experimental study on changes of the spinal evoked potential and circulatory dynamics following spinal cord compression and decompression. Spine 9, 8:800-809

Al Saadi A, Latimar F, Madercio M, Robbins T (1987) Cytogenetic studies of human brain tumors and their clinical significance. II Meningioma. Cancer Genet Cytogenet 26:127-141

Al-Mefty O (1991) Meningiomas. Raven, New York

Alcaix D, Damade R, Huchet B, Camus JP (1990) The filum terminale: an uncommon site of spinal meningioma. Rev Rhum Mal Osteoartic 57:165-166

Alexander (1939) - see: Suh and Alexander

Allen WE, D'Angel CM, Kier EL (1975) Correlation of microangiography and electrophysiologic changes in experimental spinal cord trauma. Radiology 111:107-115

Alwatban J, Tampieri D (1993) Cervical spinal meningioma. Can Assoc Radiol J 44, 2:138-140

Ambrose J, Hounsfield G (1973) Computerized transverse axial tomography. Br J Radiol 46:148-149

Ambrosetto C (1954) Istogenesi ed istopatologia delle neoplasie meningee (meningiomi). Estratto da Studi Sassaresi 32:95-171

Ambrosetto C (1961) Sull'istogenesi dei tumori meningei. G Psichiatria Neuropatol. Estratto dagli Atti della XL Riunione del Centro Triveneto Soc It Pat, pp 1-21

Amici R, Borghi GP (1959) Emorragie subaracnoidee da tumori spinali intradurali del tratto lombare. Minerva Neurochir 3:192-198

Aminoff MJ (ed) (1979) Electrophysiologic approaches to neurologic diagnosis. Churchill-Livingstone, New York

Ammermann BJ, Smith DR (1975) Papilloedema and spinal cord tumors. Surg Neurol 3:55-57

Anderson FM, Carson MJ (1953) Spinal cord tumors in children. A review of the subject and presentation of 21 cases. J Pediatr 43:190-207

Andrioli GC, Rigobello I, Iob I, Casentini L (1982) Multiple meningiomas. Neurochirurgia (Stuttg) 24:67-69

Antoni N (1936) Tumoren des Rückenmarks, seiner Wurzeln und Häute. Springer, Berlin (Handbuch der Neurologie)

Antons K (1944) Calcified spinal meningioma visible on roentgen film. Acta Psych Neurol Scand 19:5-9

Apuzzio J (1980) Spinal cord tumors during pregnancy. Int J Gynaecol Obstet 17:608-610

Arieti S (1944) Multiple meningioma and meningiomas associated with other brain tumors. J Neuropathol Exp Neurol 3:255-270

Arjundas G (1963) Intraspinal compressions. Review of 184 cases. J Physicians Assoc

Arlt HG (1936) Multiple Meningeome des Gehirns und diffuse Meningeomatosis des Rückenmarks. Z Ges Neurol Psychol 156:713-734

Arnell S, Lindström F (1931) Myelography with scadian (abrodil). Acta Radiol 12:287-288

Arnold G, Lepoire J, Barracand D (1961) Les méningiomes mains (à propos d'une observation). Rev Neurol (Paris) 105:469-479

Arseni C, Ionesco S (1958) Les compressions médullaires dues à des tumeurs intrarachidiennes. Etude clinico-statistique de 362 cas. J Chir (Paris) 75:582-594

Arseni C, Maretsis M (1967) Tumors of the lower spinal cord associated with increased intracranial pressure and papilloedema. J Neurosurg 27:105-110

Arseni C, Samitca DC (1961) Primary intraspinal tumors in children and adolescents. Report of 12 cases. J Neurosurg 18:135-138

Arseni C, Horvath L, Iliescu D (1967) Intraspinal tumors in children. Psychiatr Neurol Neurochir 70:123-133

Ashkenaze D, Mudiyam R, Boachie-Adjei O et al (1993) Efficacy of spinal cord monitoring in neuromuscular scoliosis. Spine 15, 18:1627-1633

Augenstein HM, Sze G, Becker R (1991) Imaging of spinal meningiomas. In: Al-Mefty O (ed) Meningiomas. Raven, New York, pp 603-612

Ausin G (1972) The spinal cord. Thomas, Springfield

Autori vari (1967) The evoked potentials. Electroencephalogr Clin Neurophysiol [Suppl] 26

Ayer JB (1930) Symptoms and signs of tumors involving the spinal cord. N Engl J Med 108:235

Babinski J (1923) Sur le traitment des tumeurs iuxta-medullaires. Rev Neurol (Paris) 39:695-701

Babinski J, Jarkowski J (1923) Sur le diagnostic des compressions spinales. Rev Neurol (Paris) 39:670-674

Bailey AA (1953) Changes with age in the spinal cord. Arch Neurol Psychiatry 70:299

Bailey AA, McCraig W (1950) Intraspinal meningiomas simulating degenerative diseases of the spinal cord. Mayo Clin Proc 25:233-238

Bailey OT (1940) Histologic sequences in meningioma, with a consideration of the nature of hyperostosis cranii. Arch Pathol 30:42-69

Bailey P (1903) Successful laminectomy for spinal cord tumor. J Nerv Ment Dis 30:99

Bailey P (1908) Spinal cord tumor and trauma; a report of two cases. J Nerv Ment Dis 35:316-319

Bailey P, Bucy PC (1930) Tumors of the spinal canal. Surg Clin North Am 10:233

Bailey P, Bucy PC (1931) Origin and nature of meningeal tumors. Am J Cancer 15:15-54

Bailey P, Cushing H, Heisenhardt L (1928) Angioblastic meningiomas. Arch Pathol 6:953-990

Bain GO, Shnikta TK (1956) Cutaneous meningioma (psammoma). Report of a case. Arch Dermatol 74:590-594

Baird M, Gallagher PJ (1989) Recurrent intracranial and spinal meningiomas: clinical and histological features. Clin Neuropathol 8:41-44

Banna M (1971) Intraspinal tumours in children (excluding dysraphism). Clin Radiol 22:17-32

Barber C (ed) (1980) Evoked potentials. University Park Press, Baltimore

Barbieri F, Santangelo R, Indaco A, De Furio M, Buscaino GA (1990) Neurocutaneous melanosis, neurofibromatosis and spinal meningioma: an unusual association. Acta Neurol (Napoli) 12:115-121

Barcia Goyanes JJ, Calvo Garra W (1953) Méningiomes sans attache avec l'arachnoide. Acta Neurochir (Wien) 3:241-247

Bardeci CA, Christensen JC (1954) Méningiomes multiples d'évolution maligne. Prensa Med Argent 41:487-490

Barker D, Wright E, Nguyen K et al (1987) Gene for von Recklinghausen neurofibromatosis is in the pericentromeric region of chromosome 17. Science 236:1100-1102

Barker JD, Weller RO, Garfield JS (1976) Epidemiology of primary tumours of the brain and spinal cord: a regional survey in southern England. J Neurol Neurosurg Psychiatry 39:290-296

Barr RJ, Yi ES, Jensen JL, Wuerker RB, Liao SY (1993) Meningioma-like tumor of the skin. An ultrastructural and immunohistochemical study. Am J Surg Pathol 17, 8:779-787

Barre JA (1923) Les différentes douleurs des compressions médullaires. Presse Med 40

Bassi P, Cecchini A, Dettori P, Signorini E (1982) Myelography with iopamidol, a nonionic water-soluble contrast medium: incidence of complications. Neuroradiology 24:85-90

Batson OV (1957) The vertebral vein system. Am J Roentgenol Radium Ther Nucl Med 78:195-212

Beatty RA (1970) Cold dysesthesia: a symptom of extramedullary tumors of the spinal cord. J Neurosurg 33:75-78

Beck A (1890) Determination of localization in the brain and spinal cord by means of electrical phenomena. Presented Oct. 20, 1890. Rozpr. Wydz. Mat-Przyr. Polsk. Akad. Um. Ser. II, 1, 186-232 (doctoral thesis)

Becker J (1965) Die Meningiome des Rückenmarks. Klinik und Differentialdiagnose. Inaugural Dissertation, University of Cologne

Beecher HK (1940) The first anesthesia records (Codman, Cushing). Surg Gynecol Obstet 71:689

Bello MJ, de Campos JM, Vaquero J, Kusak ME, Sarasa JL, Rey JA, Pestana A (1993) Chromosome 22 heterozygosity is retained in most hyperdiploid and pseudodiploid meningiomas. Cancer Genet Cytogenet 66, 2:117-119

Bendixen HH (1978) A foreword: the tasks of the anesthesiologist. In: Saidman LJ, Smith NT (eds) Monitoring in anesthesia. Wiley, New York, pp 227-267

Bennet M (1983) Effect of compression and ischemia on spinal cord evoked potentials. Exp Neurol 80:508-519

Bergamini L, Bergamasco B (eds) (1967) Cortical evoked potentials in man. Thomas, Springfield

Bergamini L, Bergamasco B, Fra L et al (1966) Réponses corticales et périphériques evoqueés par stimulation du nerf dans la pathologie des cordons postérieurs. Rev Neurol (Paris) 115:99-112

Berger H (1929) Über das Elektroenzephalogramm des Menschen. Arch Psychiatry 87:527-570

Beriel L (1923a) Sur la position des tumeurs intra-rachidiennes par rapport à la dure mère. Rev Neurol (Paris) 39:597-598

Beriel L (1923b) Sur certaines points d'histologie des tumeurs comprimants la moelle. Rev Neurol (Paris) 39:598

Beriel L (1932) Tumeurs intra-rachidiennes. Diagnostic General Neuvième Congrès Soc Intern Chir

Beriel L, Mestrallett A (1929) Les compressions medullaires. Baillières, Paris

Bernasconi V, Cassinari V (1961) Tumori e malformazioni vasali spinali. Acta Neurochir (Wien) 10:1-50

Bertrand I, Guillaume J, Olteanu I (1948) Etude histologique de 130 meningiomes. Rev Neurol (Paris) 80:81-99

Bharati RS, Rammamurthi B (1972) Intramedullary schwannoma. Proc Inst Neurol Madras 2:91

Bickerstaff ER, Small JM, Guest IA (1959) The relapsing course of certain meningiomas in relation to pregnancy and menstruation. J Neurol Neurosurg Psychiatry 21:89-91

Bille J, Nicolino C (1980) Reflexions à propos des compressions médullaires non traumatiques chez le sujet agé. Med Hyg Geneve 38:1817-1818

Bischoff T (1842) Entwicklungsgeschichte der Säugetiere und des Menschen. Leipzig

Black BK, Kernohan JW (1950) Primary diffuse tumors of the meninges (so called meningeal meningiomatosis). Cancer 1:805-819

Black PM (1993) Meningiomas. Neurosurgery 32:643-657

Black PM, Lisczak TM, Kornblith PL (1979) Ultrastructural and electrophysiological features of meningioma whorls in tissue culture. Acta Neuropathol (Berl) 46:33-38

Bland JC, Russel DS (1938) Histological types of meningioma and comparison of their behaviour in tissue culture. J Nath a Bakt 47:291

Blankestein MA, Van'tverlaat JW, Croughs RJM (1989) Progestin and estrogen receptors in human meningioma. Lancet 1:1381

Blaylock RL (1981) Hydrosyringomyelia of the conus medullaris associated with meningioma: case report. J Neurosurg 54:833-835

Bland-Sutton Sir J (1922) Tumors innocent and malignant. Kassel

Boccardo M, Macchia G, Carlotti G, Andrioli G (1987) The value of enhanced "dynamic" computed tomography in localizing a spinal juxtamedullary meningioma. Neuroradiology 29:313

Bodis-Wollner I (1982) Evoked potentials. Ann NY Acad Sci 388

Bogdanowitsch M (1913) Entbindung bei vollständiger Lähmung

des Rumpfes. Zentralbl Gynakol 37:809-814

Boisserie-Lacroix M, Kien P, Caille JM (1987) Imaging of intradural extramedullary tumors: neurinomas and meningiomas. J Neuroradiol 14:66-81

Bolande RP (1974) The neurocristopathie. A unifying concept of disease arising in neural crest maldevelopment. Hum Pathol 5, 4:409-429

Boldrey E (1971) The meningiomas. In: Minckler J (ed) Pathology of the central nervous system, vol 2. Mc Graw-Hill, New York, pp 2125-2144

Bondarenko ES, Malyshev II, Shoshina LM (1974) Spinal tumors in children. Zh Nevropatol Psikhiatr 74:678-682

Borghi G (1973) Extradural spinal meningiomas. Acta Neurochir (Wien) 29:195-202

Borovich B, Doron Y, Braun J, Feinsod M, Goldsher D, Gruszkiewicz J, Guilbourd J, Zaavoor M, Levi L, Soustiel J, Lemberger A (1988) The incidence of multiple meningiomas - do solitary meningiomas exist? Acta Neurochir (Wien) 90:15-22

Boudouresques J, Roger J, Bonnal J, Vigouroux R (1958) Compression médullaire à forme de pseudo-sclerose laterale amyotrophique. Rev Neurol (Paris) 98:408

Bradac GP, Riva A, Bergni M, Daniele D (1994) Meningiomi: considerazioni neuroradiologiche e neuropatologiche. Riv Neuroradiol 7 [Suppl 1]:105-110

Brechet G (1829) Recherches anatomiques, physiologiques et pathologiques sur le système veineux. Villeret, Paris

Bremer F (1958) Cerebral and cerebellar potentials. Physiol Rev 38:357-388

Bret P, Lecuire J, Lapras C, Deruty R, Dechaume JP, Assaad A (1976) Les méningiomes intrarachidiens. Reflexions à propos d'une série de 60 observations. Neurochirurgie 22:5-22

Bricolo A, Faccioli F, Signorini G et al (1975) Le risposte corticali evocate sensitive nelle lesioni midollari traumatiche acute. Riv Neurol 45:226-236

Brignolio F, Favero M (1984) Considerations on malignancy of papillary meningioma. Clinico-pathological study of eight cases. Zentralbl Neurochir 45:79-84

Broager B (1953) Spinal neurinoma. A clinical study comprising 44 cases with a discussion of histological origin and with special reference to differential diagnosis against spinal glioma and meningioma. Acta Psychiatr Scand Suppl 85:1-241

Brown MH (1941) Intraspinal meningiomas. Arch Neurol Psychiatry 47:271-292

Brown MH, Kernohan JW (1941) Diffuse meningiomatosis. Arch Pathol 32:651

Brown RH, Nash CL, Berilla JA (1984) Cortical evoked potentials monitoring: a system for intraoperative monitoring of spinal cord function. Spine 9:256-261

Buchanan D (1950) Tumors of the spinal cord in infancy. Arch Neurol Psychol 63:835

Buchstein HF (1941) Meningiomas of the spinal cord. Minn Med 24:539-545

Buckley RC, Heisenhardt L (1929) Study of a meningioma in supravital preparations, tissue cultures and paraffin sections. Am J Pathol 5:644-659

Bucy PC (1964) Some special features of tumors of the spinal cord. Memphis Mid-South Med J 173-187

Budka H (1982) Hyaline inclusions (Pseudopsammoma bodies) in meningiomas: immunocytochemical demonstration of epithel-like secretion of secretory component and immunoglobulins A and M. Acta Neuropathol (Berl) 56:294-298

Bull J (1953) Spinal meningiomas and neurofibromas. Acta Radiol 40:283-299

Bunts AT (1936) Spinal cord tumors. An analytical review of 36 cases. Surg Clin North Am 15:1047

Busch E (1935) Discussion reg the thesis of Geert-Joergensen Copenhagen

Bushong SC (1988) Magnetic resonance imaging: physical and bio-

logical principles. Mosby, St. Louis

Butti G, Assietti R, Casalone R, Paoletti P (1989) Multiple meningiomas: a clinical, surgical, and cytogenetic analysis. Surg Neurol 31:255-260

Bydder GM, Kingsley PE, Brown J, Wiendorf HP, Young IR (1985) MR imaging of meningiomas including studies with and without gadolinium-DTPA. J Comput Assist Tomogr 9:690-697

Caccia MR, Ubiali E, Andreussi L (1976) Spinal evoked responses recorded from the epidural space in normal and diseased humans. J Neurol Neurosurg Psychiatry 39:962-972

Calogero JA, Moossy J (1972) Extradural spinal meningiomas: report of four cases. J Neurosurg 37:442-447

Cambier J, Masson M, Hurth M et al (1974) Syndrome cordonal postérieur unilateral par neurinome intra-medullaire. Syncinesies homolaterales d'imitation. Rev Neurol (Paris) 130:189-199

Camp JD (1934) Significance of osseous changes in roentgenographic diagnosis of tumors of spinal cord and associated soft tissues. Radiology 22:295-303

Camp JD (1936) Multiple tumors within the spinal canal. Am J Roentgenol 36:775-781

Camp JD (1938) Roentgenologic localizazion of tumors affecting spinal cord. Am J Roentgenol Radiat Ther 40:540-544

Camp JD (1950) Contrast myelography: past and present. Radiology 54:477-506

Camp JD, Edson AW (1933) Roentgenographic findings associated with tumors of spinal column, spinal cord and associated tissues. Am J Cancer 17:348-372

Campbell EH, Whitfiel RD (1951) Tumors of spine and spinal cord with discussion of diagnostic signifiance of back pain. J Kansas Med Sci [Suppl] 52:40-45

Canale DJ, Bebin J (1975) Von Recklinghausen disease of the nervous system. In: Winken PJ, Bruyn GW, Klawans HL (eds) Handbook of clinical neurology. North Holland, Amsterdam

Cantore G, Ciapetta P, Delfini R et al (1982) Intramedullary spinal neurinomas Report of two cases. J Neurosurg 57:143-147

Capella F (1939) Contributo allo studio dei tumori intrarachidei extramidollari. Ann Ital Chir 18:445

Cappabianca P, Maiuri F, Pettinato G, di Prisco B (1981) Hemagiopericytoma of the spinal cord. Surg Neurol 15:298-302

Capponotto A, Pescarolo B (1892) Estirpazione di un tumore intradurale del canale rachideo. Riforma Med 8, 4:543-549

Caramia MD, Pardal AM, Zarola F et al (1989) Electric vs magnetic transcranial stimulation of the brain in healty humans: a comparative study of central motor tracts "conductivity" and "excitability". Brain Res 479:98-104

Cardillo F (1935) Le alterazioni radiografiche della colonna nei tumori endorachidiani. Radiat Med 22:563-579

Carella A, Federico F, di Cuonzo F, Vinjau P, Lambreti P (1982) Adverse side-effects of metrizamide and iopamidol in myelography. Neuroradiology 22:247-249

Carillo R, Matera RF, Insausti T (1946) Meningiomas multiples. Arch Neurocir Buenos Aires 3:107-128

Carman RD, Davis KF (1924) Roentgenologic evidence of spinal cord tumors: report of three cases. Radiology 3:185-188

Carrot E, Pecker J, Le Meen G (1959) Paraplégie à rechutes due à la compression de l'artère du renflement lombaire par un minuscule meningiome. Rev Neurol (Paris) 101, 4:584-586

Carta F, Silvestro C, Borzone M, Capuzzo T, Gentile S (1983) Multiple spinal meningiomas. Zentralbl Neurochir 44:3-6

Casalone R, Granata P, Simi P, Tarantino E, Butti G, Buonaguidi R, Faggionato F, Knerich R, Solero L (1987) Recessive cancer genes in meningiomas? An analysis of 31 cases. Cancer Genet Cytogenet 27: 145-159

Cassinari V, Bernasconi V (1961) Tumori e malformazioni vasali spinali. Acta Neurochir (Wien) 9:612-657

Castillo M, Quencer RM, Green BA, Montalvo BM (1987) Syringomyelia as a consequence of a compressive extramedullary lesions: postoperative clinical and radiological manifestations. AJNR

8:973-978

Caton R (1875) The electric currents of the brain. Br Med J 2:278

Cecchini A, Gozzoli L (1984) Neuroradiologia dei tumori spinali primitivi e secondari. Minerva Med 75:1345-1354

Chambers WR (1952) Hourglass tumors of the spine in children. A report of five cases. Am J Surg 84:443-448

Chang MT (1959) The evoked potentials. In: J Field et al (eds) Neurophysiology, vol 1. American Society of Physiology, Washington DC, pp 299-314 (Handbook of physiology, sect 1)

Chaparro MJ, Yung RF, Smith M, Shen V, Choi BH (1993) Multiple spinal meningiomas: a case of 47 distinct lesions in the absence of neurofibromatosis or identified chromosomal abnormality. Neurosurgery 32:298-301

Charpy A (1921) Le vaisseaux de la moelle. Traité d'anatomie humaine. Masson, Paris

Chatrian GE, Berger MS, Wirch AL (1988) Discrepancy between intraoperative SSEPs and postoperative function. Case report. J Neurosurg 69:450-454

Chavany JA, Thiebaut F (1938) Etude diagnostic des compressions médullaires. Gaz Hop 111:101

Chavany JA, David M, Thiebaut A (1936) Compression medullaire dorsale supérieure chez une femme de 73 ans atteinte de la maladie de Recklinghausen. Rev Neurol (Paris) 66:550-555

Chavany JA, Guiot B, Klein MR (1943) L'installation precipitée de certaines paraplegies par compression tumorale. Presse Med 22:308

Chee CP, Tan CT, Nuruddin R (1990) Syringomyelia associated with a cauda equina meningioma involving the conus medullaris. Br J Neurosurg 4, 6:529-533

Cheli E (1952) I meningiomi (rassegna sintetica anatomo-patologica). Boll Oncol 26:1

Cheliout-Heraut F, Marianbourg G, Fahed M et al (1991) Contribution of somatosensory evoked potentials in the surveillance of the spinal cord during spinal surgery. Rev Chir Orthop 77:344-352

Chen CN, Hoult DI (1989) Biomedical magnetic resonance technology. Adam Hilger, Bristol

Chen HJ, Lui CC, Chen L (1992a) Spinal epidural meningioma in a child. Childs Nerv Syst 8:465-467

Chen TC, Zee CS, Miller CA, Weiss MH, Tang G, Chin L, Levy ML, Apuzzo ML (1992b) Magnetic resonance imaging and pathological correlates of meningiomas. Neurosurgery 31, 6:1015-1021

Cheng MK (1982) Spinal cord tumors in the People's Republic of China: a statistical review. Neurosurgery 10:22-24

Cheng MK, Robertson C, Grossman RG et al (1984) Neurological outcome correlated spinal evoked potentials in a spinal cord ischemia model. J Neurosurg 60:786-795

Chiappa KH (1988) Evoked potentials for diagnosis of multiple sclerosis. Neurol Clin 6:861-880

Chigasaki H, Pennybacker JB (1968) A long follow-up study of 128 cases of intramedullary spinal cord tumors. Neurol Med Chir 10:25-66

Chiou SM, Eggert HR, Laborde G, Seeger W (1989) Microsurgical unilateral approaches for spinal tumour surgery: eight years experience in 256 primary operated patients. Acta Neurochir (Wien) 100:127-133

Chiras J, Merland JJ (1978) Angiographie medullaire lombosacrée. J Neuroradiol 5:303-310

Cho JH, Gong GY, Yu ES, Wang GJ, Jee KJ, Lee I (1992) Cytogenetic analysis of meningiomas. J Korean Med Sci 7(2):162-166

Christensen D, Lanrsen H, Klinken L (1983) Prediction of recurrence in meningiomas after surgical treatment. A quantitative approach. Acta Neuropathol (Berl) 61:130-134

Christiansen V (1932) Les tumeurs juxtamédullaires. Acta Psychiatr (Kbh) 12:895-947

Ciappetta P, Domenicucci M, Raco A (1988) Spinal meningiomas: prognosis and recovery factors in 22 cases with severe motor deficits. Acta Neurol Scand 77:27-30

Cioffari A (1950) I tumori delle meningi. Arch Vecchi 15:673

Cioni B, Meglio M, Moles A et al (1991) Spinal somatosensory evoked potential monitoring during microsurgery for syringomyelia: case reports. Stereotact Funct Neurosurg 57:123-129

Cirillo D, Grueff T (1952) Considerazione su due casi di tumore delle meningi spinali nei bambini. Minerva Pediatr 4:574-576

Ciuffini F (1941) Meningioma piale (emangioendoteliomatoso) maligno. Arch Vecchi 3:405

Claus D, Harding AE, Hess CW et al (1988) Central motor conduction in degenerative ataxic disorders. A magnetic stimulation study. J Neurol Neurosurg Psychiatry 51:790-795

Cleland J (1864) Description of two tumors adherent to the deep surface of the dura-mater. Glasgow Med J 11:148-159

Codegone MC, Peres B, Schiffer D (1970) Caratterizzazione istochimica dei lipidi nei meningiomi e loro raffronto con i neurinomi. Acta Neurol 25:532-534

Cohen J, Kaplan A (1943) Tumors in the region of the cauda equina. A review of 25 cases. Am J Surg 60:36-43

Cohen K (1934) Hour-glass tumors of the spine. Brain 57:49

Cohen S (1958) A nerve growth-promoting protein In: McElroy WD, Glass B (eds) The chemical basis of development. Johns Hopkins University Press, Baltimore, pp 665-676

Cohen S, Levi-Montalcini R (1956) A nerve growth-stimulating factor isolated from snake venom. Proc Natl Acad Sci USA 42:571-574

Cole GC, Wilkins PR, West RR (1989) An epidemiological survey of primary tumours of the brain and spinal cord in South East Wales. Br J Neurosurg 3:487-493

Collins J, Marcks HE (1915) The early diagnosis of spinal cord tumors. Am J Med Sci 149:103

Conrad B (1989) Changes of transcranially evoked motor responses in man by midazolam, a short acting benzodiazepine. Neurosci Lett 101:321-324

Conti P, Conti R, Lo Re F (1981) Su due rari casi di meningiomi intrarachidei dell'infanzia. Riv Neurobiol 27, 10:3-4

Conti P, Conti R, de Luca G (1983) Two rare cases of intrarachidian meningioma in infancy. Seara Med Neurocir 12:91-98

Conti P, Conti R, de Luca G (1984) Observations on some rare cases of vertebro-medullar malformations associated with tumors. J Neurosurg Sci 28:2

Conti P, Conti R, Bono P, Gallina P, Pellicanò G (1988) 344 tumori primitivi intrarachidei in 25 anni (1962-1987). Considerazioni statistiche. Atti del Convegno sui "Tumori primitivi del midollo spinale" Progressi di diagnosi e terapia, Torino (7-8 October 1988) Faccani-Lanotte, Torino

Conti P, Conti R, Lo Re F, Bono P, Gallina P, Pellicanò G (1989) Osteocondroma vertebrale e trauma: una possibile correlazione eziopatogenetica. Arch Putti Chir Organi Mov 37:2

Conti P, Conti R, Bono P, Mangiafico S, Pellicanò G (1990) Le alterazioni radiografiche nelle compressioni spinali in età infantile. Riv Neuroradiol 3:317-325

Conti P, Conti R, Lo Re F, Bono P, Mangiafico S, Giordano GP, Cappellini M, Pellicanò G (1991) Neoplasie vertebro-midollari: possibilità diagnostiche con RM e mieloTC. Atti del IX Congresso Naz dell'Ass It di Neuroradiologia, Genova, 12-14 June 1991. Il Centauro, Udine

Cooper IS (1951) Tumors in the spinal cord. Surg Gynecol Obstet 92:183-190

Corbin JL (1961) Anatomie et pathologie artérielles de la moelle. Masson, Paris

Cornil L, Mosinger M (1933) Le méningoblastome lacunaire des meninges spinales. Ann Anat Pathol 10:725

Cossa MMP, Duplay K, Martin P (1951) A propos d'une observation des méningiomes multiples. Rev Neurol (Paris) 85:552-553

Courjon J, Mauguiere E, Revol M (eds) (1982) Clinical applications of evoked potentials in neurology, vol 1. Raven, New York (Advances in Neurology, vol 32)

Courville CB, Abbot KO (1994) On the classification of meningiomas. A survey of ninety five cases in the light of existing schemes. Bull LA Neurol Soc 6:21

Coxe WS (1961) Tumors of the spinal cord in children. Am Surg

27:62-73

Cracco RQ (1973) Spinal evoked response: peripheral nerve stimulation in man. Electroencephalogr Clin Neurophysiol 35:379-386

Cracco RQ, Bodis-Wollner I (1986) Evoked potentials. Liss, New York

Cracco RQ, Cracco JB (1976) Somatosensory evoked potentials in man: far field potentials. Electroencephalogr Clin Neurophysiol 41:460-466

Cracco RQ, Evans B (1978) Spinal evoked potential in the case of asphyxia, strychnine, cord section and compression. Electroencephalogr Clin Neurophysiol 44:187-201

Crespi V, Boglium G, Delodovici MI et al (1988) Ataxic hemiparesis syndrome: sensory disturbance and somatosensory evoked potentials. Ital J Neurol Sci 9:459-466

Crock HV, Yoshizawa H (1977) The blood supply of the vertebral column and spinal cord in man. Springer, Vienna New York

Crock HV, Yamagishi M, Crock MC (1986) The conus medullaris and cauda equina in man. An atlas of the arteries and veins. Springer, Vienna New York

Croft TJ, Brodkey JS, Nulson FE (1972) Reversible spinal cord trauma: a model for electrical monitoring of spinal cord function. J Neurosurg 36:402-406

Crouzet J, Richard S, Pillet G, Muckensturm B, Srour A, Pradat P (1992) Mélanocytomes méninges ou méningiomes pigmentés multiples du canal rachidien. Revue de la litérature. Rev Rhum Mal Osteoartic 59, 11:738-743

Cruveilhier J (1829) Anatomie pathologique du corps humain ou description avec figures lithographiées et colorées des diverses alterations morbides dont le corps humain est susceptible. Baillière, Paris

Cruz Sanchez FF, Miquel R, Rossi ML, Figols J, Palacin A, Cardesa A (1993) Clinico-pathological correlations in meningiomas: a DNA and immunohistochemical study. Histol Histopathol 8,1:1-9

Culver G, Concannon JP, Koenig E (1949) Calcification in intraspinal meningiomas. Am J Roentgenol Radiat Ther 62:237-246

Cushing H (1904) Intradural tumor of the cervical meninges with early restoration of function in the cord after removal of the tumor. Ann Surg 39:934-955

Cushing H (1922) The meningiomas (dural endotheliomas): their source and favoured seats of origin. Brain 45:282-316

Cushing H, Eisenhardt L (1938) Meningiomas, their classification, regional behaviour, life history and surgical end results. Thomas, Springfield

D'Angel CM, Van Gilder JC, Taub A (1973) Evoked cortical potentials in experimental spinal cord trauma. J Neurosurg 38:332-336

Dal Pozzo G, Conti P, Conti R, Bartolozzi C, Pellicanò G (1989) Le diagnostique par imagerie des tumeurs primitives intradurales. Proceedings of the XVIIᵉ Congres International de Radiologie. Paris, 1-8 July 1989 ISR, Paris

Dal Pozzo G, Pellicanò G, Mascalchi M, Conti P, Conti R (1989) La risonanza magnetica con Gd-DTPA nella diagnostica dei tumori spinali intradurali. Atti dell'VIII Congresso Naz dell'Ass It di Neuroradiologia. Il Centauro, Udine

Dalla Palma P, Ninfo V (1977) Histogenetic study of meningiomas in tissue cultures. Lab 4:77-481

Damson GB (1954) A summation technique for the detection of small evoked potentials. Electroencephalogr Clin Neurophysiol 6:65-84

Dandy WE (1919) Roentgenography of the brain after injection of air into the spinal canal. Ann Surg 70:397-403

Dandy WE (1925) The diagnosis and localization of spinal tumors. Ann Surg 81:223

Dangaard S (1983) Ectopic meningioma of a finger. Case report. J Neurosurg 58:778-780

Danilevsky VJ (1891) Zur Frage über die elektromotorischen Vorgänge im Gehirn als Ausdruck seines Tätigkeitszustandes. Zentralbl Physiol 1

Dastur KI, Reza Raji M, Smith jr WI (1984) Pulmonary metastasis from intraspinal meningioma. AJNR 5:483-484

Daum S, Le Beau J (1961) Un cas de méningiomatose. Discussion des rapports avec la maladie de Recklinghausen. Rev Neurol (Paris) 105:349-352

Davidoff LM (1965) Tumors of the spinal cord in infancy and childhood. NY State J Med 2439-2440

Davidoff LM, Martin J (1955) Hereditary combined neurinomas and meningiomas. J Neurosurg 12:375-384

Davidoff LM, Gass H, Grossmann J (1947) Postoperative spinal adhesive arachnoiditis and recurrent spinal cord tumor. J Neurosurg 4:451-464

Davies H (1951) Discussion on myelography. Proc R Soc Med 44:881-893

Davis PA (1939) Effects of acoustic stimuli on the waking human brain. J Neurophysiol 2:494-499

Davis RA, Washburn PL (1972) Spinal cord meningiomas. Surg Gynecol Obstet 127:15-21

Dawson GD (1947) Cerebral responses to electrical stimulation of peripheral nerve in man. J Neurol Neurosurg Psychiatry 10:134-140

De Caro R, Giordano R, Parenti A, Zuccarello M (1982) Osteomatous meningioma. Report of two cases. Acta Neurochir (Wien) 60:313-317

De Gispert Cruz I (1950) Cuadro de esclerosis laterl amoitrofica per compresion medular cervical. Ann Med Barcelona 37:498-502

De Lehoczky T, Piri L (1944) Syndrome of amyotrophic lateral sclerosis caused by cervical hour-glass tumor. Confin Neurol 6:71

De Luca G, Conti P, Conti R (1984) Preliminary experiences on somatosensory evoked potentials in vertebro-medullary pathology. International Symposium on Evoked Potentials: Neurophysiological and Clinical Aspects, Roma, Palladio, Vicenza, p 40

De Luca G, Bono P, Lo Re F et al (1991a) Somatosensory and motor evoked potentials in neurofibromatosis. J Neurosurg Sci 35:4:251-252

De Luca G, Lo Re F, Conti P, et al (1991b) Intraoperative somatosensory and motor evoked potentials in lumbar canal stenosis. IX European Congress of Neurosurgery, Moscow, p 489

De Martel T (1923) Le traitement operatoire des tumeurs de la moelle et de ses enveloppes. Rev Neurol (Paris) 39:711-727

De Martel T (1928) Chirurgie médullaire en France de 1910 à 1928. XXXVII Congr Franc Chir, 960-962

De Martel T (1932) Diagnostic et traitement des tumeurs intrarachidiennes. Verhandl IX Kongress Ges Chir 2:663

De Seze S, Djian A, D'Anglejan G (1964) Rappel anatomique, physiologique et radiologique sur le rachis cervicale. Rev Prat 14:3197

De Seze S, Hubault A, Lasserre P, Monpetit G (1970) 106 cas de tumeurs intrarachidiennes dans un service de rhumatologie. Rev Rhum Mal Osteroartic 41:83-91

De Sousa AL, Kalsbeck JE, Mealey J, Campbell RL, Hockey A (1979) Intraspinal tumors in children. A review of 81 cases. J Neurosurg 51:437-455

De Vincentiis A (1935) Contributo clinico ai tumori del midollo spinale. Policlinico (Sez Chir) 52, 1

Decker K (1968) Neuroradiologia. Clinica Piccin, Padova

Deen HG, Scheithauber BW, Ebersold MJ (1982) Clinical and pathological study of meningiomas of the first two decades of life. J Neurosurg 56:317-322

Del Rio Hortega P (1930) Para el mejor conoscimiento de los meningoexoteliomas. Arch Esp Oncol 1:447

Delamarter RB, Bohlman HH, Bodner D et al (1990) Urologic function after experimental cauda equina compression: cystometrograms versus cortical-evoked potentials. Spine 15:864-870

Delbeke J, Mc Comas AJ, Kopec SJ (1978) Analysis of evoked lumbosacral potentials in man. J Neurol Neurosurg Psychiatry 41:293-302

Delitala F (1938) Paraplegia spastica da compressione del midollo. G Ital Sci Med 3:1

Demayer W (1965) Aberrant peripheral nerve fiber in the medulla oblongata of man. J Neurol Neurosurg Psychiatry 28:121-123

Depassio J, Confraveux C (1980) Les compressions médullaires lentes (causes traumatiques exceptées). Cah Med 5:1093-1105

Desmet JE (Ed) (1980) Clinical uses of cerebral brainstem and spinal somatosensory potentials. Prog Clin Neurophysiol Karger Ed., Basel, 7,1 vol.

Desproges-Gotteron R (1955) Contribution à l'étude de la sciatique paralysante. These, Paris

Deugnier Y (1979) Diagnostic des compressions medullaires lentes. Ouest Med 32:301-306

Devadiga KV, Gass H (1972) Multiple spinal cord meningiomas. Neurol India 20:142-144

Dhalin DC (1978) Bone tumors. General aspects and data on 6221 cases. Thomas, Springfield

Di Chiro G, Fisher RL (1964) Contrast radiography of the spinal cord. Arch Neurol 11:125-143

Di Lorenzo N, Giuffrè R, Fortuna A (1982) Primary spinal neoplasms in childhood: analysis of 1234 published cases (including 56 personal cases) by pathology, sex, age and site. Differences from in adults. Neurochirurgia (Stuttg) 25:153-164

Di Rocco C, Caldarelli M, Puca A, Colosimo Jr C (1984) Multiple spinal meningiomas in children. Neurochirurgia (Stuttg) 27:25-27

Di Rocco C, Iannelli A, Colosimo C Jr (1994) Spinal epidural meningiomas in childhood: a case report. J Neurosurg Sci 38:251-254

Dimitrijevic MR, Larsson LE, Lehmkuhl D et al (1978) Evoked spinal cord and nerve root potentials in humans using a noninvasive recording technique. Electroencephalogr Clin Neurophysiol 45:331-340

Dinner DS, Luders H, Lesser RP et al (1986) Intraoperative spinal SEP monitoring. J Neurosurg 65:807-814

Disertori B (1935) Compressioni del midollo spinale simulanti la sclerosi in placche. Minerva Med 1:138

Disertori B, Pezcoller A (1937) Su tre casi di tumore del midollo spinale. Riv Sper Fren 61:263

Distelmaier P, Lins E, Kolberg T (1976) Multiple meningiomas. Two patients with a spinal and intracranial meningioma. Radiological diagnosis. Neurochirurgia (Stuttg) 19:114-117

Djindjian M (1978) Spinal meningeal haemorrhage due to tumors: report of 5 cases with arteriography. Rev Neurol (Paris) 134:685-692

Djindjian R (1970) L'angiographie de la moelle épinière. Masson, Paris

Djindjian R, Houdart R (1966) Acquisitions récentes en angiographie médullaire. Rev Neurol (Paris) 115, 6:1068-1069

Djindjian R, Houdart R (1968a) La parte de l'ischémie médullaire dans les compressions de la moelle. IX journées annuelles sur la paraplégie, Paris, 14 November 1966

Djindjian R, Houdart R (1968b) Technique de l'artériographie de la moelle épinère par aortographie selective. Presse Med 76:159-162

Djindjian R, Houdart R, Julian H, Hurth M (1967a) Radiologie anatomique des artères de la moelle épinère et artériographie normale de la moelle épinère. Thomas, Nancy

Djindjian R, Julian H, Hurth M, Houdart R (1967b) Pathologie ischemique et artériographique médullaire. Rev Neurol (Paris) 117:663-664

Djindjian R, Rey A, Guilmet D, Godlewski S, Houdart R (1972) Etude des deux premiers cas operés d'ischémie médullaire par stenose ateromateuse de l' artére d'Adamkiewicz. Rev Neurol (Paris) 127, 4:471-482

Doco Fenzy M, Cornillet P, Scherpereel B, Depernet B, Bisiau Leconte S, Ferre D, Pluot M, Graftiaux JP, Teyssier JR (1993) Cytogenetic changes in 67 cranial and spinal meningiomas: relation to histopathological and clinical pattern. Anticancer Res 13, 4:845-850

Dominici L (1932) La chirurgia dei tumori spinali. IX Congr Soc Int Chir, Madrid, pp 721-809

Domino EF, Matsouka S, Waltz J et al (1964) Simultaneous recording of scalp and epidural somatosensory evoked responses in man. Science 145:1199-1200

Dommisse GF (1975) The arteries and veins of the human spinal cord from birth. Churchill Livingstone, Edinburgh

Donchin E, Lindsley DB (eds) (1969) Average evoked potentials. Methods, results and evaluations. NASA Special Publication 191

Doppman JL, Di Chiro G (1969) Selective arteriography of the spinal cord. Green, St. Louis

Dorizzi A, Crivelli G, Marra A, Scamoni C, Dario A, Bonfanti N, Brianza ML (1992) Associated cervical schwannoma and dorsal meningioma. Case report and review of the literature. J Neurosurg Sci 36:173-176

Drapkin AJ, Rose WS, Pellmar MB (1985) Chiari type I malformation with an associated intramedullary schwannoma. Surg Neurol 24:511-519

Drayer BP, Warner MA, Sudilovsky A, Luther J, Wilkins B, Allen S, Bates M (1982) Iopamidol vs metrizamide: a double blind study for cervical myelography. Neuroradiology 24:77-84

Ducker TB, Salcman, Lucus J et al (1978) Experimental spinal cord trauma: II. Blood flow, tissue oxygen, evoked potentials in both paretic and plegic monkeys. Surg Neurol 10:64-70

Dumanski JP, Rouleau GA, Nordenskjod M, Collins VP (1990) Molecular genetic analysis of chromosome 22 in 81 cases of meningioma. Cancer Res 50:5863-5867

Dyke CG (1941) The roentgenray diagnosis of disease of spinal cord, meninges and vertebrae In: Elsberg CA (ed) Surgical diseases of spinal cord, membranes and nerve roots. Hoeber, New York, pp 42-122

Dyke CG (1950) Roentgenray diagnosis of spinal cord tumors. In: Golden R (ed) Diagnostic roentgenology, chap 7. Nelson, New York

Early CB, Sayers MP (1966) Spinal extradural meningioma. Case report. J Neurosurg 25:571-573

Eccles JC (1951) Interpretation of action potentials evoked in the cerebral cortex. Electroencephalogr Clin Neurophysiol 3:449-464

Ectors L, van Bogaert L (1953) Ablation d'un méningiome du trou occipital chez un frere et une soeur. Acta Neurol Belg 53:193-204

Ectors L, Achslogh J, Saintes MJ (1960) Les compressions de la moelle cervicale. Masson, Paris

Eggert HR, Scheremet R, Seeger W, Gaitzsch J (1983) Unilateral microsurgical approaches to extramedullary spinal tumors. Operative technique and results. Acta Neurochir (Wien) 6:245-253

Eisen A, Nudleman K (1979) Cord to cortex conduction in multiple sclerosis. Neurology 29:189-193

Ekelund L, Cronqvist S (1973) Roentgenological changes in spinal malformations and spinal tumors in children. Radiology 12:541-546

Elsberg CA (1916) Disease of the spinal cord and its membrane. Saunders, Philadelphia

Elsberg CA (1923) The early symptoms and the diagnosis of tumors of the spinal cord, with remarks on the surgical treatment. Am J Med 165:719-727

Elsberg CA (1925a) Some aspects of the diagnosis and surgical treatment of tumors of the spinal cord with a study of the end results in a series of 119 operations. Ann Surg 81:1057

Elsberg CA (1925b) Tumors of the spinal cord. Hoeber, New York

Elsberg CA (1928) Extradural spinal tumors: primary, secondary, metastatic. Surg Gynecol Obstet 46:1-20

Elsberg CA (1931) Meningeal fibroblastomas. Bull Neurol Inst NY 1, 3

Elsberg CA (1933) Concerning the clinical features and the diagnosis of extramedullary meningeal and perineural fibroblastomas of the spinal cord. Bull Neurol Inst NY 3:124-137

Elsberg CA (1941) Surgical diseases of the spinal cord, membranes and nerve roots: symptoms, diagnosis and treatment. Hoeber, New York

Elsberg CA, Dyke CG (1934) The diagnosis and localization of tumors of the spinal cord by means of measurements. Bull Neurol Inst NY 3:359

Elsberg CA, Stookey B (1922) Mechanical effects of tumors of the spinal cord. Arch Neurol Psychol 8:502

Engert F (1900) Über Geschwülste der Dura Mater. Arch Pathol Anat 160:19-32

Epstein BS, Davidoff LM (1946) The myelographic diagnosis of extramedullary cervical spine tumors. Am J Roentgenol 55:413-419

Epstein BS, Epstein JA, Postel DM (1971) Tumors of spinal cord simulating psychiatric disorders. Dis Nerv Syst 32:741-743

Epstein NE, Danto J, Nardi D (1993) Evaluation of intraoperative somatosensory-evoked potential monitoring during 100 cervical operations. Spine 18, 6:737-747

Ertekin C (1976) Studies on the human evoked electrospinogram. Acta Neurol Scand 53:3-20

Ertekin C (1978) Comparison of the human evoked electrospinogram recorded from the intrathecal, epidural and cutaneous levels. Electroencephalogr Clin Neurophysiol 44:683-690

Erwin CW, Erwin AC (1993) Up and down the spinal cord: intraoperative monitoring of sensory and motor spinal cord pathways. J Clin Neurophysiol 10:425-436

Eskridge JT, Freeman L (1898) Intradural spinal tumor opposite the body of the fourth dorsal vertebra, complete paralysis of the parts below the lesion; operation; recovery with ability to walk without assistance within three months. Philadelphia Med J 2:1236-1243

Essbach H (1943) Die Meningioma. Erg Allg Pathol Pathol Anat 36:185-490

Ethier R, King DG, Melancon D, Belanger G, Thompson C (1980) Diagnosis of intra and extramedullary lesions by CT without contrast achieved through modifications applied to the EMI CT 5005 body scanner In: Post MJD (ed) Radiographic evaluation of the spine. Current advances with emphasis on computed tomography. Masson, New York, pp 377-393

Evard M, Passy V (1972) Von Recklinghausen's disease with multiple meningiomas. Laryngoscope 82:2222-2225

Fabiani A (1964) Considerazioni sul processo di ossificazione dei meningiomi con presentazione di tre casi. Riv Patol Nerv Ment 85:95-104

Fabiani A, Monticone GF (1964) Considerazioni su un raro caso di meningioma calcificato. Riv Neurobiol 10:390-397

Fabiani A, Trebini F, Favero M, Peres B, Palmucci M (1977) The significance of atypical mitoses in malignant meningiomas. Acta Neuropathol 38:229-231

Fabres A, Conocente Y, Chiorino S (1972) Neurinoma intramedullar dorsal. Presentacion de un caso. Clin Neurochir 30:100-102

Farwell JR, Dohrmann G (1977-1978) Intraspinal neoplasms in children. Paraplegia 15:262-273

Fazio C (1938) L'angioarchitettonica del midollo spinale umano ed i suoi rapporti con la citomieloarchitettonica. Riv Patol Nerv Ment 52:252

Feigin I (1978) Mixed mesenchymal tumors: meningioma and nerve sheath tumor. J Neuropathol Exp Neurol 37:459-470

Feiring EH, Barrong K (1962) Late recurrence of spinal cord meningioma. J Neurosurg 19:652-656

Feiring EH, Foer WH (1968) Meningioma following radium therapy. Case report. J Neurosurg 29:192-194

Feldman MH, Cracco RQ, Farmer P et al (1980) Spinal evoked potential in the monkey. Ann Neurol 7:238-244

Ferey D, Stabert C, Javalet A (1954) Aspects radiographiques et arteriographiques des méningiomes. J Radiol Electrol 35:634-637

Ferrante L, Aqui M, Mastronardi L, Nucci F (1987) Familial meningiomas: report of two cases. J Neurosurg Sci 31:145-151

Fischgold H, Wackenheim A (1965) La radiographie des formations intrarachidiennes. Masson, Paris

Fischgold H, Guiot C, Loeb C, Capdevielle G (1950) Etude anatomique et bioélectrique dans dix cas de méningiomes. Rev Neurol (Paris) 82:529-535

Foix C (1923a) Les compressions médullaires. Rev Neurol (Paris) 39:610-642

Foix C (1923b) Rapport sur les compressions médullaires. Rev Neurol (Paris) 30:610

Fontaine B (1993) Génétique et biologie moleculaire des neurinomes et des méningiomes. Rev Neurol (Paris) 149, 1:4-13

Fontana M, Carapella CM, Caroli F, Riccio A (1982) Spinal meningioma: an unusual radiological and clinical case. Neurosurgery 11:811-812

Foot NC (1940) Meningiomas. Arch Pathol 30:198-211

Ford FR (1952) Diseases of the nervous system in infancy, childhood and adolescence. Blackwell Scientific, Oxford

Fortuna A, Gambacorta D, Occhipinti EM (1969) Spinal extradural meningiomas. Neurochirurgia (Stuttg) 12:166-180

Fortuna A, Nolletti A, Nardi P, Caruso R (1981) Spinal meningiomas and neurinomas in children. Acta Neurochir (Wien) 55:329-341

Fournier D, Mercier P, Pouplard F, Menei P, Guy G (1993) Invasive character of an intradural spinal meningioma in early childhood. Childs Nerv Syst 9:28-31

Fox AJ, Vinuela F, Debrun G (1981) Complete mielography with metrizamide. AJNR 2:79-84

Frazier CH (1918) Surgery of the spine and spinal cord. Appleton, New York

Freedman DA, Feiring EH, Davidoff LM (1949) Carcinoma of the breast and intraspinal meningioma. A report of three cases. J Neuropathol Exp Neurol 8:85-92

Freidberg SR (1972) Removal of an ossified ventral thoracic meningioma. Case report. J Neurosurg 37:728-730

Fried H, Niebeling HG, Hohrein D (1988) Tumor induced medullary compression: experiences with 570 patients. Zentralbl Neurochir 49:270-272

Friede RL, Schachenmayr W (1978) II Fine structure of neomembranes. Am J Pathol 92:69-84

Friedmann G von, Thun F, Butzler HO (1972) Röntgendiagnostik raumfordernder, intraspinaler Prozesse im Kindesalter. Fortschr Rontgenstr 117:408-412

Friedman WA, Grundy BL (1987) Monitoring of sensory evoked potentials is highly reliable and helpful in the operating room. J Clin Monit 3:38

Fromme K, Miltner FO, Klawki P et al (1990) Spinal cord monitoring during intraspinal extramedullary tumor operations (peroneal nerve evoked responses). Neurosurg Rev 13:195-199

Frugoni P (1956) Trattamento chirurgico dei tumori del midollo. Chirurgia 11:131-149

Frugoni P (1967) Considerazioni su 43 casi di tumori intrarachidei operati d'urgenza. Minerva Neurochir 11, 2:75-83

Fujita H, Fujita S (1963) Electron microscopic studies on neuroblast differentiation in the central nervous system of domestic fowl Z Zellforsch Mikrosk Anat 60:463-478

Fujita S (1963) The matrix cell and cytogenesis in the developing central nervous system. J Comp Neurol 120:37-42

Fumarola G, Trevisini A (1936) Undici casi di tumore del midollo spinale con reperto chirurgico e anatomico. Riv Ital Endocr Neurochir 14:199

Gaidolfi E, Valentini MC, Scala A (1991) I tumori primitivi del midollo spinale. Progressi di diagnosi e terapia. Minerva Medica, Torino

Gaist G, Piazza G (1957) I tumori spinali nell'infanzia. Arch Neurochir (Wien) 4:1-24

Gaist G, Piazza G (1959) Meningiomas in two members of the same family (with no evidence of neurofibromatosis). J Neurosurg 16:110-113

Gandolfi A, Bertolino G (1978) Simultaneous cervical cord compression from herniated disk and extradural meningioma; report of a case. Acta Neurol (Napoli) 33:273-278

Ganshirt H (1965) On the clinical aspects of extra and intramedullary tumors. Radiology 5:473-477

Garcin R et al (1933) Tumeur de la moelle cervicale evolvant sous les traits d'une sclérose laterale amyotrophique. Ablation, guerison. Rev Neurol (Paris) 40:391-395

Garcin R, Godlewski S, Lapresle J, Fardeau M (1959) Syndromes vasculaires aigues probables de la partie inférieure de la moelle chez des sujets porteurs de lesions discarthrosiques du rachis dorso-lombaire (à propos de 4 cas dont un verifié anatomiquement). Rev Neurol (Paris) 100,3:212-229

Garcin R, Godlewski S, Rondot P (1962a) Etude clinique des myélopathies d'origine vasculaire. Rev Neurol (Paris) 106:506

Garcin R, Zulch KJ, Lazorthes G, Gruner J (1962b) Pathologie vasculaire de la moelle. Rapports presentés a la XXV Reunion Neurologique Internationale, Paris, 5-6 June 1962. Masson, Paris

Gasser HS, Graham HT (1933) Potential produced in the spinal cord by stimulation of dorsal roots. Am J Physiol 103:303-320

Gastaut H, Bostem F, Waltregny A et al (1967a) Les activités électriques cerebrales spontanées et evoquées chez l'homme colloque de Marseille. Monographie de physiologie causale. Gauthier Villars, Paris

Gastaut H, Regis H, Lyagoubi S et al (1967b) Comparison of the evoked potentials recorded from the occipital, temporal and central regions of the human scalp, evoked by visual, auditory and somatosensory stimuli. Electroencephalogr Clin Neurophysiol [Suppl] 26:19-28

Geisler E von, Schuck W (1963) Spinale Tumoren und das Rückenmark komprimierende Prozesse bei Kindern. Arch Kinderheilkd 169:254-266

Gelfan S, Tarlov IM (1956) Physiology of spinal cord, nerve root and peripheral nerve compression. Am J Physiol 195:217-229

Ghaly RF, Stone JL, Levy WJ et al (1990) The apport of etomidate on motor evoked potentials induced by transcranial magnetic stimulation in the monkey. Neurosurgery 27:936-942

Ghoshhajra K (1982) Blistering of the odontoid process by meningioma. Neuroradiology 23:164

Giaquinto S, Massi G, Ricolfi A, Vitali S (1984) On six cases of radiation meningiomas from the same community. J Neurol Sci 5:173-175

Giblin DR (1964) Somatosensory evoked potentials in healthy subjects and in patients with lesions of the nervous system. Ann NY Acad Sci 122:93-142

Gilligan L (1958) The arterial blood supply of the human spinal cord. J Comp Neurol 110:75-104

Ginsburg HH, Shetter AG, Raudzens PA (1985) Postoperative paraplegia with preserved intraoperative SEPs. Case report. J Neurosurg 63:296-300

Girard PF, Trillet M, Confrabeux C, Chazot G (1977) Méningiomatose multiple et familiale. Une syndrome voisine de la neurofibromatose de Recklinghausen. Rev Neurol (Paris) 133:359-362

Giuffrè R, Di Lorenzo N, Fortuna A (1981) Cervical tumors of infancy and childhood. J Neurosurg Sci 25:259-264

Glasier CM, Husain MM, Chadduck W, Boop FA (1993) Meningiomas in children: MR and histopathologic findings. AJNR 14(1): 237-241

Glauser FE (1964) Thoracic and lumbar intraspinal tumors associated with increased intracranial pressure. J Neurol Neurosurg Psychol 27:451-458

Globus JH (1937) Meningiomas: their origin, divergence in structure, and relationship to contiguous tissues in light of philogenesis and ontogenesis of meninges, with suggestion of simplified classification of meningeal neoplasm. Arch Neurol Psychol 38:667-712

Goffin J (1986) Estrogen- and progesterone-receptors in meningiomas. Clin Neurol Neurosurg 88:169-175

Goidanch IF, Battaglia L (1956) La rara varietà ossificante delle neoplasie meningee spinali. Chir Organi Mov 43:107-120

Goldhahn WE, Schmidt U (1989) Spinal meningioma. Zentralbl Neurochir 50:18-23

Gonzales MG, Allut AG, Alonso CC, Zabala AB, Rumbo RM, Oliveros FR (1985) Intramedullary spinal neurofibroma diagnosed with computed tomography: report of a case. Neurosurgery 16:543-545

Gorter CJ (1947) Paramagnetic relaxation. Elsevier, Amsterdam

Gowers WR, Horsley V (1888) A case of tumour of the spinal cord. Removal Recovery Med Chir Trans 71:377-428

Goy AM, Pinto RS et al (1986) Intramedullary spinal cord tumors: MR imaging with emphasis on associated cysts. Radiology 161:381-386

Gozzano M (1968) Trattato delle malattie nervose. Vallardi, Milano

Grant FC (1934) Notes on a series of spinal cord tumors. Am J Surg 23:89

Grant FC, Austin GM (1956) The diagnosis, treatment and prognosis of tumors affecting the spinal cord in children. J Neurosurg 13:535-545

Gravenstein MA, Sasse F, Hogan K (1984) Effects of stimulus rate and halotane dose on canine far-field evoked potentials. Anesthesiology 61:A 342

Gray ED (1942) Calcification and ossification of spinal tumors. Br J Radiol 15:365-369

Green BA, Diaz RD, Post MJD (1984) The diagnosis of spinal column and spinal cord tumors with emphasis of the value of computed tomography. In: Post MJD (ed) Computed tomography of the spine. Williams and Wilkins, Baltimore, pp 659-695

Green JR, Waggener JD, Kriegsfeld BA (1976) Classification and incidence of neoplasms of the central nervous system. In: Thompson RA, Green JR (eds) Neoplasia in the central nervous system. Raven, New York (Advances in neurology, vol 15)

Greenberg R, Ducker TB (1982) Evoked potentials in clinical neuroscience. J Neurosurg 56:1-18

Greenberg SB, Schneck MJ, Faerber EN, Kanev PM (1993) Malignant meningioma in a child. AJR 160:1111-1112

Grellier P, Duplay J, Ristori S (1982) Semiology of spinal meningiomas and neurinomas. Semin Hop Paris 58:1109-1112

Grote W, Romer F, Bock WJ, Bockhorn J, Bushe KA, Entzian W, Szepan B (1975) Langzeitergebnisse in der Behandlung spinaler Tumoren des Kindes- und Jugendalters. Monatsschr Kinderheilkd 123:112-119

Grundy BL, Villani RM (eds) (1988) Evoked potentials: intraoperative and ICU monitoring. Springer, Vienna New York

Gruner J, Lapresle J (1962) Etude anatomo-pathologique des médullopathies d'origine vasculaire probable. Rev Neurol (Paris) 106:592

Gudmondsson KR (1970) A survey of tumors of the central nervous system in Iceland during the 10 years period 1954-1963. Acta Neurol Scand 46:538-552

Guidetti B (1954) Tumori spinali. Considerazioni su 64 casi operati. Minerva Chir 9:909

Guidetti B (1967) Intramedullary tumors of the spinal cord. Acta Neurochir (Wien) 17:7-23

Guidetti B (1974) Removal of extramedullary benign spinal cord tumors. In: Krayenbuhl H (ed) Advances and technical standard in neurosurgery, vol 1. Springer, Vienna New York, pp 171-195

Guidetti B, Fortuna A (1975) Differential diagnosis of intramedullary and extramedullary tumours. In: Winken PJ, Bruyn GW, Klawans HL (eds) Handbook of clinical neurology. North Holland, Amsterdam, pp 51-75

Guidetti B, Fortuna A, Moscatelli G, Riccio A (1964) I tumori intramidollari. Lav Neuropsichiatr 35:1-409

Guilbeau JC, Morvan G, Nahum H (1982) Intraspinal calcifications. Symptomatology. Pathologic value. J Radiol 63:453-463

Guillaume J, Sigwald J (1947) Diagnostic neurochirurgical. University of France Press, Paris

Guillaume J, Oeconomos D, Mazars G (1949) Méningiome de la moelle chez une enfant de 9 ans. Ablation, guerison. Rev Neurol (Paris) 81:600-602

Guillaume J, De Seze S, Mazars G, Desproges-Gotteron R (1955) La sciatique paralysante: considerations pathologiques. Rev Neurol (Paris) 93

Guillaume J, Billet R, Caron JP, Cuccia D (1957) Les méningiomes.

Etude clinique et chirurgicale. University of France Press, Paris

Guyer RD, Collier RR, Ohnmeiss DD et al (1988) Extraosseous spinal lesions mimicking disc disease. Spine 13:328-331

Guyot JF (1970) Compression de la queue de cheval. Rev Prat 20:1843-1853

Hackney DB (1992) Neoplasms and related disorders. Top Magn Reson Imaging 4:2:37-61

Hafstrom T, Linibreg KAR (1954) Méningiomes calcifiés multiples de durée anormale. Acta Psychol Neurol Scand 29:173-179

Haft H, Shenkin H (1963) Spinal epidural meningioma: case report. J Neurosurg 20:801-804

Haft H, Ransohoff J, Carter S (1959) Spinal cord tumors in children. Pediatrics 23:1152-1159

Hallpike JF, Stanley P (1968) A case of extradural spinal meningioma. J Neurol Neurosurg Psychol 31:191-197

Hamburger V (1952) Development of the nervous system. Ann NY Acad Sci 55:117-132

Hamburger V (1975) Cell death in the development of the lateral motor column of the chick embryo. J Comp Neurol 160:535-546

Hamby WB (1938) Tumors in the spinal canal in childhood. Am J Surg 39:342-376

Hamby WB (1944) Tumors in the spinal cord in childhood. J Neuropathol Exp Neurol 111:397

Hanlon DG, Dodge JW, Siekert RG Jr (1956) Tumors of the spinal cord: occurrence in patients with pernicious anemia and subacute combined sclerosis. JAMA 162:707

Hannan JR, Hughes CR, Mulvey BE (1949) Spinal cord tumors. Radiology 53:711

Hans JS, Kauffman B et al (1983) NMR imaging of the spine. AJNR 4:1151-1159

Harkey HR, Crockard HA (1991) Spinal meningiomas: clinical features. In: Al-Mefty O (ed) Meningiomas. Raven, New York, pp 593-601

Harrington M, Bone I (1981) Spinal meningioma presenting as a focal epilepsy A case report. Br Med J 282:1984-1985

Harris AE (1965) Differentiation and degeneration in the motor horn of the foetal mouse. PhD Thesis, University of Cambridge

Harvey SC, Burr HS (1926) The development of the meninges. Arch Neurol Psychiatry 15:545-567

Hassler O (1966) Blood supply to human spinal cord. Arch Neurol 15:302

Heiskanen O (1968) Benign extramedullary tumors in the high cervical region. Ann Chir Gynaecol Fenn 57:59-62

Heiskari M, Tolonen V, Kovala T et al (1988) Somatosensory evoked potentials to posterior tibial nerve stimulation in cervical radiculopathy and radiculomyelopathy. Neuroorthop 5:78-82

Helseth A, Mork SJ, Johansen A, Tretli S (1989) Neoplasms of the central nervous system in Norway IV. A population based epidemiological study of meningiomas. APMIS 97:646-654

Henschen F (1955) Tumoren des Zentralnervensystems und seiner Hüllen. In: Henke F, Lubarsch O (eds) Handbuch der speziellen pathologischen Anatomie und Histologie, vol 13. Springer Berlin Heidelberg New York, pp 413-1040

Herdmann J, Lumenta CB, Huse KOW (1993) Magnetic stimulation for monitoring of motor pathways in spinal procedures. Spine 18, 5:551-559

Herregodts P, Vloeberghs M, Schmedding E, Goossens A, Stadnik T, D'Haens J (1991) Solitary dorsal intramedullary schwannoma. J Neurosurg 74:816-20

Herren RY (1939) Occurrence and distribution of calcified plaques in the spinal arachnoid in man. Arch Neurol 41:1180-1186

Herrmann HD, Neuss M, Winkler D (1988) Intramedullary spinal cord tumors resected with CO_2 laser microchirurgical technique: recent experience in fifteen patients. Neurosurgery 22:518-522

Herron LD, Trippi AC, Gonyeau M (1987) Intraoperative use of dermatomal somatosensory evoked potentials in lumbar stenosis surgery. Spine 12:379-383

Hicks RG, Burke DJ, Stephen JP (1991) Monitoring spinal cord function during scoliosis surgery with Cotrel-Dubousset instrumentation. Med J Aust 21, 154:82-86

Hiet C (1959) Méningiomes multiples. Theses Med Paris, N233

Hilal SK, Keim HA (1972) Selective spinal angiography in adolescent scoliosis. Radiology 102:349-359

Hinds JW (1971) Early neuroblast differentiation in the mouse olfactory bulb. Anat Rec 169:340-341

Hiramatsu K (1992) Postoperative prognostic factors in patients with spinal cord tumors. Nippon Seikeigeka Gakkai Zasshi 65, 10:862-876

His W (1890) Histogenese und Zusammenhang der Nervenelemente. Arch Anat Physiol Lpz Anat Abt Suppl 95-117

Hitchon PW, Dyste GN, Osenbach RK et al (1990) Spinal cord blood flow in response to focal compression. J Spinal Disord 3:210-219

Hoff H von, Potzl O (1937) Über Nystagmus bei Tumoren in der Höhe des Dorsalmarks. Med Klin 33:598-602

Hoff H von, Weingarten K (1952) Über spinale Tumoren im Kindesalter. Wien Klin Wochenschr 64:220-222

Hoffmann GT, Earle KM (1960) Meningioma with malignant transformation and implantation in the subarachnoid space. J Neurosurg 17:486-492

Hogenesch RI, Staal MJ (1988) Tumors of the cauda equina: the importance of an early diagnosis. Clin Neurol Neurosurg 90:343-348

Holliday PO, Davis Jr C, Angelo J (1984) Multiple meningiomas of the cervical spinal cord associated with Klippel-Feil malformation and atlanto-occipital assimilation. Neurosurgery 14:353-357

Hormes JT, Chappuis JL (1993) Monitoring of lumbosacral nerve roots during spinal instrumentation. Spine 15, 18:2059-2062

Horrax G, Poppen JL, Wu W, Weadon PR (1949) Meningiomas and neurofibromas of the spinal cord. Certain clinical features and end results. Surg Clin North Am 29:659-665

Horsley V (1890) Remarks on the surgery of the central nervous system. Br Med J 2:1286-1292

Horsley V, Gowers W (1888) A case of tumor of the spinal cord. Removal Recovery Med Chir Trans 53:377-428

Horwitz NH, Rizzoli HV (1957) Postoperative complications in neurosurgical practice. Williams and Wilkins, Baltimore, p 422

Hossmann KA, Zulch KJ (1966) Die spinalen psammomatosen Meningeome der Frau. Neurochirurgia (Stuttg) 9:106-113

Houdart R, Djindjian R, Julian H, Hurth M (1965) Données nouvelles sur la vascularisation de la moelle dorso-lombaire. Application radiologique et intérêt chirurgical. Soc Franc Neurologie, Paris, 6-7 May

Hounsfield GN, Ambrose J, Perry J et al (1973) Computerized transverse axial scanning. Br J Radiol 46:1016-1051

Huffmann G (1965) Ungewöhnliche Symptomatik raumfordernder Prozesse. Nervenarzt 36:74-77

Hughes AFW (1968) Aspects of neural ontogeny. Academic, New York

Hughes AFW (1974) Endocrines, neural development and behaviour. In: Gottlieb G (ed) Aspects of neurogenesis. Academic, New York

Huh K (1964) A study of the incidence of calcification in a histological survey of surgical biopsies of meningiomas. J Neurosurgery 21:751-757

Hume AL, Cant BR (1978) Conduction time in central somatosensory pathways in man. Electroencephalogr Clin Neurophysiol 45:361-375

Humphrey DR (1968) Re-analysis of the antidromic cortical responses Potentials evoked by the stimulation of the isolated pyramidal tract. Electroencephalogr Clin Neurophysiol 25:116-129

Hurth M (1980) Diagnostic précoce des compressions médullaires non traumatiques. Rev Prat 30:4169-4181

Hutchinson E, Yates P (1956) The cervical portion of the vertebral artery. A clinical pathological study. Brain 79:319

Ibrahim AV, Satti MB, Ibrahim EM (1986) Extraspinal meningioma. Case report. J Neurosurg 64:328-330

Iglesias JR, Esparza J, Aruffo C, Maier-Hauff K (1988) Differential diagnosis of intraspinal neurinomas and meningiomas by means of a bayesan system. Arch Neurobiol (Madr) 51:333-341

Ingebrigsten R, Leegaard T (1939) Final results in series of operated intraspinal tumors. Acta Chir Scand 82:271-281

Ingraham FD (1938) Intraspinal tumors in infancy and chidhood. Am J Surg 39:342-376

Ingram DA, Thompson AJ, Swash M (1988) Central motor conduction in multiple sclerosis: evaluation of abnormalities revealed by transcutaneous magnetic stimulation of the brain. J Neurol Neurosurg Psychiatry 51:635-642

Intrau H von, Usbeck W (1971) Komprimierende Prozesse im Wirberkanal bei Kindern. Zentralbl Chir 36:1225-1230

Iraci G (1966) Intraspinal tumors of infancy and childhood. A review of 19 surgically verified cases. J Ped Surg 1:534-545

Iraci G, Costantini FE (1963) Tumori primitivi del rachide e dello spazio epidurale: Studio di 45 casi. Ann Neurol Psich 57:211-238

Iraci G, Pellone M (1965) Tumori vertebro-midollari dell'infanzia. Ann Neurol Psich 59:529-560

Iraci G, Ruberti R (1966) Intraspinal tumors of the cervical tract. A study of 68 cases. Int Surg 46:154-167

Iraci G, Peserico L, Salar G (1971) Intraspinal meningiomas and neurinomas. A clinical survey of 172 cases. Int Surg 56:289-301

Isu T, Kunio T, Mitsumori K, Sato M, Tsuru M, Kashiwaba T (1976) A case of intramedullary spinal schwannoma. No Shinkei Geka, 9:897-901

Isu T, Kamada K, Kobayashi N, Koyanagi I (1993) Intraoperative monitoring for spinal cord tumor by spinal cord evoked potential. No Shinkei Geka 21:6:519-526

Jacquet G, Czorny A, Godard J, Steimle R, Wendling D (1992) Neurinome intramedullaire. A propos d'un cas. Revue de la littéra-ture. Neurochirurgie 38:315-321

Jain KK (1983) Handbook of laser neurosurgery. Thomas, Springfield, pp 116-123

Jeanmonod D, Sindou M (1991) Somatosensory function following dorsal root entry zone lesions in patients with neurogenic pain or spasticity. J Neurosurg 74:916-932

Jellinek D, Jewkes D, Symon L (1991) Noninvasive intraoperative monitoring of motor evoked potentials under propofol anesthesia: effects of spinal surgery on the amplitude and latency of motor evoked potentials. Neurosurgery 29:551-557

Jellinger K, Neumayer E (1962) Myelopathies progressives d'origine vasculaire. Rev Neurol (Paris) 106:107

Jellinger K, Slowik F (1975) Histological subtypes and prognostic problems in meningiomas. J Neurol 208:279-298

Jelsma F (1941) Hour-glass tumor of the cervical spine. Am J Surg 52:483-488

Jones SJ (1988) Normal and pathologic factors affecting sensory tract potentials in the human spinal cord during surgery. In: Grundy BL, Villani RM (eds) Springer, Vienna New York, pp 53-62

Jones SJ, Small DG (1978) Spinal and sub-cortical evoked potential following stimulation of posterior tibial nerve in man. Electro-encephalogr Clin Neurophysiol 44:299-306

Jorgensen J, Ovesen M, Poulsen JO (1976) Intraspinal tumours in the first two decades of life. Clinical and radiological features. Acta Orthop Scand 47:391-396

Jrasek A (1932) Diagnosis and treatment of intraspinal tumors. IX Congr Soc Int Chir (Madrid) 667-719

Julian H, Djindjian R, Caron JP, Houdart R (1968) Syndrome d'ischèmie médullaire par compression discale de l'artère du renflement lombaire. Neurochirurgie 14:163-170

Jumentie MJ (1923) Quelques remarques à propos de l'évolution des tumeurs de la moelle. Rev Neurol (Paris) 39:667-670

Kadyi H (1889) Über die Blutgefässe des menscliichen Rückenmarks. Gubynowics-Schmidt, Lemberg

Kai Y, Owen JH, Keith HB et al (1990) The use of sciatic-NMEP versus spinal potentials to predict early-onset of neurological def-

icits when intervention is still possible. J Orthop Assoc S1111

Kai Y, Owen JH, Allen BT et al (1994) Relationship between evoked potentials and clinical status in spinal cord ischemia. Spine 19,10:1162-1166

Kakigi R, Shibasaki H, Kuroda Y et al (1988) Multimodal evoked potentials in HTLV-I associated myelopathy. J Neurol Neurosurg Psychiatry 51:1094-1096

Kalkman J, Drummond JC (1994) Severe sensory deficits with preserved motor function after removal of a spinal arteriovenous malformation: correlation with simultaneously recorded somatosensory and motor evoked potentials. Anesth Analg 78:165-168

Kandel E, Sungurov E, Morgunov V (1989) Cerebral and two spinal meningiomas removed from the same patient: case report. Neurosurgery 25:447-450

Kang JK, Song JU (1983) Intramedullary spinal schwannoma. J Neurol Neurosurg Psychiatry 46:1154-1155

Kannuki S, Soga T, Hondo H, Matsumoto K, Takada K, Makino A (1991) Coexistence of intracranial and spinal meningiomas Report of two cases. Neurol Med Chir (Tokyo) 31:720-724

Kaplan A et al (1950) Cervical cord tumors simulating cerebral vascular diseases. Dis Nerv Syst 11:182

Kaplan BJ, Friedman WA, Alexander JA et al (1986) Somatosensory evoked potential monitoring of spinal cord ischemia during aortic operations. Neurosurgery 19:82

Karasick JL, Mullan SF (1974) A survey of metastatic meningiomas. J Neurosurg 40:206-212

Kasantikul V, Charuchaikul S, Shuangshoti S (1991) Extramedullary subdural meningioma after trauma. Neurosurgery 29:930-931

Katz K, Reichenthal E, Israeli K (1981) Surgical treatment of spinal meningiomas. Neurochirurgia (Stuttg) 24:21-22

Kaufman AB, Dunsmore RH (1971) Clinicopathological considerations in spinal meningeal calcification and ossification. Neurology 21:1243-1248

Kaya U, Ozden B, Turantan MI, Aydin Y, Barlas O (1982) Spinal epidural meningioma in childhood: a case report. Neurosurgery 10:746-747

Kaye AH, Giles GG, Gonzales M (1993) Primary central nervous system tumours in Australia: a profile of a clinical practice from Australian Brain Tumor Register. Aust NZ J Surg 63(1):33-38

Kearse LA Jr, Lopez-Bresnahan M, Mc Peck K et al (1993) Loss of intraoperative somatosensory evoked potentials during intramedullary spinal cord surgery predicts postoperative neurologic deficits in motor function. J Clin Anesth 5:392-398

Keegan HR, Mullan S (1962) Pigmented meningioma: an unusual variant. Report of a case with review of the literature. J Neurosurg 19:696-698

Keim HA, Hilal SK (1971) Spinal angiography in scoliosis patients. J Bone Joint Surg 5:904-912

Keim HA, Hajdu M, Gonzalez EG et al (1985) Somatosensory evoked potentials as an aid in the diagnosis and intraoperative management of spinal stenosis. Spine 10, 4:338-344

Keith RW, Stambough JL, Awender SH (1990) Somatosensory cortical evoked potentials: a review of 100 cases of intraoperative spinal surgery monitoring. J Spinal Disord 3:220-226

Keller BP, Haghighi SS, Oro JJ et al (1992) The effects of propofol anesthesia on transcortical electric evoked potentials in the rat. Neurosurgery 30 (4):557-560

Kepes J (1961a) Observations on the formation of psammoma bodies and pseudopsammoma bodies in meningioma. J Neuropathol Exp Neurol 20:255-262

Kepes J (1961b) Electron microscopic studies of meningiomas. Am J Pathol 39:499-510

Kepes J (1982) Meningiomas. Biology, pathology and differential diagnosis. Masson, New York

Kepes J (1986) The histopathology of meningiomas. A reflection of origins and expected behavior? J Neuropathol Exp Neurol 45:95-107

Kepes J, Kernohan JW (1959) Meningioma: problems of histological differential diagnosis. Cancer 12:364-370

Kernohan JW (1941) Tumors of the spinal cord; general review. Arch Pathol 32:843-883

Kernohan JW, Sayre GP (1952) Tumors of the central nervous system. Atlas of tumors pathology, sect X, Fascicle 35. Armed Forces Institute of Pathology, Washington, p 141

Kernohan JW, Woltman HW, Adson AW (1931) Intramedullary tumors of the spinal cord. Arch Neurol Psychiatry 25:679-699

Kersting G, Lennartz H (1957) In vitro cultures of human meningioma tissue. J Neuropathol Exp Neurol 16:507-513

Khan MR, McInnes A, Hughes SP (1989) Electrophysiological studies in cervical spondylosis. J Spinal Disord 2(3):163-169

Khodadad G (1973) Common errors in the diagnosis of spinal meningiomas. Geriatrics 28:143-145

Kirshnan KL, Narayanan R, Kalyanaraman S, Ramamurthi B (1978) Spinal epidural meningioma. Int Surg 63, 1:42-43

Klein M (1960) Le tumeur de la moelle chez l'enfant. Acta Neurochir (Wien) 9:69-86

Kloss K, Heppner F, Argyropoulos G (1965) Chirurgische Erfahrungen mit raumbeschränkenden Prozessen des Rückenmarks. Klin Med (Wien) 20:62

Knudson AG Jr (1985) Hereditary cancer, oncogenes and antioncogenes. Cancer Res 45:1437-1443

Kobrine AI, Evans DE, Rizzoli HV (1978) Correlation of spinal blood flow and function in experimental compression. Surg Neurol 10:54-59

Kobrine AI, Evans DE, Rizzoli HV (1979a) Experimental acute balloon compression of the spinal cord. Factors affecting disappearance and return of the spinal evoked response. J Neurosurg 51:841-845

Kobrine AI, Evans DE, Rizzoli HV (1979b) The effect of ischemia on long-tract neural conduction in the spinal cord. J Neurosurg 50:639-644

Koht A, Sloan T, Ronai A et al (1985) Intraoperative deterioration of evoked potentials during spinal surgery. In: Schramm J, Jone SJ (eds) Spinal cord monitoring. Springer Berlin Heidelberg New York, pp 161-166

Kolle K (1959) Der Psychiater. Thieme, Stuttgart

Koos W, Laubichler W (1967) Über die spinalen Geschwülste bei Kindern. Wien Z Nervenheilkd 24:247-263

Koos W, Laubichler W, Sorgo G (1973) Statistische Untersuchungen bei spinalen Tumoren im Kindes- und Jugendalter. Neuropaediatrie 4:273-303

Kordas M von, Paraicz E, Szenasy J (1977) Spinale Tumoren im Säuglings- und Kindesalter. Zentralbl Neurochir 38:331-338

Kornblum JA, Bay JW, Gupta MK (1988) Steroid receptors in human brain and spinal cord tumors. Neurosurgery 23:185-188

Kornhuber H, Deecke L (1964) Hirnpotetentialänderungen beim Menschen vor und nach Willkürbewegungen, dargestellt mit Magnetband-Speicherung und Ruckwärtsanalyse. Pfluger Arch Ges Physiol 281:52

Kostic S (1958) Observations and results in surgery of spinal cord tumors. A report based on 165 cases observed and operated on at the Neurosurgical Clinic of Belgrade. University Bull Soc Int Chir 17:387

Kozlowski K von, Michalski M (1962) Selten auftretende intraspinale Tumoren bei Kindern. Fortschr Roentgenstr 96:531-539

Krabbe KH (1947) Les tumeurs intraspinales de l'enfance. Acta Psychol 46:175

Krishnan KLM, Narayanan R, Kalianaraman S (1978) Spinal epidural meningioma. Int Surg 63:42-43

Kristiansen K (1951) Intraspinal tumors. Tidsskr Nor Laegeforen 71:790-794

Krogh E (1945) Studies on the blood supply to certain regions in the lumbar part of the spinal cord. Acta Physiol Scand 10:3-4:271-281

Kruse F Jr (1961) Hemagiopericytoma of meninges (angioblastic meningioma of Cushing and Eisenhardt): clinicopathological aspects and follow-up studies in 8 cases. Neurology 11:771-777

Kumar S, Kaza RC, Maitra TK, Chandra M (1980) Extradural spinal meningioma arising from a nerve root. Case report. J Neurosurg 52:728-729

Kunicki A, Macejak A (1964) Die Operationsergebnisse bei 154 extramedullären Meningiomen und Neurinomen. Diskussionbeitrag auf dem Symposion der Vereiningung der Neurochirurgen in der DDR. Magdeburg

Kuritzky A (1984) Cluster headache-like pain caused by an upper cervical meningioma. Cephalalgia 4:185-186

La Mont RL, Wasson SL, Green MA (1983) Spinal cord monitoring during spinal surgery using somatosensory evoked potentials. J Pediatr Orthop 3:31

Lance JW, Drummond PD, Gandevia SC et al (1988) Harlequin syndrome - the sudden onset of unilateral flushing and sweating. J Neurol Neurosurg Psychiatry 51:635-642

Landelius E (1926) Experiences of some spinal intradural tumors. Acta Chir Scand 60:180-192

Landi A, Ducati A, Cenzato M et al (1988) Somatosensory evoked potential monitoring during cervical spine surgery. In: Grundy BL, Villani RM (eds), Springer, Vienna New York, pp 63-70

Lang EF Jr, Bridge C (1959) Intramedullary spinal cord tumors. Surg Clin North Am 39:831-839

Lapresle J, Netsky MG, Zimmerman HM (1952) The pathology of meningiomas. Am J Pathol 28:757

Laquer L (1891) Über Kompression der Cauda equina. Neurol Zentralbl 10:193-204

Larionov VE (1897) On the cortical centers of hearing in dogs. Obozr Psychiat Neurol (St. Petersburg) 2, 419-424

Launay M, Chiras J, Bories J (1979) Angiographies médullaires: temps veineux. Aspects normaux. Perspectives d'application en pathologie. J Neuroradiol 6:287-315

Lazorthes G, Poulhes J, Bastide G, Roulleau J, Chancholle AR (1957) Recherches sur la vascularisation artérielle de la moelle. Applications à la pathologie médullaire. Bull Acad Nat Med (Paris) 41:464

Lazorthes G et al (1958) La vascularisation arterielle de la moelle. Neurochirurgie 4:1

Lazorthes G, Poulhes J, Bastide G, Chancholle AR, Zadeh O (1962) La vascularisation de la moelle épinière. Etude anatomique et physiologique. Rev Neurol (Paris) 106:535-557

Lazorthes G, Gouaze A, Bastide G, Soutoul JH, Zadeh O, Santini JJ (1966a) La vascularisation artérielle du renflement lombaire. Etude des variations et des suppleances. Rev Neurol (Paris) 114:109-122

Lazorthes G et al (1966b) La vascularisation artérielle de la moelle cervicale Etude de suppléances. Rev Neurol (Paris) 115:1055-1068

Lazorthes G et al (1971) Arterial vascularization of the spinal cord. J Neurosurg 35:253-262

Lazorthes G, Gouaze A, Djindjian R (1973) Vascularisation et circulation de la moelle épinière. Masson, Paris

Learmonth JR (1927) On leptomeningiomas (endotheliomas) of the spinal cord. Br J Surg 14:397

Lefebvre J, Klein MR, Lepintre J, Faure C (1956) Etude radiologique des tumeurs medullaires chez l'enfant. Acta Radiol 46:48-54

Lehmann D, Callaway E (eds) (1978) Human evoked potentials: applications and problems. Plenum, New York (NATO conference series 3, vol 9)

Lehoczky TDE, Piri L (1944) Syndrome of amyotrophic sclerosis caused by cervical "hourglass tumor". Confin Neurol 6:71-80

Leikola A (1976) The neural crest: migrating cells in embryonic development. Folia Morphol 24:155-172

Lenzi M (1960) Elementi di neuroradiologia. Minerva Medica, Torino

Lepage JR (1974) Transfemoral ascending lumbar catheterization of the epidural veins. Radiology 3:337-339

Lepoire J, Montaut J, Renard M (1966) Recidive d'un méningiome spinal 14 ans après la première intervention. Ann Med (Nancy) 5:163-171

Lesch KP, Fahlbusch R (1986) Simultaneous estradiol and progesterone receptor analysis in meningiomas. Surg Neurol 26:257-263

Lesch KP, Gross S (1987) Estrogen receptor immunoreactivity in meningiomas. Comparison with the binding activity of estrogen, progesterone, and androgen receptors. J Neurosurg 67:237-243

Lesch KP, Engl HG, Gross S (1987a) Androgen receptor binding activity in meningiomas. Surg Neurol 28:176-180

Lesch KP, Engl HG, Schott W, Gross S (1987b) Immunoreactive estrogen receptor protein in meningiomas: comparison with the androgen receptor and progesterone receptor binding activity. Zentralbl Neurochir 48:124-134

Lesch KP, Schott W, Engl HG, Gross S, Thierauf P (1987c) Gonadal steroid receptors in meningiomas. J Neurol 234:328-333

Lesoin F, Delandsheer E, Krivosic I et al (1983) Solitary intramedullary schwannomas. Surg Neurol 19:51-56

Lesoin F, Leys D, Pasquier F, Krivosic Y, Reyford H, Jomin M, Petit H (1985) Melanotic meningioma. Report of a case and review of the literature. Neurochirurgia (Stuttg) 28:205-207

Lesser RP, Raudzens P, Luders H et al (1986) Postoperative neurological deficits may occur despite unchanged intraoperative somatosensory evoked potentials. Ann Neurol 190:22-25

Levi-Montalcini R (1950) The origin and development of the visceral system in the spinal cord of the chick embryo. J Morphol 86:253-283

Levi-Montalcini R (1967) Differentiation and growth control mechanisms in the nervous system. Morphological and biochemical aspects of cytodifferentiation. Exp Biol Med 1:170-182

Levy W, Latchaw J, Hahn JF, Sawhny B, Bay J, Dohn D (1986) Spinal neurofibromas: a report of 66 cases and a comparison with meningiomas. Neurosurgery 18:331-334

Levy WJ, Bay J, Dohn D (1982) Spinal cord meningioma. J Neurosurg 57:804-812

Lhermitte F, Corbin J (1960) La circulation arterielle de la moelle et ses troubles en pathologie. Rev Prat 10:2921

Li MH, Holtas S, Larsson EM (1992) MR imaging of intradural extramedullary tumors. Acta Radiol 33:207-212

Liberson WT, Kim KC (1963) Mapping evoked potential elicited by stimulation of the median and peroneal nerves. Electroencephalogr Clin Neurophysiol 15:721

Lichtenstein BW (1941) Multiple primary tumors of the spinal cord. Arch Neurol Psychol 46:59-71

Lima A (1936) A propos de la circulation des méningiomes. Rev Neurol (Paris) 65:1412-1414

Lima A (1951) Metastase cervical de un meningioma parasagittal. Rev Esp Oto-Neuro-Oftalmol 10:313-316

Limas C, Tio FO (1972) Meningeal melanocytoma (melanotic meningioma). Its melanocytic origin as revealed by electron microscopy. Cancer 30:1286-1294

Lindgren E (1937) Skeletal changes in tumors of the spinal cord. Nervenarzt 10:240

Lindgren E (1952) Myelographie. In: Schinz, Baensch, Friedl, Hlinger (eds) Lehrbuch der Roentgendiagnostik, vol 2. Stuttgart, pp 1501-1524

List CF (1941) Intraspinal epidermoids, dermoids and dermal sinus. Surg Gynecol Obstet 73:525-538

List CF (1943) Multiple meningiomas: removal of four tumors from the region of the foramen magnum and upper cervical region of the cord. Arch Neurol Psychiatry 50:335-341

Liu HC, de Armond SJ, Edwards MSB (1985) An unusual spinal meningioma in a child: case report. Neurosurgery 17:313-316

Lombardi G (1952) La diagnosi radiologica dei tumori spinali (70 casi). Radiat Med 38:193-216

Lombardi G, Passerini A (1961) Spinal cord tumors. Radiology 76:381-391

Lombardi G, Passerini A (1964) Spinal cord diseases: a radiologic and myelographic analysis. William and Wilkins, Baltimore

Long RR, Wirth FP (1987) Reversible somatosensory evoked potential changes with neodymium: yttrium-aluminium-garnet laser use. Neurosurgery 21:465-467

Louis R (1774) Mémoire sur les tumeurs fongueuses de la dure mère. Mem Acad Roy Chir Paris 5:1-59

Louis R (1982) Chirurgie du rachis. Springer, Berlin Heidelberg New York

Low MD (1979) Event related potentials and their clinical applications. In: Klass DW, Daly DD (eds) Current practice of clinical electroencephalography. Raven, New York, pp 441-450

Low MD, Farnarier G, Purves S (1980) Les potentiels cérébraux evoqués. Encycl Med Chir Paris Neurologie 17031 A25, 10

Lu AT, Kypridakis G, Abbott KH et al (1963) Intramedullary neurofibromas of the cervical cord. Report of two cases. Bull LA Neurol Soc 28:31-36

Ludwin SK, Rubinstein LJ, Russell DS (1975) Papillary meningioma: a malignant variant of meningioma. Cancer 36:1363-1373

Lueders H, Gurd A, Hahn J et al (1982) A new technique for intraoperative monitoring of spinal cord function: multichannel recording of spinal cord and subcortical evoked potentials. Spine 7:110-115

Lumenta CB, Herdmann J, Von Tempelhoff W et al (1991) Intraoperative monitoring with evoked pootentials in spinal interventions. Zentralbl Neurochir 52:49-58

Lunardi P, Missori P, Franco C, Delfini R, Fortuna A (1992) Hard-rock spinal meningioma. J Neurosurg Sci 36:243-246

Luyendijk W (1954) Meningiomes multiples et meningiomatoses. Acta Neurochir (Wien) 3:263-274

Macdonell RAL, Donnan GA, Bladin PF (1989) A comparison of somatosensory evoked and motor evoked potentials in stroke. Ann Neurol 25:68-73

Machida M, Weinstein SL, Yamada T, et al (1985) Spinal cord monitoring: electrophysiological measures of sensory and motor function during spinal cord surgery. Spine 10:407-413

Machida M, Weinstein SL, Yamada T et al (1988) Dissociation of muscle action potentials and spinal somatosensory evoked potentials after ischemic damage of spinal cord. Spine 13:1119-1124

Macon JB, Poletti CE, Sweet WH et al (1982) Conducted somatosensory evoked potentials during spinal surgery. J Neurosurg 57:349-359

Magdalena H, Pertuiset BF, Poisson M, Martin PM, Philippon J, Pertruiset B, Buge A (1982) Progestin and estrogen receptors in meningiomas. Biochemical characterization, clinical and pathological correlations in 42 cases. Acta Neurochir (Wien) 64:199-213

Magladery JW, Porter WE, Park AM et al (1951) Electrophysiological studies of nerve and reflex activity in normal man. IV. The motoneurone reflex and identification of two action potentials from spinal roots and cord. Bull Johns Hopkins Hospital 88:199-519

Makiuchi T, Kondo T, Shinoura N, Yamakawa K, Koido T (1993) Multiple meningiomas of thoracic spinal cord: report of two cases. No Shinkei Geka 21:89-93

Maleci O (1954) I tumori spinali. Boll Oncol 28:231-312

Maleci O (1956) I tumori spinali. Riv Chir 11:97-131

Malik GM, Tomecek FJ (1991) Spinal cord meningiomas. Contemp Neurosurg 13(3):1-5

Mallory FB (1920) The type cell of the so-called dural endothelioma. J Med Res 41:349-364

Manelfe C (1992) Imaging of the spine and spinal cord. Raven, New York

Manelfe C, Lazorthes G, Roulleau J (1972) Artères de la dure-mère rachidienne chez l'homme. Acta Radiol 13 (part II): 829-841

Marchese MJ, McDonald JV (1990) Intramedullary melanotica schwannoma of the cervical spinal cord: report of a case. Surg Neurol 33:353-355

Marinaro E, Ballerini S, Mavilio N, Rosa ML (1994) Aspetti neuropatologici dei meningiomi con particolare riguardo alle basi patologiche delle immagini. Riv Neuroradiol 7 [Suppl 1]:99-103

Marks SM, Whitwell HL, Lye RH (1986) Recurrence of meningiomas after operation. Surg Neurol 25:436-440

Martuza RL (1985) Meningioma: analysis of recurrence and progression following neurosurgical resection. J Neurosurg 62:18-24

Masaryk TJ (1991) Neoplastic disease of the spine. Radiol Clin North Am 29:829-845

Mason TH, Keigher HA (1968) Intramedullary spinal neurilemomas. Case report. J Neurosurg 29:414-416

Maspes PE (1973) I tumori del sistema nervoso centrale In: Bucalossi P, Veronesi U (eds) Trattato di oncologia clinica, vol 3. Ambrosiana, Milano, pp 2333-2406

Mathew P, Todd NV (1993) Intradural conus and cauda equina tumours: a retrospective review of presentation, diagnosis and early outcome. J Neurol Neurosurg Psychiatry 56:1, 69-74

Matson DD (1969) Neurosurgery of infancy and childhood. Thomas, Springfield

Matsumoto S, Hasuo K, Uchino A, Mizushima A, Furakawa T, Matsuura Y, Fukui M, Masuda K (1993) MRI of intradural extramedullary spinal neurinomas and meningiomas. Clin Imaging 17:46-52

Mauguiere F, Fischer C (1982) Les potentiels evoqués dans les affections neurologiques. Encycl Med Chir Paris Neurologie 17031 B10, 6

Mauguiere F, Brunon AM, Echallier JF et al (1981) Intérêt des potentiels evoqués somasthesiques précoces dans l'exploration des voies de la sensibilité lemniscale mise au point à propos de 167 observations et revue de la littérature. Rev Neurol (Paris) 137:1:1-19

Mauguiere F, Ibanez V, Fischer G (1985) Somatosensory evoked potentials in intraspinal tumors. Rev Electroencephalogr Neurophysiol Clin 15:95-106

Maward ME, Rivera V, Crawford S, Ramirez A, Breitbach W (1990) Spinal cord ischemia after resection of toracoabdominal aortic aneurysms: MR findings in 24 patients. Am J Neuroradiol 11:987-991

Maxwell M, Galanopoulos T, Hedley-Wythe ET, Black PM, Antoniades HM (1990) Human meningiomas co-express platelet-derived growth factor (PDGF) and PDGF-receptor genes and their protein products. Int J Cancer 46:16-21

Maxwell RE, Chou SN (1988) Preoperative evaluation and management of meningiomas. In: Schmidek HH, Swett WH (eds) Operative neurosurgical techniques. Grune and Stratton, New York, pp 547-554

McCraig WK (1929) The use and the abuse of iodized oil in the diagnosis of lesions of the spinal cord. Surg Gynecol Obstet 49:17-28

McCraig WK (1932) The pain of tumors of the spinal cord. West J Surg 40:56

McCraig WK (1933) Experimental production of the syndrome of spinal cord tumor. Surg Clin North Am 13:915

McCraig WK (1935) Tumors of the spinal cord. Surg Clin North Am 15:1371

McCraig WK (1936) Tumors of the spinal cord and their relations to medicine and surgery. J Am Med Assoc 107:184-188

McCraig WK, Shelden CH (1940) Tumors of the cervical portion of the spinal cord. Arch Neurol Psychiatry 44:1-16

McKormick PC, Post KD, Stein BM (1990) Intradural extramedullary tumors in adults. Neurosurg Clin North Am 1:591-608

McKormick WF (1964) Intramedullary spinal cord schwannoma. A unique case. Arch Patholol 77:378-382

McPherson RW, Mahla M, Johnson R et al (1985) Effects of enflurane, isoflurane and nitrous oxide on somatosensory evoked potentials during fentanyl anesthesia. Anesthesiology 62:626-633

Mealey Jr J, Carter JE (1968) Spinal cord tumor during pregnancy. Obstet Gynecol 32:204-209

Meese E, Blin N, Zang KD (1987) Loss of heterozygosity and the origin of meningiomas. Hum Genet 77:349-351

Meinck HM, Mohlenhof O, Kettler D (1980) Neurophysiological effects of etomidate, a new short-acting hypnotic. Electroen-

cephalogr Clin Neurophysiol 50:515-522

Memon MY (1980) Multiple and familial meningiomas without evidence of neurofibromatosis. Neurosurgery 7:262-264

Milano C, Paolino G, Lotti G et al (1984) Monitoraggio della funzione del midollo spinale mediante registrazione dei potenziali evocati negli interventi sulla colonna vertebrale. Progressi in patologia vertebrale. A Gaggi Ed., Bologna, 7:217-223

Millen JW, Woollam DHM (1961) On the nature of the pia mater. Brain 84:514-520

Milz H, Hamer J (1983) Extradural spinal meningioma. Report of two cases. Neurochirurgia (Stuttg) 26:126-129

Mirimanoff RO, Dosoretz DE, Linggood RM, Ojeman RG, Moore RA, Allen MC, Wood PJ et al (1985) Peri-operative endocrine effects of etomidate. Anaesthesia 40:124-130

Mittal MM, Gupta NC, Sharma ML (1970) Spinal epidural meningioma associated with increased intracranial pressure. Neurology (Minneapolis) 20:818-820

Molaie M (1986) False negative intraoperative somatosensory evoked potentials with simultaneous bilateral stimulation. Clin Electroencephalogr 17:6-9

More RC, Nuwer MR, Dawson EG (1988) Cortical evoked potential monitoring during spinal surgery: sensitivity, specificity, reliability, and criteria for alarm. J Spinal Disord 1:75-80

Moret J, Vignaud J, Doyon D (1976) Techniques d'opacification des plexus veineux intra-rachidiens lombaires. J Radiol Electrol 57:553-560

Morioka T, Fujii K, Mitani M et al (1990) Intraoperative localization of a cervicomedullary glioma from the killed end potential: illustrative case. Neurosurgery 26:1038-1041

Morley TP (1979) Spinal subdural cyst associated with a meningioma: case report. Neurosurgery 4:256-258

Morris PG (1989) Nuclear magnetic resonance imaging in medicine and biology. Clarendon, Oxford

Mosberg Jr WH (1951) Spinal tumors diagnosed during the first year of life with report of a case. J Neurosurg 8:220

Motomochi M, Makita J, Nabeshima S, Aoyama I (1980) Spinal epidural meningioma in childhood. Surg Neurol 13:5-7

Mullan J, Evans JP (1957) Neoplastic diseases of the spinal extradural space. A review of fifty cases. Arch Surg 74:900-907

Muller J, Mealey Jr J (1971) The use of tissue culture in differentiation between angioblastic meningioma and hemangiopericytoma. J Neurosurg 34:341-348

Muller W, Iffland R, Dortmann P, Firsching R (1993) Interaction of magnesium and calcium in meningioma. Zentralbl Pathol 139(1):45-50

Muraszko KM, Antunes JL, Hilal SK, Michelesen J (1982) Hemagiopericytoma of the spine. Neurosurgery 10:473-479

Murovic J, Sundaresan N (1992) Pediatric spinal axis tumors. Neurosurg Clin North Am 3:947-958

Naffziger HC, Brown HA (1933) Hour-glass tumors of the spine. Arch Neurol Psychol 29:561-584

Nagele T, Petersen D, Klose U, Grodd W, Opitz H, Voigt K (1994) The "dural tail" adjacent to meningiomas studied by dynamic contrast-enhanced MRI : a comparison with histopathology. Neuroradiology 36:303-307

Naidich TP, Zimmerman RA, Mc Lone DG (1991) Congenital anomalies of the spine and spinal cord. In: Atlas SW (ed) Magnetic resonance imaging. Raven, New York

Nainzadeh N, Lane ME (1987) Somatosensory evoked potentials following pudendal nerve stimulation as indicators of low sacral root involvement in postlaminectomy patient. Arch Phys Med Rehabil 68:170-182

Namer IJ, Pamir MN, Benli K, Saglam S, Erbengi A (1987) Spinal meningiomas. Neurochirurgia (Stuttg) 30:11-15

Nashold BS Jr, Ovelmen-Levitt J, Sharpe R, et al (1985) Intraoperative evoked potentials recorded in man directly from dorsal roots and spinal cord. J Neurosurg 62:680-693

Nassar SI, Correll JW (1968) Subarachnoid haemorrage due to spinal cord tumor. Neurology 18:87-94

Neri V (1932) La forme ataxique initiale des compressions médullaires cervicales. Rev Neurol (Paris) 39:60-63

Neri V, Pais C (1951) I sintomi sopralesionali nelle compressioni midollari. Riv Neurol 21:137-156

Neri V, Romagnoli C (1953) Il valore semeiologico del sintomo dolore nelle compressioni midollari. G Psichiatr Neuropatol 81:453-460

Netsky NG (1957) Diffuse meningiomatosis, arachnoidal fibrosis, and syringomyelia. Arch Neurol Psychol 78:553-561

Neuss M, Westphal M, Hansel M, Hermann HD (1988) Clinical and laboratory findings in patients with multiple meningiomas. Br J Neurosurg 2:249-256

New PF (1982) Malignant meningiomas: CT and histologic criteria including a new CT sign. AJNR 3:267-276

Ng HK, Poon WS, South JR, Lee JC (1988) Tumours of the central nervous system in Chinese in Hong Kong. Aust NZ J Surg 58:573-578

Ng TH, Chan KH, Mann KS, Fung CF (1989) Spinal meningioma arising from a lumbar nerve root. Case report. J Neurosurg 70:646-648

Nicola N, Thal HU (1983) Multiple Meningiome in verschiedenen Etagen der zerebro-medullaeren Achse. Neurochirurgia (Stuttg) 26:120-124

Niebeling HG, Hohrein P (1978) 400 intraspinal space-narrowing processes: a clinical study. Zentralbl Neurochir 39:241-252

Niijima K, Peng Huang Y, Malis L, Sachdev VP (1993) Ossified spinal meningioma en plaque. Spine 18, 15:2340-2343

Niosi F (1936) Sopra due casi di tumore spinale. Minerva Med 1:513-523

Nishiura I, Koyama T, Tanaka K, Aii H, Amano S (1989) The occurrence of different types of spinal tumours in one patient. A case report and review of the literature. Neurochirurgia (Stuttg) 32, 2:52-55

Nistri M (1949) Significato ed importanza dello scompenso anatomo-funzionale in neuropatologia. Riv Patol Nerv Ment 70:203-205

Nitner K, Schiefer W (1955) Méningiomes multiples du canal rachidien. Zentralbl Neurochir 15:99-103

Nittner K (1976) Spinal meningiomas, neurinomas and neurofibromas and hourglass tumors. In: Winken PJ, Bruyn GW, Klawans HL (eds) Handbook of clinical neurology, vol 20. North-Holland, Amsterdam, pp 177-322

Novak C (1941) Contributo allo studio dei tumori intradurali. Arch Med Chir 10:55

Nystrom HM, Nyholm M (1966) Origin of calcium deposits in psammoma bodies of human spinal meningiomas. Naturwissenschaften 53:703-704

O'Brien MF, Lenke LG, Bridwell KH, et al (1994) Evoked potential monitoring of the upper extremities during thoracic and lumbar spinal deformity surgery. A prospective study. J Spinal Disord 7:4:277-284

O'Connel JEA (1962) Neurosurgical problems in pregnancy. Proc R Soc Med 55:577-582

O'Rahilly R, Miller F (1986) The meninges in human development. J Neuropathol Exp Neurol 45:588-608

Oberling C (1922) Les tumeurs des méninges. Bull Assoc Etude Cancer 11:365-394

Obrador Alcade S (1951) Aspectos neuroquirurgicos de los procesos compresivos de la medula espinal. Cir Ap Locom 8:117-130

Oddsson B (1947) Spinal meningioma. Munksgaard, Copenhagen

Odin M, Runstrom G, Lindblom A (1929) Iodized oils as an aid to the diagnosis of lesions of the spinal cord and a contribution to the knowledge of adhesive circumscribed meningitis. Acta Radiol Suppl (Stockh) 7:1929

Oganesjan SS, Oganesjan AS (1984) Extradural-mediastinal meningioma in a child. Case report. Zentralbl Neurochir 45:85-89

Ohaegbulam SC (1979) Cauda equina epidural meningioma. Acta Neurochir (Wien) 46:287-291

Ojemann RG (1985) Meningiomas. Clinical features and surgical management. In: Wilkins RH, Rengachary SS (eds) Neurosurgery. McGraw-Hill, New York, pp 635-654

Oka K, Tsuda H, Kamikaseda K, Nakamura R, Fukui M, Nouzuka Y, Sveishi K (1988) Meningiomas and hemorrhagic diathesis. J Neurosurg 69:356-360

Onofrio BM (1978) Intradural extramedullary spinal cord tumors. Clin Neurosurg 25:540

Ormos M (1939) Positive roentgen shadow of extramedullary (psammous) meningiomas. Schweiz Arch Neurol Psychol 44:309-312

Osgood EC, Arnett JH, Lewy FH (1944) Calcified spinal meningioma. Radiology 43:62-64

Owen JH (1990) Motor evoked potentials neural monitoring. In: Salzman SK (ed) Neural monitoring. The prevention of intraoperative injury. Humana, Totowa, pp 219-241

Owen JH, Bridwell KH, Shimon SM et al (1988) Sensitivity and specificity of somatosensory and neurogenic-motor evoked potentials in animals and humans. Spine 12:1111-1116

Owen JH, Jenny AB, Naito M et al (1989) Effect of spinal cord lesioning on somatosensory and neurogenic-motor evoked potentials. Spine 14:673-682

Owen JH, Naito M, Bridwell KH (1990) Relationship between duration of spinal cord ischemia and postoperative neurological deficits in animals. Spine 15:618-622

Owen JH, Bridwell KH, Lenke LG (1993) Innervation pattern of dorsal roots and their effects on the specificity of dermatomal somatosensory evoked potentials. Spine 18, 6:748-754

Pacifico A (1957) Associazione di meningiomi multipli e di pachimeningite emorragica interna. Riv Patol Nerv Ment 50:299-325

Pagni CA (1989) I meningiomi spinali. CIC Internazionali, Rome

Pagni CA, Canavero S (1993) Paroxysmal perineal pain resembling tic doloureux, only symptom of a dorsal meningioma. J Neurosurgic Sci 14, 4:323-324

Pagni CA, Regolo P (1986) Dorsal meningioma developed between two sheets of the spinal dura mater. J Neurosurg Sci 30:153-154

Pagni CA, Regolo P (1987) Sensory motor epilepsy of spinal origin. A rare first symptom of spinal meningioma. Minerva Chir 42:2003-2009

Pagni CA, Apolloni G, Favilli S, Regolo P (1985) Epidemiology of spinal cord tumors. In: Hudson AR, Hoffman H, Peerless S, Schatz S (eds) Italy Abst 8th Int Congr Neurol Surg Toronto, 131

Pagni CA, Regolo P, Baldi G, Valente G (1987) Epidural spinal meningiomas. Review of the literature and presentation of a clinical case. Minerva Med 78:751-774

Pagni CA, Naddeo M, Mascari C (1988) History of evoked potential recording in humans. In: Grundy BL, Villani RM (eds) Evoked Potentials - Intraoperative and ICU Monitoring. Springer, Vienna New York, pp 17-44

Pagni CA, Canavero S, Cento A (1990) Multiple spinal meningiomas: case report and review of the literature. Zentralbl Neurochir 51:225-228

Paillas JE (1954) Affections de la moelle et des racines. Anatomie pathologique générale des compressions (tumeurs, processus inflammatoires, lesions osteo-articulaires). Encyclopedie Medico-chirurgicale Système Nerveux 17625 A10

Pais C (1939) Tumori endorachidei. Comunic Soc Medico-Chirurgica, Venezia, 20 April 1939

Pais C, Mastragostino S (1954) Osservazioni anatomo-istologiche sui tumori endorachidei subdurali. Comunic VI Congr Soc It Radioneurochirurgica. Minerva Chir 9:909

Pais C, Mastragostino S (1955) Studio anatomo-clinico ed istogenetico dei tumori endorachidei subdurali. Neuropsychiatry 11:253-378

Pais C, Neri V (1951) I sintomi sopralesionali nelle compressioni midollari. Riv Neurol 21:1

Pansini A (1950) Variazione di rapporto tra le radici nervose spinali durante lo sviluppo ontogenetico. Soc Ital Biol Sper 26:4

Pansini A (1954) Sullo sviluppo embrionale delle meningi spinali nell'uomo. Quaderni Anat. Pratica, IX, 1-2, Lib. Scientifica Ed. Napoli

Pansini A (1991) È oggi possibile la diagnosi precoce dei tumori spinali? Atti del Convegno su I tumori primitivi del midollo spinale. Progressi di diagnosi e terapia, Torino, 7-8 October 1988. Minerva Med, Torino

Pansini A, Conti P (1981) On some rare spreading cervical lesions. J Neurosurg Sci 25:255-257

Pansini A, Conti P, Conti R, Lo Re F, De Luca G, Bono P, Gallina P, Pellicanò G (1987) Diagnostica precoce delle compressioni mieloradicolari RX - TC - RM. Piccin, Padova

Pansini A, Conti P, Pellicanò G (1988a) Prime considerazioni alla RM sugli aspetti morfologici dei tumori spinali. Atti del Convegno sui tumori primitivi del midollo spinale. Progressi di diagnosi e terapia, Torino, 7-8 October 1988

Pansini A, Lo Re F, Conti P, Conti R, De Luca G, Bono P, Gallina P, Pellicanò G (1988b) La RM con Gd-DTPA nella diagnostica dei tumori spinali. Atti del Convegno sui Tumori primitivi del midollo spinale. Progressi di diagnosi e terapia, Torino, 7-8 October 1988

Pansini A, Conti P, Conti R, Gallina P, Pellicanò G (1989) Primary intraspinal tumors: X-ray, CT, MRI. Proceedings of the XVII Int Congr on Neuroradiology, Paris, 1-8 July 1989

Pansini A, De Luca G, Lo Re F et al (1990) Somatosensory and motor evoked potentials in the spinal degenerative disc desease and stenosis at cervical and lumbar level. XII International Congress of Eletroencephalography and Clinical Neurophysiology, Rio de Janeiro, 23

Pansini A, De Luca G, Bono P, Lo Re F, Conti P, Conti R, Caprio A, Gallina P (1991) I potenziali evocati somatestesici e motori nella neurofibromatosi. XL Congresso della Società Italiana di Neurochirurgia, Perugia, 11-14 September, Minerva Med, Torino, pp 321-336

Pardatscher K, Iraci G, Cappellotto P et al (1979) Multiple intramedullary neurinomas of the spinal cord. Case report. J Neurosurg 50:817-822

Parizel PM, Baleriaux D, Rodesch G, Segebarth C, Lalmand B, Christophe C, Lemort M, Haesendonck P, Niendorf HP, Flament-Durand J et Al (1989) Gd-DTPA enhanced MR imaging of spinal tumors. AJR 152:1087-1096

Pasztor E, Paraicz E, Szenasy J (1961) Über Rückenmarksgesch-wülste im Kindesalter. Dtsch Z Nervenheilkd 182:45-59

Patronas NJ, Brown F, Duda EE (1980) Multiple meningiomas in the spinal canal. Surg Neurol 13:78-80

Paulian D, Jonesco V, Bistriceano I (1940) Contribution à l'étude anatomo-clinique des tumeurs medullaires. Arch Neurol 4:25-36

Pear BL, Boyd HR (1974) Roentgenographically visible calcifications in spinal meningioma. AJR 120:32-45

Pearce J (1967) The central nervous system pathology in multiple neurofibromatosis. Neurology 17:691-697

Pecker J, Javalet A, Simon J, Loussouarn Y (1967) Les tumeurs épidurales bénignes de la moelle. Neurochirurgie 13:647-660

Pelosi L, Caruso G, Cracco RU et al (1991) Intraoperative recordings of spinal somatosensory evoked potentials to tibial nerve and sural nerve stimulation. Muscle Nerve 14:253-258

Penfield W (1927) The encapsulated tumors of the nervous system: meningeal fibroblastomata and neurofibroblastomata of von Recklinghausen. Surg Gynecol Obstet 45:178-188

Penfield W (1932) Osteogenetic dural endothelioma. J Neurol Psychopathol 4:27-34

Percy AK, Elveback LR, Okazaki H, Kurland LT (1972) Neoplasms of the central nervous system: epidemiologic considerations. Neurology 22:40-48

Perria C, Francaviglia N, Borzone M, Chinnici A, Piano E, Pacini P (1983) The value and limitations of the CO_2 laser in neurosurgery. Neurochirurgia (Stuttg) 26:6-11

Pertuiset B, Ouvry P, Metzger J (1959) Le méningiomes rachidiens.

Etude anatomo-clinique et thérapeutique d'après 57 cas. Ann Chir 13:1073-1081

Petit H, Jomin M, Jeulin-Gaillard B, Warot P (1980) Les méningiomes rachidiens multiples "non-associés". Lille Med 25:346-349

Petit-Dutaillis D, Ectors L (1936) A propos de certaines formes des méningiomes: tumeurs multiples, tumeurs recidivantes, tumeurs infiltrantes. Presse Med 44:486-490

Philippon J (1986) Les méningiomes recidivants. Neurochirurgie [Suppl] 32:6-53

Pia HW, Djindjian R (1978) Spinal angiomas: advances in diagnosis and therapy. Springer, Berlin Heidelberg New York

Picaza JA, Baker GS (1948) Multiple meningiomas: report of a case and surgical considerations. Mayo Clin Proc 23:54-56

Pimentel J (1993) Meningiomas: presente e futuro. Acta Med Port 6, 5:199-207

Pitkethly DT, Hardman JM, Kempe LG, Earle K (1970) Angioblastic meningiomas: clinico-pathologic study of 81 cases. J Neurosurg 32:539-544

Pitlyk PJ, Dockerymb, Miller RH (1965) Hemangiopericytoma of the spinal cord. Report of three cases. Neurology 15:649-653

Pitrè D, Felder E (1980) Development, chemistry and physical properties of iopamidol and its analogues. Invest Radiol 15 [Suppl 6]:301-309

Plant G (1981) Spinal meningioma presenting as focal epilepsy. Br J Med 282:1574-1575

Ploncard P, Raposo G, Ferreira H (1974) Ablation d'un gros méningiome cervical de localisation antérieure adhérent à la moelle épinière. Révision de la littérature et discussion du cas. Neurochirurgie 20:247-262

Post MJD (1980) Radiographic evaluation of the spine. Current advances with emphasis on computed tomography. Masson, New York

Preston-Martin S (1990) Descriptive epidemiology of primary tumors of the spinal cord and spinal meninges in Los Angeles County 1972-1985. Neuroepidemiology 9:106-111

Puljic S, Schechter MM (1980) Multiple spinal canal meningiomas. AJNR 1:4:325-327

Quest DO (1978) Meningiomas: an update. Neurosurgery 3:219-225

Raclin JR, Rosenblum ML (1991) Etiology and biology of meningiomas. In: Al-Mefty O (ed) Meningiomas. Raven, New York, pp 22-37

Raimondi AJ, Beckman F (1967) Perineural fibroblastoma; their fine structure and biology. Acta Neuropathol 8:1-23

Ramamurthi B, Anguli VC, Iyer CGS (1958) A case of intramedullary neurinoma. J Neurol Neurosurg Psychiatry 21:92-94

Ramon Y Cajal (1908) L'hypothèse de Mr Apathy sur la continuité des cellules nerveuses entre elles. Anat Anz Jena 23:418-468

Ramsey EH, French JD, Strain WH (1944) Iodinated organic compounds as contrast media for radiographic diagnoses: pantopaque myelography. Radiology 43:236-240

Ramsey HJ (1966) Fine structure of hemangiopericytoma and hemangioendothelioma. Cancer 19:2005-2018

Rand RW (1952) Multiple spinal cord meningiomas. J Neurosurg 9:310

Rand RW, Rand CW (1960) Intraspinal tumors in childhood. Thomas, Springfield

Rasmussen TB, Kernohan JW, Adson AW (1940) Pathologic classification with surgical consideration of intraspinal tumors. Ann Surg 3:513-530

Rath S, Mathai KV, Chandy J (1967) Multiple meningiomas of the spinal canal. Case report. J Neurosurg 26:639-640

Rawling B (1933) Spinal tumor seen on direct x-ray examination without lipiodol. Br J Surg 20:348-349

Ray BS (1954) Cord tumors. Mississipi Doct 32:107

Ray BS, Foot NC (1940) Primary melanotic tumors of the meninges: resemblance to meningiomas. Report of two cases in which operation was performed. Arch Neurol Psychol 44:104-117

Remond A (ed) (1973) Handbook of EEG and clinical neurophysiology, vol 8. Elsevier, Amsterdam

Remond A (ed) (1975) Handbook of EEG and clinical neurophysiology, vol 9. Elsevier, Amsterdam

Resnikoff S, Verdura J, Cardenas J (1972) Multiple intraspinal meningiomas at different level. A case report. Ann Surg 176:798-800

Ricard A, Thiers F, Bovet M (1953) Résultats de 219 interventions pour tumeurs intrarachidiennes. Lyon Chir 48:527-534

Riccardi VM (1981) Von Recklinghausen neurofibromatosis. N Engl J Med 305:27, 1617-1627

Richardson FL (1960) A report of 16 tumors of the spinal cord in children. J Pediatr 57:42-54

Riggs HE, Clary WU (1957) A case of intramedullary sheath cell tumor cell of the spinal cord. Consideration of vascular nerves as a source of origin. J Neuropathol Exp Neurol 16:332-336

Riva P, Larizza L (1992) Expression of c-sis and c-fos genes in human meningiomas and neurinomas. Int J Cancer 51:873-877

Robertson PL (1992) Atypical presentations of spinal cord tumors in children. J Child Neurol 7:4:360-363

Robineau M (1923) Sur le traitement chirurgical des compressions médullaires. Rev Neurol (Paris) 39:707-710

Robineau M (1932) Diagnostic et traitement des tumeurs de la moelle. IX Congr de la Soc Int de Chir (Madrid), pp 575-662

Robinson LR, Slimp JC, Anderson PA et al (1993) The efficacy of femoral nerve intraoperative somatosensory evoked potentials during surgical treatment of thoracolumbar fractures. Spine 1, 18:1793-1797

Roda JM, Bencosme JA, Perez-Higueras A, Fraile M (1992) Simultaneous multiple intracranial and spinal meningiomas. Neurochirurgia (Stuttg) 35:92-94

Roelvinck NC, Kamphorst W et al (1987) Pregnancy-related primary brain and spinal tumors. Arch Neurol 44:209-215

Roelvinck NC, Kamphorst W, August H, Van Halphen M, Rao BR (1991) Literature statistics do not support a growth stimulating role for female sex steroid hormones in haemangiomas and meningiomas. J Neurooncol 11:243-253

Roger H (1943) Diagnostic des compressions médullaires chez l'enfant et les adolescents. Sud Med Chir 75:175-188

Rogers L (1928) A spinal meningioma containing bone. J Br Surg 15:675-677

Rogers L (1955) Tumours involving spinal cord and its nerve roots. Ann R Coll Surg 16:1-29

Rohr H, Hoffmann W (1959) Rückenmarkstumoren mit Stauungspapille. Nervenarzt 30:391-396

Rohringer M, Sutherland GR, Louw DF, Sima AF (1989) Incidence and clinicopathological features of meningiomas. J Neurosurg 71:665-672

Roka L (1951) Über Klinik und Anatomie der Tumoren der Medulla oblungata-Halsmarkgrenze. Arch Psychiatr Nervenkr 186:413-436

Romagnoli C, Dal Monte A (1964) I neurinomi intraspinali nell'infanzia. Minerva Neurochir 8:27-32

Romanes GJ (1951) The motor cell columns of the lumbosacral cord of the cat. J Comp Neurol 94:313-363

Romanes GJ (1964) The motor pools of the spinal cord. Prog Brain Res 11:93-119

Rosenbaum LH, Nicholas JJ (1983) Early diagnosis of cervical spinal cord meningioma. JAMA 249:1475-1476

Rosencrantz M, Stattin S (1972) Extradural meningiomas. Report of two cases. Acta Radiol 12:419-427

Ross AT, Bailey OT (1953) Tumors arising within the spinal canal in children. Neurology 3:922-930

Ross DA, Edwards MSB, Wilson CB (1986) Intramedullary neurilemmomas of the spinal cord: report of two cases and review of the literature. Neurosurgery 19:458-464

Rossini PM (1988) Anatomic and physiologic bases of motor evoked potentials. Neurol Clin 6:751-769

Rougerie J (1973) Le compressions médullaires non tramáutiques de l'enfant. Masson, Paris

Rouleau GA, Wertrlecki W, Haines JL et al (1987) Genetic linkage of bilateral acoustic neurofibromatosis to a DNA marker on chromosom 22. Nature 329:246-248

Rouleau GA, Merel P, Lutchman M, Sanson M, Zuchman J, Marinau C, Hoang-Xuan K, Demczuk S, Desmaze C, Pluogastel B, Pulst SM, Lenoir G, Bijlsma E, Fashold R, Dumanski J, De Jong P, Parry D, Roswell E, Aurias A, Delattre O, Thomas G (1993) Alteration in a new gene encoding a putative membrane-organizing protein cau-ses neuro-fibromatosis type 2. Nature 363:515-521

Roussy G, Cornil L (1925) Les tumeurs méningées. Ann Anat Pathol 2:63

Roussy G, Oberling C (1932) Histological classification of tumors of the central nervous system. Arch Neurol Psychol 27:1281-129

Rout D, Pillai SM, Radhakrishnan VV (1983) Cervical intramedullary schwannoma. Case report. J Neurosurg 58:962-964

Rowbotham GF (1955) Early diagnosis of compressions of spinal cord. Lancet II:1222

Roy CD (1890) Report of a case of spinal exsection and removal of a tumor from the cord. South M Rec 20:564-566

Roytta M, Wallfors P, Svedsen P, Sourander P (1982) Recurrent meningiomas. A combined clinical, neuroradiological and neuropathological study. Acta Neurol Scand 65, 91:105-106

Rubinstein LJ (1972) Tumours of the central nervous system. AFIP, Washington, DC

Russel JR, Dorothy S (1950) Meningeal tumors. J Clin Pathol 3:191-211

Russel T, Moss T (1986) Metastasizing meningioma. Neurosurgery 19:1028-1030

Russell DS (1950) Meningeal tumors: a review. J Clin Pathol 3:191-211

Russell DS, Rubinstein LJ (1972) Pathology of tumors of the nervous system 3^d. Williams and Wilkins, Baltimore

Rustichelli P, Scoditti U, Moretti G, Poletti AL, Paini GP, Baldi PG (1984) Retrospective study of 50 cases of spinal meningioma. Acta Biomed Ateneo Parmense 55:255-260

Ruttledge MH, Sarrazin J, Rangaratnam S, Phelan CM, Twist E, Merel P, Delattre O, Thomas G, Nordenskjod M, Collins VP, Dumanski JP, Rouleau GA (1994) Evidence for the complete inactivation of the NF2 gene in the majority of sporadic meningiomas. Nature Genet 6:180-184

Sackett JF, Strother CM (1979) New techniques in myelography. Harper and Row, Hagerstown

Sage MR, Wilcox J (1983) Brain parenchyma penetration by intrathecal nonionic iopamidol. AJNR 4:1181-1183

Sahar A (1965) Familial occurrence of meningiomas. J Neurosurg 23:444-445

Salah S, Horcajada J, Koos WT (1976) Microsurgery of spinal tumors. In: Koos WT, Bock FW, Spetzler RF (eds) Clinical microneurosurgery. Thieme, Stuttgart, pp 171-176

Salazar J, Vaquero J, Bravo G (1987) Diagnosis and neurosurgical treatment of intraspinal meningiomas and neurinomas. Arch Neurobiol (Madr) 50:191-205

Salcman M (1991) Malignant meningiomas. In: Al-Mefty O (ed) Meningiomas. Raven, New York, pp 75-85

Salvati M, Artico M, Lunardi P, Gagliardi FM (1992) Intramedullary meningioma: case report and review of the literature. Surg Neurol 37:42-45

Salvi G (1897) Atti Soc Toscana Sc Nat Memorie, vol 15

Salvi S, Mascalchi M, Plasmati R, Michelucci R, Calbucci F, Dal Pozzo G, Tassinari CA (1992) Multiple lesions in cerebral white matter in two young adults with thoracic extramedullary tumors. J Neurol Neurosurg Psychiatry 55:216-218

Salzman SK, Beckman AL, Mc Atee S et al (1986) False-negative results from intraoperative SSEPs. Letter J Neurosurg 64:986

Samuels MA, Kleinman GM (1979) A 51-years-old man with cervical pain, weakness of the arms and sensory deficits Meningotheliomatous meningioma. New Engl J Med 301, 3:147-154

Sarteschi M (1962) Discussion des rapports sur la pathologie vasculaire de la moelle. XXV Reun Neurol Internat Paris, 5-6 June

1962. Rev Neurol (Paris) 106:657

Sarteschi P, Giannini A (1960) La patologia vascolare del midollo spinale. Giardini, Pisa

Sartor K, Fliedner E, Pfingst E (1977) Angiographic demonstration of cervical extradural meningioma. Neuroradiology 14:147-149

Sassaroli G, Chimenz MT (1955) Neurinomi spinali: osservazioni cliniche e radiologiche. Riv Neurol 25:237

Sauer FC (1935a) The cellular structure of the neural tube. J Comp Neurol 63:13-23

Sauer FC (1935b) Mitosis in the neural tube. J Comp Neurol 62:337-405

Sauer FC (1936) The interkinetic migration of embryonic epithelial nuclei. J Morphol 60:1-11

Sauer ME, Chittenden AC (1959) Deoxyribonucleic acid content of cell nuclei in the neural tube of the chick embryo: evidence for intermitotic migration of nuclei. Exp Cell Res 16:1-6

Sawa H, Tamaki N, Kurata H, Nagashima T (1993) Complete resection of a spinal meningioma extending from the foramen magnum to the second thoracic vertebral body via the anterior approach: case report. Neurosurgery 33, 6:1095-1098

Sawaya R, Raimo OJ (1991) Systemic and thromboembolic effects of meningiomas. In: Al-Mefty O (ed) Meningiomas. Raven, New York, pp 117-135

Scaglietti O, Pansini A, Cecchini M, Simonetti E (1971) I tumori primitivi intrarachidei. Aulo Gaggi, Bologna

Scarff TB, Dallmann DE, Toleikis JR, et al (1979) Dermatomal somatosensory evoked potentials in children with myelomeningocele. Z Kinderchir 28:384-387

Schachenmayr W, Friede RL (1978) The origin of subdural neomembranes I. Fine structure of the dura arachnoid interface in man. Am J Pathol 92:53-68

Schaller A (1965) Veränderungen an der Halswirbelsäule durch ein spinales Meningioma, demonstriert an einem unbehandelten Zufallsbefund. Zentralbl Allg Pathol Anat 103:481

Scheepstra GL, De Lange JJ, Boij LDH et al (1989) Median nerve evoked potentials during propofol anaesthesia. Br J Anaesth 62:92-94

Schiffer D, Fabiani A (1975) Patologia dei tumori cerebrali. Il Pensiero Scientifico, Rome

Schiffer J, Mundel G, Lamat E, Schwartzmann H, Smental I (1980) Multiple meningiomatosis in separate neuroaxial compartments in child. Childs Brain 6:281-288

Schliack H, Stille D (1975) Clinical symptomatology of intraspinal tumours. In: Winken PJ, Bruyn GW (eds) Tumours of the spine and spinal cord. North-Holland, Amsterdam (Handbook of Clinical Neurology, vol 19)

Schmidek HH (1991) Meningiomas and their surgical management. Saunders, Philadelphia

Schmidt MB (1902) Ueber die Pacchioni'schen Granulationen und ihr Verhaeltnis zu den Sarmen und Psammomen der Dura mater. Virchows Arch Pathol Anat 170:429-464

Schmidt RC (1981) Secondary spinal cord atrophy associated with spinal meningioma. ROFO 135:737-738

Schneider R, Crosby EC (1959) Vascular insufficiency of brain-stem and spinal cord in spinal trauma. Neurology 9:10

Schonle PW, Isenberg C, Crozier TA et al (1989) Changes of transcranially evoked motor responses in man by midazolam, a short acting benzodiazepine. Neurosci Lett 101:321-324

Schramm J, Hashizume K, Fukushima T et al (1979) Experimental spinal cord injury produced slow, graded compression. J Neurosurg 50:48-57

Schroth G, Thron A, Guhl L, Voigth K, Niendorf HP, Garces LR (1987) Magnetic resonance imaging of spinal meningiomas and neurinomas Improvement of imaging by paramagnetic contrast enhancement. J Neurosurg 66:695-700

Schwartz HG (1952) Congenital tumors of the spinal cord in infants. Ann Surg 136:183

Scott M, Bentz B (1962) Intramedullary neurilemmoma of the tho-

racic cord. J Neuropathol Exp Neurol 21:194-200

Scott M, Ferrara VL, Peale AR (1971) Multiple melanotic meningiomas of the cervical cord. J Neurosurg 34:555-559

Scotti G, Scialfa G, Colombo N, Landoni L (1985) MR imaging of intradural extramedullary tumors of the cervical spine. J Comput Assist Tomogr 9:1037-1041

Scotti G, Scialfa G, Colombo M, Tampieri D (1986) Il ruolo della risonanza magnetica nella diagnosi dei tumori spinali extra ed intramidollari. In: Nacci G (ed) Neuroradiologia oggi. Laterza, Bari

Sedzimir CB, Frazer AK, Roberts JR (1973) Cranial and spinal meningiomas in a pair of identical twin boys. J Neurol Neurosurg Psychiatry 36:368-376

Seitzinger BR, Martuza RL, Gusella JF (1986) Loss of genes on chromosome 22 in tumorigenesis of human acoustic neuroma. Nature 322:644-647

Selosse P, Granieri U (1968) Méningiomes et neurinomes intraduraux spinaux. Revue de la littérature et bilan actuel. Neurochirurgie 14:135-154

Sen CN, Sekhar LN (1990) An extreme lateral approach to intradural lesions of the cervical spine and foramen magnum. Neurosurgery 27, 2:197-204

Sensing EC (1951) The early development of the meninges of the spinal cord in human embryos. Contrib Embryol 34:145-157

Serra A (1942) Considerazioni su 46 casi di tumori midollari operati. Boll Mem Soc Emiliano-Romagn Chir 335

Serra A (1947) Principi di chirurgia del cervello e del midollo spinale. Cappelli, Bologna

Shalit MN, Sandbank U (1981) Cervical intramedullary schwannoma. Surg Neurol 16:61-64

Shapiro L (1968) Myelography. Yearbook Medical, Chicago

Sheehy JP, Crockard HA (1983) Multiple meningiomas: a long term review. J Neurosurg 59:1-5

Shen WC, Lee SK (1992) MRI of concurrent spinal meningioma, ependymoma and syringomyelia. J Comput Assist Tomogr 16:665-666

Shields CB, Paloheimo M, Backman M et al (1988) Intraoperative transcranial magnetic motor evoked potentials are difficult to obtain during lumbar disc and spinal tumor operations. Muscle Nerve 11:993 (abstr)

Shimoji K, Hihashi H, Kano T (1971) Epidural recording of spinal electrogram in man. Electroencephalogr Clin Neurophysiol 30:236-239

Shuangshoti S, Netsky MG, Jane JA (1971) Neoplasm of mixed mesenchymal and neuroepithelial type, with consideration of the relationship between meningioma and neurilemmoma. J Neurol Sci 14:277-291

Shuangshoti S, Boonjunwetwat D, Kaoroptham S (1992) Association of primary intraspinal meningiomas and subcutaneous meningioma of the cervical region: case report and review of literature. Surg Neurol 38:129-134

Sicard JA (1927) Les compressions médullaires (tumeurs intrarachidiennes). Rev Neurol (Paris) 2:715

Sicard JA, Forestier J (1922) Méthode generale d'exploration radiologique par l'huile iodée. Bull Mem Soc Med Op Paris 46:463-469

Sicard JA, Forestier J (1923) Radiodiagnostic au cours des compressions rachidiennes. Rev Neurol (Paris) 39:676

Sidman RL, Miale IL, Feder N (1959) Cell proliferation and migration in the primitive ependymal zone. Exp Neurol 1:322-333

Sieb JP, Pulst SM, Buck A (1992) Familial CNS tumors. J Neurol 239(6):342-344

Siegelman ES, Mishkin MM, Taveras JM (1991) Radiologic history exhibit past, present and future of meningioma. Radiographics 11:899

Signorini E, Ciorba E, Pelliccioli GP, Caputo N, Piccinin GL (1979) First experience with the clinical use of a new hydrosoluble non-ionic contrast medium - iopamidol - in the study of the subarachnoid space. Rays 4:47-68

Singh R, Coerkamp G, Luyendijk W (1968) Spinal epidural meningiomas. Acta Neurochir (Wien) 18:237-245

Siqueira EB, Kanaan I, Ali-MA (1989) Large meningioma of the foramen magnum in a 4-year-old child. Surg Neurol 31(5):409-411

Sisti MB, Stein BM (1991) Surgery of spinal meningiomas. In: Al-Mefty O (ed) Meningiomas. Raven, New York, pp 615-620

Slager VT (1960) Arachnoiditis ossificans. Arch Pathol 70:322-327

Sloan TB, Koth A (1985) Depression of cortical somatosensory evoked potentials by nitrous oxide. Br J Anaesth 57:849-852

Sloan TB, Ronai AK, Toleikis JR et al (1988) Improvement of intra-operative somatosensory evoked potentials by etomidate. Anesth Analg 67:582-585

Sloof JL, Kernohan JW, McCarty CS (1964) Primary intramedullary tumors of the spinal cord and filum terminale. Saunders, Philadelphia, pp 165-166

Smaltino F, Bernini FP, Elefante R (1985) Neuroradiologia. Idelson, Napoli

Sobaniec W, Czerwinska-Ciechan K, Zimnoch L, Sobaniec-Lotowska M, Lewko J (1988) A case of malignant extramenigeal meningioma of tha spinal canal with multiple metastases in a 17-year-old patient. Clinical and morphologic studies. Neurol Neurochir Pol 22(5):450-453

Solero CL, Fornari M, Giombini S, Lasio G, Oliveri G, Cimino C, Pluchino F (1989) Spinal meningiomas: review of 174 operated cases. Neurosurgery 25:153-160

Solomon RA, Handler MS, Sedelli RV et al (1987) Intramedullary melanotic schwannoma of the cervico-medullary junction. Neurosurgery 20:253-258

Soo LY (1966) Spinal epidural meningioma. South Med J 59:141-144

Spiller WG (1908) The symptom complex of a lesion of the uppermost portion of the anterior spinal and adjoining portion of the vertebral arteries. J Nerv Ment Dis 35:775

Spiller WG (1909) Thrombosis of the cervical anterior median spinal artery. J Nerv Ment Dis 36:601

Spiller WG, Fraizier CH (1923) Teleangiectasis of the spinal cord. Arch Neurol Psychol 10:29-39

Spinas CR, Benini A (1992) Die multiplen intrakraniellen und spinalen Meningiome. Schweiz Arch Neurol Psychiatry 143, 5:389-456

Spittaler PJ, Johnston IH (1992) Multiple extracranial meningiomas in a child. Childs Nerv Syst 8(3):144-146

Staneczek W, Janisch W (1992) Epidemiologic data on meningiomas in East Germany 1961-1986: incidence, localization, age and sex distribution. Clin Neuropathol 11:135-141

Stechison MT, Tasker RR, Wortzman G (1987) Spinal meningioma en plaque. Report of two cases. J Neurosurg 67:452-455

Steinbok P, Cochrane DD, Poskitt K (1992) Intramedullary spinal cord tumors in children. Neurosurg Clin North Am 3,4:931-945

Stern J, Welan MA, Correll JW (1980) Spinal extradural meningiomas. Surg Neurol 14:155-159

Sterzi G (1904) Die Blutgefässe des Rückenmarks. Untersuchungen über ihre vergleichende und Entwicklungsgeschichte. Anat Hefte 24:1

Sterzi G (1915) Anatomia del sistema nervoso centrale dell'uomo. Draghi, Padova

Suh TH, Alexander L (1939) Vascular system of the human spinal cord. Arch Neurol Psychol 41, 4:659-678

Sutton S, Braren N, Zubin J et al (1965) Evoked potentials correlates of stimulus uncertainty. Science 150:1187-1188

Svien HJ, Wood MW (1957) Recurrence of a meningioma of the spinal cord after 23 years. Report of a case. Mayo Clin Proc 32:568-573

Svien HJ, Thelen EP, Keith HM (1954) Intraspinal tumors in children. J Am Med Assoc 155:959-961

Sze GK (1993) Clinical experience with gadolinium contrast agents in spinal MR imaging. J Comput Assist Tomogr 17:1:8-13

Sze G, Twohing M (1991) Neoplastic disease of the spine and spinal cord. In: Atlas SW (ed) Magnetic resonance imaging of the brain and spine. Raven, New York

Sze G, Stimac GK, Bartlett C, Gillon WP, Haughton VM, Orrison W

(1990) Multicenter study of gadopentetate dimeglumine as an MR contrast agent: evaluation in patients with spinal tumors. AJNR 11, 5:967-974

Tabaraud F, Boulesteix JM, Moulies D, et al (1993) Monitoring of the motor pathway during spinal surgery. Spine 18, 5:546-550

Tadie M, Hemet J, Aaron C, Bianco C, Huard P (1978) Les veines radiculaires de drainage de la moelle ont-elles un dispositif de securite anti-reflux? Bull Acad Nat Med (Paris) 162:550-554

Tadie M, Hemet J, Aaron C, Bianco C et al (1979) Le dispositif protecteur antireflux des veines de la moelle. Neurochirurgie 25:28-30

Tadmor R et al (1983) Advantages of supplementary CT in myelography of intraspinal masses. AJNR 4:618-631

Takemoto K, Matsamura Y, Hashimoto H, Inoue Y, Fakuda T, Shakudo M, Nemoto Y, Onoyama Y, Yasui T, Hakuba A et al (1988) MR imaging of intraspinal tumors capability in histological differentiation and compartamentalization of extramedullary tumors. Neuroradiology 30:303-309

Tanon L (1908) Les artères de la moelle dorso-lombaire. Theses Paris. Vigot, Paris

Tarlov IM (1940) Origin of perineural fibroblastoma. Am J Pathol 16:33

Taveras JM (1990) Neuroradiology: past, present, future. Radiology 175:593-602

Taylor AR, Byrnes DP (1974) Foramen magnum and high cervical cord compression. Brain 97:473-480

Tedeschi F et al (1981) On the pathology of meningiomas. A study of 412 cases. Acta Neuropathol 7:119-121

Theron J (1976) Cervicovertebral phlebography: pathological results. Radiology 118, 1:73-81

Theron J (1979) Exploration radiologique du système veineux intrarachidien. Encycl Med Chir (Paris-France) Neurologie 17032 G10, 6, 5

Theron J, Djindjian R (1973) Cervicovertebral phlebography using catheterization. A preliminary report. Radiology 108, 2:325-331

Theron J, Moret J (1978) Spinal phlebography. Springer, Vienna New York

Theron J, Houtteville JP, Ammerich H, Alves De Zouza A, Adam H, Thurel Ci, Rey A, Houdart R (1976) Lumbar phlebography by catheterization of the lateral sacral and ascending lumbar veins with abdominal compression. Neuroradiology 11:175-182

Thompson PD, Day BL, Crockard HA et al (1991) Intra-operative recording of motor tract potentials at the cervico-medullary junction following scalp electrical and magnetic stimulation of the motor cortex. J Neurol Neurosurg Psychiatry 54:618-623

Thomson AJ (1991) Misdiagnosis of intraspinal lesions in childhood. S Afr Med J 79(7):382-387

Thron AK (1988) Vascular anatomy of the spinal cord. Neuroradiological investigation and clinical sindromes Springer, Vienna New York

Thurel R (1950) Vingt cas de tumeur intra-rachidienne et laterovertebrale. Rev Neurol (Paris) 83:479-482

Thurel R (1964) Tumeurs intrarachidiennes. Bailliere, Paris

Till K (1959) Observations on spinal tumors in childhood. Proc R Soc Med 52:333-336

Till K (1970) Pediatric neurosurgery. Blackwell Scientific, Oxford, pp 193-203

Tirone P, Boldrini E (1982) Effects of iopamidol on nervous system. An experimental study. Rays 7 [Suppl 3]:61-71

Tissier H (1898) Compression lente de la moelle. Bull Soc Anat Paris 73:304

Toleikis JR, Carlvin AO, Shapiro DE et al (1993) The use of dermatomal evoked responses during surgical procedures that use intrapedicular fixation of the lumbosacral spine. Spine 18:2401-2407

Tomita T, Radkowski MA, Gonzalez-Crussi F, Zaparackas Z, Flannery A (1988) Multiple meningiomas in a child. Surg Neurol 29(2):131-136

Tonk V, Osella P, Delasmorenas A, Wiandt HE, Milunsky A (1992)

Abnormalities of chromosome 22 in meningiomas and confirmation of the origin of a dicentric 22 by in situ hybridation. Cancer Genet Cytogenet 64:65-68

Tonnis D (1965) Die Meningiome. Acta Neurochir (Wien) 13:308-310

Tonnis W, Nittner K (1959) Processi morbosi endorachidei a sviluppo espansivo. Clinica Oggi, 4:577-628

Torma T (1957) Malignant tumors of the spine and the spinal extradural space; a study based on 250 histologically verified cases. Acta Chir Scand Suppl 225:1-176

Treheux A, Picard L, Hepner H, Masingue M (1969) Méningiome dorsal calcifié. J Radiol Electr Med Nucl 50:936-937

Trofatter JA, Maccolin MM, Rutter JL, Murrel JR, Duyao MP, Parry DM, Eldridge R, Kley N, Menon AG, Pulaski K, Haase VH, Ambrose CM, Munroe D, Bove C, Haines JL, Martuza RL, Macdonald ME, Seizinger BR, Short MP, Buckler AJ, Gusella JF (1993) A novel moesin-, ezrin-, radixin-like gene in a candidate for the neurofibromatosis 2 tumor suppressor. Cell 72:791-800

Tsuji N, Mishura I, Kyama T (1986) Extradural multiple spinal meningioma. Literature review, a case report. Neurochirurgia 29:124-127

Tsuyama N, Tsuzuki N, Kurokawa T et al (1975) Clinical applications of spinal cord action potentials measurement. Hongo, Bunkyo, KU 7-3-1. 1-16

Tucker AS, Aramsri B, Gardner WJ (1962) Primary spinal tumors: a seven years study. Am J Roentgenol 87:371

Turner OA, Laird AT (1966) Meningioma with traumatic etiology. Report of a case. J Neurosurg 24:96-98

Turner OA, Mc Craig W, Kernohan J W (1942) Malignant meningiomas: clinical and pathologic study. Surgery 11:81-100

Tussen CC, Halprin MR, Endtz LJ (1982) Familial brain tumours. Developments in oncology. Nijhoff, The Hague

Twist EC, Ruttledge MH, Rousseau M, Sanson M, Papi L, Merel P, Delattre O, Thomas G, Rouleau GA (1994) The neurofibromatosis type 2 gene is inactivated in schwannomas. Hum Mol Genet 3:147-151

Tytus JS, Lasersohn JT, Reifel E (1967) The problem of malignancy in meningiomas. J Neurosurg 27:551-557

Udvarheliy GB, Teasdall RD, Shulman LE (1966) Misleading features of benign spinal tumors; report of 3 cases. JAMA 198:1057-1060

Ueta T, Owen JH, Sugioka Y (1992) Effects of compression on physiologic integrity of the spinal cord, on circulation, and clinical status in four different directions of compression: posterior, anterior, circumferential, and lateral. Spine 17 [Suppl 8]:S217-S226

Ugawa Y, Kohara N, Shimpo T et al (1988) Central motor and sensory conduction in adrenoleukomyeloneuropathy and tabe dorsalis. J Neurol Neurosurg Psychiatry 51:1069-1074

Ujiie H, Kobo O, Shimizu T, Kawamura H, Kagawa M, Ohsawa M, Maruyama S (1990) Intramedullary hemangiopericytoma of the spinal cord; case report and review of the literature. No Shinkei Geka 18(3):273-277

Umbach W (1962) Klinik und Verlauf bei 192 spinalen Prozessen mit besonderer Berücksichtigung der Gefässtumoren. Acta Neurochir (Wien) 10:167

Vagner Capodano AM, Grisoli F, Gambarelli D, Sedan R, Pellet W, De Victor B (1993) Correlation between cytogenetic and histopathological findings in 75 human meningiomas. Neurosurgery 32, 6:892-900

Vailati G, Occhiogrosso M, Troccoli V (1979) Intramedullary thoracic schwannoma. Surg Neurol 11:60-62

Valavanis A (1992) Neuroradiology of the spinal cord. Schweiz Med Wochenschr 122, 44:1649-1660

Valentino V (1965) Myelography. Thomas, Springfield,

Van Bogaert L, Martin P (1935) Méningiomatose diffuse cerebrospinale à evolution subaigue. J Belg Neurol Psychol 35:758-766

Van Duinen DM (1971) Het intramedullair neurinoom. Tijdschr Geneeskg 115:1070-1074

Vanasse M, Garcia Larrea L, Neusc,hwander P et al (1988) Evoked potentials studies in Friedreich's ataxia and progressive early onset cerebellar ataxia. Can J Neurol Sci 15:292-298

Vaughan HG (1975) The motor potentials. In: Handbook of electroencephalography and clinical neurophysiology, vol 8, part A. Elsevier, Amsterdam, pp 86-91

Virchow R (1900) Das Psammom. Virchow Arch Pathol Anat 160:32

Von Muralt RH (1949a) Zur Pathogenese der spastischen und schlaffen Lähmungen bei spinalen Kompressionen. Schweiz Arch Neurol Psychiatry 63:272

Von Muralt RH (1949b) Zur Prognose operativ behandelter spinaler Lähmungen vom spastischen und schlaffen Typ. Arch Psychiatr Nervenkr 182:140

Wackenheim A, Dietemann JL (1987) Radiodiagnostic du rachis lombaire. Masson, Paris

Wada H, Yamanouchi H, Kobayashi S, Toyokura Y (1990) Intradural extramedullary tumor of the lower spinal cord in a 89-year-old man with cervical spondylosis and lumbar spondylolisthesis. Rinsho Shinkeigaku 30,8:869-872

Waga S, Matsuda M, Handa H,, Matsushima M, Ando K (1972) Multiple meningiomas. J Neurosurg 37:348-351

Wagner W, Halbig L, Huwel N et al (1993) Intra-operative monitoring during syringo-endoscopy: results of median nerve stimulated somatosensory evoked potentials in nine patients. Acta Neurochir (Wien) 123:187-189

Walter WG (1964) Slow potentials waves in the human brain associated with expectancy, attention and decision. Arch Psychiatr Nervenkr 206:309

Wang AM, Gall CM, Shillito Jr J, Schick R, Brooks ML, Haikal N (1988) CT demonstration of extradural thoracic meningioma. J Comput Assist Tomogr 12:536-538

Wasserberg J, Marks P, Hardy D (1987) Syringomyelia of the thoracic spinal cord associated with spinal meningiomas. Br J Neurosurg 1:485-488

Watanabe E, Schramm J, Romstock J (1988) Intraoperative monitoring of cortical and spinal evoked potentials using different stimulation sites. In: Grundy BL, Villani RM (eds) Evoked Potentials. Intraoperative and ICU Monitoring. Springer, Vienna New York, 177-186

Watterson RL, Veneziano P, Bartha A (1956) Absence of a true germinal zone in neural tubes of young chick embryos as demonstrated by the colchicine technique. Anat Rec 124:379

Webb JH, Craig WK, Kernohan JW (1953) Intraspinal neoplasms in the cervical region. J Neurosurg 10:360

Weed LH (1917) Contributions to embryology. N 14 Carnegie Inst, Washington p 225

Weil SM, Gewirtz RJ, Tew Jr JM (1990) Concurrent intradural and extradural meningiomas of the cervical spine. Neurosurgery 27:629-631

Weiss A, Philippides D, Montrieul B, Steimle R (1952) Modifications osseuses accompagnant les méningiomes. J Radiol Electrol 33:701-703

Wen-Qing H, Shi-Ju Z, Qing-Sheng T, Yu-Xia L, Qing-Zhong X, Zi-Jun L, Wen-Cui Z (1982) Statistical analysis of central nervous system tumors in China. J Neurosurg 56:555-564

Wertheimer P, Dechaume J, Lecuire J, Moulin J (1957) Réflexions sur la coexistence de neurinomes multiples, de méningiomes et de gliomes encéphaliques dans la maladie de Recklinghausen (à propos des chitoneuromes). Neurochirurgie 3:145-154

Wertheimer P, Lapras A, Thierry A, Dechaume JP (1963) Les méningiomes intrarachidiens. A propos de 37 observations. Maroc Med 42:847-851

Weston JA (1970) The migration and differentiation of neural crest cells In: Abercrombie M, Brachet J (eds) Advances in morphogenesis, vol 8. Academic, New York, pp 41-114

Whittle IR, Johnston IH, Besser M (1984) Spinal cord monitoring during surgery by direct recording of somatosensory evoked potentials. J Neurosurg 60:440-443

Whittle IR, Johnston IH, Besser M (1988) Recording of spinal somatosensory evoked potentials for intraoperative spinal cord monitoring. J Neurosurg 64:601

Wise BL, Smith M (1965) Spinal arachnoiditis ossificans. Arch Neurol 13:391-394

Wolf A, Honeyman WM (1937) A note on the appearance of meningioma in tissue culture. Bull Neurol Inst NY 6:569-573

Wolff RK, Frazer KA, Jackler RK, Lansert MJ, Pitts LH, Cox DR (1992) Analysis of chromosome 22 deletions in neurofibromatosis type 2-related tumors. Am J Hum Genet 51:478-485

Wolman L (1953) The origin of the fibrous tissue in meningioma. J Neuropathol Exp Neurol 12:194

Wood EH (1949) The diagnosis of spinal meningiomas and schwannomas by myelography. Am J Roentgenol 61:683

Wood JB, Wolpert SM (1985) Lumbosacral meningioma. AJNR 6:450-451

Woods WA, Pimenta AM (1944) Intramedullary lesions of the spinal cord. Arch Neurol Psychol 52:383

Yamashita K, Akimura T, Kawano K, Adaki N, Nagamitsu T, Wakuta Y, Aoki H (1989) Multiple meningiomas of the spinal canal and posterior fossa. Case report. Neurol Med Chir (Tokyo) 29, 9:834-837

Yasui T, Yagura H, Komiyama M, Fu Y, Nagata Y, Tamura K, Khoala VK, Hakuba A (1992) Significance of gadolinium enhanced magnetic resonance imaging in differentiating spinal cord radiation myelopathy from tumor. Case report. J Neurosurg 77(4):628-631

Yniesta C (1963) Contribution a l'étude des méningiomes rachidiens. Thesis, Lyon

Young HA, Robb P, Hardy DG (1983) Large intramedullary neurofibroma of the conus medullaris: case report. Neurosurgery 13:48-51

Zang KD (1982) Cytological and cytogenetical studies on human meningiomas. Cancer Genet Cytogenet 6:249-274

Zankl H, Zang KD (1980) Correlations between clinical and cytogenetical data in 180 human meningiomas. Cancer Genet Cytogenet 1:351-356

Zappoli R, Papini M, Cabras P (1970) Spontaneous generalized and focal temporal epileptic EEG discharges and the contingent negative variation. Riv Patol Nerv Ment 91:157

Zavala LM, Adler JR, Greene CS, Winston KR (1988) Hydrocephalus and intraspinal tumor. Neurosurgery 22:751-754

Zavaleta MA (1892) Reseccion de vertebras. An Cir Med Argent 15:497-502

Zentner J, Ebner A (1988) Prognostic value of somatosensory- and motor-evoked potentials in patients with non-traumatic coma. Eur Arch Psychiatry Neurol Sci 237:184-187

Zentner J, Kiss I, Ebner A (1989) Influence of anesthetics - nitrous oxide in particular - on electromyographic response evoked by transcranial electrical stimulation of the cortex. Neurosurgery 24:253-256

Zervas NT, Shintani A, Kallar B, Berry RG (1970) Multiple meningiomas occupying separate neuraxial compartments. Case Report. J Neurosurg 33:216-220

Zimmerman RA, Bilianuk LT (1988) Imaging of tumors of the spinal canal and cord. Radiol Clin North Am 26:965-1007

Zornow MH, Grafe MR, Tybor C et al (1990) Preservation of evoked potentials in a case of anterior spinal artery syndrome. Electroencephalogr Clin Neurophysiol 77:137-139

Zulch KJ (1957) Brain tumors. Their biology and pathology. Springer, Berlin Göttingen Heidelberg New York

Zulch KJ (1961a) Die Pathogenese von Massenblutung und Erweichung unter besonderer Berücksichtigung klinischer Gesichtspunkte. Acta Neurochir Suppl (Wien) 7:51-117

Zulch KJ (1961b) Discussion Symposium sur les rammollissements médullaires. Acta Neurolol Psychol Belg 61(3):283-285

Zulch KJ (1962a) The present state of the classification of intracranial tumors and its value for the neurosurgeon. In: Fields WS, Sharkley PC (eds) The biology and treatment of intracranial tumors. Thomas, Springfield

Zulch KJ (1962b) Reflexion sur la physiopathologie des troubles vasculaires medullaires. Rev Neurol 106:632

Zulch KJ, Mennel HD (1975) The question of malignancy in meningiomas. Acta Neurochir (Wien) 31:275-276

Zumkeller M, Seifert V, Dietz H (1992) Multiple Meningiome in verschiedenen Etagen der zerebromedullaren Achse. Nervenarzt 63(12):763-767